Dentistry, Dental Practice, & the Community

THIRD EDITION

In Collaboration with

Herschel S. Horowitz, D.D.S., M.P.H.

Chief, Community Programs Section,
National Caries Program
National Institute of Dental Research
National Institutes of Health
Bethesda, Maryland

Dolores M. Malvitz, R.D.H., B.A., M.P.H., Dr.P.H.

Professor and Chairperson
Department of Dental Hygiene
College of Dentistry
University of Oklahoma
Oklahoma City, Oklahoma

Dentistry, Dental Practice, & the Community

THIRD EDITION

David F. Striffler, D.D.S., M.P.H.

Professor and Director
Program in Dental Public Health
Chairman, Department of Community Health Programs
School of Public Health
Professor of Dentistry (Community Dentistry)
School of Dentistry
The University of Michigan
Ann Arbor, Michigan

Wesley O. Young, D.M.D., M.P.H.

Professor and Chairman
Department of Community Dentistry
School of Dentistry
Professor of Public Health
School of Public Health
The University of Alabama in Birmingham
Birmingham, Alabama

Brian A. Burt, B.D.S., M.P.H., Ph.D.

Professor of Dental Public Health
School of Public Health
Associate Professor of Dentistry (Community Dentistry)
School of Dentistry
The University of Michigan
Ann Arbor, Michigan

W.B. SAUNDERS COMPANY

Philadelphia London Toronto Mexico City Rio de Janeiro Sydney Tokyo

W. B. Saunders Company: West Washington Square
Philadelphia, PA 19105

1 St. Anne's Road
Eastbourne, East Sussex BN21 3UN, England

1 Goldthorne Avenue
Toronto, Ontario M8Z 5T9, Canada

Apartado 26370—Cedro 512
Mexico 4, D.F., Mexico

Rua Coronel Cabrita, 8
Sao Cristovao Caixa Postal 21176
Rio de Janeiro, Brazil

9 Waltham Street
Artarmon, N.S.W. 2064, Australia

Ichibancho, Central Bldg., 22-1 Ichibancho
Chiyoda-Ku, Tokyo 102, Japan

Library of Congress Cataloging in Publication Data

Striffler, David F.

Dentistry, dental practice, and the community.

Rev. ed. of: The dentist, his practice, and his community/Wesley O. Young, David F. Striffler in collaboration with A. L. Russell. 2nd ed. 1969.

Includes bibliographies and index.

1. Dental public health. 2. Dentistry—Practice. I. Young, Wesley O. II. Burt, Brian Aubrey. The dentist, his practice, and his community. III. Young, Wesley O. The dentist, his practice, and his community. IV. Title. [DNLM: 1. Public health dentistry. WU 113 S917d]

RK52.S73 1983 617.6 82–40066
ISBN 0–7216–8621–4 AACR2

Dentistry, Dental Practice, and the Community ISBN 0-7216-8621-4

Last digit is the print number: 9 8 7 6 5 4 3

With respect and admiration
this book is dedicated to the memory
of the late Kenneth A. Easlick,
an inspiring teacher and critic,
and to Walter J. Pelton,
a dynamic and imaginative administrator.

Great economic and social forces flow like a tide over half-conscious people. The wise are those who foresee the coming event and seek to shape their institutions and mold the thinking of the people in accordance with the most constructive change. The unwise are those who add nothing constructive to the process, either because of ignorance on the one hand or ignorant opposition on the other.

Attributed to JOHN STUART MILL

The moral test of government is how it treats those who are in the dawn of life, the children; those who are in the twilight of life, the aged; and those who are in the shadow of life, the sick, the needy, and the handicapped.

HUBERT H. HUMPHREY

FOREWORD

This book is new, original, and significant, and not just another edition. Technically, it is the third edition and so labeled to mollify the stern guardians of library shelves who insist on serial continuity if only to preserve their own sense of well-being and the orderliness of their collections.

This series began with Pelton and Wisan's *Dentistry in Public Health* (1949 and 1955), followed by *The Dentist, His Practice, and His Community* (1964 and 1969), and now by *Dentistry, Dental Practice, and the Community*. This volume is more precise in title and has greater scope than its respected predecessor volumes. It is, in fact, a new book about the total mission of the dental profession: the provision of dental health care for all who need it.

The Preface points out that the veteran team of Striffler and Young has been joined by a new senior author, Brian A. Burt, and two collaborators, Herschel S. Horowitz and Dolores M. Malvitz. The Preface also indicates the broad scope of the changes that have been made in both presentation and content. The highly contemporary approach of the authors is demonstrated by the statement that dentistry must no longer be considered as a societal franchise *manned* solely by *males*—to commit a double effrontery in male chauvinist language. Females, who presently outnumber males in the dental work force, are now given equality with appropriate pronominal and textual changes. One does wonder how the authors would have handled "amen," if that terminal word had been needed in the text.

The broader scope of the volume is impressive. A new, first Section deals with the "sociology of dental practice." This is a proper beginning because it is about people—those who receive dental care and those who provide it. Unless these two components are brought together constructively, dental health will continue as an abstraction, along with the "conquest of poverty" and "total well-being." This Section could well stand alone as an important monograph on what dentistry is. It should be required reading for all aspirants to a career in dentistry, for all students in dentistry and related disciplines, and for all who have, or seek, certification or licensure to practice.

All of the authors are distinguished in dental public health, but this emphatically is not a textbook on that subject. It is much more than that. It explores the state of the art and problems in important areas of dental interest and concern. It presents data, opinions, judgments, and forecasts on topics such as dental personnel, "busyness," prepayment, career guidance, prevention, the attitudes of organized dentistry, dental auxiliaries, governmental roles in dental health, and a host of other issues.

The reasoned approach of the authors to these topics and issues will be heartening to many who are nettled by the currently fashionable carping at all health professionals by some opinion leaders and many government officials, and by the general lessening of public confidence in the integrity of science. The authors firmly dispatch the easy critics who propose cost-control, competition, and more regulation as "quick fixes" for the complexities of the health problem in this country.

There has been unprecedented progress in most areas of dentistry in the past three or four decades and this book confirms it.

The Section on prevention and control of oral diseases is a case in point. It could not have been written with such depth and assurance even 25 years ago because the evidence was not at hand. Today, there is a resurgent emphasis on prevention, and many dental practices are now oriented to it.

The chapters on assessing the distribution and epidemiology of oral diseases are a measure of the great progress that has been made in dental public health methodology. It is now possible to determine with considerable precision the dimensions of oral diseases and their distribution in populations. Without such data, effective planning for realistic dental health goals would not be possible. Reading this chapter would be a salutary exercise for those planning (if that is the proper word) the budgets for dental health and dental research in this country.

It is interesting to note that the authors deal with fluoridation and "other methods of prevention and control" in two separate chapters. This is a proper emphasis. Fluoridation is demonstrably the most effective public health instrument available for preventing dental caries, but its record of adoption throughout the world has been less than heartening. Political timidity at all levels and the persistence of the breed of antifluoridation folk still ensure the perpetuation of an inarticulate majority of children willfully deprived of this readily available health benefit. Only political courage and renewed public and professional support will correct this dereliction. Federal funding equal to the cost of one nuclear submarine would also be helpful.

There is an enlarged chapter on dental health education, which has made enormous advances with the collaboration of social and behavioral scientists, psychologists, and dental auxiliaries. Current practices are light years away from the misleading slogans, the mass inspections, and the teaching of dental anatomy as school "busywork." The chapter is highly recommended to all who wish to strengthen their roles in real prevention.

If this book needs a climax, it will be found in the seminal Section on "meeting the demand for dental care." After all, this is why the book was needed and written. The complex elements of this often controversial problem are handled with clarity and objectivity. The chapters on personnel, demand, prepayment, and federal gestures at funding are written forthrightly and constructively. If there are those who disagree with the authors' assessments, judgments, and projections, they have easy access to the material from which the authors derived their data and conclusions. The text is richly documented and will be a valuable reference source—until the next edition.

It must be noted that this volume is affectionately dedicated to Kenneth A. Easlick and Walter J. Pelton, two sturdy pioneers in dental public health. This last Foreword expresses serene confidence that the future editions that are inevitable will be dedicated with similar affection to the two senior authors, Striffler and Young, who announce their retirement from making new editions with this volume.

HAROLD HILLENBRAND
Executive Director Emeritus
American Dental Association

PREFACE

The second edition of *The Dentist, **His** Practice, and **His** Community* has evolved into this third edition and has been retitled affirmatively *Dentistry, Dental Practice, and the Community.*

It is hoped that similar affirmative changes have been instituted throughout the book. "His" and "hers" and "he" and "she" have become "theirs" and "they." The term "dentist" has, when possible, become "dental professional," "dental practitioner," or "dental clinician" and encompasses males and females as well as dentists, dental hygienists, and dental assistants. Also, the book deliberately is focusing on dental hygienists and dental assistants and not just dentists.

This type of change is symbolic of other changes that have taken place during the more than a decade since the second edition was published. A few examples selected at random may be indicative of the changes in the United States: The number of people covered by prepaid dental care, i.e., dental "insurance," has more than quintupled—from 12.2 million in 1970 to 68 million by 1979; the number of dental hygienists has more than doubled between 1970 and 1977; there are now more dental assistants than active dentists (in 1965, only 91 per 100 active dentists; in 1977, 123 per 100); dental schools have increased in number from 55 in 1968 to 60 in 1981; a shortage of dentists has suddenly turned into an "oversupply" or, at the least, a "maldistribution."

New acronyms and sets of initials have flourished as additional symbols of change: NHSC, EPA, OSHA, HHS, HSA, TEAM, GAO, EFDAs. . . .New or revived phrases also abound: affirmative action, capitation, cost containment, preauthorization, posttreatment reviews and audits, fluoride mouthrinses, consumerism, unnecessary radiation, mercury hygiene, scavengers, overtreatment, general practice residencies, marketing, extramural training sites. . . . And the foregoing are but a few samples.

In addition to the book's title change, the two principal authors, Young and Striffler, have become three with the addition of Brian Burt. Burt, a native of Perth, Western Australia, was graduated from the University of Western Australia with a B.D.S., from Michigan with an M.P.H., and from the University of London with a Ph.D. in oral epidemiology. He was persuaded to assume authorship of the classic chapters covering epidemiology and prevention (except for fluoridation) previously written by the now twice-retired A. L. Russell. In addition, he has taken over the chapters on the provision and financing of dental care, and dental personnel. Burt brings to the book the broad viewpoint of a dentist with international experience. It is anticipated that he will assume responsibility for the fourth and subsequent editions as the weary original authors step aside.

Assisting with this edition is Herschel Horowitz of the National Institute of Dental Research, Bethesda, Maryland, who has redone the chapter on critical appraisal of the literature. The last new author is Dolores Malvitz, Chair of the Department of Dental Hygiene at The University of Oklahoma, who has written the chapter on health education. All five authors have experience in clinical practice and all five earned the degree of Master of Public Health at Michigan (where Striffler and Burt now teach dental public health). Malvitz and Burt have doctorates beyond their M.P.H. Three currently chair their respective departments: Young, Community Dentistry at Alabama; Malvitz, Dental Hygiene at Oklahoma; and Striffler, Community Health Programs at Michigan. Young and Striffler previously occupied the first chairs of two of the pioneer departments of community dentistry: Young at Kentucky and Striffler at Michigan. Prior to those positions, Young had directed the Child Health Program of the Idaho Department of Public Health; and Striffler, the School Health Program at Dearborn, Michigan. Burt, Striffler, and Young all have been employed in state health departments in dental public health positions: Burt in Western Australia, Striffler in New Mexico, and Young in Idaho. Burt and Young also did tours of duty with the Division of Dental Health of the Public Health Service in Washington, D.C.; and all four of the dentist-authors are diplomates of the American Board of Dental Public Health.

All of the chapters have been revised and substantially rewritten. Opinion obviously has crept in despite attempts to be objective, with controversial issues presented as such and with arguments given on both (or several) sides. Many individuals have assisted with this edition. In Ann Arbor, Mrs. Arlene Fardig did the bulk of the typing and checking of references for Burt and Striffler. In Birmingham, Mrs. Muriel Wright assisted Young. The task would have been hopeless without the aid of the fine Dental Library of The University of Michigan. Head Librarian Sue Seger, herself a dental hygienist, and her staff were of help in innumerable instances. Ms. Joni Fraser, the copy editor from Saunders assigned to this edition, contributed considerably through her careful reading of the manuscript and proofs, followed by many thoughtful suggestions for improvement.

In the Foreword to the 1964 edition Dr. Harold Hillenbrand predicted ". . . that, in less time than weary authors care to contemplate, it will be high time for the [next] and 'completely revised and rewritten' edition." Almost 20 years later the "weary authors" recognize that Dr. Hillenbrand was more prophetic than had been realized. The last two decades have constituted one of the most significant periods in the history of our profession. The fatigue of the authors is the satisfying one that results from the rigors and excitement of analyzing developing trends as well as participating in and teaching about them.

DAVID F. STRIFFLER
WESLEY O. YOUNG
BRIAN A. BURT

CONTENTS

Section V
MEETING THE DEMAND FOR DENTAL CARE

Section VI
EDUCATION FOR ORAL HEALTH

I THE SOCIOLOGY OF DENTAL PRACTICE

CHAPTER 1

PRACTITIONERS, PATIENTS, AND THE COMMUNITY

Wesley O. Young
David F. Striffler

A primary purpose of a book on dental public health or community dentistry is to give dental, dental hygiene, and dental assisting students a better understanding of the patients for whom they will assume professional responsibility. Instead of emphasizing the patients and their oral disabilities as specific "cases" requiring treatment, this text will attempt to consider patients as a part of the community in which they live.* Such an approach makes it possible to measure oral health status in terms of how patients' problems are similar to those of other individuals and how they differ. The available knowledge about attitudes toward dental care and the factors that influence people to follow desirable oral health practices should give some insight into patients' motivations and provide guidance in building a practice, in planning treatment for individual patients, and in assuming the responsibilities of a professional person in the community.

The practice of dentistry involves a personal relation between the dentists, dental hygienists, and dental assistants and the patients who elect to seek professional service from them. Within the walls of the office, the "dental health team" functions in a professional world of its own. In this world, conscientious dental health practitioners continually are confronted by the problem of dental diseases. They struggle with the young child suffering from rampant caries and seek to secure the parental cooperation necessary to bring the caries attack under control. They face the discouraging prospect of attempting to restore normal function for the young adult in whom loss of teeth has destroyed the integrity of the dental arches. All too frequently they

---

*The word "community" has a variety of meanings. As used in this book, the term will ordinarily refer to the setting in which dental health practitioners live and practice.

Webster's Third New International Dictionary gives as one meaning: "A body of individuals organized into a unit or manifesting usually with awareness some unifying trait." This definition would encompass not only a city, but also would apply to a state, a region, or an entire nation. For the purposes of clarity, the writers will usually restrict the use of the term to the village, county, or city (or, in a large metropolitan area, the local neighborhood) in which the practice is located.

"Community" may sometimes be used in the broader sense of "society at large" or "people in general," as "in the interests of the community."

must try to save teeth that have lost a major portion of their supporting structures because of long neglect of periodontal diseases.

Within the limits of their ability and available current knowledge, dental practitioners attempt to conduct a practice based on regular maintenance care and the utilization of all practical preventive procedures. Both the dentist and auxiliary personnel try to emphasize health education, to correct misconceptions about proper oral health practices, and to attack apathy about dental health.

The world created within the office by the dental health team should be a creative and satisfying environment. These professionals face the challenge, and enjoy the satisfaction, of building a practice largely of congenial patients who accept professional supervision and trust the skill and efficiency with which health care is provided.

The environment in a dental office is somewhat artificial, because the patients who present themselves for treatment are not necessarily representative of the entire population. They will reflect the dentist's own age, since the younger dentists tend to serve the younger segment of the population while the older dentists see older patients. In general, the patients will be better educated and have better incomes than the population at large. There will be more women than men seeking routine care. In the older age groups, more of the patients will be those with low caries attack rates or those who consistently have received regular dental care, for the others probably will be edentulous and will seek professional service infrequently.

Consequently, one's own personal experience probably will not give an accurate indication of the occurrence of dental diseases or the full extent of the unmet dental needs in the community. Because children who experience dental caries may be the children most likely to be brought to the dentist, a practice in a fluoride area may not see, in the office, the full benefits of fluoridation in the community. Similarly, experience in a private practice may provide only a casual glimpse of the dental problems of the indigent families in the community. Patients with special problems, such as mentally retarded or cerebral-palsied children, may never appear in the dental office.

Since the patients in the practice probably will come from the segment of the population with higher income and more-than-average educational attainment, dental health practitioners are likely to underestimate the extent of general public ignorance about dental health. It is easy to assume that an individual's own interest and concern for proper oral health, or at least that of the "best" patients, is shared generally. The possibility of making this error is increased, since many patients may be reluctant to discuss their attitudes toward dental care frankly with a professional person such as a dentist or dental hygienist, who may represent "a figure of authority."

An analysis of the dental needs and the attitudes toward dental care of the entire community, therefore, provides valuable insights ordinarily not gained in private practice.

Another important objective of a book on dental public health or community dentistry is to help dental, dental hygiene, and dental assisting students understand the forces in American culture that determine the manner in which dentistry is practiced. An awareness of the way in which social factors influence methods of providing health care is necessary if the professional person is to exercise informed leadership in the community.

Because of their special education and competence, the members of the health professions alone have been accorded by the public the privilege of providing certain health services. In order to ensure the availability of quality dental service, the public has established and maintained dental schools and has set up legal restrictions to forbid the practice of dentistry by those who are not members of the dental health professions. To a large extent, the public has permitted the profession to regulate itself and to govern the practice of dentistry. Because of the unique privileges granted to them, the members of the dental professions have the responsibility of providing a high standard of service to their patients and of exercising leadership in the community in which they reside or work or both. As professional individuals, dentists, dental hygienists, and dental assistants should assume these responsibilities freely and voluntarily. In addition to the moral implications, it must be recognized that the dental profession has a selfish interest in maintaining its leadership role. The provision of dental care in American society involves a two-way relation between the dental profession as provider of service and the public as purchaser of service. The relation must continue to be satisfactory, not only to the dental health professions but also to the majority of the public if dentistry is to continue in its privileged position. In fact, the public increasingly is demanding a role as an equal partner in decisions affecting the provision of health care.

The relation of a profession to the society it serves must be an ever-changing one; as the society evolves, the profession must change and develop if it is to continue to be effective. Tremendous social changes have taken place in this country and in the world during the past half century. The luxuries of prior days have become the necessities of today. The public expectation of a minimum standard of living compatible with decency has risen constantly. Attitudes toward health care, in particular, appear to have changed quite rapidly within the last quarter century. In recent years, there has been a growing assertion that health care is a basic human right.

For one thing, the cost as well as the effectiveness of health care has increased rapidly and, as a result, the total cost of health care has become a public issue. Although not immediately in the forefront of controversies about the provision of physicians' services and hospital care, dentistry cannot remain aloof from any general changes that take place in methods of providing health care. Patterns established in relation to medical and hospital care may be expected to influence the future development of dental services. Such changes may revolutionize the practice of dentistry as it is known today.

If dental health professionals are to maintain their integrity and continue to provide a high standard of oral health care, it is important that they be prepared to provide professional leadership during this period of rapid social change. The professional individual entering practice must, therefore, be aware of the changing social scene, recognize some of the factors that are motivating changes in public attitudes, and be knowledgeable about the approaches that can be used to bring dental care to a larger proportion of the public. General ignorance of these factors on the part of the professions could well be suicidal.

The third major objective of a book on dental public health or community dentistry is to provide the dentist, dental hygienist, and dental assistant with specialized skills and knowledge that will enhance the practice of dentistry. Some acquaintance with epidemiology and clinical trials, for example, is necessary if the practitioner is to interpret research findings and make a rational selection of procedures to be used in the office. Similarly, information about the factors that influence individual attitudes toward health and about the principles of health education is useful in dealing with individual patients as well as in providing professional guidance for community efforts.

The public health approach to dental problems emphasizes the problems of dental diseases as they occur in the total population. Such an emphasis underscores the deficiencies of current efforts to maintain oral health. National surveys have consistently shown the existence of large unmet treatment needs, despite annual expenditures for dental care of more than 18 billion dollars. Members of the dental, dental hygiene, and dental assisting professions play a most important part in improving the oral health of the public. Their most basic contribution to this end is the conduct of dental practices of the highest caliber—practices that provide modern comprehensive dental care, include the use of recognized preventive procedures, are conducted in a safe environment, assume a responsibility for health education, and demonstrate a genuine concern for the patient as an individual.

Even if all dental health professionals conducted and worked toward this type of practice, only part of the goal of complete oral health care for the entire population could be attained. First, only about 25 percent of the public seeks regular dental care and is in a position, therefore, to receive full benefit from dental services. Second, there are procedures that cannot be secured as easily by individuals as by organized group action. The benefits of water fluoridation, for example, will reach a majority of children only as successful group effort results in a community fluoridation program.

The purpose of a book on dental public health or community dentistry is, therefore, to prepare practicing dental health professionals to fulfill their complete roles as professional people, both in the office and in the community in which they reside. This book should help dental health practitioners to recognize community dental health problems and to suggest sound approaches to be taken for their correction; it should help them to serve their community as sources of current and reliable information on concepts, resources, and methods related to the maintenance and improvement of oral health; it should assist them to participate effectively in the planning and promotion of dental health activities and, when necessary, in the implementation and evaluation of such activities. As a result, the professional outlook of the practitioners should advance beyond a concern with the technical aspects of restoring teeth to a concern for the total dental health of the population and the effect of dental health on its general health and well-being. Extending the sights and objectives of dental health practice should make it a more satisfying and rewarding career.

CHAPTER 2

THE SOCIAL SETTING OF DENTAL HEALTH PRACTICE

Wesley O. Young

INTRODUCTION

The interaction between an individual and the environment probably has been most memorably stated by John Donne: "No man is an island entire of itself; every man is a piece of the continent, a part of the main."[40] The phrase has become threadbare with use, yet continues to be meaningful because it highlights an important aspect of the human condition. No individual or group of people (such as dental health professionals) can stand as an island, alone and unique. All are constrained by the social, economic, and political environment of which they are a part. These factors vary with the level of interaction between practitioners and their environment. Successful promotion of community water fluoridation, for example, allows health professionals to make a major change in the patterns of dental disease in the community. On the other hand, the nature of dental health practice may be affected, for better or for worse, by law and custom or by government action either at the state or federal level. In the latter instance, the health professionals may have little influence on the intervening law or regulation.

The preceding chapter provided a brief overview of the interaction between dental health professionals and their patients as well as some of the more significant social issues facing the profession. This chapter will review in more detail many of the factors that are considered important as part of the social setting of dental health practice. Among these factors are the historic development of the dental health professions and the characteristics of dental practice that influence an individual's personal and professional satisfaction as well as the type of patient care that will be provided.

Later chapters will outline: (1) the nature of dental disease and how disease patterns are studied; (2) the prevention and control of dental disease; (3) issues involved in meeting the demand for dental care; and (4) the principles of dental health education as applied both in practice and in the community.

DEVELOPMENT OF THE PROFESSIONS

Dentistry

Early Beginning

Dental diseases, although less prevalent than today, have afflicted the human race since the earliest days. About 3,700 years before Christ, Egyptian manuscripts refer to dental problems, e.g., "blisters of the gums and gnawing teeth."[25, 102] Yet in the continuum of time from then until now, dentistry has existed as a vocation only briefly. From the ascendancy of Greece and Rome and into the Middle Ages and the Renaissance, there were those who recorded dental problems and advised means of ameliorating them. It was not until modern times that the care of the oral structures became a cohesive body of knowledge and skill. Many trace this development to 1728, when Pierre Fauchard published *Le Chirurgien Dentiste, ou Traité des Dents,* a two-volume book of more than 800 pages.[46] This was the first complete treatise on dentistry published in the Western world. It remained an authoritative document for over 100 years.

Fauchard had no formal training other than that he had worked under the chief surgeon of the French Navy, to whom he acknowledged a debt of gratitude. His genius lay in the ability to synthesize the knowledge and experience of others, to add it to the results of his remarkable powers of observation, and to record for others a systematic description of the methods of caring for the dentition—a task to which he devoted his entire professional career.

For more than another century there were no formal educational opportunities for those who wished to become dentists. Aspiring dentists were generally employed by an experienced practitioner as apprentices for a relatively brief period and then went on to establish practices of their own. According to Bremner, G. V. Black, one of the towering figures of dentistry in the latter half of the nineteenth century, possessed a formal education not exceeding 20 months and his introduction to dentistry consisted of a "few weeks" with a Dr. Speers, considered not a particularly good dentist and whose dental library consisted of one book.[25] Fortunately, Dr. Black followed the often-repeated precept that "a professional person has no choice other than to be a continuous student."

If one point in time can be identified to indicate the transformation of dentistry from a vocation to a profession, it should be the establishment in 1840 of the first dental school in the world, the Baltimore College of Dental Surgery (later the University of Maryland). The beginning was modest, but it was a start.[25] The course was 16 weeks in length after a year or more of apprenticeship; the enrollment was five; and the graduates of the session, two. At about the same time, the first national professional dental journal in the world, *The American Journal of Dental Science,* appeared and the first national professional dental organization, the American Society of Dental

Surgeons, was organized. Thus in the short span from 1839 to 1840, three major hallmarks of a profession appeared—a specialized educational institution for the development of knowledge and the teaching of students, a scientific literature for the diffusion of knowledge, and an organized society for the governance of the profession.[69]

Proprietary Schools and Licensure

It might have been anticipated that the modest beginning would have been followed by a slow but gradual increase in the numbers of formal training programs and an increasing sophistication of their curricula. In fact, a prestigious private university, Harvard, established a dental department in close association with the medical department in 1867, and a major state university, The University of Michigan, established a dental school in 1875.[63, 65, 69] However, these developments were overshadowed by a stampede to create schools to be operated for profit. Shortly after 1870 the dental engine was introduced, which revolutionized the clinical practice of dentistry. The new device made it possible to prepare cavities or to reduce teeth for crowns at a speed that previously had been unthinkable.[25] The revolution in dental practice made it more profitable and attracted more individuals to the profession. This increased demand for education made it possible for a dental school, with less than idealistic purposes, to reap large profits by maintaining a large student body and a very small faculty and by requiring the students to perform a large number of mechanical operations for which clinical patients could be charged fees—the origin of the so-called "point requirements." Bremner states, for example, that one school with 650 students employed just one instructor to teach three scientific subjects.[25] It is estimated that in the years around the turn of the century as many as 150 dental schools, both good and bad, were established.[35] Some lasted only a few years, some for extended periods, and a few with university affiliations have continued to the present.

The variation in the quality of dental education was the despair of leaders of the profession, who sought through the dual approach of accreditation and state licensing to elevate standards. From the perspective provided by time, however, the ease of entry into the profession during this period was fortuitous. It permitted dentists to match the rapid growth of the population of the United States and maintain a relatively homogeneous group of practitioners responsible for oral health care. At least in part this rapid growth allowed American dentistry to escape the division of labor between stomatologists (physicians with additional training in clinical dentistry) and dentists that has plagued some European countries.[42]

And grow the profession did. The first census in which dentists were enumerated separately (1850) showed that the population of 23 million was served by 2,900 dentists, or one for every 8,000 persons. The 1900 census identified nearly 30,000 dentists, or one for every 2,562 persons. The relative growth of the profession slowed but continued to increase through 1930. At that point the economic pressures of the depression coupled with the stiffening of requirements for accreditation reduced the number of dental graduates so that the growth of the profession did not match that of the United States population in the 1940s and 1950s.[36] The trend toward fewer dentists available in relation to the population has been reversed in recent years.[8] (For a more complete discussion of dental personnel, see Chapter 14.)

The first attempt to establish at least a minimum level of competence was the passage of state laws defining and regulating the practice of dentistry. These laws are an exercise of the police powers of the state to protect "the health, safety, welfare, and morals of its people."[76] A state board of dental examiners reviews candidates for licensure, admits those passing the examination to practice in the state, and punishes infractions of the law by suspension or revocation of the license to practice. By 1868 dental practice acts had been passed by Alabama, Kentucky, Ohio, and New York.[25, 72] Since only a minute fraction of dentists had any formal training at all, and those with training had experienced a limited education with varying degrees of adequacy, state licensing was an essential step in attempting to curtail incompetence and quackery. There are those who have questioned the relevance of dental licensure today, given the sophistication of current dental education. Others have questioned a state board's ability to guarantee the continued competence of those already licensed, since experience has demonstrated that licenses are ordinarily suspended or revoked only for gross offenses.

Around the turn of the twentieth century three groups of dental faculty were organized with the intention of upgrading the quality of dental education, primarily by encouraging university-affiliated schools that were not for profit and nonproprietary. (The three groups, together with an organization of Canadian faculties, joined in 1923 to form what is now the American Association of Dental Schools.) These efforts were successful and the last proprietary dental school became a public trust in 1929.[35, 72] During this period the number of schools dwindled to 39.

In this time of ferment, William Gies, a distinguished biochemist and dental educator, conducted a study of dental education that had a significant impact on educational patterns in the United States and Canada.[52] The study, started in 1921 and published in 1926, was financed by the prestigious Carnegie Foundation for the Advancement of Teaching, which had supported a similar survey of medical education by Abraham Flexner some years previously. When the Baltimore College of Dental Surgery was founded in 1840, it was as a separate institution. It was not added to the existing medical school for the practical reasons that there were at the time inadequate physical facilities at the medical school and internal frictions within the medical faculty. Some 86 years later, the "separate-but-equal" pattern of the relation between dental and medical education was recommended as the desirable normal by Gies. Among other recommendations made by Gies were the following:

> Dentistry, in the quality and efficiency of its service to the patient, should be made the full equivalent of an oral specialty in the practice of medicine.
>
> * * *

> Dentistry can be effectually and economically developed to the full service equivalence of an oral specialty of the practice of medicine through extension and improvement, in universities, of that system of dental education which, though separate from medical education, is closely related to it and should be more intimately associated with medical schools, hospitals, and dispensaries.
>
> * * *
>
> This extension and improvement could be accomplished without requiring the prospective general practitioner of dentistry to become a doctor of medicine before beginning his dental training, and could best be brought about by the pursuit of the following three main objects: (a) the preliminary education and instruction in the medical sciences should be practically the same in general scope and quality as for medicine; (b) the technical and clinical training, the applications of the medical sciences, and the correlations of clinical dentistry with clinical medicine should be sufficient to assure both ability to initiate safely a dependable modern general practice of dentistry and capacity to grow in proficiency; and (c) the most advanced phases of dental practice should be reserved for systematic graduate study.[52]

Dentistry in the Twentieth Century

Changes, progress, and evolution in a profession do not occur at an even pace. In some periods progress is more rapid than in others and it will be anticipated that the changes in some portions of the country will be greater than in others. Nevertheless, for organizational purposes, it is useful to divide the recent progress of dentistry as a profession into the 20 years between 1930 and 1950, the decade between 1950 and 1960, and the period from 1960 to the present.

1930 to 1950. Since the last proprietary school was converted to a public trust in 1929, it is logical to date the "roots" of present-day dentistry in the two decades starting at 1930. The major characteristic of this period was the battle for survival—of coping first with the Great Depression and second with World War II. The incomes of dentists dropped precipitously with the advent of the depression, and the economic foundations of the profession were shattered. Dentistry largely became an emergency service. Practicing dentists occupied the time between attending the few patients who came to their offices by reading or other diversions. A major study of the health professions was conducted over a five-year period by the Committee on the Costs of Medical Care (financed in part by the American College of Dentists). The survey published 28 studies, including a final report in 1932.[29] A summary of the dental aspects of the studies was prepared by Dorothy Fahs Beck and included Sinai and Mills' analysis of the adequacy of a supply of 761 dentists for the city of Detroit:

> Assuming that "needs" includes only those services for which patients are willing and able to pay, it is apparent that Detroit now has enough dentists, since three-fourths of them are devoting less than 33 hours per week to tasks for which they are paid, and since the dentists as a whole are spending one-third of their time in work for which there is no direct remuneration or in simply waiting for patients.[20]

Dental education suffered equally. The low salaries paid to teachers were cut even further and the budgets for maintenance were held to a minimum. The financial plight of the schools was compounded by a drop in enrollments caused by the financial problems of potential students.

The economy had not yet regained full prosperity when the nation underwent the shock of a long and costly war in which all matériel and personnel were in short supply. Many dentists were drafted into the armed forces and those who remained worked long hours in an attempt to provide the care that was being sought by the public, whose income rose rapidly due to the full employment resulting from the war effort. During the 1930s the dental schools had suffered from a lack of students because few could pay the tuition and costs involved. In the war years schools suffered from competition with the armed forces. As part of a total mobilization of the nation, all dental schools went on an accelerated curriculum in which the four academic years were taken in three calendar years. In addition, the majority of the students were enlisted in the Army or Navy and went into the military dental service immediately upon graduation.

The teaching of the basic sciences was perfunctory and the emphasis in the clinical sciences was almost entirely on restorative dentistry and prosthetics. Subjects such as radiology, oral diagnosis, endodontics, periodontics, and pedodontics were neglected in many dental schools. The efforts of the few full-time faculty were not devoted primarily to teaching but to supervising and attempting to coordinate the large number of part-time faculty. It was not uncommon for the latter to be at the school only for an hour or two of lecture or for a half day of clinic supervision a week. There were few educational programs for the preparation of specialists, and they varied both in quality and length.[72]

A bright spot in an otherwise rather grim picture was that of water fluoridation, one of the most remarkable preventive measures of the twentieth century. After some 40 years of research and development, fluoridation was ready for clinical trial in a community. By the end of 1945, six communities with a total population of about 232,000 were utilizing controlled fluoridation, and by 1950, 100 cities representing a total population of 1.5 million were using fluoridated water.[44]

1950 to 1960. This decade was a period of fairly rapid growth and also was the foundation for an almost explosive growth after 1960. The dental curriculum in this period was largely the traditional "horizontal" one of two years of basic science followed by two years of clinical science. However, the decade did see considerable improvement in clinical teaching. A good deal of this was related to technological advances that were available in 1950 and were spreading rapidly throughout the profession and into dental education. The availability of ultrahigh-speed cutting instrumentation and high-velocity evacuation systems changed the cutting of tooth structure from a demanding and arduous task to one of relative ease. New impression materials and prosthetic technics made practical the construction of quite elaborate restorative and fixed prosthodontic services. However, the emphasis remained on tooth-oriented or technic-centered care, rather than on comprehensive patient care. Oral diagnosis and the planning of comprehensive treatment were often neglected, and the family and community were rarely, if ever, mentioned.

The faculty remained primarily part-time. In 1950, for example, at one major university there were only about 10 full-time faculty and several hundred part-time faculty for an enrollment of 126 in a class.[80] (A comparable university dental school today would have a full-time faculty of approximately 100, supplemented by a few part-time instructors.) The basic science faculty was providing undistinguished instruction and had little involvement in research. Morris recalls that ". . . dental research was being conducted in a few isolated pockets by individuals clearly viewed as different—if not strange."[81]

In the decade following 1950 this picture would change dramatically. The first direct appropriations for dental research grants were included in the 1948 budget of the National Institutes of Health and totaled only $111,000. The National Institute of Dental Research was founded in 1950. Its first appropriation amounted to $1.78 million but in the next 25 years grew to $20.5 million. The availability of funds to support research (as well as traineeships to prepare dentists and other investigators for research careers) markedly changed the composition of the dental school faculty. Prior to 1940 there were only 20 dentists in the country with an earned Ph.D. in addition to their dental degree and that figure had reached only 47 by 1950. The figure stands at several hundred today.[80, 81]

An important aspect of this period was the definition and standardization of the education of specialists (to be described in Chapter 14). The number of persons using fluoridated water continued to grow, rising to more than 36 million by the end of the decade.[44] In the late 1940's, the first effective method for the prevention of dental caries by topical agents applied by professional personnel was developed by Knutson and co-workers.[68] Topical applications of sodium fluoride were the first in a series of methods for primary prevention* that were developed for use in the dental office and in community programs, and these became an accepted part of clinical and public health practice.

1960 to the Present. Enormous changes have taken place in dental practice and dental education since 1960. The technology of the 1950s was refined and the productivity of the dental office increased both by better management and by the expanded use of auxiliary personnel. Part of the expansion of auxiliaries was due to their informal training by dentists in dental offices. This increase in the number of office-trained personnel was paralleled by the expansion of opportunities for formal education for dental hygienists and dental assistants (which will be described later) and by dental school experimentation in the training of new types of auxiliaries (described in Chapter 14).

Experimentation extended to the dental curriculum. An early move was the replacement of the two-plus-two "horizontal curriculum" (two years of basic sciences and preclinical technics followed by two years of clinical sciences) with the so-called "diagonal curriculum." In this curriculum basic sciences were extended into the third and fourth year so that clinical sciences could

*The various levels of prevention are delineated in Chapter 8, page 202.

be introduced early in the first two years.[32] Early contact of dental students with patients seems to have had a beneficial effect on their professional development and has been extended widely throughout dental schools in the United States. Another major area of successful experimentation has been the use of various forms of packaged instruction such as programmed texts, self-pacing audiovisual packets, and computer-assisted instruction. Less successful was the attempted return to the curriculum pattern used during World War II, in which the four academic years were compressed into three calendar years. The trend apparently is for these schools to revert to the conventional four calendar years—a move made according to the Council on Dental Education ". . . primarily to relieve the pressure on faculty and students in operating on a continuous 12-month basis."[14]

A major study of the dental profession was done under the auspices of the American Council on Education at the request of the American Dental Association and published late in 1961.[62] The 600-page report was divided into sections on dental health, dental practice, dental education, and dental research and was accompanied by appendices (one of which was an early call for the entrance of more women into the profession). This report had an effect on several aspects of dentistry. One impact was on the teaching of periodontal disease control. The report highlighted the data that had recently become available indicating that after the age of 35 to 44 the loss of the vast majority of teeth was due to periodontal disease and not to dental caries.[105] The section on dental education noted that some dentists ". . . have found a way of dental practice that is extremely satisfying to them. Today they are truly combining the basic biological sciences, oral diagnosis, the treatment of soft tissue lesions, occlusion, and restorative procedures most effectively."[72] The *Survey of Dentistry* commended this development and urged that all institutions provide a predoctoral dental education to prepare students for this type of practice. A major shift in recent years has been an increase in the teaching of the prevention and control of periodontal disease and in the provision of comprehensive patient care that stresses proper oral diagnosis and the planning of total mouth rehabilitation rather than individual restorations or individual technical procedures. Along with this development has been a growing emphasis on educational experiences in hospital dentistry (made a requirement for accreditation in 1973) and in oral medicine.

The early 1960s witnessed the development of what have been termed Departments of Community or Social Dentistry or Ecological Dentistry or similar names. (The first of these units were established at Michigan and Detroit in 1962 and at Alabama and Kentucky in 1963.[65]) The objective of these departments was to bring together what Blackerby termed the "curricular orphans" that related to the nonclinical aspects of the practicing dentist's performance.[22] Among the areas of instruction often included were the history of dentistry, preventive dentistry, dental public health, epidemiology, biostatistics, health care provision, ethics and jurisprudence, and practice management. A parallel development has been the recruitment of behavioral scientists to dental faculties and the resultant teaching of the behavioral aspects of patient care. Often these faculty members are based in community dentistry departments.

Another major development has been the shift from a part-time faculty to a full-time faculty. As was indicated earlier, the number of dental faculty with advanced degrees has increased remarkably, as has the number of nondental faculty members with advanced degrees in subjects relevant to dental education. The upgrading of dental faculty has resulted, in many institutions, in a marked change in the relation between the dental school and the greater university. In the past it was not uncommon for the dental school to be physically and administratively tied to the university but, in fact, to have no basic ongoing intellectual exchange. Today a number of dental schools and the medical centers in which they are contained are the "bright jewels" of their parent university. In these institutions the dental faculty take an active role in the academic and scientific aspects of university life as well as in its governance. All these factors are related to the increase in dental research and to the strengthening of its scientific quality.[82]

Little in the increased effectiveness of the educational curriculum and the research component of the dental schools would have been possible had it not been for a major rebuilding of the physical plants of these schools. In an article aptly titled "Back from the Brink," Galagan described the problem facing dental education in the early years of this period:

> By the late 50's almost all dental schools were at least a half century old; some were built in the late 1800's. There had been no building and little renovation during the depression years of the 30's and the war years of the 40's. Schools were located in slums, often in converted factories, and other buildings never designed for dental education.[51]

Help came when the Health Professions Educational Assistance Act was passed in 1963, authorizing federal funds for construction and student aid. (This legislation was later to include per capita funding to support the basic instructional program.) In the 15 years that followed the passage of this act $250 million was put into the construction of dental schools. Matching funds of some $700 million in state, local, or private sources were added so that nearly a billion dollars was spent to reconstruct, from the ground up, the entire physical plant of dental education.[51] Funds for building and renovation of existing dental schools made expanded enrollment possible and similar funds helped to create new schools. There were 39 dental schools in 1930; the total stood at 59 in 1980.[14]

*Dental Students**

Studies of career choice patterns of the dental student (reported between 1955 and 1970) were reviewed by Fusillo and Metz.[50] In general, a significant

*This section and the later sections on hygiene students and practice organization are adapted from: Young, W. O., and Cohen, L. K. The nature and organization of dental practice. p. 193–208. (In Freeman, H. E., Levine, S., and Reeder, L. G., eds. Handbook of medical sociology. 3rd ed. Englewood Cliffs, Prentice-Hall, 1979. xi + 516 p.) During her career with the Public Health Service, Dr. Cohen, a sociologist, helped identify the behavioral and environmental aspects of dentistry, many of which are reflected in these sections.

proportion of American dentists tended to retain the occupational status level of the family origin. Their fathers were dentists or had other professional or managerial occupations. Another significant proportion of dentists were occupationally mobile, motivated to rise on the socioeconomic ladder from the backgrounds of their fathers and grandfathers.

Most dental students, as described in the literature, were predominantly from either middle or upper class family backgrounds, according to reported income and occupations of their parents. Nearly all were male and most began dental school at 21 to 22 years of age.[50] Despite active recruitment of women in recent years, the entering classes remain more than 82 percent male.[14] By the time they were juniors and seniors, most were married with no children and were still financially dependent.

Students characteristically said that they chose dentistry because of such values as the desire to "be one's own boss" and to work with one's hands, because of the prestige of the profession or the monetary advantage of the profession, as well as a desire to provide a service to other people. In the United States, relatively few dental students have actually applied to or attended medical school. According to More, the hypothesis that dentistry is a second-choice profession may not be supported. His study of applicants indicated that the "top" dental school applicant had credentials for acceptance in "most any" medical school.[78, 79] Sherlock and Cohen confirm earlier work but ingeniously describe the choice pattern as one of "minimax." The minimax strategy guides the individual to choose an occupation having minimum difficulty of access along with maximum rewards. The minimax hierarchy of six occupations, as perceived by a California dental student sample, was dentistry, law, medicine, teaching in a university, business, and accounting, thus reflecting a belief that access to dentistry was less difficult but gave rewards comparable with those of medicine. When the sample was asked to list a "maximax" occupational choice, i.e., a choice that considers both rewards and difficulty of access, the order was medicine, dentistry, law, university teaching, accounting, and business. These data suggest the predental students often entertained both the "minimax" and "maximax" stratagems of their pursuit of career choices but favored dentistry as their "minimax" choice because it combined high rewards with an easier access than medicine.[92]

Quarantelli, in proposing additional pathways to dentistry beyond the "reward-access model," states a case for a group of students for whom dentistry was "preordained"—or was their only career choice for some length of time. Another group actually attempted another field and then decided on dentistry—in an adventitious process of selection.[87]

Research on psychosocial characteristics of dental students suggests that, on average, the students tended to be pragmatic, conforming, conservative, and not academically oriented toward knowledge for its own sake. They had an ability to complete tasks, but were not high on leadership traits. The role of the dental school in altering values of students is rather bleak. Whereas most studies indicate that the faculty seems to have little influence on student ideals, at least three studies show that students appeared to become less rather than more idealistic as they progressed through four years of dental education.[50] Sherlock and Morris, moreover, note that the students they studied showed increasingly high cynicism scores over the course of their professional education.[93] A decline in "ethicalness" scores also appeared over the same period—suggesting that changes in value orientation, in fact, did occur or that the measuring instruments in other studies may not have been sensitive to these same variables.

More promising findings were reported in a study by Moody and colleagues.[77] Eron's scales of cynicism and humanitarianism were used with a wider spectrum of dental students and dental practitioners. Individuals were tested (1) the summer before entering dental schools, (2) during the dental school years, and (3) after they had been graduated and in practice for four or five years. It was concluded that shifts in "cynicism" and "humanitarianism" were apparently a temporary phenomenon resulting from the stress of the dental school environment. "Cynicism" scores of incoming students and practicing dentists were significantly lower than those of the dental students. Similarly, "humanitarian" scores of students in school were lower than those about to enter, but returned to the higher level after four or five years in practice.

Organization of the Profession in the United States

Dental students and dentists in the Federal Services may join the American Dental Association (ADA) directly. All others apply for membership in a local society (a component) representing a county, a group of counties, or a large city. If accepted at this level, the dentist automatically becomes a member of the state dental society (constituent) and, in turn, of the American Dental Association. Membership in some areas is almost automatic, but in others the membership application is passed on by a membership committee or a board of censors. Traditionally, membership standards have included graduation from an accredited dental school, a license to practice in the jurisdiction, and avoidance of unethical practices. The most common unethical practice in the past has been the advertising of dental services to the public. While some constraints on advertising remain in codes of ethics and state practice acts, recent legal decisions have made them largely inoperable.[11]

In the past, in some states, nonwhites were not allowed as members of the local dental society and were therefore ineligible for membership in the parent organization. The National Dental Association, composed primarily of black dentists, was created to fill the needs of these individuals. The American Dental Association and the National Dental Association have both stated that their objective is complete integration of the profession. Whites now may and do belong to the National Dental Association and nonwhites may and do belong to the American Dental Association, and there is a cooperative relation between the two organizations.

Membership in a medical society has an important bearing on whether or not hospital privileges are available to a physician—creating a strong incentive to hold membership in at least one medical or specialty society.

Hospital privileges have been important to the practice of only a limited number of dentists, so that this motivation has been largely absent. Membership in the national organization brings certain individuals fringe benefits, such as group insurance plans and the availability of health education materials and other aids. However, the American Dental Association serves its members—and indirectly the welfare of the public—primarily in three other areas:

1. Scientific meetings, held at the local, state, and national level, are an important mechanism for the exchange of scientific information within the profession. This exchange is enhanced by the publication of a variety of scientific journals.

2. Another significant role is that of establishing standards in important areas of practice. The establishment of standards includes the direct or indirect accreditation of professional schools for dentists, dental hygienists, dental assistants, and dental laboratory technicians. This role is indirectly supplemented by the influence of the profession acting through state licensing bodies. Standards are also established for materials, drugs, and devices used by dentists in practice and, in a few instances, for products offered for sale to the public. These standards are established by utilizing the services of experts in specialized fields as members of reviewing councils and committees.

3. Although it is less easily identifiable, an important task of a professional association in a time of rapid social change is to obtain a consensus among the profession on major issues and transmit this consensus to government agencies and others concerned with establishing social policy.[60]

Dentistry has an admirable cohesion and strength. Akers and Quinney studied the organizational patterns of the chiropractic, dental, medical, optometry, and pharmacy professions. They concluded that dentistry and medicine had resources and structures much superior to the other three. They reported:

> The American Medical Association is the largest and wealthiest association, and medical practitioners undergo the longest period of education. While the ADA is also large and wealthy, and dentists are well educated, they do not match the AMA in these respects. However, the dental profession is more tightly organized than the medical, i.e., it is more cohesive, has greater professional unity, and its major association is structurally integrated to a greater degree. Therefore, the two are placed together . . . and labelled as a profession with a degree of organization of the *first order.*[2]

The ultimate governing body of American dentistry is the House of Delegates of the American Dental Association.[15] This 417-member body is composed of elected representatives from the 50 states, the Commonwealth of Puerto Rico, and the Virgin Islands.[98] The size of delegations ranges from the smallest, which are Alaska and the Virgin Islands with the minimum number of one representative each, to the largest, which are New York with 47 and California with 44. The House of Delegates includes one representative of each federal administrative unit, including the Air Force, Army, Navy, Panama Canal Zone, Public Health Service, and Veterans Administration. (See Fig. 2–1.)

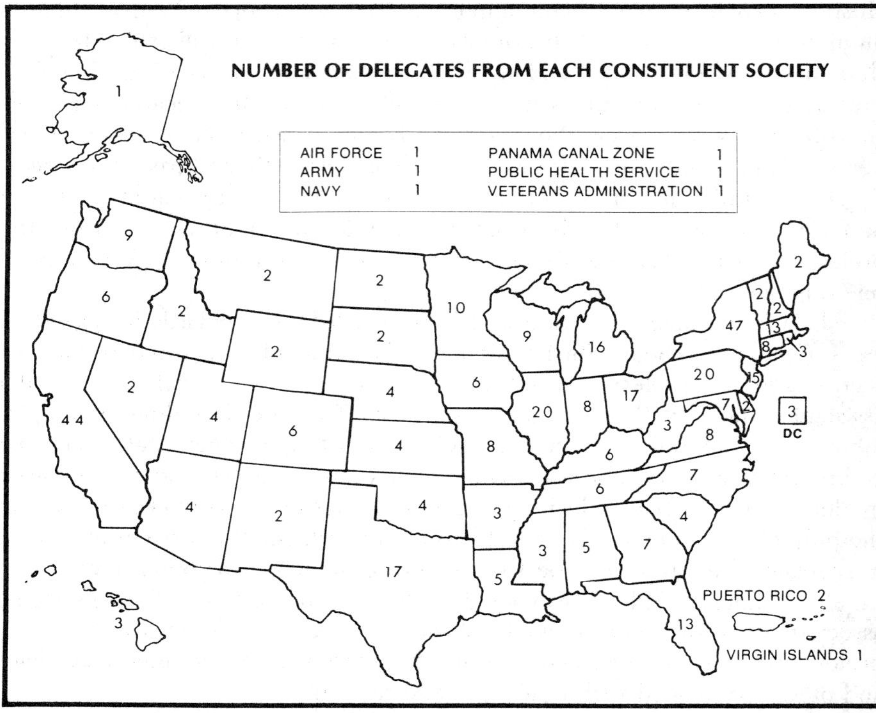

Figure 2–1. Number of delegates from each constituent society. (From American Dental Association. House of Delegates—structure and function of ADA's policy-making body. Am. Dent. A. J., 93:708–12, Oct. 1976. Copyright by the ADA. Reprinted by permission.)

The House of Delegates conducts business once a year for five days during the annual session. Resolutions may be introduced by the Board of Trustees, the 17 ADA councils, or the trustee districts or directly by delegates. Component societies may also originate resolutions that, if approved by the constituent (state) societies, are submitted to the House.

Thirty days in advance of the annual meeting a printed book of 200 to 300 pages—the *Annual Reports and Resolutions*—is transmitted to the members of the House of Delegates. Supplements to the annual reports and resolutions are mailed just prior to the annual session and supplemented again by typewritten material distributed during the session.

Resolutions, along with supporting documentation, are referred for hearing to one of eight reference committees: Budget and Administrative Matters, Dental Care Programs and Health, Dental Education and Related Matters, Legislative and Related Matters, President's Address and Miscellaneous Matters, Access to Comprehensive Dental Care, Scientific Matters, and Judicial Matters and Ethics. The hearings of the reference committees are open to all members of the Association. At these meetings members may speak their minds and advise the House of Delegates of their positions on specific issues or on the status of the Association as a whole. Those in attendance may vary from a few individuals with specific interests to as many as 500 on an issue of broad general interest. The reference committees prepare reports that are transmitted to the House of Delegates.

The efficient conduct of the business of the House of Delegates and the Board of Trustees requires logistical support of considerable magnitude. Hillenbrand, the Executive Director Emeritus, has estimated that during the five-day session a half–million pages of reports and other documents were reproduced, many of them overnight.[60] Special telephone lines are installed and often many of the hotels housing members are served by closed-circuit television reporting the events of the day. A four-page "newspaper" is available each morning.

As the House considers the issues, it usually has the original resolution and background report, the comments and recommendations of the Board of Trustees, and the report and recommendations of the Reference Committee. On the basis of this information, the House acts to accept, reject, amend, substitute, refer, or postpone.

The American Dental Association is divided geographically into 14 districts with roughly equivalent numbers of dentists. A trustee is elected from each of the districts and together with the president, president-elect, and the first and second vice-presidents, this group comprises the Board. The Board of Trustees is charged with the day-to-day responsibility for the operations of the Association and it reports on its activities to the House of Delegates. It also reviews most resolutions on their way to the House, makes comments on the validity of the action requested, and recommends action.

Dental Hygiene*

Historical Development

The first school for training dental hygienists was initiated about 70 years after the first dental school. Dental hygiene developed relatively slowly at first and was primarily centered in the northeastern United States. Around the turn of the century, preventive dentistry became of concern to leaders of the profession. It was felt that improving oral cleanliness could play a part in reducing the attack of dental caries. Although its origin is not known, a popular phrase of the time was that "a clean tooth never decays." It was felt that periodic scaling and polishing of the teeth was an important health service, but that it was time-consuming and interfered with the routine of dental

*A comprehensive history of dental hygiene has been written and should be in the holdings of the libraries of all dental and dental hygiene schools: Fales, M. J. H. History of dental hygiene education in the United States, 1913 to 1975. Doctoral Dissertation, Ann Arbor, University of Michigan, 1975. xiv + 345 p. Microfilm or microfilm-xerography copies are available from Xerox University Microfilms, 300 N. Zeeb Road, Ann Arbor, Michigan 48106. The order number is 75-29, 217.

practice. It was suggested that young women could be trained specifically for this task.

Alfred C. Fones was graduated from the New York College of Dentistry in 1890 and joined his father in practice in Bridgeport, Connecticut. During his early years in practice he perfected a technic of scaling and polishing and taught his patients how to perform necessary home care procedures. By 1906, it seemed apparent to him that the oral health of his patients was substantially improved over that of his father's patients, whose oral health had remained unchanged. In that year, the younger Dr. Fones trained his assistant, Irene Newman, to practice dental hygiene. The dental law in Connecticut recognized dental hygiene as a legal adjunct to dental practice in 1907. A number of dentists had considered the potential of creating a dental auxiliary and some had read papers on the subject. It was Dr. Fones, however, who became known as the "father of dental hygiene" by establishing the first formal school. This school started in 1913 in a carriage house on the grounds of the Fones residence.[83]

Connecticut passed legislation specifically describing the practice of dental hygiene in 1916. During the next four years dental hygiene was recognized in Maine, New Hampshire, Massachusetts, Connecticut, New York, Minnesota, Tennessee, Oklahoma, Colorado, and California. The total rose to 34 in 1935, but not until 1950 did the practice acts of all the states, the District of Columbia, and the Commonwealth of Puerto Rico include provisions for the practice of dental hygiene. The early, rather leisurely development of dental hygiene schools was largely tied to that of dental education. In 1945, of the 16 programs in existence, 13 were associated with schools of dentistry. In 1974, only 37 of 158 were so affiliated. The explosive growth experienced after 1960 centered primarily in colleges and junior colleges.[45] Federal legislation to fund vocational-technical education in health occupation training centers was a primary factor that made this expansion possible.[3] The growth continued in the next decade, and in 1980 the number of schools was 204. (See Fig. 2–2. Also see Table 14–5 and Fig. 14–7.)

During the first 30 years of the dental hygiene profession there were wide differences from school to school about both prerequisites and curriculum. This variation was due to a number of factors, including differences in state licensing acts, problems of integrating a two-year clinical program into a four-year curriculum that would meet university requirements for a baccalaureate degree, and the lack of nationally approved standards. The latter problem was remedied in 1947, when the Council on Dental Education adopted the first of a series of "Requirements for the Accrediting of a School of Dental Hygiene." In 1952, the Council on Dental Education of the American Dental Association undertook an active program in accreditation, fulfilling a long-standing goal of the American Dental Hygienists' Association.[96] A two-year curriculum must meet the standards of the Commission on Accreditation of Dental and Dental Auxiliary Educational Programs of the American Dental Association. The candidate, after passing an examination for licensure, may use the initials RDH (Registered Dental Hygienist) following the name. In all

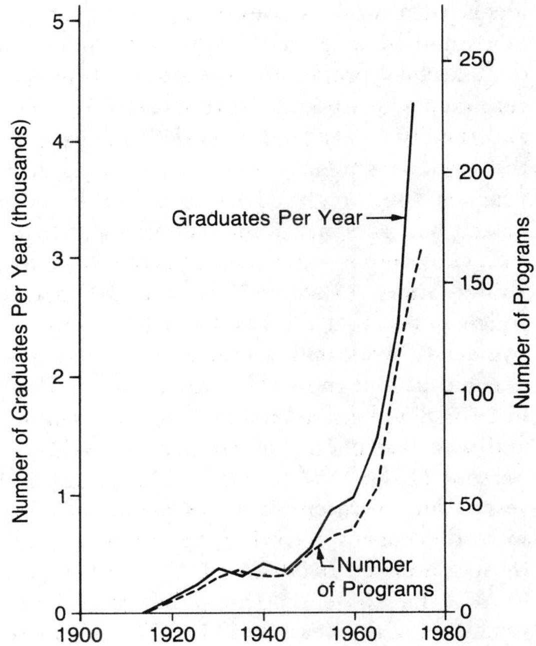

Figure 2–2. Number of dental hygiene education programs and graduates per year, 1915 to 1974. (From Fales, Martha, J. H. History of dental hygiene education in the United States, 1913 to 1975. Doctoral Dissertation, Ann Arbor, University of Michigan, 1975.)

states except Alabama (which recognizes apprenticeship, i.e., "on-the-job" training) the completion of an accredited two-year curriculum is the minimum requirement for admittance to examination for licensure by a state board of dental examiners. An individual enrolled in a four-year baccalaureate degree program must also meet university standards for that degree. Many dental hygienists earn advanced degrees (M.P.H., M.S., Ph.D., Dr.P.H.), for which the requirements of the graduate school of the university also must be met.

Dental Hygiene Students

In the late 1950s the *Survey of Dentistry* studied dental hygienists as well as dentists. Kesel reported a survey of 20,600 dental hygienists but with a response rate of only 38 percent.[66] The study found that the majority of trained hygienists who responded were not working and many who did work only devoted part-time to hygiene. They entered dental hygiene often at the behest of the family dentist, because of the promise of good salary and/or working conditions, for service to others, because of the influence of another hygienist, and because they liked working with people and the short training time required for the profession. Differences were found by Curl[31] and Hewitt[59] for hygiene students who had opted for various kinds of hygiene programs: community college, university-affiliated, and dental school-affiliated programs. In Curl's study, hygiene students in dental school settings were slightly older, had more years of schooling, and were from families of higher socioeconomic levels than were students in the other programs. All three groups were motivated by a service career with professional status, while students in the dental school programs were attracted by hygiene as a "health-oriented field." Junior college students were more likely to cite "high-financial remuneration" and the "two-year" requirement as reasons for selection. Hewitt summarized the hygiene students as of middle socioeconomic status, between 17 to 20 years of age, single, desiring a health career with professional status, and having had personal influences affecting their career choice.

The most recent count of active hygienists (1979) recorded 32,200 in the United States, or about 28 for each 100 dentists (see Table 14–4). Malvitz and Judge noted that "it has been the 'conventional wisdom' that most dental hygienists 'work only a year or two,' quit in order to rear families, and rarely become part of the work force again."[71] The writers conducted a mail survey in 1976 of all licensed dental hygienists whose mailing address was in Michigan and who had been graduated prior to May 1975. The response rate was 90 percent of the total of 2,327. The survey indicated that 76 percent of those responding were employed as dental hygienists. As might be expected, there were differences according to the year of graduation. Ninety-five percent of those graduated between 1972 and 1974 were employed. The figure dropped to 76.4 for those graduated between 1966 and 1971 and to 57.3 for the graduates of the years 1950 to 1964, but increased to 65.3 for those graduated prior to 1950. Although a proposed major study of dental hygienists in the entire United States remains unfunded, it has been anticipated that the trends identified in Michigan might be reflected in a national study.[34]

Organization of the Profession

In 1923, 46 dental hygienists representing 11 states met in Cleveland, Ohio, to organize the American Dental Hygienists' Association (ADHA) with strong support from the dental profession. The previous year the Board of Trustees of the ADA had encouraged the establishment of the Association and indicated that it would enjoy "conference relations" with the ADA. Initially, the growth of the organization was steady but not spectacular. In the 20 years following 1925, active membership went from several hundred to about 2,000. In the next 10 years (1945 to 1955) membership more than doubled to nearly 4,400 and this level of growth continued during the nine years between 1955 and 1964 to stand at approximately 8,000. In 1980 the total active membership was 22,560 and the inclusion of the junior (student) members brought the total to 28,837.[17, 97]

The organization of the profession closely parallels that of dentistry. There are seven classifications of memberships (including junior student membership for a modest fee), but the basic category of "active members" must be held through constituent and component associations if such exist. There are 53 constituent associations.[17] The House of Delegates meets once a year and is the supreme authoritative body of the Association, having all legislative and policy-making powers. The Board of Trustees is composed of the elective officers (except the Speaker of the House), 12 trustees, and the immediate past president and has responsibility for supervising the day-to-day operations. It reviews reports and makes recommendations and relates all of its activities to the House.[83, 96, 97]

A great portion of the work of the ADHA is carried out by a variety of committees. Of primary importance are the committees and staff of the Division of Educational Services and the Washington office. *The Journal of the American Dental Hygienists' Association* was established in 1927. In 1972 the name was changed to *Dental Hygiene* (the Journal of the American Dental Hygienists' Association) and in January 1975 it achieved monthly publication.[83]

Dental Assisting

The *Survey of Dentistry* study of dental assistants queried 6,011 assistants, most of whom were members of the American Dental Assistants' Association (ADAA). While the study may be outdated, the sample may not have been representative, and there was a low response rate (31 percent), it is one of the few national studies of this population.[66] Among the findings was the fact that the assistant typically is a female who is low paid and trained on the job, an office worker who performs many tasks with a high job satisfaction, but with short staying power on the job. Most have high school educations and about one quarter desire some expanded duties. A later study of vocational interests suggested that dental assistants preferred nursing, homemaking, office work, regular work hours, stability, courteous supervisors, and well-defined duties.[58]

A study of New Jersey high school females enrolled in college preparatory courses indicated that those who expressed a positive interest in dental assisting tended to come from blue-collar families with parents who were not high school graduates, and did not expect to continue their education or pursue a profession.[58] The choice of an occupation—or the matching of one's self-image with the perceived construct of an occupational role model—seems related not only to socioeconomic background but also possibly to visible career options.[58] Although experiments with expanded role models for the dental assistant have been tried, many state practice acts currently inhibit, if not specifically prohibit, the introduction of these functions into dental practice.

Clearly, more research on who enters dental assisting and how they are utilized is required, for the new entrants to this field will probably affect its role content and the remaining network of occupational groups in the dental system. With 144,700 active assistants estimated to be in practice in 1977 (see Chapter 14), a sizable labor force presents itself for study.[74]

Present trends suggest that a redefinition of the training and utilization of a variety of dental auxiliaries (including dental assistants and dental laboratory technicians) may be expected, a development outlined in Chapter 14.

CHARACTERISTICS OF DENTAL PRACTICE IN THE UNITED STATES

Nature of Dental Diseases

Medicine and dentistry share a somewhat common history, possess many similar characteristics, and share an equal basis under law. On the other hand, there are marked differences between the practices of the two professions. These differences are, in part, due to accidents of history. They are also due to the unique characteristics of dental diseases in contrast to the majority of medical conditions. The nature of these diseases would seem to be the primary factor that has determined the philosophy and emphasis of dental education, the type of student attracted to the professions, the way in which dentistry is practiced, and the types of programs that have been efficient and effective in delivering treatment to large groups of patients.

Young, an English physician, has grouped medical problems into four classes:

> The problems caused by the majority of serious medical conditions are self-limiting through cure (spontaneous or therapeutic), control, or death. A fourth category consists of those conditions which are neither fatal, controllable, nor curable. Most acute infections fall into the first category, endocrine diseases into the second, malignant diseases into the third, but chronic degenerative diseases and most psychoses fall into the last.[104]

He failed to note that, at least from birth through middle age, only a relatively small portion of the population is affected at any one time.

In contrast, common oral diseases possess quite different characteristics: (1) they occur almost universally; (2) if neglected, they accumulate a backlog of unmet needs because they do not spontaneously undergo remission or termination if untreated; and (3) they almost always require time-consuming professional treatment. Rarely do dental diseases lend themselves to control by prescription, advice, or medication or by ignoring them.

Not only do dental diseases affect almost the entire population but they also recur with periodic frequency. From the time that the teeth first erupt into the oral cavity, there will be need for periodic care as long as the patient lives, or as long as teeth remain in the mouth. If dental resources are in short supply, dental health professionals traditionally have emphasized that young children should have first priority, with the extension of programs gradually including succeeding age groups of individuals. However, given these characteristics of dental disease, the value of providing dental care to a young population, especially one without access to care in future years (as is often the case in "Headstart" programs), is likely to be of limited benefit in terms of long-term retention of the dentition.

A fact closely related to the universal and recurring nature of dental diseases is that if they are untreated, they remain in the mouth and accumulate a backlog of needs for treatment. This characteristic is reflected in the most common epidemiological measure of caries prevalence as described by Klein and Palmer in the 1930s. They pointed out that, at least in children, an examination of the mouth permitted an:

> . . . evaluation of complete caries experience. Such an evaluation requires a full consideration of what would be termed *past* and *present* caries. Present caries may be defined as actual carious lesions which are present in the mouth at the time of examination. The term past caries may be used in designating those teeth that are filled and those that are missing (extracted) because of caries.

The authors continued: "For purposes of precision and brevity, the term DMF [Decayed, Missing, and Filled] is introduced and used in this paper, therefore, to designate the complete caries experience."[67]

The characteristics of dental diseases (near universal attack and frequent recurrence) appear, on statement, simple and obvious, but their impact on dental practice and the development of effective public programs often has not been fully grasped by dentists, physicians, or the planners of health programs. Failure to recognize these characteristics of the dental problem have led to numerous failures in program planning in the United States.

More than a quarter of a century ago, the people of Great Britain enacted a National Health Service (NHS). They were determined to eliminate cost as a barrier to the receipt of physician, hospital, dental, and other health services. Unfortunately, the extent of demand was seriously underestimated. This error partly reflected a lack of understanding of the nature of chronic disease; acute disease still dominated professional thinking. This miscalculation may also have resulted from the weariness following a hard-won victory in war, the tendency of politicians to understate future costs, or the lack of technology to estimate need and demand accurately. For whatever reason, the demand for care and the resulting high cost were far greater than anticipated. All aspects of the NHS suffered, including dental services. Ignoring the problem of an accumulated backlog of need, the government had made available a full range of dental services to the entire population at state expense, and all at the same time, on July 5, 1948. The dental profession, therefore, was faced with the staggering task of treating new episodes of dental disease and, at the same time, attempting to restore the neglected defects that had accumulated over the lifetime of their patients. Providing benefits for the entire population at once created a "tidal wave" of demand, from 1948 through the early 1950s. The dislocation created by this effort has remained to plague private dental practice, the school dental service, and dental education in Great Britain to this day, despite the many achievements of the NHS.[70, 88] (For an expanded discussion of health care systems, see Chapter 12.)

Finally, the very nature of the dental services required compounds the problem. Many medical problems, it has been noted, will resolve themselves. Others can be adequately controlled by modification of the environment, changes in behavior patterns, or the use of drugs, biologicals, and devices—procedures that can often be accomplished with relatively little investment of time by the physician alone. Dental treatment, on the other hand, requires the time and professional skills of the dental professionals themselves for the surgical excising of hard and soft tissues and the replacement of defective or missing teeth.

Practice Organization

Practice Location

Decision making with regard to practice location for dental personnel has resulted in a concentration of dental professionals in areas having growing economies and easy access to metropolitan lifestyles and comforts.[23] The perception of "quality of life" offered by an area appears to play a significant role in that decision making. Qualities such as household incomes, gross rents, robbery arrests, and water fluoridation were among the more important variables in distinguishing between shortage areas and nonshortage areas.[100] Perceived advantages in living conditions, access to recreational opportunities, educational opportunities for children, opportunities to affiliate with a dental school or dental society, and access to cultural and community activities have been among the variables cited by research that influence a dental graduate to make a decision about practice location or a dental hygienist about employment location.

Glass and Baldwin, however, warn that "The decision-making process involved in this selection of a practice location is a complex phenomenon that involves many personal value judgments and little objective information."[55] The findings of their study confirm the subjective impressions of dental school faculty members with extensive experience in counseling senior dental students about choices of careers and locations for practice. The writers add that "The results of this survey suggest that many dentists are not completely satisfied with conventional methods of selecting a practice location, a significant procedure that is completely lacking in organization."

The necessity for difficult "personal value judgements" may continue to hamper rational selection of a practice location, but recent developments suggest that the availability of "objective information" will improve. In 1973 the University of Minnesota School of Dentistry, in conjunction with Minnesota's dental association and state board of dentistry, initiated a computer-based information system to aid dentists and dental auxiliaries in finding a location. The system provides statistical community profiles, a clearinghouse to match persons looking for dental personnel with personnel seeking a location, and a file of references, maps, brochures, and other descriptive information about communities. The system, with the aid of funding from the American Dental Association and the W. K. Kellogg Foundation, is being expanded to cover the United States and should improve the transmission of information about practice location opportunities and the availability of individuals seeking a location.[24]

State licensure regulations may play a significant role in such decision making, since there is only limited reciprocity among the states in this country. State board examinations sometimes have higher failure rates for out-of-state candidates than for in-state candidates. Difficulty in entry because of licensure requirements has been associated with higher dental incomes and higher utilization of auxiliaries.[73, 75]

Physical Setting

The ability to practice medicine solely with the resources of the individual practitioner (largely contained in a black bag) became obsolete with the passing of the horse and buggy. Today the ability of physicians to utilize their professional skills is largely dependent on the availability of medical and hospital facilities and resources provided by the community. Laboratory and radiographic facilities, surgical suites, complex therapeutic devices such as cobalt units and computerized tomography (CAT scan), the instrumentation of intensive care units, and a wide variety of paramedical personnel represent a major investment in health care in almost every community. The availability of these resources determines, to a large extent, the nature of medical practice in the community and the number and type (general practitioners and specialists) of practitioners that can be attracted to serve the area.

The distribution of dental professionals, on the other hand, does not reflect the availability of community health facilities, but primarily the personal choice of the practitioner. (Of course, dental personnel obviously will wish to have available good health care for themselves and their families.) The dental hygienist need only find a dental office with sufficient space and equipment and a dentist interested in prevention who wishes to employ a hygienist to share these duties. Dentists ordinarily are completely self-contained and depend on almost no outside resources, either from other practitioners or from the community. One reason is that most expensive items of equipment in the dental operatory, such as the dental chair and unit, are in almost constant use by the dental professionals themselves so there is no opportunity to share them with other health practitioners. Aside from radiographic equipment, the balance of the dentist's instrumentation is relatively inexpensive and does not create a demand for a community facility to be shared with others. Because the dentist usually does not share community-financed facilities with other practitioners, the initial cost of entering practice is significant.

Little is known about the factors involved in selection of a particular dentist by a patient. Experience suggests that it is a rather random process related to (1) the need to find a new dentist; (2) knowledge of a particular dentist's existence gained by casual questioning of friends or by seeing a professional sign in the neighborhood; i.e., usually by word of mouth and convenience; or (3) looking through the telephone directory to find a dentist in the area. The final input is any chance opportunity of finding one or more individuals who have gone to the particular dentist under consideration. It is unfortunate that this process has received scant attention, because even a fairly simplistic model would be useful to newly graduated dentists seeking a practice location, to dentists considering relocation, and to government agencies and consumer advocacy groups attempting to improve the distribution (and therefore the accessibility) of dental practice.

Organizational Structure of Dental Practice

The American Dental Association periodically surveys dentists to determine the nature, size, configuration, and productivity of dental practices. The most recent data (1977) indicate that the typical dental practice appears to be a private general practice with nearly three (2.7) treatment rooms or operatories. One or more assistants were employed by 85.6 percent of the practices. More than 90 percent of the practices employed either full-time or part-time secretaries (73.0 percent) or bookkeepers (17.8 percent). Thirty-four percent employed one or more hygienists, full-time or part-time. The average practice served nearly 80 (78.7) patient visits per week. The cost of operating a dental practice is high, with overhead consuming 46 percent of the gross in the average practice. Income and productivity of dentists vary by dentist's age—increasing up to age 34–44, leveling off in the 50s, then decreasing as retirement approaches. Utilization of auxiliaries increases as the practice develops, with the assistant the first hired and the secretary and the dental hygienist added later during higher-volume periods.[6]

Dental practices can be organized in an infinite variety of ways—matching the variety of individuals who enter practice. They may be divided into three basic types: independent solo practice (including associateships), solo with facility sharing, and partnership-group practice.

Independent solo practice reflects the personal judgment and preference of an individual practitioner. At the minimum level, such a practice may involve one practitioner who works completely alone and uses one dental operating room, a waiting room, and a small laboratory-darkroom. In this instance, the dentist carries out professional treatment, prepares filling materials, fabricates prosthetic appliances, answers the telephone, cleans up after each patient, and maintains records as necessary. These efforts may be supplemented slightly by a person—perhaps the spouse or a high school student—who comes in for a few hours a day. Archaic as they may appear, such practices still exist. In 1977, 6.3 percent of the dentists in private practice reported that they had no employees.[6] A more common pattern is for the dentist to have at least two dental operating rooms and to employ one, one and a half, or two dental assistants.

The professional tasks of the dentist may be supplemented by the skills of a dental hygienist, professionally educated and licensed to perform certain clinical procedures in the mouth. The responsibilities of the hygienist usually include patient education, radiographic and clinical examinations, and oral prophylaxes. In 1975 almost 23 percent of the dentists employed a dental hygienist on a full-time basis, and an equal number employed a part-time hygienist.[5]

A third of the dentists have gone further in refining the organization of solo practice to achieve maximum productivity. In 1977, 32.6 percent reported employing four or more auxiliaries. In such instances, auxiliaries will often include a full-time or part-time dental laboratory technician who fabricates complete and partial dentures, crowns, and fixed bridges under the professional supervision of the dentist.[6]

Older dentists, or those with unusually large practices, sometimes invite a younger dentist to join them as an "associate," a euphemistic term used to describe the employment of a dentist on a salary, or a paid percentage of the employed dentist's gross income, or a combination of these. The practice and the patients are those of the senior dentist, and it may be assumed that the characteristics of the services rendered reflect the older dentist's training, experience, and performance. For this reason, the small group of dentists who fall in the associate category (less than 3 percent) can be considered as participating in an extension of independent solo practice.[7] (The 1977 *Survey of Dental Practice* used the category of "salaried dentist" to describe employment for a salary, commission, percentage, or other compensation arrangement—*but excluded salaried dentists employed by "institutions."* The study identified 3.5 percent of dentists as being "salaried."[6])

The second organizational pattern is that of facility sharing. Again, a wide variation exists. There are offices in which all equipment and physical facilities and even auxiliary personnel are shared by two or more dentists who still maintain their individual practices. Each practice collects its own income, but costs of the shared facilities are paid jointly on a pre-agreed basis. A more common pattern is to share only a limited part of the physical facilities, such as the waiting room, laboratory, and radiographic equipment. Regardless of the extent to which costs are shared, even this small departure from complete independence has not proved to be significantly popular, since only 10 out of 100 dentists in private practice in 1972 reported that they participated in arrangements of this type.[9]

The most radical departures from tradition are the full partnerships, and "shareholder-incorporated." There have been a variety of definitions of group practice, but Sarner has pointed out that the crucial characteristic of this method of organization is that income, as well as facilities and expenses, is shared by the participants.[90] (Dentists may be employed by a group practice on a salary or commission or as junior partners. In this case they are not true "partners/owners/shareholders.") Gift and Schaid used a much more liberal definition and as a result classified a much larger number of practices as "group practice."[54] For several decades professional leaders have viewed group practice as the desirable pattern for the future. Some have said that it would be more professionally rewarding to the dentist, since one could concentrate primarily on providing those services one felt most competent to perform and could share the remainder with associates. Others have pointed to the potential of more efficient and effective use of auxiliaries, leading to an increased income or a lowering of fees, or both. Some who have been concerned with the quality of care have felt that having dentists associated with each other would reinforce professional standards and performance—either the highest or the lowest.

Despite its seeming advantages, group practice has developed only modestly. About 1.5 percent of the dentists practicing in 1952 had such an arrangement. This increased to 2.6 percent in 1958, and nine years later the percentage had risen to 4.6 percent.[10, 66] The 1972 data show an increase to 6.4 percent.[9] In 1977, 4.6 percent of dentists were identified as full members of a partnership and almost 21 percent were salaried shareholders in an incorporated practice.[6] Although the complete sharing of dental practice developed slowly at first, it has earned an established position and apparently is accelerating. Given the steady growth over the past two decades and the pressure from the public for increased productivity from the profession, there is reason to judge that full partnerships and other forms of group practice may become an important organizational pattern for dental practice in the near future. (For additional views on group practice and other types of salaried practice, see Chapter 12.)

Scope of Services

One of the major issues that has plagued medicine in recent decades has been the proliferation of specialties. This trend has been viewed by many observers as leading to a fragmentation of services, which may result in an emphasis on sporadic, episodic care of the patient. A number of leaders in the medical profession have sought ways to bring about a return to the primary physician (the so-called family physician) who could provide continuing, recurrent, preventive, and family-centered medicine. The same discussions are now occurring in dentistry to offset the kinds of problems of overspecialization that have appeared in medicine.

Most oral diseases and malconditions are treatable in contexts that do not depend on physicians' services or other members of the "medical team" such as nurses and various types of therapists. The education of a dentist supposedly includes all the technical knowledge required for treatment of dental diseases. Thus, dental care services have developed in a system usually separate from medicine. These services are provided primarily by independent solo practitioners in small general practice settings.

Although the increase in specialties has been an issue in the profession, the numbers to date have remained modest. Out of approximately 112,000 active dentists in the United States in 1975, about 10 percent (11,500) were listed as recognized specialists.[74] In the 1977 *Survey of Dental Practice*, 89.5 percent of the respondents identified themselves as general practitioners.[6]* The long-term trend in first-year enrollment in advanced educational specialty programs has remained fairly constant at around 1,200 in recent years.[8, 13]

Patterns of referral to specialists are responsive to a number of factors.

*For the same year, the Public Health Service estimated 86.3 percent (see Chapter 14, reference 103).

The age of the patient (and potential behavior problems) is a primary indication for referral to a pedodontist whose practice is basically general dentistry for children. Orthodontic practices are almost completely composed of children and young adults, but the major criterion is the presence of malpositioned teeth or dental arches. The education of many pedodontists includes the diagnosis and treatment of many of the same conditions of malocclusion, leading to "jurisdictional" disputes between the two specialties.[41]

The severity of a dental disease or condition or degree of difficulty of the treatment is the primary reason for referrals to endodontists, periodontists, prosthodontists, and oral surgeons. Oral pathologists and public health dentists are almost always on a salary in an institution such as a dental school, health agency, or hospital.

Whereas about half of the American population visit the dentist's office in a given year, two thirds visit because of a symptom related to oral disease.[88] Because of the chronic, recurring nature of dental diseases, the profession has been attempting to develop and promote preventive care rather than episodic treatment. Thus, a general family dentist who can perform preventive and restorative services is viewed as being the keystone of dental practice in the future.[18, 106]

A survey of preventive practices among dental practitioners in the United States was conducted in 1957, when a 1 percent sample of practicing dentists (758) were interviewed to determine their employment of routine "cleaning and polishing, topical fluoride treatment, x-ray examination, and periodic recall."[47] Only half of the practices at that time were moderately or highly preventive and one fourth were only negligibly preventive. Younger dentists were more likely to practice preventively, to employ office assistants, to be active to a limited extent in professional organizations, to have at least 6 percent of their patients under six years of age, and to have patients predominantly in an upper-income group. The more preventive the practice, the higher the net income. Those practices least preventively oriented reported that the reasons were lack of time, adverse patient reaction, smaller monetary return for such services, and that the procedures were not interesting for dentists to perform.

The only national study of prevention of more recent vintage (1975) was conducted by the American Dental Association at the request of and with the funding of the National Institute for Dental Research.[53] That study was able to survey 3,500 general practitioners, 250 pedodontists, and 250 other specialists by mail. In that study, although focusing on caries, a broad range of preventive procedures was measured, including diet and nutritional counseling, education for plaque control (use of the toothbrush and dental floss in a prescribed manner), oral bacteria testing, oral prophylaxis, pit-and-fissure sealant, subgingival scaling, topical fluoride applications, charting, examinations, and recall.

The intervening years since the earlier study apparently have witnessed a change in dentists' self-reported attitudes toward greater adoption of preventive measures and a broader range of preventive services. The most preventively oriented dentists tended to be general practitioners and pedodontists, while the least preventively oriented dentists tended to be specialists (other than pedodontists and orthodontists) who do not employ hygienists, whose incomes are over $20,000 a year, who are approaching retirement age, and who are open to accepting new patients in the practice.

Studies of patients' complaints about dentists suggest that there might be a great disparity between what dentists report as their practice patterns and what patients perceive as occurring.[27] Patients, for example, claim that they are being provided little information and explanation about what is to be done and why—that they are being treated as "cases" rather than as people. A limited study was conducted (1970) in which the dentist-patient interaction was monitored by tape recordings. Analysis of the tape recordings revealed that most patients could not and did not comply with dental advice because, in fact, most did not receive advice from their dentists.[33] This study may suggest that dentists overreport their provision of advice to patients, when actual transcriptions of dentist-patient interactions appear to demonstrate that relatively few of the dentists studied provided such advice. (See also Chapter 15.)

CONTINUED COMPETENCE AND QUALITY OF CARE

Freidson has pointed out that "Medicine is practice in privacy. Work in the other established professions is carried on publicly—in the court, the church, and the lecture hall—as often as in the office."[48] Because most dentistry is not usually practiced in the hospital, it is an even more private service. Only rarely will a dentist's performance be seen by any other person trained in one of the health fields. Only a small portion of dentists ever perform technical procedures in the presence of another dentist. There are few opportunities to share professional experiences and these are limited almost exclusively to discussions at dental meetings and on the golf course, which have grave drawbacks as effective methods of transmitting information. Because of the lack of these outside contacts, the continued competence of dentists has been almost exclusively their own individual responsibility. Technically speaking, there have been professional grievance committees in many dental societies, and state boards of dental examiners are supposed to be responsible for ensuring that licensed practitioners offer a quality service. Until quite recently, however, the almost complete lack of opportunities for dentists to view their colleagues at work means that these channels were rarely utilized.

The responsibilities of dentists toward patients and those who work with them in their practices are summarized in the American Dental Association's "Principles of Ethics and Code of Professional Conduct"[4].

> The dentist's primary obligation of service to the public shall include the delivery of quality care, competently and timely, within the bounds of the

> clinical circumstances presented by the patient. Quality of care shall be a primary consideration of the dental practitioner.
>
> * * *
>
> Dentists shall be obliged to report to the appropriate reviewing agency as determined by the local component or constituent society instances of gross or continual faulty treatment by other dentists. Patients should be informed of their present oral health status without disparaging comment about prior service.

The issue of the quality of dental care presents unique and sensitive problems for the dental hygienist. If defective restorations placed by an "outside" dentist are observed, they should be charted for the dentist's attention, but no comment to the patient is necessary. It is reasonable to expect the dentist to handle this rather difficult situation. It is the responsibility of the dentist to explain the necessity for replacing the restoration or restorations but at the same time hold criticism of the previous practitioner to a minimum. If the doubtful restorations have been placed by the supervisory dentist, no comment is necessary initially. Any practitioner on occasion may perform a restorative or prosthetic service that may not be up to usual standards. If a persistent trend of inadequate care is noted, the only sensible course of action probably is for the dental hygienist quietly to seek an association in another practice.*

Concern about maintenance of quality has increased in recent years, with the growth of third-party payment programs either through private groups, such as unions, or through governmental programs, such as those under Title XVIII and Title XIX (Medicaid) of the Social Security amendments. Not surprisingly, those concerned with expending large sums of money to obtain professional services feel it necessary to obtain some assurance that the services they are paying for have been, in fact, rendered, and rendered with at least an acceptable level of quality.

Audit, Assessment, and Assurance†

There are essentially three levels of review and action. The first level is a check to be certain that services for which payment is claimed have been provided. This determination is an audit, which may be done by a check of serial records by a computer program, by a clinical examination, or by an evaluation of posttreatment radiographs. (The latter method is questionable, since it may result in radiation exposure not justified by the need for diagnostic assistance.) If a discrepancy is noted, it likely is carelessness (often in recording), but could be fraud. The penalty for the latter offense may be severe, including a prison sentence, substantial fines, and loss of the license to practice. There have been publicly reported instances of fraud, but only on

*The 1982 revision of the American Dental Hygienists' Association *Manual* under the heading of "Ethics" is silent on this issue and thus provides no guidance.

†For other aspects of quality control as related to cost containment, see Chapter 13.

a limited scale. A report released in July 1979 by the then Department of Health, Education, and Welfare included the fact that only 10 dentists had been suspended for fraud in the Medicaid and Medicare programs since 1977.[99]

The second level of review is assessment of the quality of care. Some argue that this can be accomplished without actually examining patients, with the use of posttreatment radiographs and records.[49] Others have argued that, in addition to causing unnecessary radiation, a method of this type does not provide adequate information to judge quality. Several systems have been developed for the clinical assessment of dental care. Among these systems are those of Ryge and Snyder,[89] Cons,[30] Soricelli,[95] Bailit and colleagues,[19] Friedman,[49] and the Indian Health Service of the U.S. Public Health Service.[37] Schonfeld has reviewed most aspects of evaluating "oral care systems."[91] Several component or constituent organizations of the American Dental Association have developed similar systems, the best known probably being the product of the California Dental Association.[26] In addition to clinical standards, the California system includes an evaluation of program design covering priorities, administration, benefit packages, and other aspects. The American Academy of Pedodontics (AAP) and the American Society of Dentistry for Children (ASDC) have jointly published three editions of a *Manual for Children's Dental Care Programs.*[86] This document outlines specific dental services that should be provided for children and a ranking by priority. The AAP/ASDC manual includes in the section on "Assessment of Clinical Quality" consideration of the management of the child and the control of pain and anxiety.

Audit and the assessment of the quality of care are steps toward the ultimate goal—the *assurance* of quality. To be more specific: "Quality assessment + action = quality assurance."[101] A more detailed definition is provided by a report of the American Dental Association's Quality Assurance Project:

> Quality assurance is the assessment or measurement of the quality of care and the implementation of any necessary changes to either maintain or improve the quality of care rendered.[16]

The third level, thus, is implementation of necessary changes. Varying "actions" may be taken to maintain or improve the quality of care but they vary in effectiveness. Continuing education to eliminate the lack of skill or knowledge identified by quality assessment is one course of action thought by many to be most appropriate. This is currently being done by some agencies that employ clinical dentists on a salary. For the programs operated by institutions or agencies, further actions may involve censure, probation, or dismissal.

The assurance of quality is not as simple a task for programs (either private or public) dependent on the purchase of care from private practitioners who function essentially as private contractors. Again, continuing education opportunities are an appropriate place to start. Unfortunately, although the value of continuing education is part of the "common wisdom" of the profession, little is known of its effectiveness in modifying behavior. Practitioners who are aware of gaps in their knowledge and are motivated to improve their clinical skills will profit from continuing education, but they are not likely to be the individuals for whom "quality assurance" efforts are appropriate. State dental practice acts technically provide avenues for legal recourse to bar inept dentists from practice. Practically, experience indicates that a jury is not likely to remove or suspend a license except for the most gross misconduct, such as sexual abuse in the office, drug addiction, or fraud. Jurors are not likely to deprive a "poor dentist" and family of their living.

The American Dental Association has strongly urged state and local dental societies to replace or supplement existing grievance committees with a peer review system to provide objective answers to questions or complaints that may originate from a patient, a practicing dentist, or a third party that is being asked to pay for the cost of dental treatment. This effort has included the development of a structured training program for local dental society members, the production of a film, and the publication of a *Peer Review Procedure Manual.*[12]

Apparently, the profession has reacted sufficiently early in its development of systems of peer review of continuing competence and the quality of care to meet the demand for such systems before their absence became a threat to the integrity of the profession. It could be wished that these developments had occurred earlier, but the climate of professional attitudes only recently shifted from the traditional desire to maintain the total independence of the practitioner from outside forces. The shift has been remarkable. A summary of the 1975 *Survey of Dentists* indicated that 83 percent of the practitioners responding believed peer review (including the quality of care) should be a permanent program of dental societies and 85 percent stated that corrective action should be taken against a dentist found to be repeatedly practicing at an unacceptable level of quality.[56]

Professional Standards Review Organization (PSRO)

Evaluation of the quality of dental care is not new and has been done by state boards of dental examiners and dental schools for many years, although in a relatively unstructured way and often with little attempt at standardization. These assessments related, moreover, to individual procedures performed for individual patients. As early as 1949, in the first version of this text (then titled *Dentistry in Public Health*), Wisan reported that the New Jersey State Health Department employed part-time consultants to ". . . periodically check the work of the participating dentists by examining groups of treated children."[103] Most of the quality review systems cited in the previous section, however, evolved in the 1960s and the early 1970s.

The Social Security Amendments of 1972 (P.L. 92-603) created a heightened sense of urgency by mandating a national system for the review of health services provided under Social Security, primarily Medicare and Medicaid.[84] The Department of Health and Human Services has divided the country into more than 200 Professional Standards Review Organization (PSRO) areas. In each area a panel of physicians (and osteopaths) are to evaluate whether services ". . . conform to appropriate professional standards, are medically necessary, and are provided in the most economical setting appropriate for effective care."[84] The first priority will be hospital-based physicians' services; the second, outpatient physicians' services. It is anticipated that eventually outpatient dental services will be added to the system despite the fact that dentists currently can be used only as advisors or "contractors" to review dental care—a discriminatory act, since dentists cannot currently serve on the basic PSRO review body. The American Dental Association has strongly opposed this discrepancy.

The PSRO concept has drawn strong opposition from both the current Department of Health and Human Services and the American Medical Association—an unusual alliance, even though the basis for the opposition is quite different. (The Department's opposition is based on the cost, while the medical profession resents further government intrusion.) Because of the controversy, the PSRO program may not survive in its present form. If the PSRO does not survive, the principle that health professions must be accountable to the agency that pays for the care will probably surface in another form. It might be said that "accountability" will be a major characteristic of health practice in the last two decades of the twentieth century.

Peer Review

There is apparently confusion about the use of the term "peer review" in relation to quality assessment and assurance, since sometimes the three terms are used as though they were interchangeable—*which they are not*. It has been noted previously that assessment is only part of the effort to ensure quality. Assessment may be done by "peers" or those who are not. *Webster's New Third International Dictionary* defines "peer" as "belonging to the same group in society, especially when membership is determined by age, grade, or status."[57] The peer of a dentist is another dentist with similar education and experience, and the peer of a dental hygienist is another dental hygienist with similar training and experience.

"Peer review" does not necessarily refer to judgments about fees, the relevance of patient complaints, or the appropriateness of a particular course of treatment, but it can apply to any or all of these judgments. In other words, "peer review" means *only* that some type of judgment is made by one's peers. More precise use of the term should reduce confusion in terminology.

TOWARD THE TWENTY-FIRST CENTURY

At the beginning of this century, the elements of a strong and useful profession were present, although some were in embryonic form. The last 80 plus years have seen dentistry's growth, differentiation, and maturation.

What of the future? With the research arm of the profession greatly strengthened in the recent past, both scientific and technical breakthroughs may be anticipated. A vaccine against dental caries, sought for some 50 years,[64] may become a reality as the oral flora becomes more clearly understood. The attack of periodontal diseases can be modified by meticulous oral hygiene to control plaque formation. Although effective, the procedure is time-consuming and requires a high degree of motivation. Perhaps this can be more easily accomplished in the future by a mouthrinse or a specially formulated toothpaste.

Enormous advances have been made in restorative and prosthetic technics that have made possible more efficient restoration of tissue, with less stress to the patient and the dentist. Dental auxiliaries are playing an increasing role in dental practice, as dental offices and clinics become increasingly sophisticated. In the long term, new auxiliaries will probably be formally designated and with them will come a reallocation of professional responsibilities within a "dental practice team."

The demand for dental care will continue to rise if the number of government and other third-party payers and if what Pelton and Bothwell[85] have termed the "automatic market" resulting from rising income and education continue to increase. A minimum measure of effective demand, the number of persons who reported visiting a dental office within a 12-month period, rose from 42 percent in 1963–1964 to over 50 percent in 1975,[38, 39] but then leveled off (see Chapter 11).

Probably the most dramatic changes will come in public attitudes toward and expectations of dental care. Words heard often today—cost-containment, accountability, accessibility, patient-oriented care—will be heard with increasing frequency in the future. All aspects of health care have become the topics of debate. And in recent years consumers have achieved a forum in which to express their views; for example, as members of advisory councils, state and regional health planning boards (Health Systems Agencies), and state boards of dental examiners.

References

1. Ahlberg, J. E. The effect of plaque control in Sweden: a preventive experience. p. 215–24. (In Ingle, J. I., and Blair, Patricia, eds. International dental care delivery systems: issues in dental health policies. Cambridge, Mass., Ballinger, 1978. xxi + 263 p.)
2. Akers, R. L., and Quinney, Richard. Differential organization of health professions: a comparative analysis. Am. Sociol. Rev., 33:104–21, Feb. 1968.
3. American Association of Dental Schools, Administrative Board, Council of Auxiliaries. Allied dental educator preparation; a guide to program planning. [Chicago, The Association, 1978.] 15 p. draft, duplicated.
4. American Dental Association [Council on Bylaws and Judicial Affairs]. ADA principles of ethics and code of professional conduct; with official advisory opinions revised to July 1982. Am. Dent. A. J., 105:493–5, Sept. 1982.
5. American Dental Association, Bureau of Economic and Behavioral Research. Personal communication, June 29, 1979.
6. ———. The 1977 survey of dental practice. Chicago, The Association, c1978. 99 p.
7. American Dental Association, Bureau of Economic Research and Statistics. The 1975 survey of dental practice. Chicago, The Association, c1977. 41p.

8. ——. Growth in population and number of dentists to 1985. Am. Dent. A. J., 87:901–3, Oct. 1973.
9. ——. The 1973 survey of dental practice. Chicago, The Association, [1973]. 39 p.
10. ——. The 1968 survey of dental practice, II. Income of dentists by location, age, and other factors. Am. Dent. A. J., 78:342–6, Feb. 1969.
11. American Dental Association [Council on Bylaws and Judicial Affairs]. Truth in advertising tenets bind dentists. Am. Dent. A. J., 96:397–8, Mar. 1978.
12. American Dental Association, Council on Dental Care Programs. Peer review procedure manual. Chicago, The Association, 1975. 18 p.
13. American Dental Association, Council on Dental Education. Trend analysis 1977–78; supplement 11 to the annual report 1977–78. Dental Education. Chicago, The Association, [1978]. 26 p. duplicated.
14. ——. Summary of the 1979–1980 annual report on dental education. Am. Dent. A. J., 100:926–30, June 1980.
15. American Dental Association. House of Delegates: structure and function of the A.D.A.'s policy-making body. Am. Dent. A. J., 93:708–12, Oct. 1976.
16. American Dental Association. Quality assurance project: executive summary, parts 1–3. Am. Dent. A. J., 98:81–5, Jan.; 98:261–7, Feb.; 98:429–35, Mar. 1979.
17. American Dental Hygienists' Association, Membership Services. Chicago, Ill., Personal communication, Aug. 21, 1980.
18. Ast, D. B. Oral health delivery systems: changes resulting from more efficient preventive measures and use of auxiliaries. p. 129–86. (In Brown, W. E., ed. Oral health, dentistry, and the American public; the need for an improved oral care delivery system. Norman, Okla., University Oklahoma Press, 1974. vx + 372 p.)
19. Bailit, Howard, et al. Quality of dental care: development of standards. Am. Dent. A. J., 89:842–53, Oct. 1974.
20. Beck, Dorothy F. A preliminary summary of the facts pertaining to dentistry contained in the published reports of the Committee on the Costs of Medical Care. Am. Dent. A. J., 19:230–51, Feb. 1932.
21. Bellin, L. E., and Kavaler, F. Policing publicly funded health care for poor quality, overutilization and fraud: the New York City Medicaid experience. Am. J. Pub. Health, 60:811–20, May 1970.
22. Blackerby, P. E., Jr. Why not a department of social dentistry? J. Dent. Educ., 22:322–8, Nov. 1958.
23. Born, D. O. Dental manpower planning and distribution; a survey of the literature. p. i–xxvi. (In Koehler, H. M., ed. 1975, Advances in socio-dental research. Chicago, American Dental Association, 1975. xxxi + 218 p.)
24. Born, D. O., and Burton, Kristine. Impact of a computerized placement service on practice location of recent graduates. Am. Dent. A. J., 97:175–8, Aug. 1978.
25. Bremner, M. D. K. The story of dentistry; from the dawn of civilization to the present. 3rd ed. Brooklyn, Dental Items Interest, c1954. xv + 462 p.
26. California Dental Association. Quality evaluation for dental care. Los Angeles, The Association, 1976. v + 93 p.
27. Carlos, J. P., ed. Prevention and oral health. Washington, Department Health, Education, and Welfare, Public Health Service, National Institutes Health, 1973. xii + 90 p.
28. Cohen, Lois K. and Knott, E. M. Interest of high school girls in dental auxiliary careers. J. Dent. Educ., 31:20–7, Mar. 1967.
29. Committee on the Costs of Medical Care. Medical care for the American people; the final report. Chicago, University Chicago Press, 1932. xvi + 213 p.
30. Cons, N. C. Method for posttreatment evaluation of the quality of dental care. J. Pub. Health Dent., 31:104–8, Spring 1971.
31. Curl, D. M. A comparative study of dental hygiene educational environments and student preference. Master's Thesis, Iowa City, University Iowa, 1966.
32. Dachi, S. F. Basic health sciences and correlated dental sciences. p. 360–92. (In Durocher, R. T., ed., The Kentucky conference on dental curriculum. J. Dent. Educ., 26:303–488, Dec. 1962.)
33. Davis, Milton. Patients' compliance with dental advice. Los Angeles, University of Southern California School Medicine, 1970. 49 p. processed. (Not generally available, Division of Dental Health, U.S.P.H.S., Research Grant DH00160-01.)
34. Department of Health, Education, and Welfare, Public Health Service, Division of Health Manpower (James Ake). Personal communication, Nov. 12, 1980.
35. Department of Health, Education, and Welfare, Public Health Service, Division of Dental

Resources. A study of dental manpower requirements in the West. Boulder, Colo., Western Interstate Commission Higher Education, 1956. ix + 247 p.
36. Department of Health, Education, and Welfare, Public Health Service, Division of Dentistry. Unpublished estimates, 1976.
37. Department of Health, Education, and Welfare, Public Health Service, Indian Health Service. Dental staff development criteria and standards. Rockville, Maryland, Dental Services Branch, The Service, n.d. Various paging.
38. Department of Health, Education, and Welfare, Public Health Service, National Center for Health Statistics. Current estimates from the Health Interview Survey, United States—1975, by Drury, T. F. DHEW Publ. No. (HRA) 77-1543, Series 10-No. 115. Washington, D.C., Government Printing Office, Mar. 1977. iv + 74 p.
39. ——. Dental visits; volume and interval since last visit, United States—1969, by Wilder, C. S. DHEW Publ. No. (HSM) 72-1066, Series 10-No. 76. Washington, D.C., Government Printing Office, July 1972. iv + 37 p.
40. Donne, John. Meditation XXVII. p. 1214–5. (In Abrams, M. H., et al., eds. The Norton anthology of English literature. New York, Norton, c1974. xxxii + 1521 p.)
41. Doyle, W. J., examining member, American Board of Pedodontics. Personal communication, June 12, 1977.
42. Ennis, John. The story of the Federation Dentaire Internationale. London, The Federation, 1967, 238 p.
43. Ertel, P. Y., and Aldridge, M. G., eds. Medical peer review; theory and practice. St. Louis, Mosby, 1977. xvi + 421 p.
44. Estimates of the effects of fluoridation, improved equipment, and additional auxiliary personnel on dental manpower requirements. p. 475–82. (In Hollinshead, B. S., The survey of dentistry; the final report. Washington D.C., American Council Education, c1961. xxxiv + 603 p.)
45. Fales, Martha J. H. History of dental hygiene education in the United States, 1913 to 1975. Doctoral Dissertation, Ann Arbor, University Michigan, 1975. xiv + 345 p.
46. Fauchard, Pierre. Le chirurgien dentiste, ou traité des dents. Paris, Mariette, 1728. 2 vols., 802 p.
47. Freeman, Beatrice R., and Colett, Patricia C. Factors associated with preventive dental practice: report no. 69. Chicago, National Opinion Research Center, University Chicago, 1959. 160 p., processed, not generally available.
48. Freidson, Eliot. The organization of medical practice. p. 343–58. (In Freeman, H. E., Levine, S., and Reeder, L. G., eds. Handbook of medical sociology. 2nd ed. Englewood Cliffs, New Jersey, Prentice-Hall, 1972. xxiv + 588 p.)
49. Friedman, J. W. A guide for the evaluation of dental care. Los Angeles, University California, School Public Health, 1972. 93 p.
50. Fusillo, Alice E., and Metz, A. S. Social science research on the dental student. p. 15–67. (In Richards, N. D., and Cohen, L. K., eds. Social sciences and dentistry; a critical bibliography. London, Federation Dentaire Internationale, c1971. 381 p.)
51. Galagan, D. J. Back from the brink: how and why U. S. dental schools were rebuilt. Dent. Surv., 54:14–18, May 1978.
52. Gies, W. J. Dental education in the United States and Canada. New York, Carnegie Foundation Advancement Teaching, 1926. xxi + 692 p.
53. Gift, Helen C. A study of the role of the practicing dentist in the delivery of caries prevention. Chicago, American Dental Association, 1975. 21 p. processed.
54. Gift, Helen C., and Schaid, K. A. Patterns of dental practice in the United States: solo vs. group practice. Am. Dent. A. J., 91:148–52, July 1975.
55. Glass, R. L. and Baldwin, D. C. Factors influencing the selection of dental office location. Am. Dent. A. J., 81:1337–41, Dec. 1970.
56. Goldberg, H. J. V., et al. Survey of dentists' opinions on issues facing the profession. Am. Dent. A. J., 93:348–54, Aug. 1976.
57. Gove, P. B., ed. Webster's third new international dictionary of the English language, unabridged. Springfield, Mass., Merriam, 1961. 56a + 2662 p.
58. Harmon, L. W., and Campbell, D. P. Use of interest inventories with non-professional women—stewardesses versus dental assistants. J. Counseling Psych., 15:17–22, 1968.
59. Hewitt, J. L. A survey of psychosocial characteristics of students in two-year programs of dental hygiene. Master's Thesis, Iowa City, University Iowa, 1967.
60. Hillenbrand, H. H. Structure and functions of the American Dental Association. Birmingham, University Alabama, 1972. videotape.
61. Hillsman, J. T. Quality assurance in dentistry. Am. Dent. A. J., 97:787–90, Nov. 1978.

62. Hollinshead, B. S. The survey of dentistry: the final report. Washington, D.C., American Council Education, c1961. xxxiv + 603 p.
63. Horner, H. H. Dental education today. Chicago, University Chicago Press, c1941. viii + 420 p. (p. 113)
64. Jay, P. Professor of Dentistry, School of Dentistry, University Michigan. Seminars on dental caries. 1951.
65. Kelsey, C. C. The School of Dentistry—1952–71. Mich. Univ. Sch. Dent. Alumni. Bul., n.v.:99–120, 1972.
66. Kesel, R. G. Dental practice. p. 95–238. (In Hollinshead, B. S. The survey of dentistry; the final report. Washington, D.C., American Council Education, c1961. xxxiv + 603 p.)
67. Klein, Henry, and Palmer, C. E. The dental problems of elementary school children. Milbank Mem. Fund Quar., 14:267–86, July 1938.
68. Knutson, J. W., and Scholtz, Grace C. The effect of topically applied fluorides on dental caries experience. VII. Consolidated report of findings for four study groups, showing reduction in new decay by individual tooth and by tooth surface, and frequency distribution of newly decayed teeth in treated and untreated mouth halves. Pub. Health Rep., 64:1403–10, Nov. 11, 1949.
69. Koch, C. R. E., ed. History of dental surgery. 2 vols. Chicago, National Art Publishing, 1909. vol 1, xxiv + 1186 p.
70. Lindsey, Almont. Socialized medicine in England and Wales; the National Health Service, 1948–1961. Chapel Hill, University North Carolina Press, 1962. xii + 561 p.
71. Malvitz, Dolores, and Judge, Susan. Employment patterns of dental hygienists in Michigan. Dent. Hyg., 50:463–8, Oct. 1976.
72. Mann, W. R. Dental education. p. 239–422. (In Hollinshead, B. S., The survey of dentistry; the final report. Washington D.C., American Council Education, c1961. xxxiv + 603 p.)
73. Maurizi, A. R. An economic analysis of the dental profession. Doctoral Dissertation, Palo Alto, Stanford University, 1967. (67–17463) Ann Arbor, University Microfilms, Inc.
74. Meskin, L. H., Loupe, M. J., and Mecik, Rudolph, eds. Current and future dental roles in primary care. Minneapolis, Division Health Ecology, University Minnesota, 1976. 152 p.
75. Milgrom, Peter. Regulation and the quality of dental care. Germantown, Maryland, Aspen Systems, 1978. xv + 251 p. (p. 17–51)
76. Miller, S. L. Legal aspects of dentistry. New York, Putnam, 1970. xi + 428 p.
77. Moody, P. M., Van Tassel, Carol, and Cash, D. M. Cynicism, humanitarianism, and dental career development. J. Dent. Educ., 38:646–9, Nov. 1974.
78. More, D. M. The dental student. Am. Col. Dent. J., 28:5–93, Mar. 1961.
79. ——. Social origins of future dentists. Midwest Soc., 21:69–76, July 1959.
80. Morris, A. L. Personal communication. July 15, 1978.
81. ——. Dentistry: retrospect and prospect. Am. Dent. A. J., 87:992–7, Oct. 1973.
82. Morris, A. L., and Greulich, R. C. Dental research: the last two decades. Science, 160:1081–8, June, 1968.
83. Motley, Wilma E. Ethics, jurisprudence, and history for the dental hygienist. 3rd ed. Philadelphia, Lea & Febiger, c1976. x + 185 p.
84. O'Donnell, J. F. Contending with P.S.R.O. Am. Dent. A. J., 89:836–7, Oct. 1974.
85. Pelton, W. J., and Bothwell, Ruth. The dental profession in the Great Lakes region. Am. Col. Dent. J., 26:3–27, Mar. 1959.
86. Posnick, W. R., and Young, W. O., eds. Manual for children's dental care programs. 3rd ed. Chicago, American Academy Pedodontics and American Society Dentistry Children, 1978. 27 p.
87. Quarantelli, K. L. The career choice patterns of dental students. J. Health Human Behav., 2:124–31, Summer 1961.
88. Richards, N. D. Utilization of dental services. p. 209–40. (In Richards, N. D., and Cohen, L. K., eds. Social sciences and dentistry; a critical bibliography. London, Federation Dentaire Internationale, c1971. 381 p.)
89. Ryge, Gunnar, and Snyder, Mildred. Evaluating clinical quality of restorations. Am. Dent. A. J., 87:369–77, Aug. 1973.
90. Sarner, Harvey. Methods of group practice. Am. Col. Dent. J., 36:206–14, July 1969.
91. Schonfeld, H. K. Evaluation of the quality of oral care systems. p. 229–78. (In Brown, W. E., ed. Oral health, dentistry, and the American public; the need for an improved oral

health care delivery system. Norman, Okla., University Oklahoma Press, 1974. vii + 372 p.)
92. Sherlock, B. J., and Cohen, A. The strategy of occupational choice: recruitment and dentistry. Social Forces, 44:303–13, Mar. 1966.
93. Sherlock, B. J., and Morris, R. T. Becoming a dentist. Springfield, Ill., Thomas, 1971. 138 p.
94. Slack, G. L., and Burt, B. A., eds. Dental public health; an introduction to community dentistry. Bristol, Eng., Wright, 1974. ix + 338 p. (p. v–vii, 113–59)
95. Soricelli, D. A. Methods of administrative control for the promotion of quality in dental programs. Am. J. Pub. Health, 58:1723–37, Sept. 1968.
96. Steele, Pauline F., and Charchut, Eleanor V. Dental hygiene profession. p. 389–433. (In Steele, Pauline F., ed. Dimensions of dental hygiene. 2nd ed. Philadelphia, Lea & Febiger, 1975. 447 p.)
97. Swanson, Margaret E. History and organization of dental hygiene. p. 483–505. (In Steele, Pauline F., ed. Dimensions of dental hygiene. Philadelphia, Lea & Febiger, 1966. 520 p.)
98. Swanson, R. K., Secretary, Hospital and Institutional Dental Services, American Dental Association. Personal communication, June 27, 1979.
99. Ten suspended dentists named in Medicare, Medicaid program fraud. Am. Dent. A. News, 10:1, July 9, 1979.
100. Tiede, J. W., and Born, D. O. Delineating dental manpower shortage areas. St. Paul, Minneapolis Dental Association, 1974. n.p.
101. University of Tennessee, Child Development Center, Department of Dentistry. Proceedings of a conference on quality control in dentistry. Memphis, June 21–23, 1979. In press.
102. Weinberger, B. H. An introduction to the history of dentistry, with medical and dental chronology and bibliographic data. St. Louis, Mosby, 1948. xv + 514 p.
103. Wisan, J. M., State dental programs. p. 298–328. (In Pelton, W. J., and Wisan J. M., eds. Dentistry in public health. Philadelphia, Saunders, 1949. xi + 363 p.)
104. Young, K. Heads you win—tails I lose. Royal Soc. Health J., 98:112–5, June 1978.
105. Young, W. O. Dental health. p. 5–94. (In Hollinshead, B. S., The survey of dentistry; the final report. Washington D.C., American Council Education, c1961. xxxiv + 603 p.
106. ———. Dentistry looks toward the twenty-first century. p. 3–49. (In Brown, W. E., ed. Oral health, dentistry, and the American public; the need for an improved oral care delivery system. Norman, Okla., University Oklahoma Press, 1974. xv + 372 p.)

CHAPTER 3

CAREER PERSPECTIVES

Wesley O. Young

INTRODUCTION

At first glance it is easy to conceive of a dentist, a dental hygienist, or a dental assistant as a professional person with a single specified and defined function in society. In reality the dental health practitioner fulfills many functions or "roles" in society.* Among the roles that may be assumed (in no particular order) are those of neighbor, health care provider, teacher, parent, clinician, healer, researcher, scientist, spouse, business person, advisor, and citizen.[2] In the long term, the effectiveness and satisfaction of a professional career will largely be determined by the degree to which the roles appropriate to the individual are developed, balanced, and integrated. Such planning should start as early in a professional career as possible and, ideally, would be a long-range and probably continuous process. Unfortunately, " . . . most people are so busy living from moment to moment that they rarely take stock of where they really want to go."[10] This situation may be true particularly for students in professional schools, because external pressures are sufficient in themselves to discourage students from taking time to establish long-term and short-term goals. Yet decisions must be made—decisions that may establish long-term goals reaching many years ahead.

Planning for the future should consider the full range of appropriate roles—personal, social, private, and public—as well as the traditional professional ones. Storrow has indicated that an individual should set aside a specific period of time for the development of goals. He has suggested that the answers to the following questions be written on a sheet of paper:

1. How would you like to live your life if you knew you had only six months to live?
2. How would you like to be spending your time five years after graduation?
3. What are your lifetime goals?[10]

The answers to the last question should fill at least one page. The next step

*Two definitions given for the word "role" are "a socially prescribed pattern of behavior corresponding to an individual's status in a particular society" and a "function performed by someone or something in a particular situation, process, or operation."[7]

is to review potential goals for incongruities and inconsistencies. If a major personal goal is to live and rear a family in a rural area, for example, and a major professional goal is to limit oneself to an endodontic practice, the two goals are probably mutually exclusive. It is to the future practitioner's advantage if conflicting goals can be identified and resolved early in the period of professional development. The final step in the initial process of establishing lifetime goals is to rank them in order of relative priority.

SHORT-TERM VS. LONG-TERM GOALS

In general, it is useful if long-term, lifetime goals can be developed early in a professional career. Some dental health students may be unable to identify the location and character of practice that would be most rewarding. Others may have established at least tentative long-term objectives but can defer pursuit of these goals in order to sample the variety of experiences that can be enjoyed by a dental health professional. The period immediately after graduation provides, for many, the best opportunity to "see the world" and to experience the provision of health care under unusual, even exotic, circumstances. Later in this chapter a variety of opportunities for salaried employment in the United States will be explored. There are also some opportunities for service in other countries. Although an American dental degree is not accepted in most developed countries, there are opportunities in some dental schools in Great Britain and in some areas of Australia. (All United States dental degrees are accepted in Canada as are all Canadian degrees in the United States.) Millions of individuals in the rural areas and urban slums of less-developed countries are without any dental care. Extractions for the relief of pain and infection are a desperately needed and sometimes lifesaving service. The need for restorative care is equally great. A variety of charitable organizations and churches organize public health programs to bring American dentists to areas of greatest need. Such assignments may be for a month or two or for a year or longer. Many health professionals have found service in these programs to be both personally and professionally rewarding.

The first goal of a professional person should be to serve the public by providing health care of a high quality with efficiency, holding cost at an acceptable level. This objective can be achieved in a variety of settings. Another worthy objective is to provide leadership to the health care community and to the community at large. Having completed from 18 to 20 or more (in the case of specialists) years of education, dentists may strive to assume a leadership role in community affairs—and many have. In general, these opportunities may be more common in small towns and cities than in major metropolitan areas.

Dental auxiliaries have also assumed leadership roles in their communities. Their special training and preparation have enabled them to make significant contributions to their communities, especially in activities related to dental health. Some examples are organizing programs for the custom-fitting of mouthguards for athletes engaged in contact sports, campaigning to remove "junk foods" from schools, and helping to bring dental care to the homebound, bedridden, or institutionalized chronically ill, aged, or handicapped.

PROFESSIONAL ROLES

Primary

Private Clinical Practice

The majority of dental graduates traditionally enter private solo practice. The dentist has an almost unlimited choice of where to locate his or her practice, subject to the constraint of securing a license to practice in the state of choice. The wide freedom of choice is a relatively rare opportunity, but it presents hazards to those who are unable or unnecessarily fearful of thinking about the future. Webber, writing for business executives, stresses that they ". . . need to value today less and tomorrow more."[11] He admitted, however, that thinking about the future is a little frightening: "It's unstructured, wide open, like outer space." The establishment of a dental practice is a major commitment—one that is frequently for life. Even if space is rented, the cost of equipping a dental office may well require an investment of fifty thousand dollars or more. If the initial choice of a community in which to practice is in error, for either personal or professional reasons, the subsequent or resulting change of location may approach a financial disaster.

The choice of community in which to practice is not an easy subject on which to give advice—especially in times of a perceived oversupply of dentists. However, many successful practitioners emphasize that the choice should be influenced primarily by personal preference of the dentist and spouse as to where they would like to live and rear a family. Dunlap,[5] in an excellent book, *The Beginning Dental Practice: The First Year*, offers many helpful suggestions on locating.

The majority of dental graduates remain in the state of their birth, which is usually also the location of their education. Many also return to their "home towns" or to areas near them. For many, remaining with or returning to their "roots" may be a wise strategy. It obviously simplifies the process of making a decision, since it is the election of a known set of circumstances. To do so as blindly as a robot, without carefully considering the alternatives, could be a tragic mistake—and the stakes are too high to take such a risk. Because many dentists come from upwardly mobile families, they may achieve an occupational status different from that of their parents. This change could make the surroundings of their youth uncomfortable or inappropriate in adult life.

A serious consideration of alternatives requires careful delineation of the characteristics of "where one wants to live." It has been suggested that these specifications be written down after leisurely meditation or discussion. The more distant the community, the more difficult it will be to determine the degree to which it may possess desirable characteristics. The dental professional looking for a location will want to examine the standard references and other sources of information: an atlas, an almanac, and the current *American Dental Directory* of the American Dental Association (ADA); phone books from the localities under consideration; chamber of commerce promotion pieces and brochures; and, as the choice narrows down, perhaps even a subscription to the local newspaper. The national placement service operated through the ADA also can be of help. If the dental professional represents one of two incomes in the household of a married couple, location will be determined by the job opportunities of both or a reconciliation of the pros and cons of both.

Once several tentative sites for the location of a practice have been identified, an attempt should be made to visit the communities. (One of several reasons why the process of finding a practice location should start early in the professional school years is that students have relatively little free time and if the process is left until the senior year there will be only a few days available to visit communities for observation.)

When visiting a community it is wise to attempt to make appointments to see several individuals. Obviously, the opinions of dentists practicing in the community should be solicited, although their opinions should be measured with some skepticism. Younger dentists with full practices may subconsciously fear competition and imply that near starvation is their lot, while the older dentists who may have slightly more patients than they desire may give the erroneous impression that there are large numbers of people actively seeking dental care. A key individual in most communities is an officer of a bank, since it is the bank's job to put its finger on the pulse of the business and financial aspects of the community. This individual should be able to provide information about the city's financial basis, population changes, and potential for new industry and the availability of homes and business and professional buildings that might be used for a dental practice.

Another important source of information is the local health department—county, city, or regional. The health officer (often a physician), public health nurse, or sanitarian usually knows the area intimately, especially its health and social service aspects. A few minutes or an hour spent in conversation with these health professionals can be most illuminating.

Ultimately some decisions will need to be made about the extent of need for additional dentists in the area. This judgment ordinarily must be made against the background of the financial resources of the new practitioner. A person who is heavily in debt may be compelled to find a location in which the need for a dentist is clearly evident and there is reassurance that a new practitioner will be busy almost from the start. If finances are not a major factor, a more attractive location may be one where a reasonable load of patients may be anticipated from the start, with a full practice perhaps not realized for two or three years. With the increasing number of dentists in the United States, unusually attractive areas probably should not be considered unless an individual has the resources to go without significant practice income for a considerable length of time.

The relative supply of dentists in an area has traditionally been expressed as the number of persons per dentist. This figure varies widely (see Chapter 14), ranging from roughly one to 1,368 in Connecticut (a state with one of the highest per capita incomes of the contiguous 48 states), to close to one in 3,067 in Mississippi, one of the poorest states. The national average stands at approximately one dentist for every 1,828 persons. The dentist-to-population ratio is a useful method of making crude comparisons, but it must be recognized as a rough measure. In many ways it disguises as many elements of the actual circumstances as it illuminates. In the first place, the ratio must be related to a frequently arbitrary jurisdiction such as a city, county, or state, and rarely is available for a realistic trade area. A rural county may show a large number of persons per dentist but is obviously not representative if the county is just across the state line from a major city in an adjoining state. Similarly, the number of persons per dentist in a county may not be useful in defining the relative status of a situation in a city at an extreme end of one county, in which most of the patients may come from the adjoining county. In the latter circumstance it is wise for potential practitioners to combine county data to develop their own counts of the number of persons per dentist.

Furthermore, the number of persons per dentist does not take into consideration variations in the productivity of dentists or the social and economic characteristics of the population. Younger dentists and those over the age of 55 tend toward relatively lower productivity. A community of 10 dentists in which six are 55 years of age and over is obviously quite a different community from one with an equal number of dentists, most of whom are 45 years of age or younger. Chapter 11 describes the powerful influence of the patient's social and economic status on the desire for dental care and ability to pay for care. Economic summaries based on the findings of the decennial census and other business and economic surveys are available for most states. They are usually published by the school of business of a state university or by a planning office of the state government and should be available by consulting the reference librarian in the dental school or public library. An important characteristic for study is population trends, since a city with a declining population may represent a dying community while a population that has shown sustained growth indicates strong economic capacity and a regular infusion of new potential patients. In addition, these publications provide data on annual mean income, median years of school completed by those 25 years of age and older, race, occupation of the head of the household, and other important methods of classifying population characteristics.

Most dental hygienists will enter practice in the offices of private practitioners, on either a straight salaried basis or a combination of a salary and a commission. Graduating dentists may find opportunities to associate with established practitioners. An associateship may represent a relatively short-term form of salary (or salary-percentage of gross) and a way to improve clinical skills before establishing a practice on one's own. On the other hand, it may be a form of establishing a private practice but in conjunction with another individual rather than completely "solo."

Determining opportunities for locating a dental specialty practice presents unique problems. The choices for the two types of specialists who usually work only in salaried positions—oral pathologists and public health dentists—are limited to the cities where positions are available. Likewise, individuals (both dentists and dental hygienists) who wish to pursue careers in dental education and research will have a limited choice of places to live. For other specialists, the process of choosing a practice location parallels that for general practitioners, with two important exceptions: first, that the choice usually is limited to the larger population centers and second, that the referral potential of the practitioners in the area, as well as the number of specialists located there, must be assessed. In the early years of a specialty practice the supply of patients is dependent primarily on referrals from the other dentists. (Later, self-referrals may become common as the specialist establishes a reputation in the community.) A group of mature dentists with busy, established practices may be anxious to refer almost all children or most extractions, for example. If the same number of dentists includes a large proportion of young, "hungry" dentists attempting to establish their own practices, referrals may be few and limited to the most extreme problems. Orthodontists have the least competition from general practice, but they have problems of their own. The number of orthodontists has increased considerably in recent years, and it has become increasingly difficult to find a location that will support a new full-time practice.

The problem of establishing a location for a dental hygienist or a dental assistant may be either considerably more complex or considerably more simple than for the dentist. Ten or 15 years ago it could generally be said that dental hygienists were in demand throughout the United States, outside of the Northeast, and thus hygienists were in a position to choose, with considerable discrimination, the dental practice with which they wished to become affiliated. With the rapid expansion of dental hygiene training opportunities in the last 15 years (see Chapter 14), this situation has been reversed in many states. There are large areas of the country in which employment opportunities in metropolitan areas are quite limited. In smaller communities, dental hygienists may remain in considerable demand. In general, the process of choosing a community in which the dental hygienist wishes to live will parallel the suggestions that have been made previously for choosing the location for a dental practice. Once the community has been selected, the employment opportunities within that community must be assessed in terms of the professional goals of the dental hygienist and the extent to which an individual dental practice meets the expectation of providing a preventively oriented, patient-serving, professional service of a high quality that will be personally rewarding.

Salaried Clinical Practice

It has previously been noted that although private solo practice has been the mode of choice of the vast majority of practitioners, it is not necessarily the right choice for new graduates. Salaried practice offers a number of immediate advantages, including the opportunity to reduce debts incurred in dental school before borrowing money to establish a practice, an immediate specified income, a "breathing spell" before making a commitment to a private practice location, and the opportunity to develop additional clinical experience and speed of operation. For others, salaried practice may be attractive as a life career. A reasonably good salary (although not as high as private practice at its peak) plus fringe benefits, such as a good retirement plan, often combine to make the long-term financial prospects of salaried employment very attractive. Advanced education opportunities are frequently available for career development.

Dentists in the U.S. Public Health Service, a component of the Department of Health and Human Resources, serve as commissioned officers of the federal government and enjoy essentially the same pay, rank, and privileges as their counterparts in the Army, Navy, and Air Force.[8] Although it is the oldest health service of the federal government (tracing its origin as the Marine Hospital Service to 1798 and its Commissioned Corps to 1873), it may not be as well known as the Commissioned Corps of the Armed Forces.

Dentists in the other uniformed services support the military mission of the service of which they are members. The U. S. Public Health Service carries a broader mission related to the health of the entire nation, in recognition of which its chief officer is commissioned as Surgeon General of the United States. The Public Health Service carries out major responsibilities in health research and in the promotion of health through public health efforts. Direct clinical care is provided primarily to five groups: the merchant seamen, the Coast Guard, American Indians and Alaskan natives, residents of federal prisons, and certain other special populations denied ready access to care because of special health problems, geographical location, or poverty. The National Health Service Corps (described in Chapter 14) is the most recent of the programs to serve special populations. It includes provisions for dentists to serve in private practice settings in communities that have been designated as critical shortage areas—both rural and central city. Public Health Service dental officers serve in a wide variety of assignments in all the contiguous states, plus Alaska, Hawaii, and Puerto Rico. The clinics of the Indian Health Service, for example, range from Point Barrow, Alaska (the farthest northern point of the United States above the Arctic Circle), to clinics in Arizona just north of the Mexican border, and from clinics in California on the West Coast to North Carolina with clinics in the Appalachian Mountains.

Other major federal dental services are the dental corps of the Army, Navy (which also serves the Marine Corps), and Air Force.* These components

*If representatives of the federal dental services are not available at one's dental school, inquiries can be made by letter. Requests for information about opportunities may be addressed to: (1) Chief, Commissioned Personnel Operations Division, Office of Personnel Management OM/PHS, Room 4–35 Parklawn Building, 5600 Fishers Lane, Rockville, Maryland, 20857; (2) Assistant Surgeon General for Dental Services, Office of the Surgeon General, HQ, U.S. Air Force, Washington, D.C. 20314; (3) Assistant Surgeon General for Dental Services, Office of the Surgeon General, Department of the Army, Washington, D.C. 20310; and (4) Dental Division, Bureau of Medicine and Surgery, Department of the Navy, Washington, D.C. 20372.

of the Department of Defense have absorbed large numbers of new dental graduates during periods of military activity. At other periods, with reduced levels of military personnel to be served and a better retention rate for dental officers on active duty, the number of openings available is more limited, although always present. The usually favorable retention rate is convincing evidence of the attractiveness of a reasonably good income, generous fringe benefits, usually excellent clinical facilities, and rewarding professional opportunities. Because of the world commitments of the United States, assignments are available in a variety of locations. Dentists serve throughout the contiguous states, Alaska, Hawaii, and Puerto Rico, and many countries overseas. In the Navy, duty is also available on ships.

For the graduating dentist interested in going into general practice, a general practice residency offers a form of short-term "salaried practice" that combines advanced educational opportunities with the ability to earn. There are more than 250 accredited general practice residencies, usually of 12 months in length and offering stipends in the range of ten to twenty thousand dollars.* They generally include rotations through such areas as medicine, emergency care, anesthesia, and various special areas of clinical dentistry. Unfortunately, they more often than not ignore social, community, public health, and preventive aspects of dentistry.

Another major federal dental service, the Veterans Administration (VA), is a major participant in postdoctoral dental education and it offers, in addition to specialty programs, more than half of the general practice residencies available in the federal services. There are nearly 150 affiliations between VA institutions and dental schools. The Veterans Administration was established in 1920 to improve services to veterans of American wars. Care is provided in VA hospitals and outpatient clinics or, in some rare instances, is purchased from private practitioners. Employment as a clinical dentist is sometimes available to the new graduate. However, the retention rate for VA dentists is high and the vacancies that do occur tend to be filled from the Administration's own educational programs. All federal dental programs offer equal employment opportunities for male and female dentists. Under some circumstances they have been able to accommodate the special problem of married couples in which both are health professionals.

In the Army, Navy, and Air Force, the major share of clinical procedures ordinarily performed by hygienists are carried out by specially trained enlisted personnel. The federal civil service offers employment opportunities for dental hygienists, but these are usually limited in number and salary. Dental hygienists are employed by the U.S. Public Health Service both through Civil Service and the Commissioned Corps. Expanded opportunities for employ-

*The Council on Dental Education of the American Dental Association (211 East Chicago Avenue, Chicago, Illinois 60611) annually publishes a *Directory of Accredited Advanced Dental Education Programs*, which includes general practice residencies as well as approved specialty training programs in both the United States and Canada. This directory lists all such programs, including those in the Veterans Administration. Requests for information about VA programs should be directed to the individual VA hospital.

ment may be available for dental hygienists who have advanced degrees such as a Master's in Public Health.

Outside of the federal dental services there are other opportunities for salaried employment. Dentists and dental hygienists are employed by state and local health departments, group dental practices, prepaid dental programs, industry-sponsored clinics, and institutions such as hospitals, prisons, and schools for the mentally retarded and the mentally ill. These positions may involve public health activities or clinical practice or a combination of both. The availability of these types of opportunities varies widely from area to area and can be determined only by making local inquiry.

Developments in the last decade have seen an increasing number of "department store" or "shopping mall" group practices, which are often franchised or operated on a contract with a parent company doing business in one or more states. An increasing number of recent graduates of dental professional education programs are being recruited to these groups. Some groups are associated with health maintenance organizations (HMOs); others are operated by insurance carriers; some are run by unions; and still others are freestanding. Because of the newness and varied sponsorship of these groups, the recent graduate is cautioned to evaluate them carefully before signing an employment contract. They can be quality groups of fine reputation or fly-by-night operations with dubious sponsorship. A carefully selected salaried position in a quality group practice can be a rewarding and wise beginning for the new graduate.

Dental Specialties

Over 10 percent of dentists choose to specialize. In order to prepare to do so, the minimum period of additional postdoctoral education required is at least two years. Either an advanced degree, usually a master's degree, or a certificate is awarded at the successful completion of the graduate curriculum. A significant number of dentists are now securing a second doctorate, either a Ph.D. or a Dr.P.H., especially those planning to teach and to conduct research. There is increasing concern in dental circles that too many dentists are going into a specialty, resulting in increased fragmentation of the profession. What is recommended instead is one or two years of a general practice residency. (See Chapter 14.)

Dental Public Health

Since many positions for salaried clinical practice occur in agencies whose titles include a variation of the phrase "public health" (such as the U.S. Public Health Service, the Michigan Department of Health, the Detroit City Health Department, or the Jefferson County Health Department, for example), new graduates accepting positions of this type often assume that they are "going into public health." This can be true only in a very loose sense, since, like their classmates, they are entering the clinical practice of dentistry or dental hygiene; the only major difference is that they will do so under the auspices of a public health agency.

Confusion also often exists in the minds of dental professionals about "The Public Health Service" (the U.S. Public Health Service) and "public health service." Whereas one may serve the public either in the U.S. Public Health Service or in service in public health, only if one is actually employed by the federal U.S. Public Health Service is one "with or in the Public Health Service." As will be outlined in Chapter 4, "public health" as such refers to the health of an entire population and not just an individual patient, important as that patient is.[1] Treatment of an individual is an important part of a community-wide approach to improving health, but it is only a part. Dental public health is one of the eight specialties recognized by the American Dental Association. The specialty is defined in full in Chapter 4.

Dentists or dental hygienists may be said to have entered the field when they occupy a position in which they are concerned full time with public health administration, health promotion, epidemiology and research, community prevention programs, the study of community oral health problems, or teaching. Dentists may become recognized specialists when, in addition to full-time employment in the fields mentioned, they have satisfied the educational requirements of the Council on Dental Education of the ADA—two years of accredited advanced graduate education in the specialty. The ultimate certification of specialty status is to become a diplomate of the American Board of Dental Public Health.

The specialty of dental public health is relatively small, engaging perhaps less than 300 individuals, but for these individuals it has provided a challenging and rewarding career. Public health almost always involves a team effort with a multiplicity of professional persons including physicians, nurses, engineers, social workers, and nutritionists. The field of operation is not confined to a single dental office but to the wider horizons of a city, county, or state, or even a nation. Among the rewards is the ability to bring about improvement of the oral health status of large groups of individuals rather than single patients. Public health dentists serving in the Indian Health Service of the Public Health Service, for example, have been able to demonstrate in some 30 years their ability to increase dental care for several million American Indians and Alaskan natives from almost nothing except emergency treatment to comprehensive care for school children and services for selected adults. Similarly, a dental public health professional who successfully wins a fluoridation campaign or institutes a mouthrinse program for the use of topical fluorides can demonstrate improvements in the oral health of thousands of persons in a relatively short period.

Despite their small numbers, dental public health professionals have played an important role in advances in dentistry. Epidemiological studies have demonstrated the value of water fluoridation, developed and demonstrated a variety of other uses of fluoride applied topically, defined the problems of periodontal disease in mass populations, and pointed a way toward better control of periodontal disease. This group of individuals has demonstrated the value of dental care provided on a routine basis and implemented in a logical, sequential way for large population groups. They have demonstrated the increases in productivity that can be brought about by the use of multiple auxiliaries in the dental clinical setting. Dental hygienists are valued members of a team conducting oral examinations in epidemiological surveys to assess the prevalence of oral disease or to evaluate the success of an educational program. They may organize, conduct, and evaluate school health education programs or direct preventive efforts such as the use of fluoride mouthrinse in schools.

Dental Education and Research

Similar comments might be made about those who seek careers in dental education and research. A certain number of new graduates will accept positions as full-time or part-time teachers in dentistry and dental hygiene, but their preoccupation initially will be with the clinical supervision of students. This is an opportunity to gain additional clinical experience, to earn money following graduation, and to determine whether or not full-time careers in education might be considered. Generally, the individual pursuing a career in dental education will obtain an advanced degree either in the basic sciences or in one of the clinical specialties. Dental hygienists will ordinarily achieve advanced degrees in education, public health, or related fields. The future of the profession rests with its dental education institutions and research institutes. Those employed in these institutions have the rewards and challenges of being on the "cutting edge" of the profession, of interacting with talented fellow faculty members, and of relating to dental, dental hygiene, and dental assisting students who will be the future members of the profession.

Collateral Roles

Progress in dentistry has always required the leadership provided by its members operating outside of their primary professional function. Pierre Fauchard, an early example, took time from the practice of dentistry to collate the knowledge about dental treatment that was available in the 1700s and write *The Surgeon Dentist (Le Chirurgien Dentiste).*[3] Many of the important technics developed by G. V. Black in the 1800s came about while he was in full-time dental practice. Chapter 7 outlines the development of water fluoridation as a near ideal preventive procedure and the central role of a general practitioner from Colorado Springs—Dr. F. S. McKay—in its development. These examples are only three of many that could be cited. In more recent times, much of the equipment needed to practice sit-down-four-handed dentistry has been developed by full-time practitioners, just as methods for the efficient use of chairside assistants are also largely the products of their pioneering efforts.

Other dentists have given their time and effort to support and guide the activities of the American Dental Association, the National Dental Association, and the many other related dental organizations. Dental hygienists have fulfilled similar roles in the American Dental Hygienists' Association and its component groups, as well as such organizations as the American Public Health Association and the American Association of Public Health Dentists.

A limited number of dental professionals have served in positions of leadership outside of organized dentistry, even outside of the field of health. Boards of health, at the city, county, and state levels, have often had dental professionals as members. Dental professionals have served on city councils, in state legislatures, as governors of states, and as members of the U.S. Senate, House of Representatives, and the President's Cabinet. These individuals have served their communities well, have been a credit to the profession, and have often been in a unique position to advance dental health by direct governmental action. Leadership in fields outside of dentistry might be said to have been a commendable luxury in the past but it is increasingly becoming a matter of practical necessity. More and more decisions about the provision of health services are being made by persons who are not health professionals and by agencies that are outside of the traditional health agencies.

The most notable of the new groups for the establishment of health policy are the health systems agencies (HSAs). These agencies, mandated and funded by Congress, divide the United States into multicounty health planning areas. They employ a professional staff (often with a clinical health background) and are governed by a voluntary board, the majority of which must be composed of those who are consumers and not providers of health services; the consumers may be housewives, politicians, attorneys, businessmen, and labor leaders. The HSA develops an overall health plan for the area and encourages other agencies to tailor their programs to achieve the objectives of the plan. The agencies are required to review applications for most federal health grants submitted from the area and to approve or disapprove. Only in extraordinary circumstances will a grant be funded by the federal government without the approval of the local HSA. In addition, the HSA must review and approve any proposed construction or renovation (over a certain dollar amount) of health facilities such as hospitals and nursing homes. If the project is approved, the agency grants a certificate of need (CON). Even if nongovernmental funds are available for health facilities construction, the lack of a CON is a fatal defect for most projects, since it prohibits the use of federal funds (such as Medicaid and Medicare) to pay for health care. (For further discussion of HSAs, see Chapters 12 and 13.)

The rationale for the drastic change in the planning for health care is to improve the distribution of health care facilities and to reduce costs by minimizing the duplication of facilities. Desirable as the objectives may be, they place the health professions on an entirely new basis in planning for the future. The certificate of need device is currently applied only to institutions that are used jointly by groups of health personnel to serve the public (such as hospitals and nursing homes) and affect private practices only marginally. (A heart surgeon, for example, would not be expected to locate in a community in which the facilities are not available for that type of specialized service.) It is conceivable, however, that in the future the use of a certificate of need to govern the establishment of a new medical or dental practice may be used, particularly if other methods for improving the distribution of practitioners (such as the National Health Service Corps) are not successful.

It appears certain that dental professionals should actively seek representation on the governing body of every health systems agency. If representation is achieved, the dentists or dental hygienists who are chosen will bear a serious responsibility. The individual who attends meetings only sporadically, or who participates actively only when dental projects are considered, is not likely to earn the respect of the group and to have clout when issues important to dental health are decided. Since a dental health practitioner is only one of the health providers and health consumers constitute a majority of the governing body, influence must come from respect. The health systems agencies are only one example of a variety of new demands on the leadership potential of members of the dental health profession who are able and willing to function professionally outside of the confines of their own clinical practice. Freidson and other students of the sociology of the health professions have classified medicine (and dentistry) as members of the "consulting professions," in contrast to scholars and others classified as members of the "learned professions."[6] Because of the very technical nature of dental health, the consulting role of the dentist has been less significant than, for example, that of the pediatrician, the internist, or the psychiatrist. This aspect of dentistry will become more important in the future, in part because of the increasing role of preventive dentistry and in part because of the increased need for the expertise of dental health personnel as knowledgeable consultants in fields outside the confines of the dental office.

This chapter has outlined the spectrum of a wide variety of opportunities for the primary professional roles that may be sought by the dental health practitioner. It has suggested ways in which professional goals can be matched and integrated with personal goals. Finally, it has pointed out the opportunities for and the necessity of practitioners to function in "collateral" professional roles, such as consultant and advisor on health matters outside of their practice. The next chapter will outline some of the ways in which the practitioner can function in a community setting.

References

1. American Board of Dental Public Health Incorporated. Informational brochure. (Chapel Hill), the Board, 1981. 8 p.
2. Bodden, R. W., Chairman, Department of Oral Diagnosis, University of Alabama-Birmingham. Presentation at a faculty retreat, May 1979.
3. Bremner, M. D. K. The story of dentistry; from the dawn of civilization to the present. 2nd ed. Brooklyn, Dental Items Interest, 1946. xiii + 336 p.
4. Dieter, Leslie, Engineer, Mountain States Telephone and Telegraph. Personal communication, July 1980.
5. Dunlap, J. E. The beginning dental practice; the first year. Tulsa, Dental Economic/PPC Books, c1978. xiii + 250 p. (p. 19)
6. Freidson, Eliot. Profession of medicine; a study of the sociology of applied knowledge. New York, Dodd Mead, 1970. xiv + 409 p. (p. 6)

7. Gove, P. B., ed. Webster's third new international dictionary of the English language, unabridged. Springfield, Mass., Merriam, c1961. 56a + 2662 p.
8. Robertson, Jack, Deputy Chief Dental Officer, U. S. Public Health Service. Personal communication, August 28, 1980.
9. Sherlock, B. J., and Morris, R. T. Becoming a dentist. Springfield, Ill., Thomas, 1972. vi + 138 p. (p. 13–31)
10. Storrow, H. A., Chief, Adult Psychiatric Clinic, University of Kentucky College of Medicine. Goals for living inventory. Distributed to medical students, Sept. 1979.
11. Webber, R. Time and management. New York, Van Nostrand Reinhold, 1977. 190 p.

CHAPTER 4

WHAT IS PUBLIC HEALTH?*

David F. Striffler

INTRODUCTION

Before attempting to answer the question that is the title of this chapter—"What is public health?"—dental professionals should ask another question: "Why do we need to know about public health anyway?" The first three chapters of this book have provided the answer indirectly, if not directly. Chapter 1 discussed the dental health professional's leadership role and responsibility to the community. The transition from the private clinical setting to the community and the dental health professional's obligation to serve the total health of the community were explored.

Chapter 2 pointed out the problems inherent in the traditional self-selection attributes of dental professionals when working as "lone wolves" in small group settings and the need for them to grasp the significance of the extent of dental disease in the community, for example, in planning. The changing scene of dental practice, with outside forces seeming to intrude more and more into the traditional small dental practice setting, the increasing role of third-party payment, and the demand for accountability to beneficiaries for what is purchased were also covered.

Chapter 3 addressed dental career perspectives, dental professionals' roles in society, collateral professional roles, and careers in public health. Because the balance between demand and supply of dental services apparently is coming closer to equilibrium, more and more dental professionals are looking toward practice settings other than the traditional choices, at least immediately upon graduation, when they are getting started.

Therefore, given all of the foregoing considerations, it might be well to know what the field of public health is all about and the role of dental practitioners therein. Even if the dental practitioners decide on solo practice, they still need to know what public health is. If the local health agency has no dental component, they need to determine if and what type of dental

---

*This chapter has drawn largely on the contribution of the late John W. Knutson, written for the second edition of *Dentistry in Public Health*.[5] In addition, the programmed paperback, *Introduction to Dental Public Health: A Self-Instruction Course*, developed by R. L. Weiss, the late D. W. Podshadley, and Peter Pipe,[8] had a significant impact.

public health program is needed and how to help establish one. They also need to know how a public health agency can be of help to them. Contrary to the all too often carelessly or thoughtlessly expressed notion of "big government" and "them" as "being on our backs," it is not always "them" who are at fault. "Them" is "us"; "they" are "we." After all, "that government" and its public health division with its dental public health arm are our government and our health department. As Pogo once said, "We have met the enemy and they is us." Thus, it just might be wise to learn what public health is all about.

Among the many definitions of public health that have been formulated, Winslow's is most widely accepted and quoted by public health workers. Winslow defined public health as "the science and art of preventing disease, prolonging life, and promoting physical health and efficiency through organized community efforts . . . ."[9] This definition is comprehensive and encompasses aims that are noble indeed. "Health" itself is an elusive concept, just as is "public health." The World Health Organization (WHO) definition,[10] while well known, holds perhaps unrealistically that health comprises complete physical, mental, and social well-being and is not merely the absence of disease. Sociologist Talcott Parsons,[7] at the other extreme, states pragmatically that health is merely "a state of optimum capacity for the performance of valued tasks." Nevertheless, it is generally agreed that human health is much more than just the absence of disease and that attaining or preserving health is a common goal.

Thus the generality of Winslow's definition of public health had much to do with its widespread acceptance among the public health profession. It is doubtful, however, that it gives private dental practitioners or the students of dentistry, dental hygiene, or dental assisting a working knowledge of public health. A clear understanding, not just a general or vague concept, is essential if dental practitioners are to fulfill with competence their direct and indirect roles in shaping the community's public health programs.

The American Board of Dental Public Health developed a further refinement of Winslow's definition, which was subsequently approved by the American Association of Public Health Dentists, the Dental Health Section of the American Public Health Association, and the American Dental Association. The definition, mentioned in Chapter 3, is stated in full here:

> Dental public health is the science and art of preventing and controlling dental diseases and promoting dental health through organized community efforts. It is that form of dental practice which serves the community as a patient rather than the individual. It is concerned with the dental education of the public, with applied dental research, and with the administration of group dental care programs as well as the prevention and control of dental diseases on a community basis.[1, 2]

Implicit in this definition is the requirement that the specialist have broad knowledge and skills in public health administration, research methods, the prevention and control of oral diseases, the provision and financing of oral health care, and the study and development of resources.

Dental Practitioners' Roles in Public Health

Perhaps a student's most common aim is to become a successful practitioner. Because of the personal nature of the services rendered in a dental setting, success ordinarily will be related directly to the number of people in the community who place confidence in the dental practitioner's abilities. That confidence will not be limited to technical dental services but will extend over a broad scope of day-to-day community affairs. These community affairs may include proposals to build a new school building or to close an underused one, fluoridate the drinking water supply, expand the recreational facilities for children, build a community health center, construct a new water treatment plant, or help settle a salary dispute of school teachers or other public employees. Whatever the proposal at issue, many persons seek the advice and guidance of their family dental practitioner. In particular, they will expect expert advice on community proposals for health improvement. Moreover, they will not understand nor be satisfied with a disclaimer of competency to advise because a particular proposal is of a nondental nature. The patient seeking the advice is usually not a health professional. The patient may even be a consumer member of an agency such as the local health systems agency (HSA), which has been charged with the responsibility of considering a particular proposal and of making specific recommendations for its approval or rejection (see Chapter 12).

A prominent characteristic of successful public health administrators or elected officials is their ability to stimulate broad discussion of community health problems by local civic, social, and professional groups and organizations and to encourage wide participation in designing plans and providing continuous financial support for an organized community program. An evasive reply arising from the dental professionals' lack of knowledge in these matters will be interpreted by the patients as indifference. It may inadvertently influence the patients to assume a similar attitude. On the other hand, a response based on inaccurate information is likely to be poor advice. In either event, the dental professionals have materially, although indirectly, shaped the pattern of their community's action on a public health problem. Therefore, the responsibility of being an adviser or counselor on community affairs resides with the practicing dental professionals, whether they will it or not.

The dental practitioners' opportunities to exercise their responsibilities as professional persons directly are also great. The chances are excellent that, if they so agree, they will be appointed to community health committees of civic, social, or voluntary organizations or to school, industrial, city, county, or regional health councils. How well and how long they serve will depend on the quality of knowledge, advice, and guidance that they bring to such councils. Furthermore, their own professional organizations, at the local, state, or national level, will have councils on dental health. Here, too, effective participation requires a clear concept of public health and the procedures employed in solving public health problems. Thus the opportunities of dental professionals to serve their communities and their professions will inevitably arise. Whether or not their professional lives are enriched by active participation in community affairs will be determined by the manner in which these opportunities are rejected or accepted and handled.

Public Health Is People's Health

Since "public" means "of or pertaining to the people of a community, state, or nation," the simplest yet most comprehensive definition of public health might be the literal one—*public health is people's health.* Indeed, there is a book entitled *Public Health Is People.*[4] Public health is concerned with the aggregate health of a group, a community, a state, a nation, or groups of nations. Public health, in accord with this broad definition, is not limited to the health of people on welfare, or by methods of rendering health services, or by the nature of health problems. Nor is it defined by the method of payment for health services or by the type of agency responsible for supplying those services. It is simply concern for and activity directed toward the improvement and protection of the health of a population group in the aggregate.

Leavell and Clark attempted to clarify the meaning of public health by pointing to the essential *differences* between the public health director and the private practitioner in the exercise of their professions.[6] The opposite approach will be adopted in this chapter, emphasizing the marked *similarity* in methods and procedures employed by family dental practitioners and by public health professionals. Dental professionals receive intensive preparation to equip them to care for their patients effectively and efficiently. They are encouraged to develop patterns of thinking and methods of approach that, when followed, are most likely to lead to desirable results. If it is recognized that the same patterns of thinking and the same methods of procedure are employed in public health, comprehending the meaning of public health should be greatly simplified. In one instance, the individual patient is the object of concern. In the other, it is all the people of a community. Although the tools employed in handling each may vary somewhat, the basic procedural patterns are virtually identical.

PERSONAL VERSUS COMMUNITY HEALTH

Examination/Survey

When patients come to a dental office or clinic, the first thing the dental professional does is to perform a careful *examination.* The examination ordinarily starts with a health and personal history, which may be obtained in many ways. One way (for new patients, not recalls), is to ask the patients what the difficulty is or what problem brought them into the office. If the patient has a chief complaint, the time of onset, mode of development, and symptoms are determined. The history also will include identifying data such as name, age, sex, address, occupation, and previous health experience. The dental examination may be simple or complex, but it usually includes examination of lips, oral mucosa, tongue, pharynx, and teeth. The examiner will, among other things, note the occlusion; any signs of abnormal functional stresses; lost, carious, and devitalized teeth; the condition of restorations; and the arch relations. A series of dental radiographs, a blood analysis, a urinalysis, or biopsy studies may be indicated. The regional lymph nodes should be examined and information of a general medical nature that has a bearing on the patient's health or ability to undergo successful treatment should be elicited. Modern chemical and laboratory aids may be employed in arriving at a correct diagnosis.

The first step in modern public health procedure parallels that used by the dental clinician, only here it is the community that must be examined. It is called a *survey* instead of an *examination*; nevertheless, it is an examination, and the technics and purposes of the survey are similar. Furthermore, the survey or examination of the community may be initiated by a chief complaint. One of the school teachers or school nurses may complain that there are no facilities for caring for the toothaches of children of indigent parents. The school health committee, after studying reports of experiences with a new preventive measure applied in a neighboring community, may raise the question, "Why aren't we doing something about it in our community?" Whatever the specific health problem, the initial approach to its solution should involve an examination to determine its dimensions and particular characteristics.

If, for example, the health problem is infectious hepatitis or a particular type of cancer, one might obtain information first on the size of the population involved, its age and sex distribution, its occupational composition, its mortality rates, the number of positive diagnoses, and the frequency of hospitalization. One may augment this information by conducting a community screening program for selected groups of the population. Such a survey is designed to determine the amount of disease in a community and to screen out or identify cases that have not been diagnosed or recognized. The survey would include an examination of the economic status of the community, the nature of the distribution of the community's wealth, and the community's resources for doing something about the problem (for example, hospital facilities, physicians, nursing care, and facilities of modern therapeutic treatment). Perhaps a clue or two as to the source of the problem and to its elimination or prevention can be identified.

The problem may be the widespread occurrence of mottled enamel, and the survey might be limited to a diagnostic verification of the condition and determination of the degree of mottling. The survey would include a review of records of chemical analyses of the local water supply to determine the fluoride content. If fluoride is being added, the check would be in the nature of surveillance. Also to be checked are other uses of fluoride in the community, such as inappropriate prescription of supplements. But the purpose of this survey in either instance would be to determine the nature and extent of the problem, just as is done when a patient comes to the dental office or clinic with a complaint.

Diagnosis/Analysis

The *examination* or the *survey* is not an end in itself. It is an important beginning—an essential component—that, when taken carefully, increases the likelihood that subsequent action will be correct and effective. The second component is *diagnosis*. An accurate diagnosis is essential if a proper course of treatment is to be prescribed. The need for additional information or supplementation in order to make a differential diagnosis may not become apparent until the data initially collected have been analyzed. This analysis also may indicate a need for the services of expert consultants or specialists.

The same methods are used in public health. In public health, however, the *diagnosis*, or second component, is referred to frequently as *analysis* of the survey data. Information collected in the survey is analyzed in order to define the characteristics of specific community health problems. Here one is dealing with groups of people instead of with an individual, and it becomes necessary in most instances to organize the data in such a way as to obtain meaningful figures. Electronic data processing (EDP) tools such as computers are frequently brought into play. The organized data can then be used for comparisons and to help simplify the description of the situation at hand. For this purpose, statistical tools may be used in order to derive such common descriptive constants as the mean, the median, the range, and the standard deviation. Rates may be calculated to determine the number of times an event occurs among the number of persons exposed to the risk of its occurrence during a given interval of time. Examples would be birth, death, and sickness rates. Ratios, or relative figures in fractional form, are used to indicate the relations of two factors to each other. These elementary examples are but some of the means of converting raw data, or absolute numbers collected in an examination or survey, into meaningful figures or statistics. They are the material that the public health workers use to obtain a description of the problem and its characteristics. They are the material that the public health professionals use to arrive at a correct diagnosis or analysis, just as dental clinicians use their examination data to guide them to an accurate diagnosis.

More and more frequently, clinical data, gathered as part of the patient's record by the clinician or for third-party prepaid group purchasers of care, are being used by the public health analyst, administrator, epidemiologist, or researcher for a variety of purposes. These purposes may range from pretreatment review to posttreatment quality assurance and to alerting appropriate officials of a group's special treatment needs for planning purposes.

Treatment Planning/Program Planning

Once the diagnosis has been made, one can proceed to make plans for effective treatment. The job of *treatment planning* may be simple or extremely complex, though more frequently the latter than the former. To most persons in need of dental treatment the cost of treatment is an important factor, and in many instances alternative methods of treatment at varying costs must be considered. In fact, the problem may be resolved in a variety of ways, ranging from the patient's refusal to undergo treatment because of a lack of appreciation of its importance, to acceptance of an ideal solution recommended by the dental professional who made the examination and diagnosis and designed the treatment plan. For example, the ideal treatment plan may call for balancing of occlusion, construction of one or more dental bridges, restoration of several carious teeth, treatment of gingivitis, changes in diet, and institution of a specific home care regimen. Porcelain fused to metal may have been prescribed as the ideal restorative materials for the anterior teeth. The reaction of the individual patient can vary widely, however. As previously suggested, patients may decide to do nothing or they may decide to have the carious anterior teeth restored and "let the rest go till later." They may choose a temporary appliance instead of a fixed bridge. They may accept the advice on dietary changes, but the length of time they adhere to the change may vary widely. Similarly, the instructions given for home care may be followed explicitly, they may be carried out indifferently, or they may be ignored completely.

The broad range of factors that influence the reaction of the patient to treatment plans has been emphasized to point out the need for considering alternative methods of treating a patient's problem. The patient becomes an active party in making the decision. After all, it is the patient's decision. Financial resources, health habits, the value placed on health services, and the whole background of correct and incorrect health information will affect the decision.

The same factors influence the third aspect for the public health worker, *program planning*, in a similar fashion. Both dental clinicians and public health workers desire to have the optimum treatment or program plan accepted without question. However, the community's reaction to such a plan, like that of the patient, may be to do nothing, to carry out only part of the plan, or to adopt an alternative, less comprehensive, and probably less costly program. It is the community that makes the decision either directly or indirectly through its administrative and elective officials. The decision will reflect the relative value that the community places on solving the particular health problem in comparison with the many other community problems in need of attention. Therefore, if the community's decision is to be a reasonable one, it must be based on community-wide knowledge of the survey findings, on an understanding of the analysis of these findings, and on a familiarity with proposals for a control program. Each of these areas of need for information can be filled by appropriate health education technics.

The increasing emergence of consumer groups of various types representing diverse and sometimes conflicting interests has forced public health workers to go much slower and to plan and work *with* and not do *for* and *to*. Consumerism also affects individual clinicians' practices, but perhaps not so obviously. For example, union representatives on a Blue Cross/Blue Shield or a Delta Dental Plan Board have a strong influence on the type of dental benefits chosen and methods of cost containment pursued. No longer will what was thought of by dental professionals as strictly a professional decision be made only by dental professionals—be they public health workers or individual providers.

Nevertheless, the most certain and effective way of ensuring not only that the community will be informed, but also that the facts will be understood correctly and a wise decision made, is through broad community participation in the conduct of the survey (insofar as it can), in the analysis, and in the program planning.

Treatment/Program Operation

When the plan has been accepted by the patient, the dental clinician arranges a specific schedule for *carrying out* the indicated *treatments*. If the treatment plan is rather difficult and complex, it may require referring the patient to an oral surgeon for needed extractions, to a prosthodontist for partial dentures, or to a periodontist for treatment of the supporting tissues of the teeth. A variety of specialists within the field of dentistry may be called upon to participate in the treatment plan. However, responsibility for coordination of these efforts will rest with the patient's primary dentist, who is responsible for successful administration of the plan. In the instance of the team treatment of the child with a cleft palate, not only a variety of dental specialists but also other health and medical specialists make up the team. The entire program for children and families challenged by such a disability may be managed and coordinated by a public health specialist. In this instance, clinical practice of a variety of disciplines and public health practice have come together, working for the well-being of patients.

Similarly, when a specific community public health program has been adopted, a varied group of disciplines, which constitutes a public health team, may be called upon for *execution of the program*. If, for example, the program is water fluoridation, local dental professionals may be asked to collect baseline data of the prevalence of dental caries, engineers will determine the type of equipment needed to carry out the fluoridation procedure, chemists will make water analyses, and the waterworks operators will be given the job of adding the proper amounts of fluorides to the water supply. Since fluoridation is a continuing program, there will be the overall problem of administration, including surveillance and quality control—that is, the responsibility for seeing that the work of the different specialists is coordinated and carried out effectively and efficiently on a regular routine basis.

Payment/Financing

Mutually agreeable methods of *payment* for dental services usually are arranged between the patient and the dentist or office staff before the treatment plan is undertaken. (Two thirds of the public still do not have dental insurance and those that do rarely have complete coverage.) The arrangement may vary, but the traditional patterns provide for payment on a monthly billing or a cash down payment, with subsequent payments to be made at the time of each clinic session in the course of treatment. The latter arrangement assures the dentist payment for services rendered and ensures against non-payment in case dental service is terminated prior to completion of the treatment plan. For many reasons, it is not uncommon for the patient to decide to discontinue treatment before it has been completed. Unforeseen or emergency demands on financial resources may be one cause for discontinuance. Dissatisfaction with the treatment may be another. A lower value on dental service may have been engendered by competing desires for such items as a new car or a new television set or maybe even paying the rent. In many instances the successfully competing value may realistically require a higher priority of attention than the dental treatment, such as satisfying one's own basic economic wants.

Usually, community public health programs are *financed* by funds appropriated by the governing body of the community. Local funds are often supplemented by state or federal funds or by funds provided by voluntary agencies such as a local service club. Frequently, the program plan may be approved, but funds are not appropriated for carrying out the activity and the program may die aborning. Since appropriations are made usually on an annual or biennial basis, the program may get under way only to be terminated through lack of subsequent appropriations. If this occurs, it should be clear that competing needs have been given a higher priority. However, funds for supporting a community health program also may be derived from contributions by local civic, social, or voluntary organizations. But whether the program is dependent for support on official or voluntary agencies of the community, continuance of that support will, in each case, be determined by community awareness of a real need.

Evaluation/Program Appraisal

Evaluation of the treatment rendered may begin during the course of treatment or be made at subsequent intervals of time, depending on the conditions under treatment. Evaluation by the patient actually begins much earlier with the initial selection of the dental professional before ever seeking care. Evaluation continues with each subsequent procedure—during examination, upon diagnosis, and with acceptance, partial acceptance, or rejection of the treatment plan. How well a simple restorative procedure was carried out will depend on subsequent observations to determine whether or not the cavity was prepared properly so that the carious process was interrupted, whether or not the preparation was extended sufficiently to deter recurrence of caries, and whether or not the occluding and contact portions of the tooth were restored properly so that the tooth does not suffer from traumatic occlusal forces. These observations can be evaluated from time to time on recall, when the patient returns for periodic examination and service. The evaluation can be an objective one only if careful examination records of initial conditions were made and are available for study and comparison.

Similarly, data collected in the initial survey by the public health worker for community program planning purposes must serve as the baseline against which *appraisals* can be made to assess the effectiveness of the program. Public health workers are accountable to the community for a periodic appraisal of their performances, just as dental clinicians are accountable to their patients for the effectiveness of the course of treatment rendered. There are other dimensions of evaluation than just *effectiveness*. Also to be considered are *efficiency, appropriateness, adequacy,* and possible *side effects*—good or bad. For instance, a simple Class I restoration could be quite *effective* in arresting the progress of a carious lesion and could be carried out *efficiently* with a minimum expenditure of time and resources. It would not be *appropriate* were the tooth indicated for extraction for other reasons, nor would it be *adequate* if there were a carious lesion elsewhere on the tooth. In each instance, the evaluation by the dentist, staff, and patients or the appraisal by the public health worker, program recipients, governing body, and other taxpayers should be performed in a spirit of self-discipline and for one's own guidance in developing competence. But it is the value assigned by the patient or the community that will ultimately determine the confidence placed in the individual dental practitioner or the public health worker.

As mentioned earlier, consumer groups will have their impact, especially in evaluation. They will evaluate regardless of the providers' wishes, whether the providers are public health professionals or individual practitioners or both. Therefore, including them at the beginning by inviting their participation, although seemingly time-consuming, may well save time in the long run.

Procedural Pattern

The foregoing analogy between the procedures employed by the dental clinician and the public health worker was summarized by Knutson as follows:

PATIENT	*COMMUNITY*
1. Examination	1. Survey
2. Diagnosis	2. Analysis
3. Treatment planning	3. Program planning
4. Treatment	4. Program operation
5. Payment for services	5. Finance
6. Evaluation	6. Appraisal

As with most analogies, some caveats are in order. First, while the analogy implies sequential steps and it lists "payment/finance" as step 5 and "evaluation/appraisal" as step 6, both "steps" are much more likely to be applied during or before all other procedures. For example, it has been pointed out earlier that some degree of evaluation takes place before a patient selects a dentist. Paradoxically, not bothering to evaluate is a form of evaluation. Evaluation also takes place before an acceptance of a treatment plan. Often payment is required at each appointment. In the instance of prepaid plans, payment takes place in the form of premiums paid in advance. Delayed payment or no payment is certainly out of step and might even be a form of evaluation. Obviously, slow payers or nonpayers may be telling the dentist what they think of the quality of care.

In public health programs, evaluation should be "built in" to the program. For example, the initial survey is often of a pilot nature for the exact purpose of deciding whether to go ahead with a full survey; then evaluating, on the basis of findings of the full survey, whether to go ahead with planning the program and then whether to carry out the plans. Thus evaluation is inherent each step of the way, consciously or unconsciously. Just so with payment and financing. The initial survey costs somebody some money. It is often the cost of the program that is the crucial factor in evaluating whether the program should continue or stop.

Tied inextricably to evaluation/appraisal and to payment/finance and, for that matter, to all of the other procedures as well is *education*—both in community programs and in individual personal health care. Education is necessary to get a patient into a dental setting and to get the patient to accept a treatment plan, to complete a course of treatment, and to come back for recall (evaluation).

Even initiating a pilot survey in a community program requires education—education of the public health decision-making authorities: the health commissioner, the board of health, advisory councils, appropriating and budget-making financial authorities, the intended recipients of the program, and ultimately other taxpayers as well. The educational process continues with each aspect of the program. Failure to inform, failure to secure cooperation and compliance, failure to secure support for the program to whatever degree—all indicate a measure of evaluation of the program or phase of the program, whether the program is one of individual health care in a personal setting or a larger community effort.

Thus a seventh component, *education*, must be added, perhaps as a vertical component. If so, *financing* and *evaluation* also should be inserted as vertical components operating at all stages. The modified procedural pattern appears on the top of page 69.

Although the terms used to describe the public health worker's approach to community health problems differ from those used to describe the dental practitioner's approach to individual patients' dental problems, the procedures are similar. Thus the training in procedural skills received by dental professionals provides a basic pattern of approach to problems, which should be

PERSONAL				*COMMUNITY*
Examination	E	F	E	Survey
	D	I	V	
	U	N	A	
Diagnosis	C	A	L	Analysis
	A	N	U	
	T	C	A	
Treatment planning	I	I	T	Program planning
	O	N	I	
	N	G	O	
Treatment			N	Program operation

helpful in enabling them to fill with competence and distinction the role of advisers and counselors on community health problems.

Another caution is in order. Even with the foregoing modified procedural pattern showing the similarities between individual or personal health care and community or public health programs, there are *differences,* as Leavell and Clark attempted to show.

DIFFERENCES IN PERSONAL AND COMMUNITY HEALTH CARE

Probably the most fundamental difference between personal and community health care is that individual dental practitioners usually deal with one patient at a time in relatively confining cubicles with a relatively few fellow workers. Typically there is one dentist, a part-time dental hygienist, one or two dental assistants and perhaps a receptionist. Rarely are they associated in group practices; hospital-based activities are perfunctory and occasional. Therefore, they seem to work in a microculture, with little contact with the outside world. The patients come to the dental practitioner. Those who do come usually can and do pay. More often than not the situation is controlled by the dentist who examines, diagnoses, prescribes treatment, and quite often provides it that same day or at the next appointment. The dentist makes the decisions. Patients who disagree usually express that disagreement by not returning rather than by straightforward discussion of their concerns. Those patients who do return thus are conforming patients who accept the dental recommendations. Private dental patients tend to be similar to the dentist and the dental office personnel in age, education, and socioeconomic status. There are relatively few external controls in personal health care despite the complaints of dental practitioners that "big government" or third-party carriers are intruding in their practices.

In contrast, the public health professional is a salaried employee who works both for an immediate supervisor and for the taxpayers, who are usually represented in the form of a board of health, an advisory council or two, and a governing legal body—the Congress, a state legislature, a county commission, or a city or town council. Rarely is a decision made on one's own; usually it is in concert with several other groups and made over a considerable period of time. Sometimes a year can pass before a decision is made and then another year before a program is actually put in operation. In some instances the program is set aside or delayed because the problem the program proposes to address is not determined to be a "public health" problem. For example, the direct provision of health care for many years was not considered to be a function of public health agencies. The limited care that was provided at public expense was reserved to welfare agencies. Such is the public policy and practice in some regions of the country to this day. Other areas are more liberal in their interpretation of what constitutes a public health problem and thus will design a public health program to attack it.

Over the years some criteria have emerged to help determine what constitutes a public health problem. The first mention in print[3] that could be located delineated these criteria as:

1. A condition or situation that is a widespread actual or potential cause of morbidity or mortality.
2. There is a body of knowledge about this situation that, if applied, would prevent, ameliorate, or cure this condition or situation.
3. This body of knowledge is not being applied.

A later textbook modified these criteria to " . . . help determine what priority public health officials allocate a given health problem . . . [as]:

1. A disease or other threat to health is widespread.
2. It is known how to prevent, alleviate, or cure this condition.
3. Such knowledge is not being applied."[8]

The text goes on to add that these three criteria should not be regarded as the complete and final test of what problems should be tackled by public health officials and agencies.

Clearly other criteria must be considered. For example, if the survey turned up a deadly—that is, high mortality—disease, even if it were not widespread, its threat to life would enter into the decision making and program planning as a major factor. Also, if the governing authority decided a problem deserved attention and assigned it to the public health agency, the problem would become, ipso facto, a "public health" problem. The respective governing authority could be the board of health, the state legislature, a town council, or the Congress. By the same token, an executive officer—whether the President, a governor, or a mayor—can issue executive orders, which by decree declare a problem a "public health" problem. Often these latter two types of decision, i.e., legislative mandate and executive order, disturb the orderly program planning process and take financial precedence over more traditional issues.

Another difference between the public health professional and the individual private practitioner is that the focus of the former is on *groups* of people, often in communities with special characteristics and often different from the public health professional serving them. Different cultures, different languages, different socioeconomic status, and different education all too often tend to separate the professional public health provider and the recipient. Public health workers often must care for those outside the mainstream. Lower socioeconomic status, different ethnic backgrounds, and special problems make some groups of people more difficult and often more expensive per capita to reach (see Chapter 12). In addition, the public health professionals and their work are visible and they are publicly accountable.

Usually the public health workers' system of rewards varies from that of individual private practitioners. Public health professionals are rewarded directly, of course, by a regular salary check. Although take-home pay does not on the average match that of private dental professionals, fringe benefits—retirement, sick leave, insurance, and paid vacation, for instance—are quite generous. Other benefits, mostly intangible ones, play a major role. For example, seeing the benefits of fluoridation come to thousands of children after a physically and emotionally exhausting election battle is a reward that cannot be measured. Knowing that one was quietly instrumental in bringing a health care program to an isolated community—isolated geographically or because of special problems such as being bedridden—is another example. Community-active private practitioners, of course, also share in such intangible rewards.

Thus it can be seen that there are differences between the public health professional and the individual practitioner just as there are similarities. All of these go to make up "what public health is."

References

1. American Board of Dental Public Health, Incorporated. Informational brochure. (Chapel Hill), The Board, 1981. 8 p.
2. American Dental Association, Commission on Dental Accreditation. Requirements for advanced specialty education programs [dental public health]. Rev. ed. Chicago, The Association, 1980 i + 33 p. (p. 14) duplicated.
3. Blackerby, P. E., Jr. Treatment in public health dentistry. p. 187–221. (In Pelton, W. J., and Wisan, J. M., eds. Dentistry in public health. Philadelphia, Saunders, 1949. xi + 363 p.)
4. Ginsburg, E. L. Public health is people. New York, Commonwealth Fund, 1950. xiv + 241 p.
5. Knutson, J. W. What is public health? p. 20–9. (In Pelton, W. J., and Wisan, J. M., eds. Dentistry in public health. 2nd ed. Philadelphia, Saunders, 1955. x + 282 p.)
6. Leavell, H. R., and Clark, E. G. Preventive medicine for the doctor in his community; an epidemiologic approach. 3rd ed. New York, McGraw-Hill, c1965 and 1978. ix + 684 p. (p. 7–13).
7. Parsons, Talcott. Definitions of health and illness in light of American values and social structures. p. 165–87. (In Jaco, E. G., ed. Patients, physicians, and illness. Glencoe, Ill. Free Press, 1958. viii + 600 p.)
8. U. S. Public Health Service, Division of Dental Public Health and Resources, Dental Health Center. Introduction to dental public health; a self-instruction course, by Podshadley, D. W., Weiss, R. L., and Pipe, Peter, PHS Publ. no. 1134, Washington, D.C., Government Printing Office, 1964. vii + 183 p.
9. Winslow, C.-E.A. The untilled fields of public health. Mod. Med., 2:183–91, Mar. 1920.
10. World Health Organization. Constitution of the World Health Organization. Geneva, The Organization, 1946. 18 p. (p. 3)

Additional Readings

Breslow, Lester, Fielding, J. E., and Lave, L. B., eds. Annual review of public health. Vol. 1. Palo Alto, Annual Reviews, 1980. xiii + 411 p.

Brown, W. E., ed. Oral health, dentistry, and the American public; the need for an oral care delivery system. Norman, Okla., University Oklahoma Press, 1974. vii + 372 p.

Dunning, J. M. Principles of dental public health. 3rd ed. Cambridge, Mass., Harvard University Press, 1979. xiv + 655 p.

———. Dental care for everyone: problems and proposals. Cambridge, Mass., Harvard University Press, 1976. 228 p.

Hanlon, J. J., and Pickett, G. E. Public health: administration and practice. 7th ed. St. Louis, Mosby, 1979. x + 787 p.

O'Shea, R. M., and Cohen, Lois K., eds. Toward a sociology of dentistry. Milbank Mem. Fund Quar., 49:1–336, July 1971.

Richards, N. D., and Cohen, Lois K., eds. Social sciences and dentistry; a critical bibliography. London, Federation Dentaire Internationale, c1971. 381 p.

Silberman, S. L., and Tryon, A. F., eds. Community dentistry; a problem-oriented approach. Littleton, Mass., PSG, c1980. xvii + 331 p.

Slack, G. L., and Burt, B. A., eds. Dental public health; an introduction to community dentistry. 2nd ed. Bristol, Engl., Wright, 1981. ix + 343 p.

II THE ASSESSMENT OF THE PROBLEM OF ORAL DISEASES

CHAPTER 5

METHODS FOR ASSESSING THE DISTRIBUTION OF ORAL DISEASES

Brian A. Burt

EPIDEMIOLOGY—AN INTRODUCTION

The more thoughtful dental practitioners will wonder why they see such a variety of disease patterns among their patients. Why, for example, do some patients have rampant caries while others living under apparently the same conditions and lifestyles do not? Sometimes there may be fairly obvious answers to these and similar questions, but for many other questions there appear to be none. When answers can be found or even suggested, dentists can approach diagnosis and treatment with more confidence.

The branch of scientific inquiry that attempts to determine some order among these seemingly haphazard patterns of disease in population groups is called *epidemiology*. Although many definitions have been suggested, epidemiology can perhaps be most simply described as the study of health and disease in defined populations and of how these states are influenced by heredity, environment, and ways of living.

The methods of inquiry in epidemiology have much in common with those used in other physical, biological, and social sciences. The basis of all scientific investigation is methodical and disciplined observation. Analysis of these observations can lead to the establishment of a *hypothesis*, defined as a suggestion regarding the way in which facts are linked together. A hypothesis can be tested experimentally, and if found to be true, the proof of the subsequent scientific proposition is predictability. A high degree of confidence in the predictability of the laws of gravity, for example, allowed men to fly to the moon and return safely to earth. The goal of the scientific investigator is to find some basis for estimation of the regularity with which specific events or reactions may be expected to occur and under what conditions.

There is an important difference, however, between research in the physical and that in the biological sciences. Physical laws tend to be more universally true than biological laws. The set of circumstances that will lead to a heart attack, cancer, or tooth decay in one person will not necessarily produce these conditions in another person of the same age, sex, or race. The reasons for these differences between two similar individuals may be rooted in the genetic endowment of the individuals, in the environment in which they live, in particular aspects of their lifestyles, or perhaps in a combination of these and other factors. These differences between individuals are examples of *biological variation.* While the concept of biological variation is implicitly understood by the clinician, the epidemiologist attempts to find patterns among people who can be grouped by particular characteristics (such as age, sex, race, marital status, socioeconomic status, place of residence, diet, smoking or drinking habits, occupation, or exposure to specific environmental factors, for example) and the occurrence of disease among the groups. If clear differences are found between different groups with respect to the occurrence of a disease, hypotheses can be set up that seek to explain a cause-and-effect relation. Of course, some biological variation will still occur, but the study of groups rather than individuals will allow its influence to be "averaged out."

Environment and Lifestyle

Epidemiology seeks to relate factors affecting health and disease in populations to factors in the environment or in the population's way of living. The term "environment" can have either a wide or a narrow definition, depending on the context in which it is used. It can be as broad as housing conditions if relating to a disease such as tuberculosis, or it can be as narrow and focused as the inner surface of adherent dental plaque if the microbiology of dental caries is being studied. Environmental conditions in the middle of the nineteenth century, for example, were clearly important in determining the main causes of death at that time. Poor sanitation and squalid housing were factors directly contributing to the high mortality from typhoid fever, cholera, tuberculosis, and dysentery. Changes in the environment in economically developed countries, as a result of public health legislation over the last 100 years, have now made these diseases uncommon in those countries. But other diseases of a more chronic nature have arisen to take their place as causes of death and disability: the occurrence of conditions such as cancer and the cardiovascular diseases is related to modern factors in the environment and to lifestyles. Smoking, alcohol, mobility, leisure time, affluence, diet, moral standards, occupational hazards, environmental pollutants, chemical contaminants, and drugs (both legal and illicit) can all play a part in the occurrence of disease in economically developed countries.

Epidemiology is also related to *ecology,* that branch of biology dealing with the interrelation of organisms with their environment. Ecology has contributed to epidemiology the concept of multifactorial causes of disease—a model in which the host, the agent of disease, and the environment are inextricably linked in a certain balance.

The Epidemiology of Chronic Diseases

Chronic conditions such as rheumatoid arthritis, the cardiovascular diseases, many cancers, mental illnesses, and periodontal diseases are highly complex and often poorly understood morbid diseases. In most chronic illnesses, the dividing line between health and disease is not as clear-cut as it is in the acute infectious diseases; it is rather a matter of definition. A given clinical state in a noncommunicable condition may be the result of an intricate interaction among a number of causal factors, none of which produces disease when acting alone, opposed by a complex of protective factors. Months or years may pass before an effect of an agent becomes obvious in a person or population, whereas in acute diseases the onset of symptoms is more rapid. In addition, a given agent may produce a variety of clinical effects under different conditions. The search for a single cause and a single effect therefore must be superseded by the concept of a *multifactorial* causation of disease.[88]

Epidemiology is a fundamental discipline in research into the control of these chronic diseases. For example, chemical contaminants and potential carcinogens appear to be becoming more common in the environment, and epidemiological inquiry is needed to determine what the effects of these agents might be. Living habits are changing, often at a bewildering speed, and their effects on disease status also must be studied.

The conditions that the dental practitioner treats fall predominantly into the category of chronic diseases. Their etiologies, while not yet fully understood, are clearly multifactorial. Dental practitioners can only develop a rational basis for prevention and control of these diseases among their patients if they have an understanding of the epidemiology of these conditions. The purpose of this chapter is to describe the methods used in the measurement of oral diseases so that the practitioner may better develop that understanding.

THE EPIDEMIOLOGICAL METHOD

Early Studies

Epidemiology was learned and practiced empirically long before it was named. Many early civilizations understood from experience that malaria is a disease of wet lowlands. Even now, people in some economically underdeveloped countries continue to make their homes on the higher slopes to escape malaria, even though this practice involves an arduous daily journey into the valley to work their fields or to draw water. Despite the fact that these customs grew haphazardly, much of this sort of learning led to improvements in the way of life of the people concerned. On balance, however, humans were wrong more often that they were right in their speculations about the conditions that favored disease. Periodic epidemics of plague, for example, swept Europe from the Middle Ages until fairly recent times, and the populations of the countries concerned were quite helpless to do much about it.[25] These diseases struck so suddenly and so universally that it was no wonder that religious significance was often ascribed to them.[53]

It was from the more rational study of these epidemics that epidemiology evolved to its present form. Samuel Pepys, author of *The Diary of Samuel Pepys*, that marvelously vivid chronicle of life in seventeenth-century London, was able to use the Bills of Mortality, the forerunner of modern death certificates, to measure the progress of an outbreak of plague in London in 1665. Later works showed the beginning of a more analytical approach. For example, in England, Dr. Percival Pott wrote his *Treatise of the Chimney Sweep's Cancer* (1775), in which he described the unusually high occurrence of scrotal cancer among chimney sweeps. Pott's careful work is probably one of the first scientific descriptions of an occupational hazard.

One of the best-known examples of early epidemiology is that of John Snow and the Broad Street pump. In 1854, John Snow, a medical practitioner in the Soho area of London, went so far as to control an outbreak of cholera by the application of his epidemiological conclusions. In his efforts to determine the cause of the outbreak, Snow set about trying to find what features were held in common by those who had died from the disease. He mapped out, on a map of the city, the residences of those who had died (see Fig. 5–1).

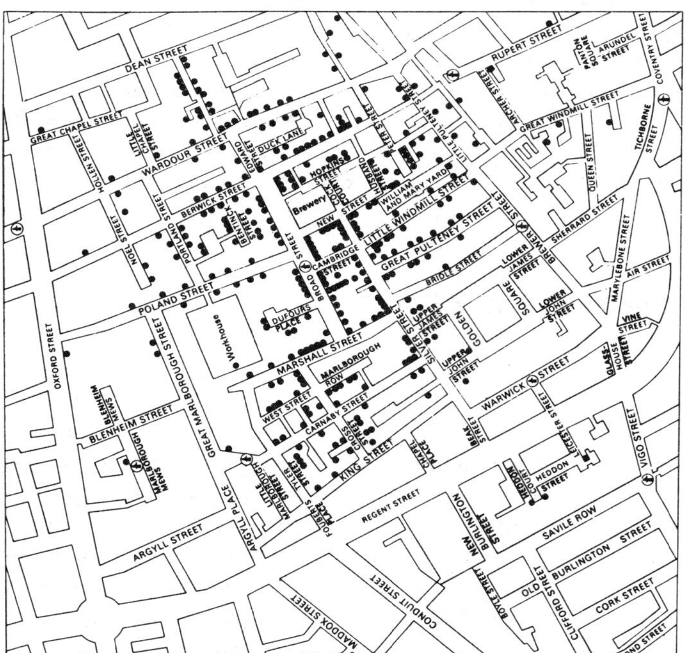

Figure 5–1. John Snow's map of the Soho area of London, showing deaths from cholera during the epidemic of 1854. (From Longmate, Norman. Alive and well; medicine and public health 1830 to the present day. Harmondsworth, England, Penguin Books, 1970, p. 46. Copyright Norman Longmate, 1970. Reprinted by permission of Penguin Books Ltd.)

In his methodical follow-up investigations, he found that the most common feature was that all of the victims had used water from the same source. That source, in the days before household municipal water supplies, was a public pump in Broad Street (now Broadwick Street). Although this investigation took place some years before the germ theory of disease was understood and generally accepted, Snow concluded rationally that some agent in the water was responsible for the spread of the disease. Snow's method of preventing people from using the contaminated water was to persuade the authorities simply to remove the handle of the pump. The epidemic soon subsided.

Snow's subsequent investigations on the relations between cholera and the source of water supply are classics in the history of epidemiology.[88] The results of his brilliant and patient work, along with some parallel efforts by other investigators of his time, benefit present-day society. Their investigations led to gradual but immense improvements in sanitation, in living conditions, and in the development of public health codes affecting housing, water supply, and food processing that are now taken for granted. But it should be remembered that diseases such as cholera, typhoid, yellow fever, plague, and relapsing fever are rare in developed countries today largely because of the pioneering work of these early epidemiologists. Their work continues; perhaps the best recent example of how these methods can be successful was the 1978 announcement by the World Health Organization that smallpox had been eradicated throughout the world.[95]

Types of Epidemiological Studies

An often used and simple classification of epidemiological studies refers to them as *descriptive* or *analytical* studies. A *descriptive* study is one that attempts to do no more than describe the pattern of occurrence of a condition relative to other characteristics of the population. For example, a study that attempted to measure the degree of dental caries in a school district relative to the age, sex, and socioeconomic characteristics of the children, without attempting to explain why those particular distributions were found, would be a descriptive study. It would also be a *prevalence* study, in which prevalence is the number of persons in a population affected by the condition at any one time.

An *analytical* study, on the other hand, is one that attempts to explain the distribution of a condition relative to some other factor. A study that measures the influence of water fluoridation on the distribution of dental caries in a population, while allowing for any expected differences in characteristics such as age, sex, or socioeconomic status, would be an analytical study. Analytical studies frequently, though not always, require at least two series of measurements at different times to determine what the progress of the condition has been in the intervening time period. Such a study could also be called an *incidence* study, in which incidence is the change in prevalence of a condition over a given period of time. Incidence can only be assessed accurately when the same group of subjects is examined at two different times.[74]

Other related terms used to describe types of epidemiological studies are *cross-sectional* and *longitudinal.* A cross-sectional study is one in which a sample of a population (a "cross section") is assessed at one time, whereas a longitudinal study is one in which the same group of people is studied on two or more occasions. It follows that a longitudinal study must be an incidence study, and it is usually (though not always) an analytical study. Sometimes an analytical study can be cross-sectional, too, in those instances in which several cross-sectional studies are made over a period of time for analytical purposes. An examination of mortality from a particular disease over a period of time, for example, must be cross-sectional (obviously it cannot be the same people who die on several different occasions!). A comparison of the prevalence of dental caries in today's sixth-graders with that of 10 years ago must be a cross-sectional study, though it could also be an analytical one; again it is obvious that different persons are studied each time. But if all the children originally in first grade in a school system are studied periodically until they finish sixth grade some years later, the study would be longitudinal because the same children would be seen on several occasions.

Readers of the dental literature will also find reference to *prospective* and *retrospective* studies. A prospective study is one in which the planning of the entire study is carried out before the data are to be collected. If the study is intended to determine the effect of a fluoridated dentifrice in reducing the incidence of dental caries, for example, a prospective study is typically designed in which similar groups of children are selected, only one of which receives the dentifrice during the period of the study. Measurement of caries at the beginning and the end of the study period allows the incidence of the disease to be determined for each group and to be compared for differences. This basic design of the *clinical trial* or *field trial* is also seen to be an analytical study, an incidence study, and a longitudinal study.

A retrospective study, on the other hand, is one in which the planning for the study takes place after the data have been collected. If the researcher wishes to find out what dental services a practice has provided for its patients over a year, one way the information could be collected is to abstract it from the clinical records of the practice. While this approach would be easier and cheaper than planning a prospective study to run for a year hence, retrospective studies do have potential problems, usually stemming from the possibility that the data available may not always be exactly the kind of data the researcher wants. However, so long as these problems are recognized, much useful information can be gathered from retrospective studies.

Uses of Epidemiology

The various ways in which the epidemiological method can be used can be conveniently grouped under the following headings.

Collection of Data to Describe Normal Biological Processes. Examples are height at various stages of growth, blood groups, and times and order of tooth eruption.

An Understanding of the Natural History of Diseases. Observations of disease progression and outcome in populations have enabled investigators to distinguish those diseases that are fatal or disabling from those that will resolve satisfactorily. The diagnosis of most forms of cancer requires that some intervention be made if the disease is not to progress inevitably to a fatal outcome. On the other hand, a diagnosis of chicken pox means that no intervention is called for, because knowledge of the natural history of the disease indicates that it will resolve satisfactorily. An examination of the natural history of disease by an epidemiologist can also lead to the development of hypotheses intended to explain the disease occurrence and distribution relative to specific characteristics in populations.

Testing of Hypotheses for the Prevention and Control of Disease through Special Studies in Populations. This use of the epidemiological method is the clinical trial, or field trial, in which potential agents, regimens, or procedures for the prevention and control of disease are put to experimental testing. As an example, the Salk vaccine was subjected to rigorous and controlled testing on a large population group before it could be accepted as effective in the prevention of poliomyelitis. In dentistry, the various uses of fluorides to prevent and control dental caries have nearly all been subject to similar clinical trials in human populations.

Planning and Evaluating Health Care Services. This application is a relatively recent development of the epidemiological method. Data that describe (a) the distribution of disease, both treated and untreated, in the population under study; (b) the population's utilization of health care services; and (c) the availability and productivity of health care services can all be employed. New and still developing statistical technics can then be used to describe and predict what the services required to treat the population might be and what types of personnel and facilities are required.

A related application is in the validation of the effectiveness of treatment technics, both new and traditional, and in the determination of the quality of treatment provided.

Epidemiology and the Practitioner

Practitioners may still ask how knowledge of health and disease tendencies in a particular group of people can help them to diagnose and treat the individual patient. After all, biological variation being what it is, the individual patient may or may not be typical of the group. The answer is that the epidemiological findings can define *risk factors,* meaning that the patient is more likely to exhibit a particular disease if he fits into a defined category than if he does not. For example, a man who smokes may or may not have lung cancer, but he certainly runs more risk of developing lung cancer than if he does not smoke.[69, 90] The examining physician would take this fact into account during his examination and diagnosis. Similarly, an elderly man who both smokes and drinks heavily is more at risk of oral cancer than a person who does not.[3] Again, the examining dentist should consider that fact during examination and diagnosis. Practitioners who group their patients in various ways can add to their practice this useful "third dimension," which can help them treat each individual more completely.

There are numerous other risk factors with which physicians and dentists are now so familiar that they may not realize that epidemiological research first identified them. Two factors that pertain to dentistry are that the patient who receives nonfluoridated water is more at risk of dental caries than the patient who drinks fluoridated water,[76] and that the patient with subgingival calculus is more at risk of having periodontal pockets than is the patient without it.[96]

Application of the epidemiological method in clinical trials has also given dentistry much of its knowledge of preventive technics. The practitioner who applies a topical fluoride for a young patient and the hygienist who carries out a deep scaling for an older one are both secure in the knowledge that they are using proven technics to help prevent the onset of further oral disease.[40, 96] This knowledge has come from controlled studies in which groups of people received the treatment regimen and were compared with similar groups who did not. (Because practitioners need to be able to make their own assessments of clinical trials that test a preventive or treatment regimen, some of the fundamentals of clinical trials will be described later in this chapter.) Of course not everyone in the tested group showed the same degree of improvement in the condition being studied or the same degree of resistance to the onset of a new disease. Other factors in the life of each individual in the group, such as diet, toothbrushing habits, or unknown factors in biological variation, could influence whether each received a great deal of benefit or little benefit. The clinical trial shows the benefits (or absence of them) to be derived *on average* for the group under study. Some grasp of epidemiological principles and clinical trial procedures also helps a practitioner determine the quality of the evidence favoring a procedure.

Biological variation also presents problems if the practitioner attempts to apply the results of an individual patient's history to the population at large. While individual case histories do have their place in defining certain syndromes and identifying specific reactions, the practitioner can never know whether the individual under study is representative of a population or not. On the other hand, the results of epidemiological research provide a great deal of assistance to the physician or dentist in treating individual patients because they help to define the individual at risk of a particular disease.

THE MEASUREMENT OF DISEASE

The good clinician thinks in qualitative terms. During a diagnostic examination the dental practitioner not only looks for existing disease but also tries to look ahead for possible areas of future disease. Will that stained fissure become carious? Would it be better to remove that tooth, or should it have endodontic and restorative treatment? The practitioner thinks in terms of the quality of the patient's oral condition and then bases the treatment plan on the best interests of that particular patient.

However, this approach is not adequate for quantifying disease, for there are too many areas of subjective judgment involved. The clinician can also quite correctly be influenced by particular demands from a patient, by the degree to which a particular patient may cooperate in self-care, and perhaps by the patient's ability to pay for treatment received. The measurement of the degree of disease in a given population, therefore, requires technics that are much more standardized and objective. Established and standarized criteria for determining whether a carious lesion is present or not, or whether a periodontal pocket is present or not, replace the judgment of the practitioner. The dental epidemiologist judges the condition of the oral tissues as they are at a particular time, not on how they might be in the future. This application of standard criteria, which can require suppression of intuitive clinical judgment, is the most important philosophical difference between the clinical and the epidemiological examination.

It is important to point out that the application of standard criteria in a dental practice is not tantamount to treating patients impersonally. Indeed, the practitioner who standardizes criteria for diagnosis of disease is likely to provide a higher quality of care.

Another distinction between the technics of the two examinations is that the epidemiological examination rarely attempts to establish the absolute prevalence of a condition. This is because for most epidemiological purposes the extent of disease in the group under study is used for a comparison with the prevalence in some other group, rather than for establishment of a treatment plan for an individual patient. In that instance, so long as the same criteria to define disease are being used in the two situations, the *relative* difference in disease prevalence will still be valid.

While an accurate count of cases is theoretically possible in an acute disease such as measles, chronic conditions such as dental caries and periodontal disease present a more difficult problem in counting. The lesion of dental caries is characterized by a long preclinical stage during which the lesion cannot be diagnosed in the living human by clinical methods.[85] Periodontal diseases represent a slow and subtle alteration of tissue quality from health to an end point—the loss of function. An absolute count of lesions of these diseases could always be challenged by a new count based on better diagnostic skill, or an improved diagnostic aid, or by the inadvertent inclusion of a number of normal areas as lesions, an error that in statistical terms is called the "inclusion of false positives."

Figure 5–2 provides a representation of the different approaches required for quantifying acute and chronic diseases. Acute diseases, such as measles, are characterized by a sudden onset of symptoms, so that the patient rapidly progresses from a state in which the disease is clearly absent to one in which

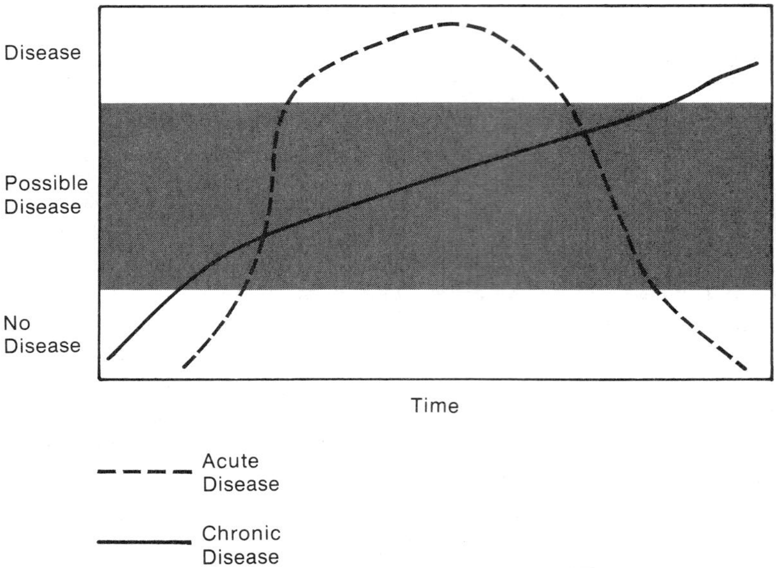

Figure 5–2. A representation of the difference in time, between acute and chronic disease, in the clinical manifestation of disease.

the disease is clearly present. There is little time spent in the "gray areas." Remission of the acute phase of the disease is equally rapid. At any given time, therefore, measles is likely to be either clearly absent or clearly present in the members of a population group, thus making its quantification fairly straightforward. Chronic diseases, on the other hand, are usually characterized by a much slower time of onset. It is difficult to establish exactly when arthritis, alcoholism, mental illness, dental caries, and periodontal diseases become definitely established; as shown in Figure 5–2, there is a relatively greater "gray area," where it cannot be stated with certainty whether the disease is established or not. Quantification in such cases is difficult.

In these instances, when the absolute total prevalence of lesions is unknown, it is more helpful to count all lesions that meet some specific criterion, such as disclosure by a given diagnostic apparatus or technic or, in the case of dental caries, by counting those lesions clearly large enough to require treatment. Again, the crucial point to be determined is whether or not there is more disease in one group than in another. A difference, if found, can be tested by professional and statistical logic. This requirement clearly demands use of a quantitative estimate, that is, for the disease to be expressed in numerical rather than purely clinical terms.

THE MEASUREMENT OF ORAL DISEASES

The principal focus of oral epidemiology has traditionally been on dental caries; more recently, periodontal diseases have received similar attention.

The tissues involved in these diseases are readily accessible to direct examination by a variety of methods: by inspection with reflected or transmitted light, by probing with an appropriate instrument, by palpation, and by radiographic examination. Both diseases are chronic and progressive to the point at which, lacking treatment, they can be identified in unequivocal fashion by the simplest of diagnostic methods. The ready access of the oral cavity to examination gives the oral epidemiologist an advantage not enjoyed by most medical colleagues. As a result, oral diseases can be quantified more precisely than can most other chronic conditions.

The simplest form of measuring any disease is by a count of the number of cases of its occurrence. Diagnosed causes of death, for example, can be determined from a study of death certificates. The number of persons admitted to and discharged from hospitals can be determined by institutional records. But with the oral diseases simple counts of cases are often of limited use because of the high prevalence of these conditions in many of the world's populations.

The simple count can be made more useful by turning it into a proportion, which is done by providing a denominator to the count. Knowledge of the occurrence of various cancers, for example, is increased by knowing the proportionate prevalence in the population. In these cases, the count can be divided by the total population or by some subgroup within it, such as males aged 55 to 64. In oral diseases, proportions are useful when looking at those conditions that occur relatively uncommonly, such as cleft lip and palate and the oral cancers. But with the more prevalent conditions of dental caries and periodontal diseases, proportions are of limited use except in those populations or subgroups in which the conditions occur less frequently. As an example, a measure of the proportion of the population suffering from dental caries in many parts of India is a useful measure, because caries is still relatively infrequent there. In Western countries, the proportion of first-grade elementary schoolchildren free of caries can be a useful measure for the same reason.

A *rate* is a proportion that uses a standarized denominator. A widely used rate in health statistics is infant mortality, which is almost universally measured by the number of deaths of newborn infants within the first year of life per 1,000 live births. In the United States, the infant mortality rate has been reduced from 24.7 per 1,000 live births in 1965 to 15.2 in 1976.[92] As well as being a source of useful comparisons, such rates can be used to establish or evaluate social policy. The prevalence of a condition can also be expressed as the *percentage* affected by a condition, which is really another way of expressing a rate. In oral epidemiology, the percentage is a useful way of measuring conditions such as the proportion of edentulous persons in a population or the proportion of five-year-old children affected by dental caries.

However, the measurement of the more commonly occurring oral diseases, that is, dental caries and periodontal disease, usually requires that they be measured by the degree of intensity and not just simply the prevalence of the condition. While the disease can be present in two individuals, meaning that both would be included in a prevalence count, the intensity of the condition can vary greatly between them. Clearly, the individual who suffers from dental caries in only two of a complement of 32 teeth has a much lower intensity of disease than does the person who has carious lesions in 16 of 32 teeth. A simple prevalence count would not discriminate between these two degrees of intensity. Such differences usually can only be determined by use of an index.

An *index* has been defined by Russell[78] as a numerical value describing the relative status of a population on a graduated scale with definite upper and lower limits, which is designed to permit and facilitate comparison with other populations classified by the same criteria and methods. Both proportions and rates would be classified as indexes* under this definition. Indeed, the word index is often used to apply to the simplest form of quantification of disease. Russell's definition is useful in helping researchers remember how indexes should be developed and applied.

Ideally, an index should possess the following properties:

1. Clarity, simplicity, and objectivity. The examiner should be able to carry the rules of the index in his head, and the index should be reasonably easy to apply so that there is no undue time lost during field examinations. The criteria for the index should be clear and unambiguous, with mutually exclusive categories.
2. Validity. The index must measure what it is intended to measure, so it should correspond with clinical stages of the disease under study at each point. To illustrate, the number of bacteria in a sample of saliva is not a valid measure of bacteria in dental plaque, nor is the number of missing teeth in an adult necessarily a valid measure of caries activity, because the teeth can be lost for reasons other than caries.
3. Reliability. The index should measure consistently at different times and under a variety of conditions. The term "reliability" is virtually synonymous with *reproducibility,* which means the ability of the same or different examiners to interpret and use the index in the same way.
4. Quantifiability. The index should be amenable to statistical analysis, so that the status of a group can be expressed by a number that corresponds to a relative position on a scale from zero to the upper limit.
5. Sensitivity. The index should be able to detect reasonably small shifts, in either direction, in the group condition.
6. Acceptability. The use of the index should not be painful or demeaning to the subject.

Probably no index used in oral epidemiology completely meets all of these conditions, but choice of an index in any given situation should be made on the basis of how closely the index approximates them and by the requirements of the study in which the index is being used.

There are a number of other terms describing indexes that the reader will come across in the dental literature and that should be defined here. One

*Both "indexes" and "indices" are acceptable plural forms of the word "index."

is the distinction between a *reversible* and an *irreversible* index. An irreversible index is one that measures cumulative conditions that cannot be reversed. Dental caries, for example, is usually regarded as an irreversible condition. Once the lesion of caries has reached a clinically discernible stage, the lesion either continues or it is treated by restoration or extraction. Clinically established caries, therefore, leaves a permanent scar. On the other hand, gingivitis, an inflammatory condition in soft tissue, is reversible. Healthy gingival tissues can become inflamed and then, under certain conditions, can return to a state of health again. An index of gingivitis, therefore, is considered a reversible one.

An *ordinal* scale is a scale of measurement that lists conditions in some sort of order; for example, classifying the condition of gingival tissues as good, fair, or poor. Use of this sort of scale merely attempts to order a condition progressively, without attempting to define any mathematical relation between the categories defined. A *nominal* scale is even less rigidly defined; it simply gives names to different conditions and therefore is not strictly a scale at all. An example is Angle's Classification of Malocclusion,[4] which merely attaches names to variously defined conditions of malocclusion. An *interval* or a *ratio* scale (a ratio scale has a true zero point, an interval scale does not) is one in which the numbers used in the measuring scale purport to have a mathematical relation to each other. If, for example, the number "1" is used to describe a degree of gingivitis that meets certain criteria, the condition that receives the number "2" is considered to be twice as bad, that which receives the number "3," three times as bad, and so on, until the upper limit of the scale is reached. Although many indexes used in oral epidemiology are considered to be interval or ratio scales, the validity of this claim can be questioned in almost every case. However, for practical purposes, the difference between an interval and an ordinal scale as used in oral epidemiology can become more academic than practical, although it can affect the choice of statistical methods used in the analysis of the data and therefore the conclusions reached. (Further discussion of measurement scales is given in Chapter 10.)

Indexes Used in Measuring Dental Caries

Measurements of the intensity of dental caries, such as the proportion of first molars lost through caries[42, 43] and the percentage of permanent teeth affected by caries,[2, 62] have been in use since the earlier years of the twentieth century. Both of these methods provide useful comparative information but are too crude for many applications. At the other extreme, the Bodeckers' index, described in 1931,[8] was sensitive but too complex for use in epidemiological surveys. The approach to measuring caries by counting the numbers of teeth in the mouth visibly affected by caries was used in a systematic manner by Dean and colleagues in their historic studies of the dental caries/fluoride relation.[22] However, the first systematic description of what is now known as the **DMF** index is usually attributed to Klein, Palmer, and Knutson in their studies of dental caries in Hagerstown, Maryland, in the latter part of the 1930s.[48] Since then, the DMF index has received practically universal acceptance and is probably the best known of all dental indexes. The DMF index is applied only to permanent teeth. As described by the authors, **D** is used to describe decayed teeth; **M**, teeth missing due to caries; and **F** for teeth that have been previously filled. DMF can therefore be defined as an irreversible index on a ratio scale. The DMF score from any one individual can range from 0 to 32, in whole numbers. The DMF values for a group studied in an epidemiological survey constitute the total of the individual values divided by the number of subjects examined, so a DMF group score can have decimal values. The DMF index can be applied to whole teeth or to surfaces of teeth. Modifications can be made to account for such factors as teeth that have been filled and have redecayed on another surface, secondary caries around an existing restoration, crowned teeth, bridge pontics, and any other particular attribute that is required for the purposes of a survey. DMF can also be used in a half-mouth fashion in which opposite diagonal quadrants of the mouth are examined.

The DMF index as applied to the permanent dentition is always used with capital letters. The equivalent index for measuring caries in the primary dentition is the **def** index, described by Gruebbel in 1944.[37] As defined by Gruebbel, **d** stands for decayed teeth, **e** means indicated for extraction, and **f** stands for filled teeth. It should be noticed that in the def index teeth missing due to caries are not recorded because of the difficulty, in many children, of distinguishing between extracted and naturally exfoliated primary teeth. Modifications of this index are (1) **dmf** for use in children before ages of exfoliation, (2) dmf applied only to the primary molar teeth, and (3) the **df** index in which missing teeth are ignored. Close observation shows that df and def should be numerically the same; def allows for two grades of caries and neither counts missing teeth. Both def and df may therefore understate the true extent of the carious attack and thus lose validity. For comparative purposes, however, the greater reliability gained by ignoring missing teeth can make both indexes more useful.

The DMF index has been extraordinarily valuable in increasing knowledge of the distribution of dental caries throughout the world and by demonstrating how caries distribution within any one population is influenced by the demographic variables of age, sex, race, and socioeconomic status. (This distribution of disease will be discussed more fully in Chapter 6.) However, no index is perfect, and the DMF, like all other indexes, does have some limitations. These limitations can be described as follows:

DMF Values Are Not Related to the Number of Teeth at Risk. DMF scores are a simple count of those teeth that in the examiner's judgment have been affected by caries. There is no denominator to an individual's DMF score. As a result, the DMF scores do not directly give an indication of the intensity of the attack in any one individual. A seven-year-old child with DMF score of 3.0 may have only nine permanent teeth in the mouth; thus one third of these teeth have already been attacked by caries in a short space of time. An adult may have a DMF score of 16.0 from a full complement of 32 teeth;

thus over a longer period of time half of the teeth have been affected by caries. One cannot always tell from simply looking at the DMF scores which individual has been affected most by the disease.

The DMF Index Can Be Invalid in Older Adults Because Teeth Can Become Lost for Reasons Other Than Caries. It has been suggested by the World Health Organization that the **M** component of average DMF scores over age 30 might be more appropriately called the *tooth mortality score,* because tooth loss over this age represents teeth lost for reasons of dental caries, periodontal disease, accidents, cultural reasons, and perhaps others. In other words, the **M** count is not necessarily a valid reflection of tooth loss because of dental caries.

The DMF Index Can Be Misleading in Children Whose Teeth Have Been Lost Due to Orthodontic Reasons. Just as in adults over 30 in whom teeth can be lost for periodontal reasons, in some child populations there can be a heavy loss of bicuspids in the course of orthodontic treatment. Inclusion of these teeth in the M component of the DMF score would obviously give misleading results.

The DMF Index Can Overestimate Caries Experience in Teeth in Which "Preventive Fillings" Have Been Placed. Some dentists place restorations in teeth that although not yet carious they think may decay in the future. In an epidemiological survey, such teeth must be included in the F component of DMF, although had they not been filled in the first place, the survey examiner might have diagnosed them as sound teeth. Again, in highly treated populations where many such "preventive fillings" have been placed, the DMF scores will tend to be inflated.

The DMF Index Is of Little Use in Studies of Root Caries. Root caries is that particular form of the disease seen in older populations in Western countries, and in some younger populations in developing countries, in which the lesion begins below the cementoenamel junction following recession of the gingivae.

Other methods of measuring dental caries using a different philosophical base from that of the DMF index have been suggested. One is Grainger's Hierarchical Method, an ordinal scale designed to simplify the recording of the caries status of a population, which uses five zones of severity of the carious attack.[33] Tests of its validity and applicability indicate it may be useful,[46, 47, 64,] but it has not yet received wide acceptance.

One continuing source of potential differences between oral epidemiologists is the establishment of criteria for diagnosing the early carious lesion. As discussed earlier in the chapter, dental caries as a chronic disease has a particular period in its development when it enters the "gray area," where it is difficult to tell whether the disease is irreversibly established or not. It is known that by the time caries can be clinically detected by either visual or radiographic methods, a lesion is histologically well established.[84] Referring to Figure 5–2, the detection of the completely sound tooth is not difficult, nor is detection of the obvious lesion that has visible cavitation. Between these two extremes, however, there is difficulty in diagnosis. It is here that careful definition of criteria and the ability of the examiner to adhere to them during many examinations becomes critical, for consistency of diagnosis is clearly necessary in an epidemiological examination if data are to be valid. However, the determination of criteria for what is to be regarded as caries can also affect the final results. Examiners tend to be more consistent when the criteria are "liberal," that is, tending toward clear and unequivocal detection of a lesion and not scoring "borderline" lesions. The cost of using such criteria, however, is that many established lesions may be passed over and called sound; hence, there could be a significant underestimate of the extent of disease in particular populations where there are many lesions.

Criteria for diagnosis of caries used in North America, Britain, and the other English-speaking countries tend to be of the more liberal variety.[39] However, some European investigators use much stricter criteria in which grades of carious lesions are diagnosed.[5, 72] (Examples of these two sets of criteria are shown in Table 5–1.) Use of these "European" criteria requires a longer, more meticulous survey examination and could lead to a greater degree of examiner inconsistency because of the increased number of diagnostic decisions that have to be made. However, if applied reliably, "European" criteria may give a more accurate estimate of disease progression.

The principal point made in the preceding descussion is that the type of criteria used in any one epidemiological examination can influence the values obtained regarding the extent of dental caries in a population. Clearly, an examiner using the "European" criteria shown in Table 5–1 would be likely to find more carious lesions in a population than would an examiner using the "Anglo-Saxon" criteria. This point should be borne in mind when comparisons are made between different studies. In the same way, of course, use of

Table 5–1. Different Criteria for Diagnosing Pit-and-Fissure Caries by "Anglo-Saxon" System* and the "European" System†

Anglo-Saxon (Liberal)	European (Conservative)
Pits and fissures on the occlusal, vestibular, and lingual surfaces are carious when the explorer "catches" after insertion with moderate to firm pressure *and* when the "catch" is accompanied by one or more of the following signs of decay:	In upper molars, mesio-occlusal and disto-occlusal-palative fissures assessed separately. In lower molars, the occlusal fissures and the buccal pits are assessed separately. Teeth are dried, sharp new explorers used. Caries diagnosed in four categories:
1. Softness at the base of the area. 2. Opacity adjacent to the area provides evidence of undermining or demineralization. 3. Softened enamel adjacent to the area that may be scraped away by the explorer.	C I. Minute black line at base of fissure. C II. In addition, a white zone along margins of fissure (dark in transmitted light). C III. The smallest perceptible break in the continuity of the enamel. C IV. Large cavity, more than 3 mm wide.
Note: These areas should be diagnosed as sound when there is apparent evidence of demineralization, but no evidence of softness.	

*Described by Horowitz.[39]

†Described by Backer-Dirks, Houwink, and Kwant.[5]

radiographs will tend to show more lesions in a population than a survey procedure in which radiographs are not used. However, the possibility of inconsistencies is also more likely.

Indexes Used in Measuring Periodontal Disease

Clinical diagnosis of gingivitis depends on the examiner's determination of changes in color, shape, and texture of the papillary and marginal tissues. Diagnosis of more destructive periodontal disease is based on similar factors, together with clinical and radiographic observations of pocket deepening and bone loss. Since gingivitis is an inflammatory condition, the disease is reversible in its early stages, and even a moderate degree of advanced periodontal disease can be reversed with appropriate treatment.[55] However, the line of demarcation between normal tissue and a periodontal lesion is even more difficult for examiners to judge than is the case with caries. Gordon's principle of the "biological gradient of disease"[32] becomes even more important in population estimates of periodontal disease than it does in estimates of dental caries.

Some periodontal indexes developed for use in epidemiological surveys can measure the reversible effects of the disease (gingivitis), while some others measure the irreversible effect, that is, bone loss. Some of the most commonly used indexes measure both irreversible and reversible effects.

Many early epidemiological studies of periodontal diseases were based on radiographic surveys of alveolar bone loss.[26, 79, 80, 86] But radiographic studies, a standard procedure in diagnosis and treatment planning of the individual periodontal patient, now find little application in field studies of periodontal disease because of (1) the frequent impracticability of bringing x-ray equipment into field situations, (2) the fact that adequate epidemiological information can be obtained without x-rays,[73] and (3) growing public and professional sensitivity about radiation. A useful estimate of bone loss in a group can be obtained, without the use of radiographs, by counting the average percentage of teeth per person with gingival recession exposing the cementoenamel junction.[86] Since bone loss is a relatively late development in destructive disease, these cumulative measures are not very discriminatory in young persons, and their use requires a long time span to demonstrate a change for the better following treatment. For these reasons, several reversible indexes with scores that can diminish as the tissue condition improves were developed.

The oldest reversible index is probably the **P-M-A**, developed by Schour and Massler,[54, 81] based on the concept that the extent of inflammation serves as an indicator of the severity of the condition. The presence or absence of inflammation is recorded in the papillary tip (**P**), the marginal (**M**), or the attached (**A**) areas of the gingiva around the teeth. Criteria for the P-M-A require positive scoring for any deviation from a stringently defined ideal condition of the tissues. More detailed knowledge has cast doubt on the validity of this index, and it has not received much use in recent years.

Probably the most frequently used index of gingivitis at the present time

Table 5–2. Criteria for the Gingival Index (GI)*

Score	Criteria
0	Normal gingiva.
1	Mild inflammation—slight change in color, slight edema. No bleeding on probing.
2	Moderate inflammation—redness, edema, and glazing. Bleeding on probing.
3	Severe inflammation—marked redness and edema. Ulceration. Tendency to spontaneous bleeding.

*As described by Löe and Silness.[52]

is the Gingival Index, the **GI**, of Löe and Silness.[52] The GI judges the conditions of the gingiva on the mesial, distal, buccal, and lingual surfaces of the teeth. Each area is scored on a scale from 0 through 3 according to the criteria shown in Table 5–2. The GI can be used on selected teeth in the mouth as well as on all erupted teeth;[51] in fact it was first described for use on six selected teeth.[52] As can be seen from the criteria listed in Table 5–2, the GI is purely an index of gingivitis and takes no account of deeper changes in the periodontium. The GI is probably as sensitive an index as could be devised for any gingival index based on clinical examination, but its use can still present some problems. While on a group basis it distinguishes clearly between those with little or no gingivitis and those with severe gingivitis, it is often difficult to tell whether it discriminates adequately between the middle ranges of the conditions. Examiners find that the difference between scores of 0 and 1, and 1 and 2, are often difficult to judge. Although the GI, when used by a skilled examiner, is quite sensitive enough to detect differences in gingival status between groups, some investigators still find it to be insufficiently sensitive in determining the initial stages of gingivitis. As a result, Mühlemann and Son[56] developed an index that they called the Sulcus Bleeding Index, the **SBI**, which takes the GI score of 0 and splits it into two zones. In other words, the SBI adds an extra demarcation zone of incipient gingivitis. While this index may indeed provide a more sensitive measure of the condition, it also, as discussed earlier in this chapter, introduces further consistency problems for the examiner and perhaps increases the degree of inconsistent scorings.

A good discussion point, though perhaps a little academic, is whether the GI and the SBI are interval or ordinal scales. While their statistical treatment is usually based on the assumption that they are interval scales, a close examination of the criteria for the GI shown in Table 5–2 could lead one to conclude that it is, in reality, an ordinal scale. It cannot be said, for example, that the condition scored as 2 is twice as bad as that scored as 1.

Probably the most widely used periodontal index in epidemiological surveys around the world has been the **PI**, the Periodontal Index devised by Russell in 1956.[73] The PI is a composite index because it records both the reversible changes due to gingivitis and the more destructive and presumably

Table 5–3. Scoring and Criteria for the Periodontal Index (PI)*

Score	Criteria
0	*Negative.* There is neither overt inflammation in the investing tissues nor loss of function due to destruction of supporting tissue.
1	*Mild gingivitis.* There is an overt area of inflammation in the free gingivae, but the area does not circumscribe the tooth.
2	*Gingivitis.* Inflammation completely circumscribes the tooth, but there is no apparent break in epithelial attachment.
6	*Gingivitis with pocket formation.* The epithelial attachment has been broken and there is a pocket (not merely a deepened gingival crevice due to swelling in the free gingivae). There is no interference with normal masticatory function; the tooth is firm in its socket and has not drifted.
8	*Advanced destruction with loss of masticatory function.* The tooth may be loose; may have drifted; may sound dull on percussion with a metallic instrument; and may be depressible in its socket.

*As described by Russell.[73]

irreversible changes wrought by deeper periodontal disease. The reason for its widespread use and popularity is to be found in its ease of use, the clarity of the criteria (shown in Table 5–3), and the reasonable comparability of results obtained. This index has probably had more attention paid to its validity than most others. Russell chose the scoring values (0,1,2,6,8,) in order to relate the stages of the disease scored in an epidemiological survey to the clinical conditions observed. The jump from 2 to 6 in the scale, for example, recognizes the change in disease condition from a severe gingivitis to an overt destructive periodontal disease with obvious loss of attachment. In that sense, the PI can be considered a true interval scale. Although the PI is not designed for diagnosis of the individual patient, there is a general correspondence between the clinical status and the average PI score for a group. Most persons judged to be negative for periodontal disease, for example, have PI scores in the neighborhood of 0 to 0.2. Most individuals in the terminal stages of disease have scores approaching the upper limit of the scale, that is between 6 and 8. A summary of the relation between clinical conditions and group PI scores[77] is shown in Table 5–4.

Table 5–4. The Relation Between Scores on the Periodontal Index (PI) and Clinical Conditions*

Most People With	Score in the Range of:
Clinically normal tissues	0–0.2
Gingivitis	0.1–1.0
Incipient destructive periodontal disease	0.5–1.9
Established destructive disease	1.5–5.0
Terminal stages of periodontal disease	4.0–8.0

*As described by Russell.[77]

Another composite index of periodontal disease utilizing both reversible and irreversible signs is the Periodontal Disease Index (**PDI**) of Ramfjord.[67] Six specified teeth are examined in each mouth: the maxillary right first molar, the maxillary left central incisor, the maxillary left first bicuspid, the mandibular left first molar, the mandibular right central incisor, and the mandibular right first bicuspid. The gingiva surrounding each tooth is scored on a scale running from 0 to 3 according to the degree of inflammation observed. The gingival crevices on the mesial and buccal areas of the assigned teeth are then probed and a score of 4, 5, or 6 assigned, depending on the distance from the cementoenamel junction to the bottom of the crevice. The criteria used for the PDI are shown in Table 5–5. The PDI is likely to be more sensitive than the PI and is also more meticulous and time-consuming. Unlike the PI, it is intended for use in scoring conditions for individual patients and is therefore a useful index for the general practitioner to use in measuring progress in periodontal patients. In epidemiological work, Ramfjord stated that it is more suitable for clinical trials than for surveys of populations.[68] Both the PI and the PDI originally allowed for radiographic examination, but it has been shown that radiographs add little to the accuracy of results gained from clinical examinations alone.[82]

An adaptation of the PDI index called the Gingival Periodontal Index (**GPI**) has been used by O'Leary in screening Air Force personnel to determine those in need of periodontal treatment. Both gingivitis and pocket depth are scored in six segments in the mouth. The worst condition found in any one

Table 5–5. Criteria for the Periodontal Disease Index (PDI)*

Score	Criteria
0	Absence of inflammation.
1	Mild to moderate inflammatory gingival changes not extending all around the tooth.
2	Mild to moderately severe gingivitis extending all around the tooth.
3	Severe gingivitis, characterized by marked redness, tendency to bleed, and ulceration.
4	Gingival crevice in any of the four measured areas (mesial, distal, buccal, lingual), extending apically to the cementoenamel junction but not more than 3 mm.
5	Gingival crevice in any of the four measured areas extending apically to the cementoenamel junction 3–6 mm.
6	Gingival crevice in any of the four measured areas extending apically more than 6 mm from the cementoenamel junction.

*As described by Ramfjord.[67]

segment is taken as the score for that segment.[50, 59] The GPI can be used either for determining a group score or for monitoring the status of an individual patient.

The indexes described are not the only ones suggested for measuring gingival and periodontal conditions.[44] Probably the relative proliferation of indexes for gauging periodontal disease, when compared to the relative isolation of the DMF in measuring caries, is itself an indication of the uncertainty involved in quantifying the condition.

All of the indexes of periodontal disease have been useful in epidemiological surveys and yet all have their problems. They require reasonably well-trained examiners for reliable use. All are designed as quantitative measures of disease, rather than as indicators of treatment requirements once the disease is present.

In an effort to reduce possible inconsistency when making distinctions between varying grades of gingivitis, an extraoral colorimetric test for gingivitis has been tried.[10] The test relies for its validity on the presence of reactive inflammatory cells in the saliva. A sample of saliva from a patient with periodontal disease is mixed with some of the test material, and the degree of color change supposedly indicates the degree of gingivitis present in the mouth. The test material is insufficiently reliable for widespread use, but the idea may be worth further development.

Several epidemiological methods for determining treatment needs in populations have also been suggested and tried. One is the Periodontal Treatment Need System (**PTNS**), developed and used in a number of studies in Norway.[7] The PTNS is based on categorizing patients into certain levels of treatment need and assigning times for the type of treatment required. The World Health Organization[94] recommends a similar system: a present or absent approach to scoring intense gingivitis and advanced periodontal involvement of teeth in six segments in the mouth. These types of assessments of treatment needs, although seemingly crude by clinical periodontal standards, may be useful for planning personnel requirements to treat population groups.[6]

The World Health Organization (WHO) is continuing to develop more refined methods of assessing periodontal diseases—methods that are still suitable for epidemiological use. Approaches in the early 1980s center around testing a method[96] that examines the same teeth as in the PDI in four age groups. Examination is for calculus, depth of pocket, and presence and absence of bleeding. Further development of this method can be expected.

It must be remembered that the more sensitive an index, the greater the degree of information likely to be obtained, but at a cost of possible inconsistency of recording and, hence, unreliability of results. Cruder measures, such as those just described, do not provide the same depth of information, but the data obtained may be detailed enough and should be of a more reliable nature. Much depends on what the purpose of the information-gathering exercise is.

Indexes Used in Measuring Plaque and Calculus

It has been learned by experience that periodontal data, expressed by whatever index, are often more useful when the state of oral hygiene is also taken into account. This is because of the close causal association between the two (to be discussed in Chapter 6). An index of oral hygiene which has had wide use in field surveys of periodontal disease is the Simplified Oral Hygiene Index (**OHI–S**).[35, 36] This is a quick and practical index that has proved itself extremely useful in large-scale epidemiological surveys. Its lack of sensitivity, however, makes it less useful in the individual patient. It is applied to six tooth surfaces in the mouth; four posterior and two anterior. Two scores are given for each tooth examined; one for the amount of debris on the tooth and the other for calculus. Both debris and calculus are scored on a scale from 0 to 3. Results can be expressed separately for either debris or calculus; the two added together give the total OHI–S score.

An index that the dental practitioner will find more useful for monitoring the individual patient, as well as one which has been used in epidemiological studies, is the Patient Hygiene Performance Index (**PHP**) of Podshadley and Haley.[63] This index is carried out with the same teeth and surfaces that are used in the OHI–S. Soft deposits are scored according to the stain left after the patient has used a disclosing tablet. To use the index the examiner must mentally divide the surface of the tooth examined into five segments, as shown in Figure 5–3. Each of the five subdivisions is scored for presence or absence of pink-stained plaque; a score of 0 is assigned to each section if no stain is detected; a score of 1 is assigned if any plaque at all is present. The debris score for each tooth is determined by adding the values of each of the five subdivisions. The PHP score for the patient is the sum of the scores for each of the six teeth divided by the number of teeth scored.

Silness and Löe have developed a plaque index (**PlI**)[83] designed to be used along with their GI. The same surfaces of the same teeth are scored as in the GI and the same scoring system of 0 to 3 is used. The principal difference between the PlI and the OHI–S approach is that the plaque index scores the plaque present according to its thickness at the gingival margin rather than its coronal extent. It has been claimed that measuring plaque thickness is a more valid gauge than measuring coronal extent of plaque.[1]

The WHO also has suggested, for its basic assessment of disease, a simple approach comparable to its assessment of periodontal status.[94] The only instrument used is a mouth mirror. If soft deposits are clearly visible to the unaided eye on the gingival margin of one or more teeth within the segment, a score of 1 is given for the segment. If no soft deposit is evident, a score of 0 is given. The same approach is taken for calculus, the only distinction being that an obvious deposit suspected of being calculus, as determined by direct inspection with the aid of a mouth mirror, should be tested with a periodontal probe to determine that it is indeed calcified. If so, a score of 1 is given; if not, a score of 0.

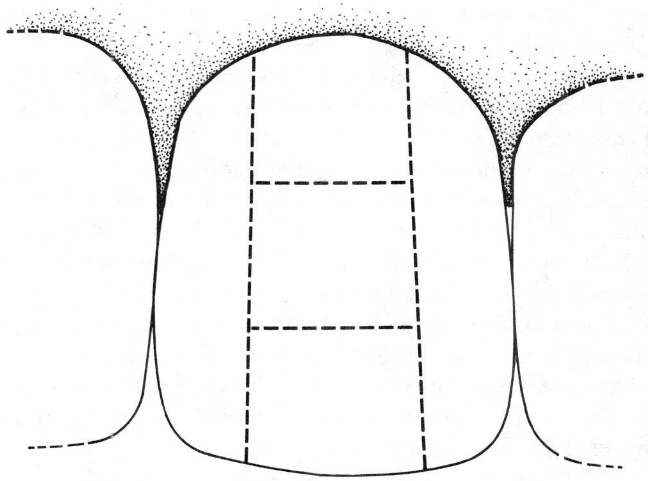

Figure 5–3. A representation of the five divisions of a tooth surface as used in the Patient Hygiene Performance Index (PHP) of Podshadley and Haley. (Data from Podshadley, A. G., and Haley, J. V. A method for evaluating oral hygiene performance. Pub. Health Rep., 83:259–264, Mar. 1968.)

Indexes Used in Measuring Malocclusion

Malocclusion has proved to be a difficult entity to define, because individual perceptions of what constitutes a malocclusion problem differ widely. As a result, no generally accepted epidemiological index of malocclusion has yet been devised. Thoughtful commentaries on the problems of classifying and scoring malocclusions have been provided by Jago[45] and Foster.[31]

The best known classification of malocclusion conditions is that of Angle, which dates from the nineteenth century.[4] While Angle's classification is still useful in determining the kind of treatment a patient should receive, it is of virtually no use in epidemiological surveys because it is a nominal classification and would not provide useful information applicable to a population. A number of indexes of malocclusion, however, have been proposed and used. Most record specific conditions. The Malalignment Index[93] assesses rotation and tooth displacement, whereas the Occlusal Feature Index[65] records crowding and cuspal interdigitation and vertical and horizontal overbite. The **HLD** Index[24] has been used for assessing treatment needs in New York state. Grainger developed the Treatment Priority Index (**TPI**) for the same purpose, and this index has been used in national studies of orthodontic needs of children.[91]

The Occlusal Index (**OI**) of Summers[87] now seems one of the better accepted orthodontic indexes. It makes measurements of nine characteristics: dental age, molar relation, overbite, overjet, posterior crossbite, posterior openbite, tooth displacement, midline relations, and missing permanent maxillary incisors. Its validity has been checked on several occasions by Summers and its reliability is said to be high. A fair degree of examiner skill and training, however, is still required for the application of this index.

The *Fédération Dentaire Internationale* (FDI) attempted to develop its own internationally accepted and simplified method of determining malocclusion.[28] The result, however, was a carefully qualified description of a method of measuring occlusal traits. It has been applied on at least one occasion in New York state by Cons and associates,[13] though the precise application of the results obtained remains to be determined.

The WHO, continuing its efforts to provide simplified, standardized basic methods of recording oral disease, bases its assessment (as it did with gingival disease and plaque) on a "present/absent" basis. The WHO suggests[94] that a dentofacial anomaly be recorded as present if in the judgment of the examiner one or more of the following criteria is met:

1. It has a significant and unacceptable effect on facial appearance.
2. It causes a significant reduction in masticatory function or results in significant impairment of speech.
3. There is a gross defect such as cleft lip, cleft palate, or pathological or surgical injury that unquestionably has high priority for treatment.
4. It constitutes an occlusion predisposing to tissue destruction in the form of periodontal disease or caries.

The WHO recommends that this approach be used, pending the development of a generally acceptable system for assessing dentofacial anomalies. The organization continues to work jointly with the FDI for the development of such a system. In view of the nature of the condition, however, it must be questioned whether such a system will ever be developed and whether the WHO approach, which is admittedly highly subjective, is not as near to this ideal as one is ever going to get for most field studies. The growing importance of orthodontic treatment programs in third-party and other public programs, however, provides a stimulus for continuing the search for a suitable index of malocclusion.[31] At present, the OI and the WHO indexes seem to be the two best choices.

Measurement of Oral Cancers and Clefts

Oral cancer is usually measured in terms of a rate, as are other cancers. The age-adjusted death rate from oral cancer among male Americans, for example, was 4.8 per 100,000 in 1975–77.[3] Five-year survival rates are a common measurement in the epidemiology of cancers; patients with localized lesions of the oral cavity have a five-year survival rate of 67 percent.[3] The occurrence of cleft palate is also usually expressed as a rate; about one birth in 700 exhibits this condition.[34] Soft tissue abnormalities of various kinds, as well as the more rare types of oral pathoses, are also most suitably expressed as rates.

The Measurement of Dental Fluorosis

Dental fluorosis is a hypoplasia of the dental enamel caused by excessive ingestion of fluoride during the period of tooth calcification. Depending upon the quantity of fluoride ingested over a period of time during calcification, the degree of hypoplasia can range from barely noticeable to a severe and ugly brown stain with pitting and even flaking of friable enamel. The historical importance of dental fluorosis and its role in the discovery of fluoridation as a public health measure are discussed in Chapter 7. With the continuing political agitation concerning water fluoridation in the United States and other countries, however, the ability of dentists to recognize, diagnose, and classify dental fluorosis is clearly of importance.

The discovery in 1931 that fluoride in drinking water was the causative agent of enamel fluorosis led to the assignment of H. Trendley Dean of the U. S. Public Health Service to work on determining the prevalence of fluorosis in the United States. Dean's epidemiological studies during the years 1933 to 1946 are superb examples of a patient and methodical use of the epidemiological method to define a problem and develop hypotheses from that definition. His early investigations showed that the condition was widespread in many areas of the United States and also, according to clinical observations, was of varying severity.[14] With both prevalence and severity to be measured, his first task was to develop an index of dental fluorosis. This he did in 1934.[15] The Fluorosis Index set criteria for the categorization of dental fluorosis on a seven-point scale: normal, questionable, very mild, mild, moderate, moderately severe, and severe. This first description of the Fluorosis Index could be considered an ordinal scale; although no numbers were used, the conditions were ordered in degree of severity. Dean continued to use the seven-point scale for his Fluorosis Index for some time,[16, 19] but by 1939 he had combined the moderately severe and severe categories into a single category called "severe."[21] By 1942, Dean had revised his Fluorosis Index into the six-point scale (including "normal") that is still used today.[17] Dean apparently considered this revision necessary because experience had shown some deficiencies in the original 1934 index. The criteria for this revised version of the Fluorosis Index are shown in Table 5–6.

A logical development from the Fluorosis Index was Dean's use of the Community Fluorosis Index (**CFI**), which in 1935 he arbitrarily defined[20] on a seven-point ordinal scale, again ranging from negative and borderline to marked and very marked. Figure 5–4 is an example of Dean's charting of the CFI, using a number of towns he examined in Texas and elsewhere before 1935.[20] Later, however, he added a numerical weight to these categories and thus was able to derive a numerical CFI.[17] Table 5–7 is an example of how the

Table 5–6. Criteria for the Fluorosis Index*

Diagnosis	Criteria
Normal	The enamel represents the usual translucent semivitriform type of structure. The surface is smooth, glossy, and usually of a pale creamy white color.
Questionable	The enamel discloses slight aberrations from the translucency of normal enamel, ranging from a few white flecks to occasional white spots. This classification is utilized in those instances where a definite diagnosis of the mildest form of fluorosis is not warranted and a classification of "normal" not justified.
Very mild	Small, opaque, paper white area scattered irregularly over the tooth but not involving as much as approximately 25 percent of the tooth surface. Frequently included in this classification are teeth showing no more than about 1–2 mm. of white opacity at the tip of the summit of the cusps of the bicuspids or second molars.
Mild	The white opaque areas in the enamel of the teeth are more extensive but do not involve as much as 50 percent of the tooth.
Moderate	All enamel surfaces of the teeth are affected, and surfaces subject to attrition show marked wear. Brown stain is frequently a disfiguring feature.
Severe	Includes teeth formerly classified as "moderately severe" and "severe." All enamel surfaces are affected and hypoplasia is so marked that the general form of the tooth may be altered. The major diagnostic sign of this classification is the discrete or confluent pitting. Brown stains are widespread and teeth often present a corroded appearance.

*As defined by Dean in 1942.[17]

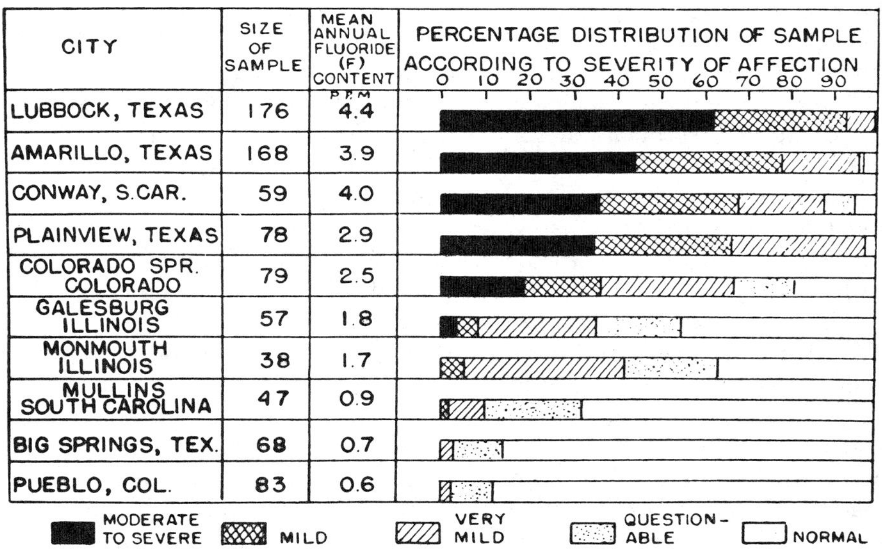

Figure 5–4. Dean's use of the Community Fluorosis Index (ordinal scale) from his examinations in 10 communities. (From Dean, H. T., and Elvove, Elias. Further studies on the minimal threshold of chronic endemic dental fluorosis. Pub. Health Rep., 52:1249–64, Sept. 1937.)

Table 5–7. Derivation of the Community Fluorosis Index. The Example of Amarillo, Texas, where Drinking Water Averages 3.9 ppm Fluoride*

Fluorosis Category	Numerical Weight	Frequency†	Frequency × Weight
Normal	0	9	0
Questionable	0.5	19	9.5
Very mild	1	44	44
Mild	2	81	162
Moderate	3	98	294
Severe	4	38	152
Total		289	661.5

$$\text{Community Fluorosis Index} = \frac{661.5}{289} = 2.3$$

*As defined by Dean.[17]
†Number of children in each category.

CFI of 2.3 was derived for Amarillo, Texas. Having now a quantifiable CFI, Dean related this index to the concentration of fluoride in a water supply and was able to show a linear correlation as shown in one of his original charts (Fig. 5–5).

The use of a numerical scale permitted statistical analysis relating the degree of fluorosis in a community to the concentration of fluoride in the

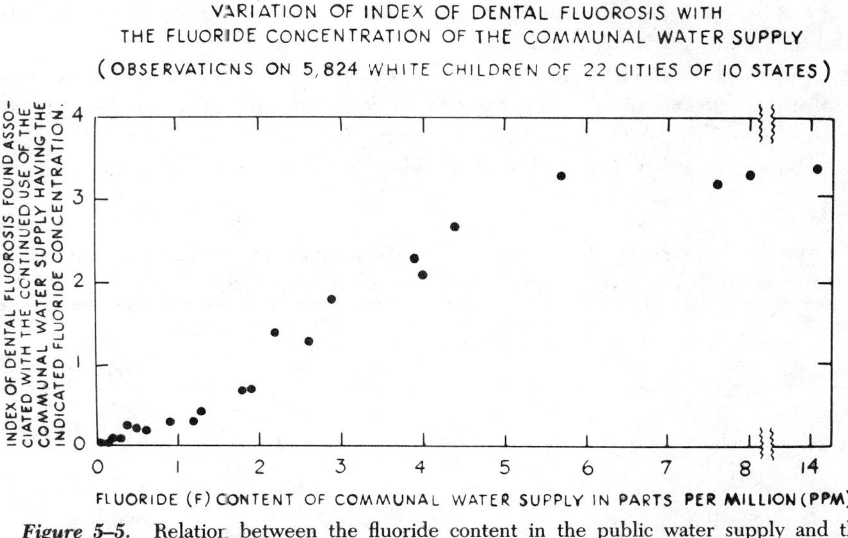

Figure 5–5. Relation between the fluoride content in the public water supply and the Community Fluorosis Index (interval scale). (From Dean, H. T. The investigation of physiological effects by the epidemiological method. [In Moulton, F. R., ed. Fluorine and dental health. AAAS Publication No. 19. Washington, D.C., American Association Advancement Science, 1942. 101 p. Copyright 1942, AAAS])

Table 5–8. Public Health Significance of Community Fluorosis Index Scores*

Range of Scores for Community Fluorosis Index	Public Health Significance
0–0.4	Negative
0.4–0.6	Borderline
0.6–1.0	Slight
1.0–2.0	Medium
2.0–3.0	Marked
3.0–4.0	Very marked

*As defined by Dean.[18]

water supply. It was also necessary to demonstrate the subsequent finding—namely, the relation between the concentration of fluoride in the water supply and the prevalence of dental caries. However, a number is an abstract thing; it says nothing about the clinical importance of the condition found. Dean therefore related his numerical CFI scale to what he termed "the public health significance" of the fluorosis problem,[18] as shown in Table 5–8. It can be seen that Dean also considered the severity of the public health problem to increase as the CFI increases. Of course, the levels of importance that Dean attached to the numerical scale represented his personal judgment. While his experience with fluorosis makes his opinion worthy of attention, the gradings of public health significance may not be quite the same today because much has changed since the 1930s.

As a result of grading the public health significance of the fluorosis problem, Dean was able to categorize various communities as having different degrees of the problem. Table 5–9, for example, shows four of the many cities that Dean studied in the 1930s, displaying the water fluoride concentration,

Table 5–9. Levels of Fluoride in the Drinking Water, the Community Fluorosis Index (CFI), and the Public Health Significance of That Index*

City	Water Fluoride Concentration (ppm.)	Community Fluorosis Index	Public Health Significance
Amarillo, Texas	3.9	2.3	Marked
Colorado Springs, Colorado	2.6	1.3	Medium
Galesburg, Illinois	1.9	0.69	Slight
Lima, Ohio	0.3	0.09	Negative

*As judged by Dean.[17]

Table 5–10. Differential Diagnosis between Milder Forms of Dental Fluorosis (Questionable, Very Mild, and Mild) and Nonfluoride Opacities of Enamel*

Characteristic	Milder Forms of Fluorosis	Nonfluoride Enamel Opacities
Area Affected	Usually seen on or near tips of cusps or incisal edges.	Usually centered in smooth surface; may affect entire crown.
Shape of Lesion	Resembles line shading in pencil sketch; lines follow incremental lines in enamel, form irregular caps on cusps.	Often round or oval.
Demarcation	Shades off imperceptibly into surrounding normal enamel.	Clearly differentiated from adjacent normal enamel.
Color	Slightly more opaque than normal enamel; "paper-white." Incisal edges, tips of cusps may have frosted appearance. Does not show stain at time of eruption (in these milder degrees, rarely at any time).	Usually pigmented at time of eruption; often creamy-yellow to dark reddish-orange.
Teeth Affected	Most frequent on teeth that calcify slowly (cuspids, bicuspids, second and third molars). Rare on lower incisors. Usually seen on six or eight homologous teeth. Extremely rare in deciduous teeth.	Any tooth may be affected. Frequent on labial surfaces of lower incisors. May occur singly. Usually one to three teeth affected. Common in deciduous teeth.
Gross Hypoplasia	None. Pitting of enamel does not occur in the milder forms. Enamel surface has glazed appearance, is smooth to point of explorer.	Absent to severe. Enamel surface may seem etched, be rough to explorer.
Detection	Often invisible under strong light; most easily detected by line of sight tangential to tooth crown.	Seen most easily under strong light on line of sight perpendicular to tooth surface.

*Russell.[75]

the CFI, and the public health significance of the CFI values. In the examples shown in Table 5–9, it can be seen that while Amarillo, Texas, had a marked fluorosis problem, Lima, Ohio, had none.

The development of the Fluorosis Index has been discussed at length not only because of its intrinsic importance but also because it illustrates, as few other examples do, the development of an epidemiological study from clinical observations to a quantifiable status of a public health problem. The end result of Dean's work was that his index was of vital importance in the establishment of water fluoridation as a public health measure. Dean's Fluorosis Index has been modified by some investigators in order to increase its sensitivity at higher levels of fluoride concentration,[89] but its principles are still the basis of recent investigations into the epidemiology of this condition.[38, 60]

Fluorosis is not always an easy condition for dental practitioners to differentiate from other enamel hypoplasias. Indeed, various forms of enamel hypoplasia have been wrongly called fluorosis at different times in the past. In order to assist dental practitioners in their diagnosis, Table 5–10 shows Russell's description[75] of some distinguishing features between milder forms of fluorosis and nonfluoride enamel opacities. Of course, an accurate water intake history is also important in making a diagnosis.

The Measurement of Oral Health

Although epidemiology was defined as the study of health and disease in populations, all of the indexes described have been used for the determination of disease or treatment needs rather than for the measurement of health.

What is health? *Dorland's Illustrated Medical Dictionary* uses the same definition as that given by the World Health Organization:

> A state of optimal, physical, mental and social well-being, and not merely the absence of disease and infirmity.[23]

This definition is not very helpful to those who are seeking to develop a quantitative measure of general health or oral health, for it refers to a vague ideal state rather than a quantifiable condition. Health remains an elusive entity to define. It is a dynamic state influenced by such factors as genetic endowment, nutrition, housing and environment, life habits, personal attitudes and beliefs, and medical care received—probably in that order of importance.

When definition of a concept is difficult to state, so is its measurement. The task of developing an index for oral health, therefore, at some point requires making value judgments as to which state of health or disease is better or worse than another. For example, is the young adult with a full complement of sound teeth but with early periodontal disease in better or worse health than a young adult who has lost several teeth but has a complete absence of periodontal disease? Is the young adult with a full complement of caries-free teeth and an absence of periodontal disease, but who is bothered by a malaligned central incisor, in better or worse oral health than another adult who has lost the upper central incisors and remains unworried by it? The need to come to grips with questions such as these brings a whole new dimension into oral epidemiology: the social area. An excellent commentary on the need for dentistry to develop sociodental indicators, as well as a recognition of all the complex problems involved in so doing, has been presented by Cohen and Jago.[12]

Bulman and co-workers[9] made an effort to develop what they modestly described as an oral health grading rather than an oral health index. They considered oral health under three major headings: dental, periodontal, prosthetic. They deliberately excluded orthodontic and assigned an examined subject three grades within each of the three divisions. Bulman and his group were able to condense the number of possible grades into seven and therefore suggested a seven-point ordinal scale with which to grade adults. They recognized that the grading still tended to measure oral neglect rather than oral needs and also that it was not possible to differentiate between denture wearers and others by this scale. In addition they pointed out that, with the exception of the extreme scores 1 and 7, the measure would give little indication of treatment needs. However, in a comparative study of the oral health of adults in two English cities they were studying, the index was sensitive enough to show a difference between the two groups.

Nikias and colleagues used an empirical approach to link clinical measures of eight separate oral conditions into multidimensional profiles of oral status.[57] This set was later collapsed into 42 profiles based on four conditions. These conditions were: numbers of missing and unreplaced teeth divided into four levels of severity; periodontal disease in four levels; decayed teeth in two levels; and oral hygiene in two levels. To answer the questions posed at the beginning of the section, that is, which type of oral condition was better or worse than another type, Nikias asked a group of 29 dentists from a number of different professional specialties to rank them. While obviously there were some differences between the dentists in regard to which of the profiles was considered better than others, there was a reasonable level of agreement—enough to give some hope that this approach could be developed even further.[58] However, the authors themselves consider this effort no more than a starting point toward development of a true oral health index.

If a true and useful index of oral health is ever to be developed, it is likely to be a sociodental type of indicator of the kind described by Cohen and Jago.[12] The information obtained by such an index would give some indication not only of need for dental care, but also likely demand levels. Information like this could be useful to policy planners, but may be of limited use to the dental practitioner in treating the individual patient.

THE CLINICAL TRIAL

Most of the discussion in this chapter has been in terms of the observational study, otherwise called field epidemiology, which is used to detect relations between one factor and another. The clinical trial, however, is used to determine whether a known or suspected relation is one of cause and effect. There are some essential differences between the two types of study despite the fact that similar indexes and methods may be employed.

A basic procedure in many field studies is the comparison of findings from studies of two or more independent populations. Comparison is likewise the fundamental objective in the clinical trial, but the comparison is of two or more segments of a *single* population theoretically divided in such a way as to be essentially similar in all pertinent characteristics except for the use or avoidance of the agent under test. The group (or groups) receiving the agent or regimen under study is often called the *test* group (or *study* group, or *experimental* group). The comparable group not subject to the agent or regimen is usually called the *control* group.

A clinical trial can be defined as a controlled experimental study of group comparison, based on epidemiological principles and designed to test the hypothesis that a particular agent or procedure favorably alters the natural history of a disease. The FDI has called the clinical trial "an epidemiological experiment."[29]

Factors Affecting the Validity of Clinical Trials

To produce valid results, certain principles in the conduct of clinical trials must be adhered to by investigators. Over the years these principles have become refined.[27, 30] The major ones are described as follows:

Choice of Population Group in Which the Trial Will Be Conducted. If the purpose of the trial is to test whether a particular agent is effective in preventing disease, the project should be conducted with subjects who are susceptible to the disease. Geographical area and age of subjects therefore need to be chosen carefully, and the subjects in this group need not be representative of the population from which they come. If, however, the purpose is to assess the effectiveness of a proven agent under real-life conditions, then representative populations should be chosen.

Comparability of Study and Control Groups. The randomized clinical trial, considered the most elegant form of such a study,[11] is one in which the similarity of the groups is achieved by randomly assigning subjects to the study and control groups. Statistical probability is such that the assumption can then be made that the groups differ from each other only in terms of the agent under study. Any uncontrolled variables influencing the outcome of the study are therefore likely to affect subjects in both groups equally, because the essence of the clinical trial is *relative* difference between the groups.

The principle of random assignment of subjects to groups is simple, though it is important to note that it is a carefully planned and controlled procedure rather than a haphazard assignment or one based on volunteering or self-selection. The allocation procedure should be such that each subject has an equal chance of being assigned to study or control groups. In practice, the procedure may be intricate and should wherever possible be left in the hands of a capable statistician. The statistician can further improve the probability of establishing comparable groups by a process of *stratification*, which means that before allocation the base population can be stratified by those factors known or thought to influence disease occurrence. The most obvious factors are those of age, sex, race, socioeconomic status, and previous disease experience. Subjects from each stratum are then randomly allocated to study and control groups.

Nonrandomized designs for clinical trials have also been used.[70, 71] While the randomized design is ideally preferable, sometimes practical considerations preclude its use. For example, a school system in which a proposed caries preventive agent is going to be tested may insist that there be no control group because school administrators want all children taking part in the study to receive any possible benefit. In such cases a before-and-after design can be used. In this design, children are examined at the beginning of the trial, the agent or regimen is applied, and then cross-sectional groups of children of similar ages are examined periodically until the completion of the trial. Differences between caries status at the beginning and the end of the trial are then judged for children of similar age or grade levels. While such studies usually can be controlled, the danger is that some untoward event may have occurred during the duration of the trial, which could affect the disease status of the study groups. In other words, results obtained may not be entirely due to the agent being tested. Without a true control group it is impossible to tell if beneficial effects obtained were due entirely to the agent or at least in part to the outside possibilities. Probably the greatest threat to the validity of a before-and-after design comes from sociodemographical change in the population under study during the period of the trial.

Adequate Numbers of Subjects. Any longitudinal prospective study like a clinical trial will have subjects dropping out over time—that is, attrition. Though undesirable, such an occurrence is a fact of life and must be allowed for at the planning stages. The danger is that if the numbers of subjects in the groups are not big enough to begin with, at the end of the trial the researcher will be left with too few subjects to be able to show by statistical logic whether a difference exists between the groups. The result may then be that a real difference cannot be detected, and an agent that in fact is effective will not seem to be so.

Consistency in Examination Diagnosis. The examiner in a clinical trial, whether it be for dental caries, periodontal disease, or soft tissue lesions, must record disease (at the second and subsequent examinations) that has developed over a relatively short period of time. This requirement forces the examiner to diagnose disease at an early stage of its development at the cost of increased error by the classification of the marginal or doubtful lesions. In clinical trials for dental caries, the most troublesome form of error is that a lesion classed as carious at the first round of examinations may be classified as sound in subsequent examinations. This kind of error is most common at the early stages of development of the carious lesion, especially in pit-or-fissure caries of molars where the lesion is at a borderline level. This kind of error is referred to as a *reversal* and is practically unavoidable in the present state of the art of detection of clinical caries.[66]

The validity of the results of the clinical trial depends heavily on the reliability of the examiner. This factor is usually referred to as *intraexaminer consistency* — that is, the ability of the examiner to record consistently the same lesions and conditions the same way over a period of time. Most examiners with training and experience develop an acceptable degree of intraexaminer consistency. Consistency between different examiners, that is, *interexaminer consistency*, is a different matter. Even though the same written criteria may be used, different examiners can see things in different ways, an inescapable fact of clinical trials that has to be dealt with. Ideally it is best to use one well-qualified examiner, but the size and scope of some studies require that more than one be used. In such cases, the examiners should undergo a period of training to bring their diagnostic standards as close together as can possibly be managed. This training procedure is referred to as *calibration* or *standardization*.

Radiographs have been used in many clinical trials in the past, especially in trials for dental caries. The obvious advantage is that approximal lesions may be detected that may not be detectable visually by clinical means, and they can also be seen in a presumably shorter period of time. Because one object of a clinical trial is to detect newly occurring lesions over a relatively short space of time, radiographs can be of help. However, there are also problems connected with their use. One is that problems of diagnosis still arise; many clinicians have looked at shadows in a radiograph and found it difficult to determine whether a lesion was present or not. Intraexaminer and interexaminer consistency can be just as, if not more, difficult to maintain with radiographs as with clinical examinations. In addition, use of radiographs adds extra time and cost to a study, because equipment must be taken to the field and personnel must be available to expose and develop the radiographs. Most of all, there is growing public and professional concern about the whole subject of radiation; current attitudes dictate that human subjects should not be exposed to radiographs unless there is a direct diagnostic necessity to do so.[41]

Duration of the Trial. Clinical trials must be continued long enough to be able to detect the development of new disease or extension of lesions already present during the period of the trial. For clinical trials for caries, the minimum period of a trial is now considered to be at least two years,[27] and a minimum of three years is considered preferable. Conducting clinical trials for this length of time obviously makes them more expensive than those lasting, say, six months. However, until more certain methods of detection of early carious lesions are developed, dentistry is dependent on clinical and/or radiographic examination to determine when the lesions are present.

Clinical trials for gingivitis can be quite short because of the nature of the condition. The FDI[30] has suggested that in the absence of other oral hygiene procedures, studies of plaque-inhibiting agents last between eight and 21 days. They have also suggested that studies of agents for the prevention of calculus should last 90 days for supragingival calculus and longer for subgingival calculus. Studies involving the prevention of gingivitis following a prophylaxis should include the time necessary (two to three weeks) for the effect of the prophylaxis to subside as well as the time required to demonstrate any prevention of gingivitis by the agent or procedures. Such studies should be at least 90 days in duration.[30] Motivational or educational studies requiring the cooperation of subjects should be of not less than six months' duration to show short-term effectiveness, and a year or longer to determine continued effectiveness of the motivational regimen or procedures. A two- or three-year follow-up evaluation should be considered if the experimental groups remain reasonably intact.[30]

Longitudinal studies looking at agents or procedures for the prevention of chronic, destructive periodontal disease, however, should be considerably longer because of the nature of that disease. Trials of five to seven years' duration have been suggested, provided that the sample size is large enough to allow for attrition and that the trial is started prior to the age when the destructive process usually becomes evident.[30] The FDI has also suggested that demonstration of positive effects might require studies of longer duration (10 to 15 years), though the practicality of conducting studies for such length of time is dubious.

Efficiency in Clinical Trials for Caries

The expense of running a clinical trial for two or three years has been mentioned before, so trials for caries must be run as efficiently as possible. Some past inefficiency is thought to have come from the confusion of objectives, in particular distinguishing between *efficacy* (whether the agent will work at all, even under ideal conditions) and *effectiveness* (whether it will work in everyday use).

To deal with this problem, O'Mullane has suggested that clinical trials be divided into two kinds, which he calls the *experimental clinical trial* and the *community clinical trial.*[61] By an experimental clinical trial he means that a highly artificial situation can be constructed in order to give the agent every chance to show its efficacy. This could involve selection of highly caries-susceptible subjects to be randomized into study and control groups. It could also involve use of the agent in a rather artificial manner. The object is that if the agent is indeed efficacious, a trial constructed this way will show it. The next step, assuming the agent is shown to be efficacious, is the community clinical (or field) trial in which the agent is applied in what might be called real-life conditions. A randomized clinical trial is again set up, but in this case there is no selection of a special (e.g., caries-susceptible) population for study, and personnel applying the preventive agent or supervising its use may have had little special training. The object of this division is that efficacious agents can perhaps be identified in a reasonably short period of time by use of the experimental clinical trial. Then, with efficacy demonstrated, the community clinical trial is set up to judge their general effectiveness in real-life use. If an agent is not efficacious, it can also be identified more readily through the experimental clinical trial, thus reducing the expense of a subsequent field trial.

There have been a number of "demonstration" preventive programs conducted in the United States, some combining different forms of preventive therapy.[49] A demonstration program is intended to apply accepted preventive procedures in a real-life situation in order to "demonstrate" the feasibility of preventive programs. In this sense, a demonstration program may be more analogous to a community clinical trial or field trial than to an experimental clinical trial.

Preventive dentistry is progressing at such a rate that clinical trials of preventive agents are certain to continue to be needed in the future. With the increasing cost and difficulty of running such trials, improved and more efficient methods of determining the effectiveness of preventive agents must be sought. Means for earlier detection of lesions, perhaps with totally different methods based on microbiological tests for detection of caries or periodontal lesions, need to be developed and refined. Refinements in study design and methods of statistical analysis may also help make clinical trials more efficient. Even if such advances are accepted, however, it is difficult to see that the basic principles of clinical trial design will be altered.

SUMMARY

The epidemiological method has undergone a great deal of refinement over the years, and its application to dental and oral disease continues to progress. New frontiers for the epidemiological method lie in better use of available service statistics (including treatment records), development of new indexes to answer present-day problems of health planning and policy development, and continued refinement of clinical trial technics.

The material in this chapter is introductory in nature and is not intended to be an instruction manual for persons who wish to employ these indexes and procedures in actual practice. Individuals who wish to conduct epidemiological studies are strongly advised to gain some experience with an experienced investigator or research group before forging out on their own.

References

1. Ainamo, J., and Bay, I. Problems and proposals for recording gingivitis and plaque. Internat. Dent. J., 25:229–35, Dec. 1975.
2. Ainsworth, N. J. Mottled teeth. Brit. Dent. J., 55:233–50, 274–6, Sept. 1, 1933.
3. American Cancer Society. 1980 cancer facts and figures. New York, The Society, 1979. 31 p.
4. Angle, E. H. Classification of malocclusion. Dent. Cosmos, 41:248–64, Mar. 1899.

5. Backer-Dirks, O., Houwink, B., and Kwant, G. W. The results of 6½ years of artificial drinking water in the Netherlands; the Tiel-Culemborg experiment. Arch. Oral Biol., 5:284–300, Dec. 1961.
6. Barmes, D. E. What a public health planner wants from a periodontal assessment. Internat. Dent. J., 26:429–34, Dec. 1976.
7. Bellini, H. T., and Gjermo, P. Application of the Periodontal Treatment Need System (PTNS) in a group of Norwegian industrial employees. Community Dent. Oral Epidemiol., 1:22–9, Jan. 1973.
8. Bodecker, C. F., and Bodecker, H. W. C. A practical index of the varying susceptibility to dental caries in man. Dent. Cosmos, 73:707–16, July 1931.
9. Bulman, J. S., Richards, N. D., Slack, G. L., and Willcocks, A. J. Demand and need for dental care; a socio-dental study. London, Oxford University Press, 1968. viii + 103 p.
10. Burt, B. A., Roder, D. M., Cecil, J. C., and Eklund, S. A. Saliva-based colorimetric test as an index of gingival inflammation in eqidemiologic studies. Community Dent. Oral Epidemiol., 6:290–5, Nov. 1978.
11. Cochrane, A. L. Effectiveness and efficiency; random reflections on health services. London, Nuffield Provincial Hospitals Trust, 1971. xi + 92 p. (p. 20–25)
12. Cohen, Lois K., and Jago, J. D. Toward the formulation of sociodental indicators. Internat. J. Health Services, 6:681–98, 1976.
13. Cons, N. C., Mruthyunjaya, Y. C., and Pollard, S. T. Distribution of occlusal traits in a sample of 1,337 children, ages 15–18, residing in upstate New York. Internat. Dent. J., 28:154–64, June 1978.
14. Dean, H. T. Distribution of mottled enamel in the United States. Pub. Health Rep., 48:703–34, June 23, 1933.
15. ———. Classification of mottled enamel diagnosis. Am. Dent. A. J., 21:1421–6, Aug. 1934.
16. ———. Chronic endemic dental fluorosis (mottled enamel). p. 387–414. (In Gordon, S. M., ed. Dental science and dental art. Philadelphia, Lea & Febiger, 1938. 731 p.)
17. ———. The investigation of physiological effects by the epidemiological method. p. 23–71. (In Moulton, F. R., ed. Fluorine and dental health. Washington, D.C., American Association Advancement Science, 1942. 101 p.)
18. ———. Epidemiological studies in the United States. p. 5–31. (In Moulton, F. R., ed. Dental caries and fluorine. Washington, D.C., American Association Advancement Science, 1946. 111 p.)
19. Dean, H. T., and Elvove, Elias. Further studies on the minimal threshold of chronic endemic dental fluorosis. Pub Health Rep., 52:1249–64, Sept. 1937.
20. Dean, H. T., Dixon, R. M., and Cohen, Chester. Mottled enamel in Texas. Pub. Health Rep., 50:424–42, Mar. 1935.
21. Dean, H.T., Elvove, Elias, and Poston, R. F. Mottled enamel in South Dakota. Pub. Health Rep., 54:212–28, Feb. 10, 1939.
22. Dean, H. T., Arnold, F. A., Jr., and Elvove, Elias. Domestic water and dental caries. V. Additional studies of the relation of fluoride domestic waters to dental caries experience in 4,425 white children aged 12–14 years of 13 cities in 4 states. Pub. Health Rep., 57:1155–79, Aug. 7, 1942.
23. Dorland's Illustrated Medical Dictionary. 26th ed. Philadelphia, Saunders, 1981. (p. 583) xxix + 1485 p.
24. Draker, H. L. Handicapping labio-lingual deviations proposed for public health purposes. Am. J. Orthodont., 46:295–305, Apr. 1960.
25. Dubos, Rene. The mirage of health. New York, Doubleday, c1959. 230 p.
26. Dunning, J. M., and Leach, L. B. Gingival-bone count: a method for epidemiological study of periodontal disease. J. Dent. Res., 39:506–13, May–June 1960.
27. Fédération Dentaire Internationale, Commission on Classification and Statistics for Oral Conditions. Horowitz, H. S., Baume, L. J., Backer-Dirks, O., Davies, G. N., and Slack, G. L., eds. Principal requirements for controlled clinical trials of caries preventive agents and procedures. Internat. Dent. J., 23:506–16, Sept. 1973.
28. ———. A method for measuring occlusal traits. Internat. Dent. J., 23:530–7, Sept. 1973.
29. ———. Classification of epidemiologic studies of dental caries and definitions of related terms. Internat. Dent. J., 25:79–87, Mar. 1975.
30. ———. Principal requirements for controlled clinical trials in periodontal diseases. Internat. Dent. J., 27:62–76, Mar. 1977.
31. Foster, T. D. The public health interest in assessment for orthodontic treatment. J. Pub. Health Dent., 39:137–42, Spring 1979.

32. Gordon, J. E. Dental problems in an epidemiological perspective. Am. J. Pub. Health, 49:1041–9, Aug. 1959.
33. Grainger, R. M. Epidemiological data. p. 311–53. (In Chilton, N. W. Design and analysis in dental and oral research. Philadelphia, Lippincott, 1967. 365 p.)
34. Greene, J. C. Epidemiology of congenital clefts of the lip and palate. Pub. Health Rep., 78:589–602, July 1963.
35. Greene, J. C., and Vermillion, J. R. The oral hygiene index: a method for classifying oral hygiene status. Am. Dent. A. J., 61:172–9, Aug. 1960.
36. ———. The simplified oral hygiene index. Am. Dent. A. J., 68:7–13, Jan. 1964.
37. Gruebbel, A. O. A measurement of dental caries prevalence and treatment service for deciduous teeth. J. Dent. Res., 23:163–8, June 1944.
38. Hollis, M. J., and Malaki, T. Fluorosis and dental caries in the Ellice Islands. N. Z. Dent. J., 70:181–4, July 1974.
39. Horowitz, H. S. Clinical trials of preventives for dental caries. J. Pub. Health Dent., 32:229–33, Fall 1972.
40. ———. Fluoride research on clinical and public health applications. Am. Dent. A. J., 87:1013–8, Oct. 1973.
41. ———. Ethical considerations of study participants in dental caries clinical trials. Community Dent. Oral Epidemiol., 4:43–50, Jan. 1976.
42. Hyatt, T. P. Report of an examination made of two thousand one hundred and one high school pupils. Dent. Cosmos, 52:507–11, Apr. 1920.
43. ———. Prophylactic odontotomy. Dent. Cosmos, 65:234–41, Mar. 1923.
44. Jackson, D. The measurement of gingivitis. Brit. Dent. J., 118:521–7, June 15, 1965.
45. Jago, J. D. The epidemiology of dental occlusion; a critical appraisal. J. Pub. Health Dent., 34:80–93, Spring 1974.
46. Katz, R. V., and Meskin, L. H. Testing the internal and external validity of a simplified dental caries index on an adult population. Community Dent. Oral Epidemiol., 4:227–31, Dec. 1976.
47. Kingman, Albert. A method of utilizing the subject's initial caries experience to increase efficiency in caries clinical trials. Community Dent. Oral Epidemiol., 7:87–90, Apr. 1979.
48. Klein, Henry, Palmer, C. E., and Knutson, J. W. Studies on dental caries: I. Dental status and dental needs of elementary school children. Pub. Health Rep., 53:751–65, May 13, 1938.
49. Klein, S. P., and Bohannon, H. M. The first year of field activities in the national preventive dentistry demonstration program, prepared under grants from the Robert Wood Foundation to the Rand Corporation and the American Fund for Dental Health. Santa Monica, Calif., Rand Corporation, 1979. xiv + 100 p.
50. Lightner, L. M., O'Leary, T. J., Drake, R. B., Crump, P. P., Jividen, G. J., and Junghans, J. J. The periodontal status of incoming Air Force Academy cadets. Am. Dent. A. J., 75:111–7, July 1967.
51. Löe, Harald. The gingival index, the plaque index, and the retention index systems. J. Periodont., part II, 38(Suppl.):610–6, Nov.–Dec. 1967.
52. Löe, Harald, and Silness, J. Periodontal disease in pregnancy. I. Prevalence and severity. Acta Odont. Scand., 21:533–51,Dec. 1963.
53. Longmate, Norman. Alive and well; medicine and public health from 1830 to the present day. Harmondsworth, England, Penguin, 1970. 108 p.
54. Massler, Maury, Schour, Isaac, and Chopra, Baldev. Occurrence of gingivitis in suburban Chicago schoolchildren. J. Periodont., 21:146–64, 196, July 1950.
55. Morrison, Edith C. The effect of professional prophylaxis and personal oral hygiene on the severity of periodontitis. Doctoral Dissertation, Ann Arbor, University Michigan, 1977. vii + 106 p.
56. Mühlemann, H. R., and Son, S. Gingival sulcus bleeding — a leading symptom in initial gingivitis. Helvetia Odont. Acta, 15:107–13, Oct. 1971.
57. Nikias, Mata K., Sollecito, W. A., and Fink, Raymond. An empirical approach to developing multidimensional oral status profiles. J. Pub. Health Dent., 38:148–58, Spring 1978.
58. ———. An oral health index based on ranking of oral status profiles by panels of dental professionals. J. Pub. Health Dent., 39:16–26, Winter 1979.
59. O'Leary, Timothy. The periodontal screening index. J. Periodont., part II, 38(Suppl.):617–24, Nov.–Dec. 1967
60. Olsson, Berit. Dental findings in high-fluoride areas in Ethiopia. Community Dent. Oral Epidemiol., 7:51–6, Feb. 1979.

61. O'Mullane, D. M. Efficiency in clinical trials of caries preventive agents and methods. Community Dent. Oral Epidemiol., 4:190–4, Sept. 1976.
62. Pedersen, P. O. Dental disease in Europe and Greenland. Royal Soc. Health J., 91:23–7, Mar.–Apr. 1971.
63. Podshadley, A. G., and Haley, J. V. A method for evaluating oral hygiene performance. Pub. Health Rep., 83:259–64, Mar. 1968.
64. Poulsen, S., and Horowitz, H. An evaluation of a hierarchical method of describing the pattern of dental caries attack. Community Dent. Oral Epidemiol., 2:7–11, Feb. 1974.
65. Poulton, D. R., and Aaronson, S. A. The relationship between occlusion and periodontal status. Am. J. Orthodont., 47:690–9, Sept. 1961.
66. Radike, A. W. Examiner error and reversals in diagnosis. p. 92–5. (In Proceedings of the conference on the clinical testing of cariostatic agents. Chicago, American Dental Association, 1972. viii + 117 p.)
67. Ramfjord, S. P. Indices for prevalence and incidence of periodontal disease. J. Periodont., 30:51–9, Jan. 1959
68. ———. The periodontal disease index. J. Periodont., part II, 38(Suppl.):30–7, Nov.–Dec. 1967.
69. Reif, A. E. Public information on smoking: an urgent responsibility for cancer research workers. J. Nat. Cancer Inst., 57:1207–10, Dec. 1976.
70. Ringleberg, M. L., Conti, A. J., and Webster, D. B. An evaluation of single and combined self-applied fluoride programs in schools. J. Pub. Health Dent., 36:229–36, Fall 1976.
71. Ripa, L. W., Leske, G. S., and Levinson, A. Supervised weekly rinsing with a 0.2% neutral NaF solution: results from a demonstration program after two school years. Am. Dent. A. J., 97:793–8, Nov. 1978.
72. Rugg-Gunn, A. J., Holloway, P. J., and Davies, T. G. H. Caries prevention by daily fluoride mouthrinsing. Brit. Dent. J., 135:353–60, Oct. 16, 1973.
73. Russell, A. L. A system of classification and scoring for prevalence surveys of periodontal disease. J. Dent. Res., 35:350–9, June 1956.
74. ———. Longitudinal technics in the study of oral disease. Am. J. Pub. Health, 46:728–35, June 1956.
75. ———. The differential diagnosis of fluoride and nonfluoride enamel opacities. Pub. Health Dent., 21:143–6, Winter 1961–2.
76. ———. World epidemiology and oral health. p. 21–39. (In Kreshover, S. J., and McClure, F. J., eds. Environmental variables in oral disease. Washington, D. C., American Association Advancement Science, Publ. no. 81, 1966. xii + 311 p.)
77. ———. The periodontal index. J. Periodont. part II, 38(Suppl.):13–9, Nov.–Dec. 1967.
78. ———. Epidemiology and the rational bases of dental public health and dental practice. p. 35–62. (In Young, W. O., and Striffler, D. F. The dentist, his practice, and his community. 2nd ed. Philadelphia, Saunders, 1969. xvi + 346 p.)
79. Sandler, H. C., and Stahl, S. S. Measurement of periodontal disease prevalence. Am. Dent. A. J., 58:93–7, Mar. 1959.
80. Schei, Olav, Waerhaug, Jens, Lovdal, A., and Arno, A. Alveolar bone loss as related to oral hygiene and age. J. Periodont., 30:7–16, Jan. 1959.
81. Schour, Isaac, and Massler, Maury. The P–M–A index of gingivitis. Abstr. J. Dent. Res., 28:634, Dec. 1949.
82. Sheiham, Aubrey, and Striffler, D. F. A comparison of four epidemiological methods of assessing periodontal disease. II. Test of periodontal indices. J. Periodont. Res., 5:155–61, 1970.
83. Silness, J., and Löe, H. Periodontal disease in pregnancy. II. Correlation between oral hygiene and periodontal condition. Acta Odont. Scand., 22:112–35, Jan. 1964.
84. Silverstone, L. M. Structural alterations of human dental enamel during incipient lesion development. p. 3–49. (In Rowe, N. H., ed. Proceedings of a symposium on incipient caries of enamel, held at The University of Michigan, Nov. 11–12, 1977. Ann Arbor, University Michigan Press, 1977. iv + 169 p.)
85. ———. Preventive dentistry. London, Update Books, 1978. 168 p.
86. Stahl, S. S., and Morris, A. L. Oral health condition among Army personnel at the Army Engineer Center. J. Periodont., 26:180–5, July 1955.
87. Summers, C. J. The occlusal index; a system for identifying and scoring occlusal disorders. Am. J. Orthodont., 59:552–67, June 1971.
88. Susser, Mervyn. Causal thinking in the health sciences: concepts and strategies of epidemiology. New York, Oxford University Press, 1973. xviii + 181 p.

89. Thylstrup, A., and Fejerskov, O. Clinical appearance of dental fluorosis in permanent teeth in relation to histologic changes. Community Dent. Oral Epidemiol., 6:315–28, Nov. 1978.
90. U. S. Public Health Service. The health consequences of smoking 1975. DHEW Publ. no (CDC) 76-8704. Washington, D. C., Government Printing Office, 1975. xi + 235 p. (p. 44–7)
91. U. S. Public Health Service, National Center for Health Statistics. Orthodontic treatment priority index, by Grainger, R. M. PHS Publ. No. 1000-Ser. 2-No. 25. Washington, D. C., Government Printing Office, 1967. vi + 49 p.
92. U. S. Public Health Service, National Center for Health Statistics. Facts of life and death. DHEW Publ. No. (PHS) 79-1222. Washington, D. C., Government Printing Office, 1978. iv + 47 p.
93. Van Kirk, L. E., Jr., and Pennell, E. H. Assessment of malocclusion in population groups. Am. J. Orthodont., 45:752–8, Oct. 1959.
94. World Health Organization. Oral health surveys; basic methods. 2nd ed. Geneva, The Organization, 1977. 68 p.
95. ———. Decisions of the health assembly. WHO Chron., 32:270–9, July 1978.
96. ———. Epidemiology, etiology, and prevention of periodontal diseases; report of a WHO Scientific Group. Tech. Rep. Series No. 621. Geneva, The Organization, 1978. 60 p.

CHAPTER 6

THE EPIDEMIOLOGY OF ORAL DISEASES

Brian A. Burt

Dental practice is concerned with the prevention and treatment of oral diseases and their sequelae. Practitioners, therefore, should be familiar with the epidemiology of the conditions they treat, because the type of treatment services provided obviously relates to the diseases prevalent in the community. As described in Chapter 5, practitioners can apply the epidemiological method in their own practices to provide a "third dimension" to help them evaluate the impact of their services.

This chapter describes the distribution of the major oral diseases in the United States and elsewhere and the factors influencing that distribution.

DENTAL CARIES

Caries in Ancient Man

Limited knowledge of the distribution of dental caries in earlier ages has come from examination of ancient skulls. Dental caries has afflicted man to some extent from the time that agriculture replaced hunting and gathering as the principal source of food. However, the prevalence of the condition in ancient times was considerably less than that of today. Examination of skulls in Britain indicates that caries prevalence changed little from the Anglo-Saxon period (fifth to seventh centuries A.D.) to the end of the Middle Ages, approximately 1500 A.D.[84, 85, 87] The diet for most people during this period was coarse, and there was little in the way of food preparation. Dental attrition was marked and occurred early in life. The lesions of caries that have been found in skulls dating from this period are most commonly cervical or root caries; coronal caries was relatively uncommon. The disease seems to have been uncommon in the primary dentition, although some lesions in younger persons seem to have begun in the occlusal fissures but developed no further because the rate of attrition was faster than the rate of progression of the lesions. The modern pattern of caries in Western society,* in which the disease usually begins in pit and fissure surfaces and develops later on proximal surfaces, does not appear to have become common in Britain until the Tudor period—that is, around the sixteenth century.[86] Changes in dietary habits during the seventeenth century—principally increased refinement of the diet and greater use of sucrose as sugar became more available—are considered chiefly responsible for the development of the modern pattern of caries.[87] Import duties on sugar in Britain began to be removed in 1845 and were completely eliminated in 1875.[87] During this period the prevalence of caries greatly increased.[20, 60] By the end of the nineteenth century, dental caries was well established as an endemic disease of massive proportions not only in Britain, but also in most countries of the Western world.[16]

Since ancient times, therefore, three distinct changes in caries occurrence in Western countries can be identified from the limited evidence available:

1. The prevalence of caries and the intensity of its attack have increased greatly, although caries did exist in ancient times. The prevalence of caries remained virtually unchanged until about the seventeenth century, when it began to increase. The rate of increase accelerated during the nineteenth century, until by the early twentieth century peak prevalence was reached.
2. Marked attrition, universal in ancient times, has practically disappeared in economically developed countries.
3. The pattern of the carious attack has changed from one usually beginning in root and cervical areas to the present pattern beginning in fissures and contact areas. The rate of development of lesions has almost certainly increased over many centuries.

Current Global Distribution

Some of the ancient patterns of high attrition, low prevalence of coronal caries, and moderate-to-high prevalence of root caries can still be found in remote parts of the world in the twentieth century.[112, 113] However, such patterns are fast disappearing as isolated populations become infected with the organisms of dental caries and develop more contact with cariogenic diets and the Western way of life.[81]

In the past, dental caries was often referred to as "a disease of civilization." Without going into a philosophical discussion of who is civilized and who is not, this expression has been used to describe the prevailing pattern of caries observed during the twentieth century—high prevalence in those countries with a greater degree of economic development and higher socioeconomic status (for example, Western Europe, North America, Australia, New Zealand,

*"Western" populations, in this context, refers to the citizens of those countries that can be described as "economically developed." In the dental context, these countries have at least reasonably well-developed dental services and their citizens subsist to a considerable extent on a refined, processed diet, with foods often distributed far from their point of origin. "Western" countries are thus at the other end of the spectrum from "developing" countries.

and Japan); low prevalence in those countries with less economic development and a lower material standard of living (such as countries of Central Africa and the Indian subcontinent). Caries can be described as a disease of affluence.

There are probably a number of interrelated reasons why this pattern developed. One reason could certainly be related to diet; the high level of consumption of refined carbohydrates in economically developed countries has long been synonymous with the "good life." Poorer societies, on the other hand, tend to survive on hunting and on subsistence farming, both of which provide diets low in fermentable carbohydrates. A related reason concerns the evolution and proliferation of cariogenic bacteria under the selective pressure of suitable diets, which is clearly a widespread phenomenon in those societies where caries is endemic.[21]

There is now evidence, however, that this traditional pattern may be changing to some extent. Certainly the prevalence and intensity of dental caries in many developing countries are rising at an alarming rate, as is shown in Table 6–1. These data show that within this century, and in some cases quite recently, caries in many such countries (at least in their urban areas) has advanced from negligible proportions to a public health problem of the first order. At the same time, there is some reason to think that in those countries traditionally having a high prevalence of dental caries some kind of "saturation" level may have been reached and that prevalence is going no higher and in some instances may be diminishing.[16, 109] Again, the reasons for this turnabout in traditional trends could be highly complex.[16]

But even among the economically developed countries, there are quite distinct differences from one country to another and from region to region within a country. In the early 1970s a study was launched by the World Health Organization (WHO), with funding and close cooperation from the U.S. Public Health Service and the participating countries of the International Collaborative Study (WHO/USPHS/ICS). The object of this study was to examine the structure of various dental care systems and to measure their effectiveness and efficiency in terms of oral health, services available and received, and social and economic costs of achieving any given level of oral health. This challenging goal required considerable planning. Initially, five

Table 6–1. Data to Show the Increase in Prevalence of Dental Caries in Children Aged 10–14 From Selected Countries*

Country	Increase in DMF *From*	*To*	Within Number of Years
Ethiopia	0.2	1.6	17
Kenya	0.1	1.7	21
Iraq	0.7	3.5	9
Thailand	0.7	4.5	15
Vietnam	2.0	6.3	11
French Polynesia	negligible	7.5	50
Greenland	1.5	10.4	20

*World Health Organization, Oral Epidemiological Data Bank.[81]

nations took part in the study (Australia, Federal Republic of Germany, Japan, New Zealand, and Norway); the United States and Canada later joined and several other countries have subsequently taken part.

Data from the first seven countries in the WHO/USPHS/ICS project, gathered in the years 1973 to 1975, are displayed in Figures 6–1 to 6–3. Figure 6–1 shows the average decayed, missing, and filled primary teeth for children aged 8–9 from seven countries. It can be seen that df scores are considerably higher in Norway and Japan than they are in the United States, and that only in New Zealand is most of the caries in the primary dentition treated. In the other countries the "d" component is relatively high.

Figure 6–2 shows average DMF values for children aged 13–14 in the same seven countries, and Figure 6–3 shows similar data for adults aged 35–44.

It should be understood that these data are not from nationally representative population samples of each country, but rather from selected communities in which the dental care system was thought to typify the national system. The data from the United States, for instance, came from the

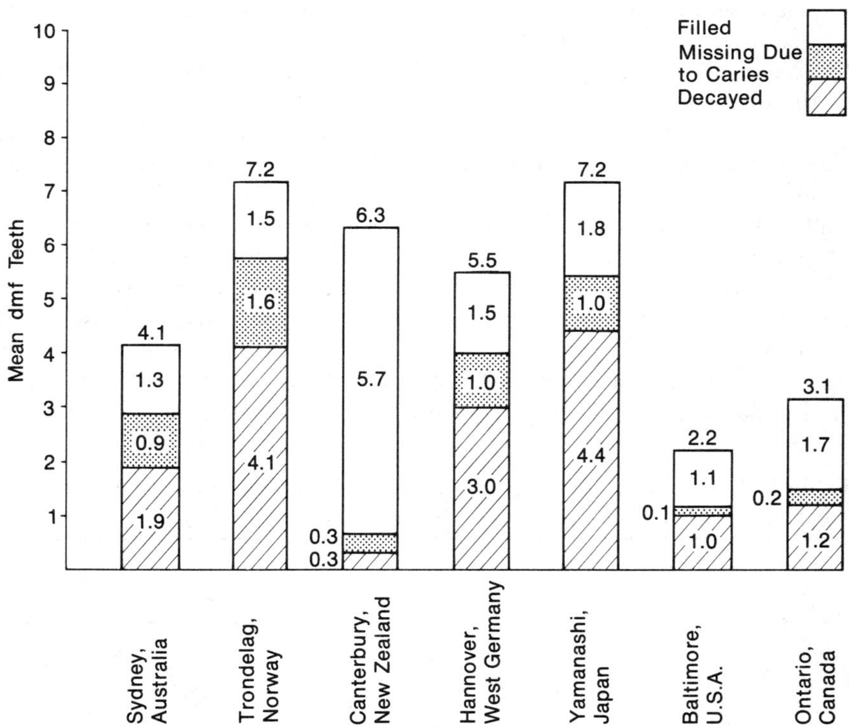

Figure 6–1. Decayed, missing, and filled primary teeth in children aged 8–9 in seven countries. Data from the World Health Organization, U.S. Public Health Service, International Collaborative Study [WHO/USPHS/ICS], 1973, and replicative studies in the United States [1975] and Canada [1977].[7, 13, 30]

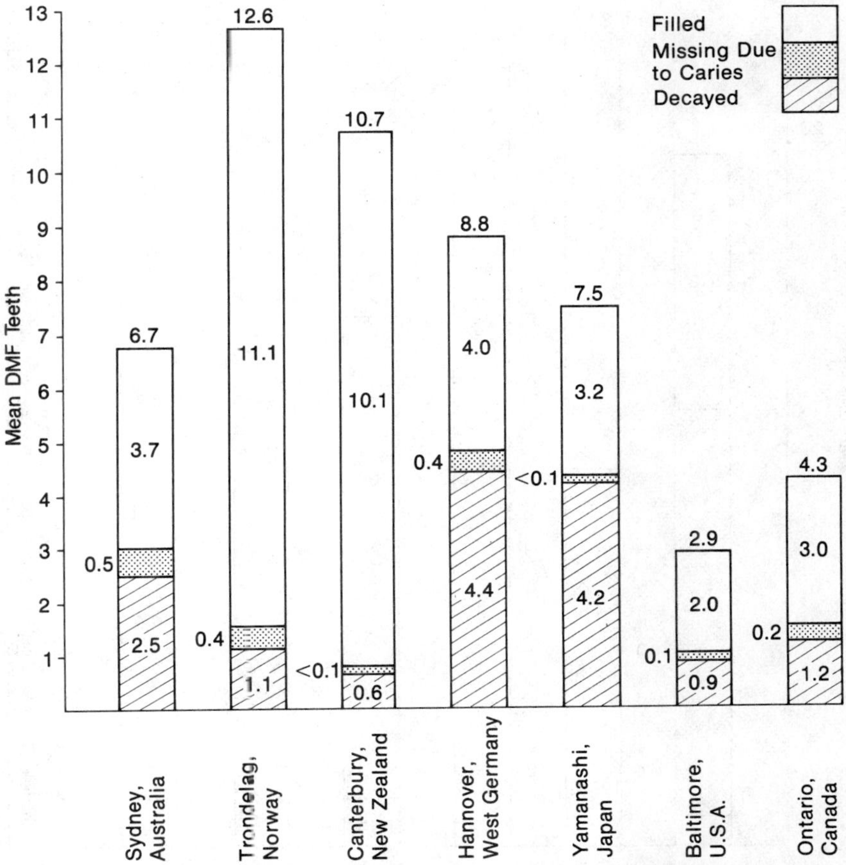

Figure 6–2. Decayed, missing, and filled permanent teeth in children aged 13–14 in seven countries. Data from the World Health Organization, U.S. Public Health Service, International Collaborative Study [WHO/USPHS/ICS], 1973, and replicative studies in the United States [1975] and Canada [1977].[7, 13, 30]

metropolitan area of Baltimore, a city fluoridated since 1952. The areas chosen for examination in Australia and Canada also had been fluoridated for some years.

Caries Prevalence in the United States

Regional variations in the prevalence of caries exist within the United States. These differences had been observed for some time, but were well documented with the examination of entrants into the Armed Forces during World War II.[91, 116, 117] These surveys were in general agreement that the highest prevalence of dental caries was seen in recruits from New England,

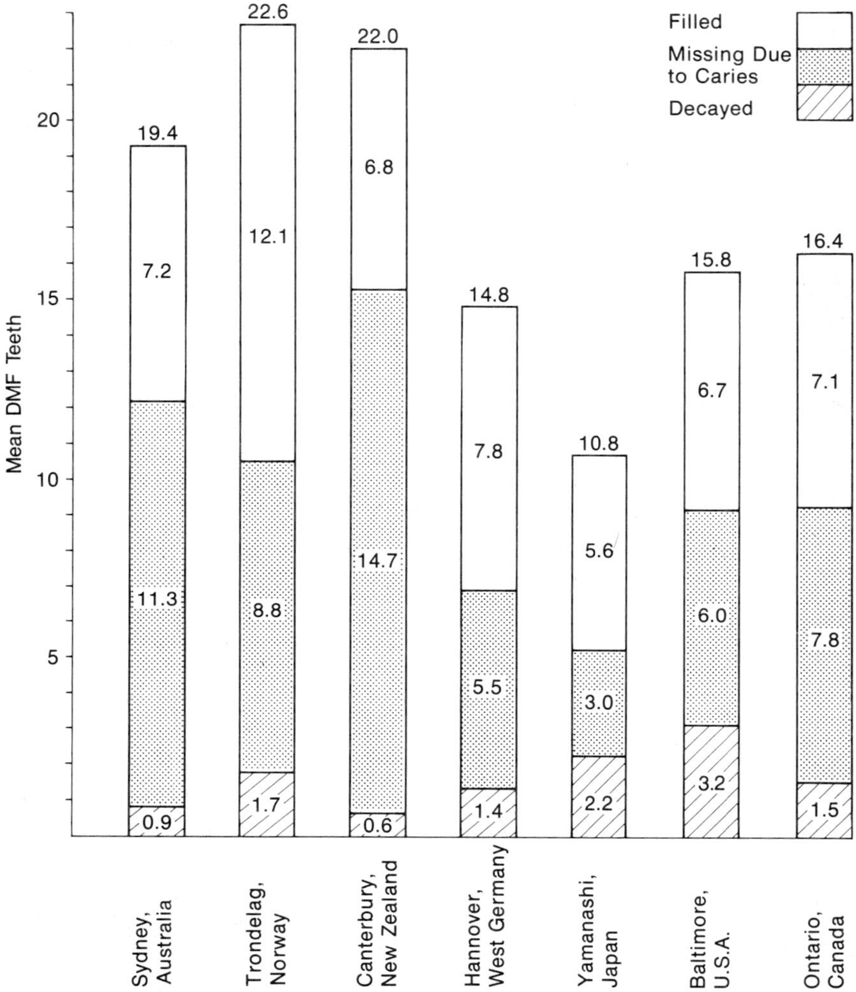

Figure 6–3. Decayed, missing, and filled teeth in adults aged 35–44 in seven countries. Data from the World Health Organization, U.S. Public Health Service, International Collaborative Study [WHO/USPHS/ICS], 1973, and replicative studies in the United States [1975] and Canada [1977].[7, 13, 30]

the Pacific Northwest, and the Great Lakes area, with distinctly less prevalence seen in young men from the South, the Southwest, and the Mountain states. In the years since World War II, some of these differences have been obscured by the spread of water fluoridation, but they were still quite apparent in the 1966–1970 survey of a representative sample of youths in the United States aged 12–17.[138] These regional differences are illustrated in Figure 6–4 and are quite marked. Other studies have indicated the differing prevalence of caries even within subregions.[67] Interestingly, regional differences in caries preva-

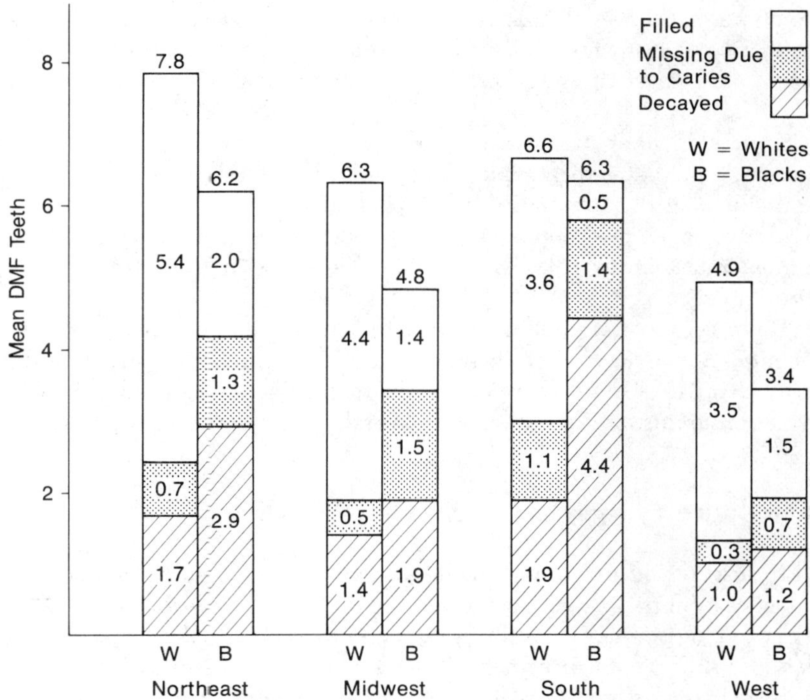

Figure 6–4. Decayed, missing, and filled teeth in whites and blacks, aged 12–17, in four geographic areas of the United States, 1966–1970.[138]

lence among different tribes of American Indians were demonstrated in the early 1930s.[51] A higher prevalence was found among tribes in the Northwest than among those in the Southwest.

By the end of the 1970s there was evidence that the prevalence of caries in the United States was declining, and at quite a sharp rate among young persons. This development, if indeed it is true, is likely to have the most profound implications for the practice of dentistry and the education of dental professionals.

The evidence to suggest a decline in caries prevalence in the United States has come from several sources. In a report of a clinical trial conducted in North Dakota in the mid-1970s it was noted that the increment of caries in the control group had dropped by 38 percent since the completion of a similar study in 1969.[94] A sequence of studies in Columbus, Ohio, from 1967 to 1973 indicated that the caries prevalence in children entering school dropped considerably, even over that short period.[147] The results of statewide surveys in Tennessee[15] and North Carolina[42] in the late 1970s showed that caries prevalence among children in those states also had dropped substantially since earlier surveys conducted some 20 to 30 years previously. Additional evidence from Massachusetts shows that age-specific DMF values in 1979 were generally

30 to 50 percent lower than they were in the same areas during the 1950s.[25, 32] Results of a nationwide study of children during the 1978–79 school year substantiated these findings gathered from particular areas in the United States.*

Similar declines in prevalence of caries have been reported from other countries,[16, 43, 68, 109] indicating that this trend could be a fairly widespread phenomenon in the Western world. When allied to the previously described increases in caries prevalence in developing countries, the indications are that the global distribution of caries could be shifting in the latter part of the twentieth century.

There are several possible reasons for the decline in caries prevalence in the United States. The most likely reasons are the spread of water fluoridation, the widespread use of fluoride supplements and organized school-based fluoride programs, and the almost universal use of fluoride dentifrices.

Dental Caries by Age, Sex, and Race

In susceptible communities, dental caries begins early. Studies from a number of countries, including the United States, show that some 25 to 80 percent of children between the ages of one to five have already suffered from caries.[10, 41, 59, 97, 126, 144] Caries begins in the permanent dentition soon after the first permanent molars erupt, usually in the pit and fissure surfaces of those teeth.

Teeth vary in their susceptibility to caries, though most teeth that develop the disease usually do so within two to four years after eruption.[18] The pioneering Hagerstown studies of Klein and Palmer ranked the susceptibility of teeth to caries in the following order:[54]

1. Mandibular first and second molars.
2. Maxillary first and second molars.
3. Mandibular second premolars, maxillary first and second premolars, maxillary central and lateral incisors.
4. Maxillary canines and mandibular first premolars.
5. Mandibular central and lateral incisors, mandibular canines. (Third molars had not erupted in the children studied.)

Although the Hagerstown studies were carried out in 1937, this ranking of tooth vulnerability has probably not changed. It is also similar in less susceptible communities, though caries may begin in the second molar rather than the first. Some evidence suggests that second molars may be more susceptible to caries than first molars.[48]

Caries experience as measured by the DMF index continues to increase steadily with age. Figure 6–5 shows that DMF values increase most sharply

*U.S. Public Health Service, National Institute of Dental Research, National Caries Program. The prevalence of dental caries in United States children 1979–1980; the national caries prevalence survey. NIH Publ. No. 82-2245, Washington, D.C., Government Printing Office, 1981. iv + 159 p.

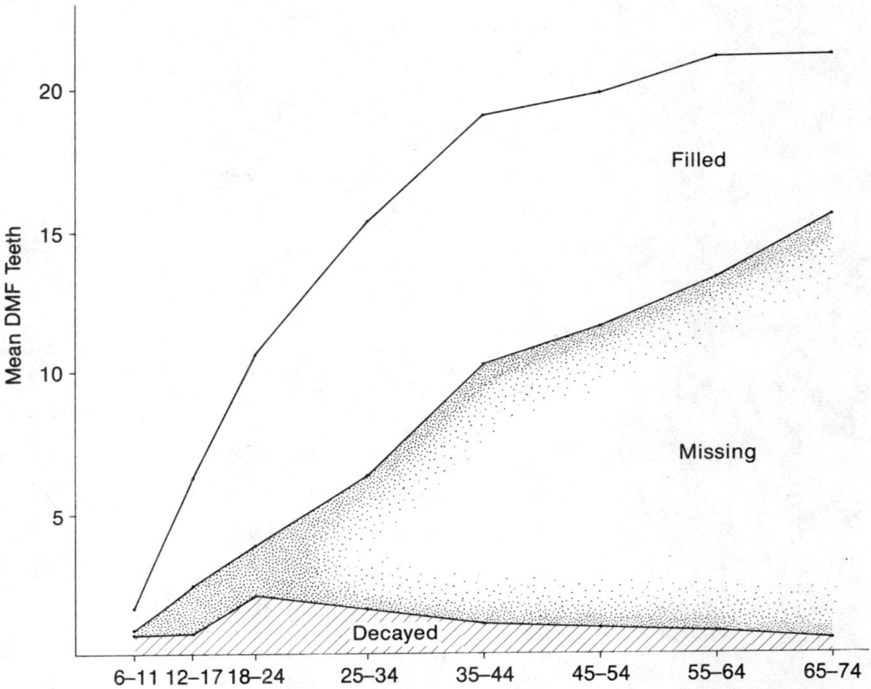

Figure 6–5. Decayed, missing, and filled teeth, by age, United States, 1971–1974.[144]

in youth and early adult years and more slowly in the later years of life. It is important to note that the increasing domination of the DMF by the missing teeth component (discussed in Chapter 5) may not all be due to caries. The pattern of DMF by age shown in Figure 6–5 is fairly typical of information obtained in any cross-sectional survey in caries-susceptible, highly treated societies. The apparent slowdown in the caries attack rate, which is seen to occur in the early adult years, is due largely to the fact that nearly all susceptible surfaces are likely to have been attacked by that time. Other factors contributing could be the buildup of fluoride in outer layers of enamel over time and possibly the change in dietary habits assumed to come with adulthood.

One age-related problem is root caries, found where gingival recession has led to exposure of the roots and to the accumulation of bacterial plaque around these exposed roots. Root caries is found both in Western and non-Western societies.[6, 112] The root caries seen in a remote society in New Guinea[112] apparently bears a great similarity to the forms of caries seen in ancient man, which were described earlier. Root caries may be more prevalent in older persons in Western countries than was previously thought.[6] Dental practitioners are likely to have to spend more of their time dealing with this problem, both its prevention and treatment, as more people keep their teeth into older age and the number of older people increases.

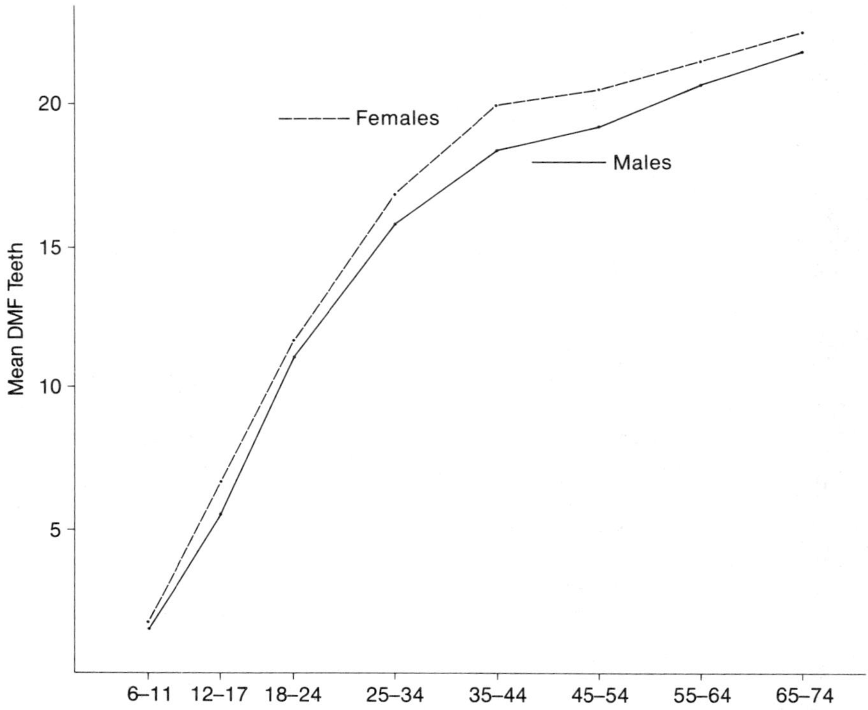

Figure 6–6. DMF values, by age, for males and females, United States, 1971–1974.[144]

Females generally appear to develop higher DMF scores than do males,[23, 140] although this finding is not universal. The difference is small enough to be explained by the earlier eruption of teeth in females;[53, 126] their teeth are at risk in the oral environment for a longer time. Figure 6–6 shows the DMF curves by age for males and females in the United States in the early 1970s; it will be noticed that the values for females are higher than those for males at all ages. It cannot be assumed from these data alone, however, that females are more susceptible to caries than are males, for other factors weigh on the DMF values. Females generally tend to have a better state of oral hygiene than males[134, 140] and they also visit the dentist more frequently.[131] Thus a "treatment factor" is likely to be involved in the DMF figures seen in Figure 6–6. Probably these factors plus the earlier eruption of teeth in females noted previously are sufficient to explain the observed differences in DMF values between males and females.

Contentions that certain races enjoy an immunity or at least a high degree of resistance to dental caries have been evident in dentistry for a long time. They probably stemmed from the earlier observations that certain non-European races, such as those in Africa and India, seemed to enjoy a much greater freedom from dental caries than did Europeans. These assertions have faded in recent years, as the evidence mounts that global differences in caries prevalence are more a result of environment than they are of inherent racial attributes. One convincing piece of evidence is the observation that certain racial groups, once thought to be resistant to caries, seemed to become more susceptible to the disease when they moved to more economically developed societies or to areas with different cultural and dietary patterns.[12, 82, 106]

In the United States, the National Health Survey conducted in 1960–62 showed a marked difference in DMF scores between white and black adults of the same age group—a difference that remained even when the groups were standardized for income and education.[135] Data from the National Health and Nutrition Examination Survey (NHANES I), conducted on a representative sample of the U.S. population in 1971–74, are shown in Table 6–2. It can be seen that whites still register higher DMF scores than blacks, although in younger age groups this difference is small. Surveys conducted in particular localities in the United States have usually shown whites to have higher DMF scores than blacks of the same age, although again this pattern is not universal.[5] Figure 6–4, presented earlier to show differences in geographical distribution of caries in the United States, also shows that there is a considerable difference in DMF patterns between blacks and whites in each of the areas examined. However, Figure 6–4 also gives a clue as to why these differences should exist: examination of the components of the DMF index clearly indicates that treatment patterns are quite different. Given the long-standing socioeconomic differences between blacks and whites in the United States, it is likely that many of the observed differences in caries patterns in the past could be attributed to socioeconomic and cultural differences, especially those related to dietary practices and the availability and receipt of dental care.[55, 78, 138] Whites in the United States have better access to dental care than blacks, in general.

The overall pattern that emerges from the evidence presented is that there is little basis for believing in inherent differences between blacks and whites in terms of susceptibility to dental caries. If socioeconomic differences between the races narrow further in the United States, differences in DMF experience can be expected to diminish also.

Table 6–2. Mean DMF Values for Blacks and Whites, United States, 1971–74*

Age	Black Males	Black Females	White Males	White Females	All Blacks	All Whites
1–5	0.1	0.2	0.1	0.1	0.1	0.1
6–11	1.5	1.8	1.6	1.7	1.6	1.7
12–17	5.1	6.0	5.8	6.7	5.5	6.3
18–44	11.8	12.8	14.8	15.7	12.4	15.3
45–64	12.7	15.7	20.7	21.6	14.2	21.2
65–74	19.5	20.3	22.3	22.7	19.9	22.5

*U.S. Public Health Service.[140]

Familial and Genetic Patterns

Familial tendencies ("good or bad teeth run in families") are seen by many dentists and have been demonstrated by dental research.[31, 52, 56, 99] However, whether such tendencies have any genetic basis or whether they only represent bacterial transmission or continuing familial dietary or behavioral traits is difficult to ascertain. Husband-wife similarities clearly have no genetic origin, and intrafamilial transmission of cariogenic flora has also been shown to occur.[58, 100]

Examination of the evidence of a possible connection between race and prevalence of dental caries seems to weaken the case for genetic inheritance of a susceptibility or resistance to caries, though Klein concluded that the similarities within families involved " . . . strong familial vectors which very likely have a genetic basis, perhaps sex-linked."[50] Mansbridge[75] compared pairs of identical twins with matched but unrelated pairs of children and concluded that whereas genetic factors could affect caries experience to some extent, the influence of environmental variables was stronger. Jackson[46] has argued for some years in favor of a genetic basis for the prevalence of caries, but his argument seems to have gained few adherents.

Until further evidence is forthcoming, Mansbridge's conclusions on the minor influence of genetics on caries seem to be those most accepted.

Diet, Nutrition, and Dental Caries

The word *diet* refers to the total oral intake of substances that provide nourishment and/or calories, whereas *nutrition* refers to the absorption of nutrients.

In view of the fundamental role of nutrition as a determinant of human health, it is natural that its role in the etiology of caries should receive a lot of attention. However, despite many investigations, no links have been demonstrated between nutritional deficiency in childhood and subsequent development of dental caries. (The exception to this statement is the benefit derived from the ingestion of fluoride during the time of dental development—see Chapter 7). Mellanby, in 1934, suggested that a deficiency of vitamin D was a causative factor in subsequent hypoplasia and development of dental caries.[79] Mellanby's theory emanated from research with beagle dogs and may have been influenced by contemporary findings on the importance of vitamins in human health. There are more recent suggestions from animal studies that nutritional imbalances may affect postdevelopmental resistance to caries.[1, 24] However, although certain nutritional deficiencies during developmental periods can lead to hypoplasia of enamel,[1] epidemiological evidence cannot show any relation between nutritional status (other than fluoride-ingestion) and subsequent development of caries.

To review this epidemiological evidence: it has already been stated that the prevalence of caries is lowest in those countries where living standards are also lowest; where generalized malnutrition is the norm, dental caries is uncommon. Even in those developing countries where caries prevalence is increasing, as mentioned earlier, this increase is largely confined to urban populations in which dietary and cultural changes are occurring rapidly. Traditional village populations in Africa and India still show little sign of dental caries, although many of these populations are in a chronic state of malnourishment.

A series of studies conducted in the late 1950s for the Interdepartmental Committee on Nutrition for National Defense (ICNND) examined, among other things, the relation between nutritional deficiencies and dental caries.[102, 104, 105] These studies were conducted in a number of countries where some grave, widespread nutritional deficiency was either known or suspected to exist. In practically all of these populations studied, caries prevalence was extremely low despite the documented nutritional deficiencies. The Ethiopian diet, for example, was deficient in vitamin A and caloric intake and critically low in ascorbic acid. The diets in Burma, Thailand, and South Vietnam depended heavily upon highly polished rice. Thiamin was dangerously low in South Vietnam and riboflavin was also deficient. The principal deficiency in Lebanon was riboflavin. The diet of Alaskan natives was low in vitamin A and very low in ascorbic acid, particularly in the more remote villages that were the homes of most of the older men with low caries experience. It is apparent that in these countries the traditional diets, even though deficient in certain basic nutrients, had not proved cariogenic. The reports confirmed the results of earlier studies[26, 74, 76, 125] in which very low caries prevalence had been reported in populations of various parts of the world suffering from osteomalacia, rickets, or pellagra.

This failure to demonstrate an effect of "protective" nutrients (except fluoride) on dental caries is the usual finding in studies with human beings, though not necessarily with animals. However, it does not follow that starvation or malnourishment is necessarily a caries-inhibitory condition. If it were, one would expect that within malnourished populations people with caries would be better fed than people without caries, but this is not so. In the ICNND study, groups of Vietnamese children who were either caries-free or who had experienced caries showed similar levels of serum ascorbic acid, vitamin A, carotene, urinary thiamin, riboflavin, hemoglobin, and hematocrit and similar heights and weights.[102] Similar findings had earlier been reported from a study of children in five Guatemalan villages where children with dental caries and those without dental caries had about the same average values of serum protein, riboflavin, ascorbic acid, carotene, vitamin A, vitamin E, and alkaline phosphatase. The customary diet of these children was deficient in vitamin A, riboflavin, and animal protein.[44]

Finally, the evidence from the NHANES I survey in the United States, 1971–1974, bears out the results of these previous studies. The NHANES I survey collected a considerable body of data on many aspects of health, including dietary and nutritional intake, from a representative sample of the population of the United States. In the analysis of data from the NHANES I survey, each of a series of nutritional variables was related to DMF values and examined within various age, sex, and racial groups, both individually and using multiple regression statistical technics. The nutritional variables examined were protein, fat, carbohydrate, vitamin A, riboflavin, thiamin, niacin, vitamin C, calcium, and iron. No relation of any kind could be demonstrated between these nutritional variables and DMF values.[17]

Although additional research may always throw new light on this area, which is difficult to study in humans, current epidemiological evidence from human populations favors the conclusion that *nutritional* status does not influence the prevalence of dental caries.

While nutritional status is essentially unrelated to caries, *dietary* factors have a most profound influence on caries prevalence. In particular, the relation between the intake of dietary sugars and other refined carbohydrates on the one hand, and the prevalence and severity of caries on the other, is so strong that sugar is clearly a major etiological factor in the causation of caries.[72, 73, 89] The observed link between the consumption of sweets and the development of dental caries goes well back into history. In this case, the time-honored observation has been shown to be correct, even though the complex mechanisms involved have only recently been described and are still not completely understood.[88]

Sugar is not the only dietary factor likely to be involved in the etiology of caries, because a limited degree of caries occurs in populations that do not eat refined carbohydrates.[114] Current evidence, however, clearly shows it to be a major factor in caries prevalence.

Early Theories on Diet and Dental Caries

Throughout the Middle Ages and Renaissance dental caries was predominantly a disease of royalty and other nobles. It became more widespread, however, during the seventeenth century as sugar began to become more widely available.[86] The great voyages of exploration of the seventeenth and eighteenth centuries led to the discovery of peoples previously unknown to Europeans, such as the islanders of the South Pacific, who appeared to enjoy a way of life free of the diseases that afflicted European society at the time. It is perhaps not surprising that the concept of the "noble savage"[27] developed during the latter part of the eighteenth century. An understandable offshoot from this ideal was the belief that the apparent freedom from caries enjoyed by so-called primitive races could be attributed to the "natural" diet on which they existed. Eating hard, fibrous, and unprocessed food, so the theory went, led to better development of the jaws and teeth and helped to clear food debris from the surfaces of the teeth. By contrast, Western man even at that time was eating a lot of processed food, high in fermentable carbohydrates, which was thought to exercise the masticatory apparatus insufficiently and lead eventually to tooth decay. It was against the background of these beliefs that Miller, in the late nineteenth century, put forward his chemoparasitic theory of the development of dental caries. Miller's theory, developed in the

"Golden Age of Bacteriology," was based on the action of microorganisms upon fermentable carbohydrates that adhered to the tooth's surface.[80]

Theories about the preventive value of hard and fibrous foods became more widespread in the early twentieth century. Wallace[146] was a firm proponent of "cleansing foods." He followed Miller in stating that accumulations of fermentable carbohydrates were the cause of caries. In addition, he believed that such deposits could be removed by eating hard and fibrous foods, the so-called cleansing or detersive foods. Pickerill[95] stated that if a meal was finished with a salivary stimulant such as an apple, the mouth would be kept free of fermentation both by the physical cleansing effect of the fibrous food and also because of the salivary flow induced by it.

It is possible that the unrefined diet of ancient man and the "noble savage" may have contained some ill-defined factors that protected the teeth against ravages of caries.[73] It is more likely, however, that the low cariogenicity of these diets was attributable not to the *presence* of hard and fibrous foods but to the *absence* of fermentable carbohydrates in the diet.

Epidemiological Studies on Diet and Dental Caries

The complexities of the human diet and eating habits are such that epidemiological studies are difficult to conduct with the necessary degree of control over extraneous factors, such as can be attained in the laboratory. Even so, the relation between dental caries and the ingestion of carbohydrates was well demonstrated before World War II by Bunting, Jay, and others. Their work and the subsequent control measures they developed are described in Chapter 8. Further evidence of the major etiologic role played by sugar in the causation of caries came from countries that suffered major social disruption during World War II.[124, 128, 129, 130]

Norway was occupied for much of World War II, and during this period of five to six years strict food rationing was enforced. Protein intake for all age groups remained adequate, but carbohydrate and fat intakes were greatly reduced. General mortality rates increased during this period, although mortality from diabetes and circulatory disorders fell from prewar levels. Among children aged 8–14, average height and weight were reduced.

Dental effects included delayed eruption of teeth, which began to be seen a year or two after rationing began and reached a peak after the war, only returning to normal in the 1950s.[128] Caries in the permanent dentition was drastically reduced, even after allowance for the effects of delayed eruption, with the number of caries-free children aged 7–8 increasing three- to fourfold between 1941 and 1946.[129] Caries prevalence returned to 1941 levels by 1949, after rationing had ended.[130] In Japan, strict food rationing made sugar virtually unobtainable during World War II. By the end of the war the mean DMF for 10-year-old children in 1950 was considerably below values recorded in 1940. By 1957, DMF values had come back to just higher than 1940 levels.[124]

A unique site for the long-term study of the effects of dietary changes on dental health has been the island of Tristan da Cunha in the South Atlantic, a remote community composed of people of principally European descent who for years lived undisturbed by the rest of the world. The community's limited contacts with the outside world gradually increased as modern communications improved. Then a volcanic eruption in the early 1960s led to the temporary emigration of the entire community to England. The islanders returned when the island was habitable again, and in recent years the establishment of some industry has created an economy and a demand for consumer goods. Much of the diet now consists of processed food.

The islanders were dentally examined on the island in 1932, 1937, and 1953; in England in 1962; and again on the island in 1966. The results show that the prevalence of caries in the first permanent molars of 6- to 19-year-olds was zero in 1932 and 1937, increasing to 50 percent in 1962 and to 80 percent in 1966.[29]

Hopewood House, an institution in the Australian state of New South Wales, provided an opportunity for a 15-year study of a group of children living on a basically vegetarian diet that also was severely restricted in sucrose intake. The study began with 81 children, aged 4–9, of whom 63 (77.8 percent) were caries-free.[61] Fifty-three percent of the children were still caries-free at age 13, compared with 0.4 percent of the local noninstitutionalized population of the same age.[123] Over the years some of the dietary restrictions in the institution were relaxed, but at the conclusion of the study 34.7 percent of 13-year-olds remained caries-free.[38] While this study used small numbers and lacked a rigid research design, it was one of those occasions where advantage could be taken of a real-life situation. In any event, the differences between the Hopewood House children and the nearby population were so profound that the dental value of dietary control was difficult to question.

Probably the best-known attempt to conduct an experimental study on the effect of diet on dental decay in humans was the Vipeholm study, conducted in Sweden between 1945 and 1952.[36] The study was conducted in a mental institution and was so ethically controversial that it is unlikely to be repeated. However, the results from it are conclusive enough to have profoundly affected the thinking of dentistry about the role of sugar in dental decay. The inmates of the institution were divided into groups that had different amounts of refined sugar intake varying from none to 24 sticky toffees per day. Despite some observed flaws in the research design, the differences between the groups were so conclusive that they are difficult to argue away. The conclusions from the Vipeholm study still hold up in the light of present day evidence. They are that:

1. Sugar consumption increases caries activity.
2. The risk of increased caries activity is greater if the sugar is in sticky form.
3. The risk is greatest if the sugar is taken between meals and in a sticky form.
4. The increase in caries under uniform conditions shows great individual variation.

5. The increase in caries disappears upon withdrawal of sticky foodstuffs from the diet.
6. Caries can still occur in the absence of refined sugar, natural sugars, and total dietary carbohydrates.

In addition to these studies, there are numerous instances reported of the disastrously rapid increase in caries prevalence that occurs when a previously remote society comes in contact with a Western diet and way of life. While the changes in such people's lifestyles are often so profound and so abrupt that it is difficult to state from the evidence presented that all changes in caries prevalence are due to diet, there is little question that the dietary factors are important. Examples of such instances have been reported from Polynesia,[10] Ghana,[69] and Greenland,[47, 83, 92] among Eskimos,[22] and among children in a remote Scottish island where a twentieth-century lifestyle has replaced traditional ways.[37]

The subject of sugar and other refined carbohydrates in relation to dental decay has also been dealt with in a series of reviews of the literature. All have concluded that sugar ingestion has a profound influence on the prevalence of dental caries.[3, 28, 39, 77, 118] Additional evidence of an intriguing variety comes from the study of the few persons who have a rare hereditary disease called Hereditary Fructose Intolerance (HFI). This condition requires that people who have it greatly minimize their sugar intake on a lifelong basis. Studies of persons with HFI show that they experience virtually no caries compared with normal subjects without HFI.[90]

While the sugar/caries relation is universally accepted in dentistry, there is less unanimity about the strength of this relation. For example, while Newbrun and colleagues[90] state that "caries is initiated when the sucrose content of the diet and frequency of ingestion exceed a low limit," Jackson argues that the importance of sugar has been overemphasized.[46] What is true is that the sugar/caries relation is not a simple linear one, though it is a direct relation. In other words, it cannot be stated that an individual who eats twice as much sugar as another will experience twice as much caries, although populations with a high sugar consumption tend to have a high prevalence of caries. Dental caries is a complex disease, and other factors related to sugar consumption—for example, the physical form of sugar and frequency of ingestion—have also been shown to be of great importance.[36] In the NHANES I survey in the United States, the relation between DMF values and total sugar consumption was weak, as it was in a Finnish study.[49] However, DMF values in the NHANES I study were strongly related to the reported consumption of sweet snacks between meals and even more strongly related to the frequency of consumption of such snacks.[17] Caries (especially root caries) also occurs in populations who eat no refined carbohydrates,[108, 114] although the prevalence of coronal caries in such populations tends to be low.

In summary, it can be said that although many questions still remain to be answered about the sugar/caries relation, there is no doubt that it is one of profound importance, even if sugar is not the only food involved in caries etiology. Much research remains to be done, such as further development of the pioneering methods to determine the cariogenic potential of foodstuffs and dietary patterns.[14] The full extent of the sugar/caries relation should be made clearer in the future by a combination of controlled animal studies, basic research into the ecology of dental plaque, and epidemiological studies in humans.

PERIODONTAL DISEASE

Anthropological evidence indicates that periodontal disease, like dental caries, was present in ancient peoples, but it seems to have afflicted them more seriously, for ancient skulls even of quite young persons show considerable bone loss.[84, 85] Periodontal disease has been a remarkably persistent disease throughout human history, without the secular variations that characterize dental caries.

The term "periodontal disease" is generally recognized as a generic term used to describe a group of diseases.[98] Other texts describe in detail the clinical manifestation of these conditions. In this context, "periodontal disease" refers to gingivitis and the chronic long-term loss of attachment and bony support.

There is less information available on the epidemiology of periodontal disease than there is on that of caries. The dental profession has been largely caries-oriented for much of its short history; consequently, the necessary level of consciousness of periodontal disease for the development of indices (see Chapter 5) has only been achieved in the post–World War II era. Nonetheless, sufficient research has been carried out in that time to provide a substantial body of information on the epidemiology of periodontal disease; knowledge that provides a basis for applied research into the etiology of the disease and its subsequent control.

Geographical Distribution

Periodontal disease is almost universally prevalent, with over 70 percent of adults in all countries affected.[8] In many nations the disease is widespread in much younger persons.[107] However, there is considerable variation in the intensity of the disease in different parts of the world.

By and large, the prevalence and severity of periodontal disease on a global basis are inversely related to the degree of economic development of the country concerned. In other words, periodontal disease is more severe, particularly at an early age, in countries lacking economic development and is relatively more moderate in countries of the Western world.[107] This pattern differs from that found with dental caries, as described earlier. Figure 6–7 shows the severity of periodontal disease in several population groups around the world, gathered in ICNND surveys. The trend illustrated in Figure 6–7 is

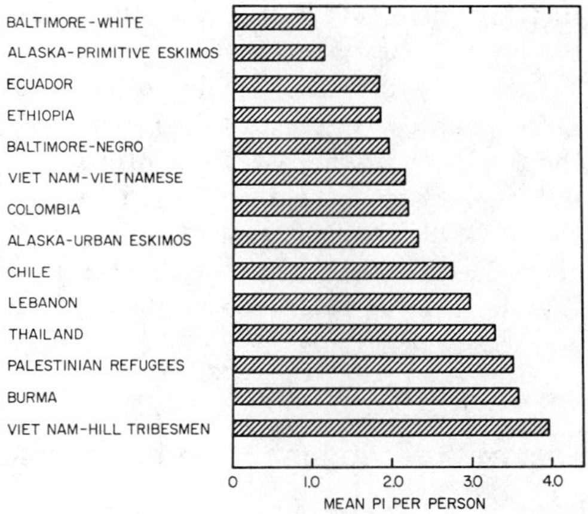

Figure 6–7. Mean Periodontal Index scores for civilian groups aged 40–49 years. (From Russell, A. L. World epidemiology and oral health. [In Kreshover, S. J., and McClure, F. J., eds. Environmental variables in oral disease. AAAS Publication No. 81. Washington, D.C., American Association Advancement Science, 1966. xii + 312 p. Copyright 1966, AAAS].)

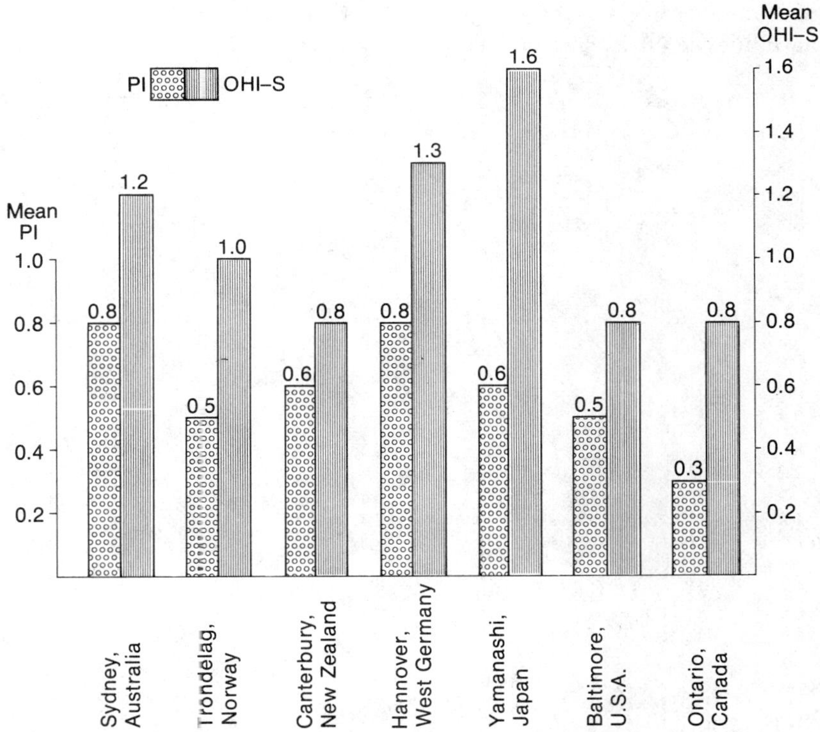

Figure 6–8. Periodontal Index (PI) scores and Simplified Oral Hygiene Index (OHI–S) scores in children aged 13–14 in seven countries. (Data from the World Health Organization, U.S. Public Health Service, International Collaborative Study [WHO/USPHS/ICS], 1973, and from replicative studies in the United States [1975] and Canada [1977].[7, 13, 30])

that the most severe periodontal disease is found among those groups with the lowest material standards of living.

Even within the economically developed countries, however, there is quite a range in the severity of periodontal disease recorded. Figure 6–8 shows the Periodontal Index (PI) scores as well as Simplified Oral Hygiene Index (OHI–S) scores for children aged 13–14 in seven countries examined during the WHO/USPHS/ICS surveys. Figure 6–9 presents similar data for adults aged 35–44. Just from the PI scores alone, it is evident that periodontal disease, even in the economically developed countries, is common at an early age and can become severe by adulthood.

Factors Affecting the Severity of Periodontal Disease

Age and oral hygiene are the two predominant variables associated with the severity of periodontal disease. Sex and race do not seem to be related to the distribution of the disease independently. No nutritional or dietary factors have been shown to be directly related to the prevalence or intensity of periodontal disease, although the possibility that generalized malnutrition may be an influence on its severity cannot be ignored.[105]

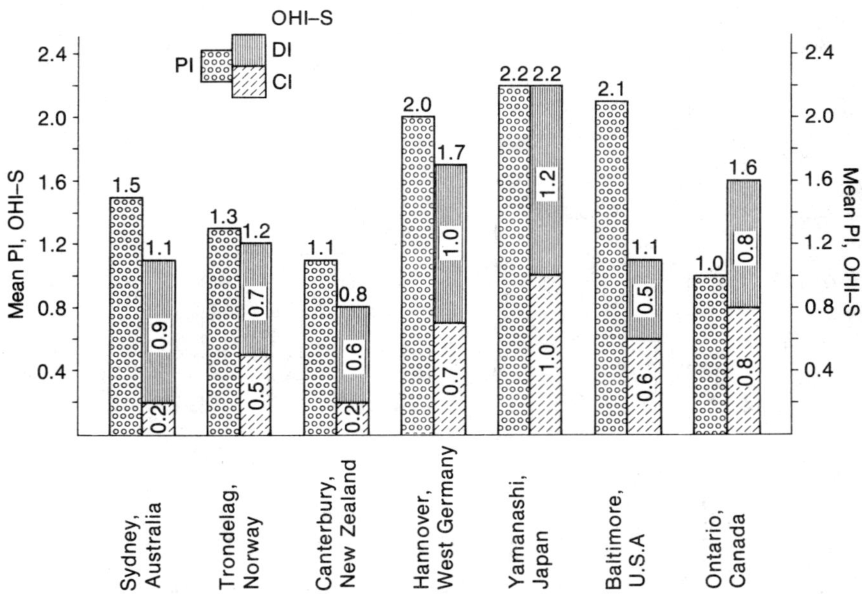

Figure 6–9. Periodontal Index (PI) scores and Simplified Oral Hygiene Index (OHI–S) scores in adults aged 35–44 in seven countries. (Data from the World Health Organization, U.S. Public Health Service, International Collaborative Study [WHO/USPHS/ICS], 1973, and replicative studies in the United States [1975] and Canada [1977].[7, 13, 30])

Table 6–3. Percent Distribution of Children (1963–65), Youths (1966–70), and Adults (1960–63), by Status of Periodontal Disease and Age, United States, 1960–70*

Status	Children 6–11	Youths 12–17	Adults 18–79
Without periodontal disease	61.3%	32.1%	26.1%
With periodontal disease	38.7	67.9	73.9
Without pockets	37.9	62.1	48.5
With pockets	0.8	5.8	25.4

*U.S. Public Health Service.[137]

Age

Periodontal disease increases in prevalence and severity with increasing age. Table 6–3 presents data from the National Health Survey of the United States, conducted during the years 1963 to 1970.[133, 136, 137] From the NHANES I survey of 1971–74, similar information on the distribution of periodontal disease by age is shown in Figure 6–10. Both Table 6–3 and Figure 6–10 show that the proportion of persons without periodontal disease diminishes steadily with age and that the severity of the disease, as represented by numbers of periodontal pockets, increases with age. Similar data have been shown from other countries.[107] Comparison of Table 6–3 and Figure 6–10 seems to indicate an improvement in periodontal conditions in the United States in recent years. For example, 32.1 percent of those aged 12–17 were free of disease in 1966–70, whereas 60 to 72 percent were classified as free of periodontal disease in 1971–74. This apparent improvement seems rather dramatic over such a short time and may be due in part to examiner differences.

Even when groups are equalized for sex, race, and oral hygiene, age appears to be an independent variable related to an increasing intensity of periodontal disease. This relation is shown in the long-term study conducted by Löe and colleagues on the natural history of periodontal disease in man.[4, 63, 64, 65] Löe selected two groups for long-term study. One comprised college students and professors in Oslo, Norway, a group highly motivated, dentally aware, and of high socioeconomic status. By contrast, his second group comprised tea workers in Sri Lanka, poorly educated and of low socioeconomic status. The Oslo group had received a significant amount of dental treatment; the Sri Lankans, virtually none. The oral hygiene status of the Oslo group was excellent, with no increase in the prevalence and severity of gingivitis from the late teenage years to around 40 years of age. There was little loss of gingival attachment in this group, and what loss was recorded progressed at a slow rate Among 31-year-olds in Oslo, mean loss of attachment was 0.98 mm; for those aged over 37, it was 1.66 mm. The mean annual loss of gingival attachment in this group was 0.07 to 0.13 mm. By contrast, the Sri Lankans had plaque on virtually all surfaces of all teeth by age 15 and no significant improvement in oral hygiene status occurred up to age 40. By age 17, only a few of the Sri Lanka group showed normal periodontal support,

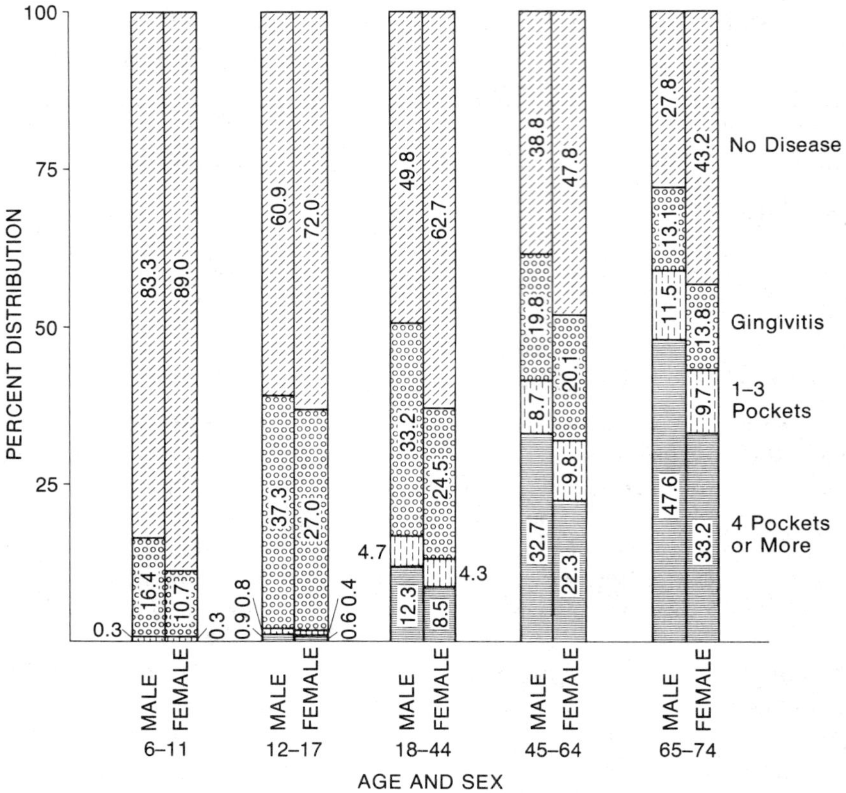

Figure 6–10. Percent distribution of males and females by periodontal classification, United States, 1971–1974. Classified by age.[140]

and all those above age 21 had lost some support. By age 31, the mean loss of attachment in the tea workers was 3.11 mm, and the mean annual loss was 0.2 to 0.244 mm per year. It should be noted that the researchers went to great pains to ensure the reliability and precision of their measurements.

Several interesting points are illustrated by this study, which confirms other observations concerning the natural history of periodontal disease. One is that *some* loss of attachment occurs with age, even with excellent oral hygiene, although the loss of attachment is considerably more rapid in conditions of poor oral hygiene. This study also showed that tooth loss was greater among the Sri Lankans than among the Oslo group. Among the Sri Lankans, nearly all teeth with a loss of attachment of 10 mm or greater at the beginning of the study were lost in the next seven years. There were no teeth with this degree of attachment loss in the Norwegians; in fact, the Oslo group lost no teeth to periodontal disease throughout this study. Interestingly, more teeth, especially premolars, were lost in the Oslo group before age 17 than in the ages 17 through 40—a result of orthodontic treatment. Among the Sri

Lankans, the mortality rate for those teeth that had lost 10 mm or more of support at the beginning of the study was 0.6 per year, compared with 0.03 per year for teeth having a greater amount of support.

Oral Hygiene

The close relation between periodontal disease and level of oral hygiene has been demonstrated many times, both in the United States and in other countries.[17, 66, 101, 103, 115, 119, 120, 126, 133] Waerhaug, in his review of the literature in 1966,[145] concluded that no differences in levels of periodontal disease among different races can be detected if the groups are balanced for age, sex, and socioeconomic status. Indeed, much of the difference in periodontal disease levels between peoples of developed and developing countries shown in Figure 6–7 can be attributed to differences in oral hygiene levels.[106]

Table 6–4 shows the PI values by age and sex in the United States as found in the NHANES I survey in 1971–74. These data show that blacks at practically all ages have higher PI levels than do whites, and that males, at all age levels, have higher PI levels than do females. However, as pointed out earlier, when blacks and whites are balanced within each age group by oral hygiene levels, the differences in PI values disappear.[101]

Figure 6–11, from the same NHANES I survey in 1971–74, shows the OHI–S values for males and females in different age-groups. The OHI–S values are higher at all levels for males, largely accounting for the differences in PI scores between males and females shown in Table 6–4. Again, when men and women are balanced by age and similar oral hygiene levels, differences in PI scores disappear.

Russell considered his findings on periodontal disease in South Vietnam to be representative of the findings on periodontal disease for the whole ICNND series of surveys.[103] In South Vietnam, Russell found that the combined effects of age, oral debris, and calculus accounted for some two thirds of the total variance in PI scores.

Diet, Nutrition, and Periodontal Disease

No single dietary factor has been discovered to influence periodontal disease in a manner analogous to the effect of sugar on dental caries. It was

Table 6–4. Mean Periodontal Index (PI) Values for Blacks and Whites, United States, 1971–74*

Age	Black Males	Black Females	White Males	White Females	All Blacks	All Whites
6–11	0.2	0.1	0.1	0.1	0.1	0.1
12–17	0.6	0.5	0.4	0.2	0.5	0.3
18–44	1.6	1.0	0.8	0.6	1.3	0.7
45–64	3.2	2.4	1.6	1.2	2.8	1.4
65–74	4.2	3.4	2.6	1.8	3.8	2.2

*U.S. Public Health Service.[140]

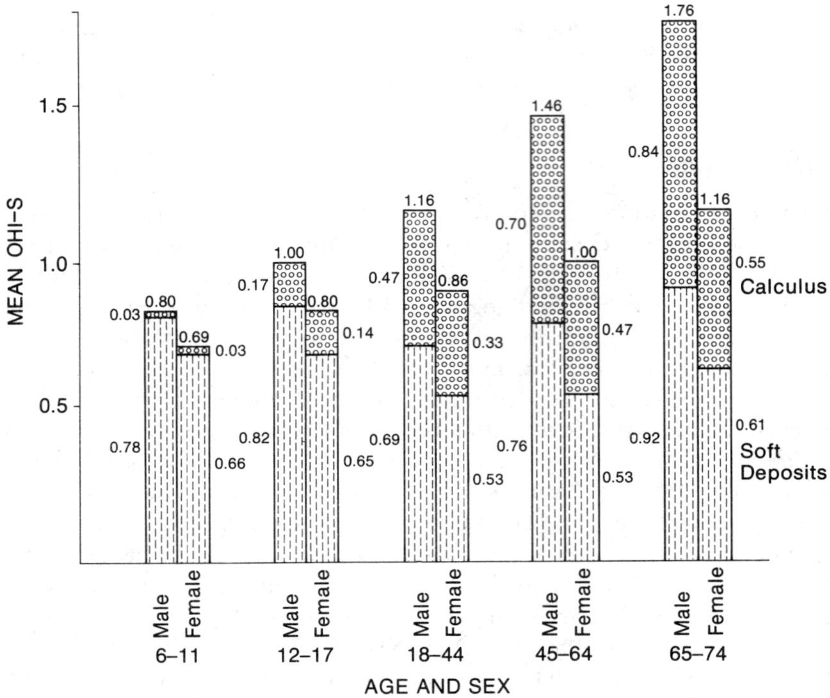

Figure 6–11. Mean Simplified Oral Hygiene Index (OHI–S) values for males and females by age, United States, 1971–1974.[140]

natural, however, for early researchers to think that there was a nutritional component in periodontal disease. Observations such as the bleeding gums noted among early sailors who suffered from scurvy (severe deficiency of ascorbic acid) naturally led to such a view.

While there is little firm evidence to support such a contention, the picture is not entirely clear, for there is a possibility that generalized malnutrition may have some influence on the prevalence and intensity of periodontal disease.[107] Again, pioneering work in this area was carried out by Russell in the ICNND surveys. Russell found that in South Vietnam, with the statistical effects of age and oral hygiene status held constant, there were slight but significant residual associations between the disease, deficiency in serum vitamin A, and low hematocrit levels. Little or no effect could be ascribed to hemoglobin levels, serum ascorbic acid, serum carotene, serum protein, thiamin, riboflavin level in urine, height-weight ratios, skin thickness, or physical signs of malnutrition such as cheilosis or loss of the ankle or knee-jerk reflex. Neither vitamin A nor hematocrit levels were found to be associated with periodontal disease in other studies in the ICNND series.[103]

Some limitations of this type of analysis were pointed out in Chapter 5, and Russell's data from Vietnam would have limited value if they were not consistent with other results from other populations. Major reviews of the literature[19, 145] conclude that researchers have been unable to find any correlation between intake levels of particular nutrients and periodontal disease.

These results do not rule out diet or nutrition as contributory factors in periodontal disease. They do indicate it is extremely unlikely that there is a primary etiological role for dietary vitamin A, ascorbic acid, thiamin, riboflavin, or niacin in periodontal disease.[104] By contrast, dental plaque is invariably found to be the most dominant factor associated with periodontal disease, and this association becomes stronger as the age of studied groups advances. Indeed, with the establishment of experimental gingivitis in man by Löe and his colleagues,[62] a cause-and-effect relation was first demonstrated between the presence of dental plaque and periodontal disease. The causative agents are largely bacteria, with perhaps other mitigating agents, found in dental plaque.

The fact remains that the greatest prevalence and intensity of periodontal disease are found in areas of the world where generalized malnutrition is common, so the possibility exists that there are nutritional factors affecting the severity of the disease. Other systemic factors, such as certain hormones, are known to influence severity, though they are not primary etiological agents.[121] Considerably more research is needed in this particular area. When studies are carried out among populations enjoying a good level of nutrition, however, the dominance of oral hygiene and to a lesser extent age as determining factors in the prevalence of periodontal disease is unquestioned.[17]

Relation between Dental Caries and Periodontal Disease

A long-established belief among some dentists is that caries and periodontal disease are inversely related—a patient with severe caries is less likely to develop periodontal disease. Data from the NHANES I survey of 1971–74 show that there is no basis for this belief. Among persons with poor oral hygiene in that survey, there was a slight positive association between the severity of the two diseases.[17] Among persons with good oral hygiene, there appeared to be no relation of any kind.

TOOTH LOSS

The end result of untreated dental caries and periodontal disease is tooth loss. The data relating to tooth loss in a community are a reflection of both the extent of disease and the adequacy of treatment for established disease.

In the United States, as shown by the NHANES I survey of 1971–74, fully 29.8 percent of youths aged 12–17 had lost one or more permanent teeth and 4.8 percent had lost four or more teeth.[144] Given modern treatment methods and the trend toward declining caries prevalence in the United States described earlier, these figures are far from satisfactory, though they are an improvement on tooth loss figures from earlier days. For example, in 1920, Hyatt reported that 13.5 percent of first molars in a group of Brooklyn girls, aged 13–17, had been lost,[45] and in the Hagerstown studies of 1938, Knutson and Klein reported that 15-year-old children had lost, on average, 1.1 permanent teeth per child; 94 percent of the lost teeth were first molars.[57] In the NHANES I survey of 1971–74, 15-year-olds had lost an average of 0.1 permanent teeth each,[144] so there has clearly been some improvement over time.

In Britain, the situation on tooth loss seems to be less favorable among children at present than in the United States. The national survey for British children in 1973 showed that 23 percent of 12-year-olds had lost at least one permanent tooth and that 6 percent had lost four or more permanent teeth.[126] (Tooth loss rates for different age-groups in different countries drawn from the WHO/USPHS/ICS study are given in Figures 6–1 to 6–3.)

Loss of permanent teeth in childhood is usually attributable to advanced dental caries. In adults aged 35 years and over, however, periodontal disease is universally regarded as the principal cause of tooth loss. Evidence for this statement comes from surveys of dental practitioners, such as those shown in Figure 6–12, seeking the reasons given for loss of teeth among patients of different ages.[93] Results similar to those in Figure 6–12 come from a survey conducted in Denmark.[11] Figure 6–12 shows that although caries is the major reason for tooth loss in younger years, periodontal disease increases significantly as a reason for tooth loss with advancing age. For all ages combined, these data indicate that more teeth were extracted because of periodontal disease than for other reasons. Although these results come from a survey in the 1950s, they are still generally regarded as valid.

Löe and his colleagues have stated that by age 40, some 8 to 10 percent of teeth are lost because of periodontal disease. Their studies on the natural history of periodontal disease indicate that without intervention, tooth loss from periodontal disease increases rapidly after that age.[64]

Total tooth loss not only represents the results of oral disease, but it also reflects the availability and type of dental treatment in the community and attitudes toward that treatment and to dental health in general.[16] There is considerably less total tooth loss in higher socioeconomic groups than in lower socioeconomic groups. Women suffer a greater degree of total tooth loss than do men and also tend to become edentulous at a younger age.[33, 127, 132] In the United States, total tooth loss is related to race; a higher proportion of white people suffer total tooth loss than do blacks.[132] Differences by sex and race might be attributable to the socioenvironmental contexts of these groups.

Table 6–5 shows the extent of total tooth loss in eight countries. Much of the data comes from the WHO/USPHS/ICS survey. The range in degrees of edentulousness by country is considerable and is difficult to explain solely in terms of dental disease. Attitudes are important—there is still quite a high proportion of adults in New Zealand, for example, who attach no stigma to the wearing of full dentures.[23]

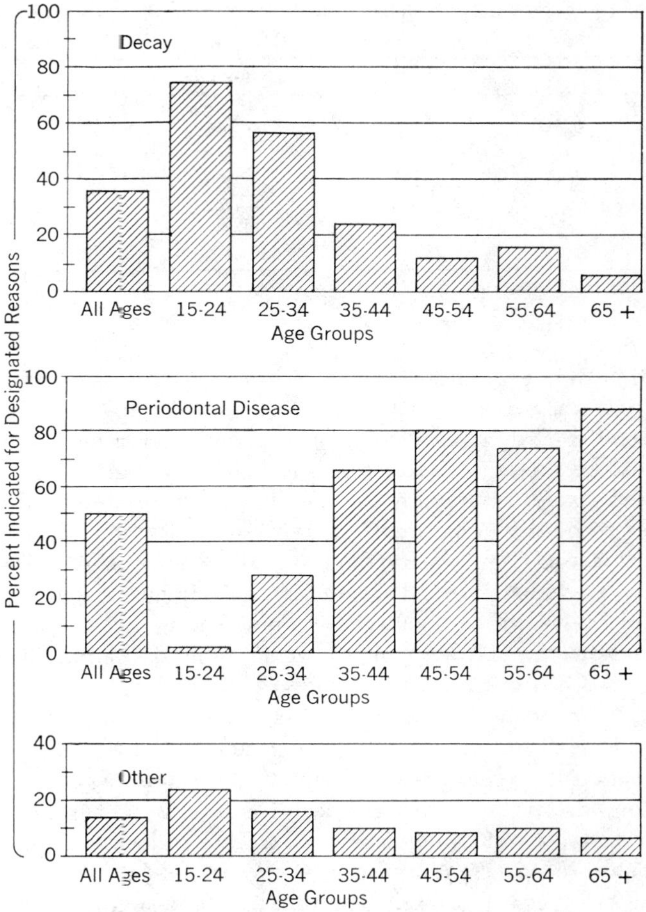

Figure 6–12. Teeth indicated for extraction because of decay, periodontal disease, and other reasons. (From Pelton, W. J., Pennell, E. H., and Druzina, A.: Tooth morbidity experience of adults. Am. Dent. A. J., 49:439–45, 1954. Graph from Young, W. O.: Dental health. *In* Hollinshead, B. S., The survey of dentistry; the final report. Washington, D.C., American Council Education, copyright 1961.)

Table 6–5. Percent of Persons Aged 35–44 Who Are Edentulous, for Eight Countries, 1968–77

Community	Percent Edentulous
Yamanashi, Japan[9]	0.0
Hanover, West Germany[9]	1.6
Trondelag, Norway[9]	6.4
Ontario, Canada[30]	8.7
Baltimore, U.S.A.[15]	10.6
Sydney, Australia[9]	13.2
England and Wales[33]	22.0
Scotland[127]	35.0
Canterbury, New Zealand[9]	35.7

Table 6–6. Percent of Persons Edentulous by Age and Sex, United States, 1971–74*

Age	Males	Females	All
6–11	0.0%	0.0%	0.0%
12–17	0.0	0.3	0.1
18–44	3.4	4.7	4.1
45–64	22.5	24.9	23.8
65–74	43.6	47.0	45.5
6–74	9.5	11.8	10.7

*U.S. Public Health Service.[144]

Table 6–6 shows the proportion of persons edentulous by age and sex in the United States as reported in the NHANES I survey, 1971–74. In particular, the sharp trend toward increasing loss of teeth with increasing age is apparent, and it can also be seen that females tend to be more subject to total tooth loss at all ages than males. However, the degree of total tooth loss in the United States seems to be declining; a 1971 survey showed that 11.2 percent of the total population was edentulous, compared to 13 percent in 1957–58.[132] It is interesting to note that in the 1971 survey 8.2 percent of males and 10.4 of females aged 35–44 were totally edentulous. These data seem to correlate fairly closely with the 10.6 percent shown in Table 6–5 for Baltimore in the WHO/USPHS/ICS project.

It is expected that total tooth loss in the United States will continue to decline with time, even though the number and proportion of older persons in the population is increasing (see Chapter 14). Tooth loss because of caries has diminished drastically, although there is still some uncertainty about the extent to which tooth loss from periodontal disease is declining from the levels shown in Figure 6–12. Dental personnel should not be lulled into thinking that because preventive methods against caries appear to be working well, the problem of tooth loss has diminished. It is possible that much of the problem is simply being transferred from the younger end of life to the later years, and dental practitioners may need to adapt their treatment methods increasingly to counter that possibility.

ORAL CANCER

It is fortunate that oral cancer is a relatively unusual disease, because once contracted, its effects for the individual and the family concerned are catastrophic. Age-adjusted death rates for cancer of the buccal cavity and pharynx in the United States seem to have declined slightly since the early 1960s. At that time, the age-adjusted death rate was about 3.4 deaths per 100,000,[141] whereas in 1970 it was 3.1, and in 1976, 3.0.[143]

The occurrence of oral cancer and its site distribution within the mouth varies widely in different parts of the world.[96, 122] These differences appear

Table 6–7. Estimated New Cancer Cases and Deaths, by Sex, for All Cancers and for Cancer of the Oral Cavity, 1977*

Site	New Cases Total	New Cases Male	New Cases Female	Deaths Total	Deaths Male	Deaths Female
All Cancers	690,000	347,000	343,000	385,000	210,500	174,500
Cancers of the Oral Cavity	23,900 (3.5%)	17,000 (4.9%)	6,900 (2.0%)	8,450 (2.2%)	6,000 (2.9%)	2,450 (1.4%)

*American Cancer Society.[2]

chiefly due to the environmental factors with which they are linked. The most persistent environmental factor on a global basis, according to Pindborg,[96] is the use of tobacco in its various forms, although others reported are exposure to sunlight and consumption of alcohol.[2]

Table 6–7 shows the extent of the problem of oral cancer within the United States. It can be seen that cancer of the oral cavity constitutes about 3.5 percent of all new cases reported and 2.2 percent of all cancer deaths. It is two-and-a-half times more prevalent in males, and twice as many deaths occur in males as in females. There is considerable difference, however, between males and females in the specific sites within the oral cavity in which oral cancer is found (see Table 6–8). There are no specific reasons that can be given for these differences.

As described in Chapter 5, one of the measures of the severity of cancer is the five-year survival rate; that is, the proportion of people still alive five years after the cancer has been diagnosed. Table 6–9 shows that oral cancer has a 67 percent five-year survival rate for localized cancer, and a 30 percent rate when there already is regional involvement at diagnosis of the initial lesion. Table 6–9 also shows that a considerable number of other types of cancer have better survival rates than oral cancer, which underlines even further the need for vigilance on the part of dental personnel in the early detection and diagnosis of suspicious oral lesions.

Table 6–8. Site Occurrence of Oral Cancer, for Estimated New Cases and for Deaths for Men and Women, United States, 1977. Expressed as Percent of All Oral Cancers*

Site	New Cases Total (n = 23,900)	New Cases Male (n = 17,000)	New Cases Female (n = 6,900)	Deaths Total (n = 8,450)	Deaths Male (n = 6,000)	Deaths Female (n = 2,450)
Lip	17.2	22.4	4.3	2.7	3.3	1.0
Tongue	18.8	18.2	20.3	23.7	23.3	24.5
Salivary Gland	36.4 (Salivary Gland, Floor of Mouth, Other and Unspecified combined)	30.6 (combined)	50.7 (combined)	7.7	6.7	10.2
Floor of Mouth				6.2	6.7	5.1
Other and Unspecified				14.8	13.4	18.4
Pharynx	27.6	28.8	24.6	45.0	46.6	40.8

*American Cancer Society.[2]

Table 6–9. Five-Year Survival Rates for Selected Cancer Sites, Adjusted for Normal Life Expectancy, United States, 1977. Expressed as Percent of All Diagnosed Cases*

Site	Localized Cancer	With Regional Involvement
Breast	84%	56%
Uterus	82	44
Larynx	79	38
Bladder	71	21
Colon/Rectum	71	43
Prostate	68	57
Oral	67	30
Lung	33	10

*American Cancer Society.[2]

Oral cancer is closely related to increasing age. Of the 8,114 deaths from oral cancer registered in 1976, almost 81 percent (6,550) were persons aged 55 and over.[142]

Oral cancer, then, clearly emerges as a disease chiefly of older men, particularly those who are heavy users of tobacco and alcohol and who may be exposed to sunlight. Whereas the causes of oral cancer, as with many other types of cancer, cannot be stated with any certainty, the risk factors have been fairly well described by epidemiological surveys. Dental personnel should be aware of these factors and include them when taking the medical histories of new patients.

CLEFT LIP AND PALATE

Greene has estimated that about 6,000 children are born alive in the United States each year with cleft lip or palate or both,[34] a rate of about one to 700 live births. This distressing condition is predominantly of genetic origin, although there is evidence that some environmental factors also play a role in its etiology.[111]

Attempts to isolate some of these environmental variables have proved difficult for several reasons. One is that the relatively low occurrence of the condition means that a large number of birth records need to be examined in order to establish statistical correlations. Second, although cleft lip and palate as a congenital malformation is supposedly recorded on birth certificates in the United States, it is likely that some cases are not.[71] In spite of these difficulties, some of the epidemiological correlations reported from several studies are as follows:[35, 110]

1. More facial clefts appear in boys, but more isolated cleft palates appear in girls.
2. Cleft lip and palate appear more frequently in plural births than in single births.

3. Babies with clefts generally are of lower birth weight, and a relation has been found between clefts and prematurity. Possibly this correlation is also associated with the high infant mortality rate for children born with cleft lip and palate, found to be some five times greater than it is for normal children.[70]

Clefts are associated with:

1. Threatened spontaneous abortion during the first and second trimester of pregnancy.
2. Influenza and fever in the first trimester.
3. Maternal drug consumption during the first trimester, particularly opiates, penicillin, and salicylates.

Greene's study, conducted in four states of the United States, found that ethnically, the lowest reported prevalence was among blacks and the highest among persons of Japanese ancestry.[35]

Greene also found a relation between advancing age of parents and cleft lip and palate, although this relation was not confirmed in Saxén's study in Finland.[110] No correlation has been reported between birth order and clefts.

Saxén's studies do indicate that chance correlations can occur in individual studies of cleft palate, meaning that the associations described need to be replicated in other studies before they can be fully accepted. More epidemiological knowledge of associations between possible etiological factors and the occurrence of cleft lip and palate is required in order to increase knowledge of this disfiguring condition.

MALOCCLUSION

The difficulties of quantifying malocclusion were described in Chapter 5. Consequently, the distribution of this dentofacial abnormality is not well understood. Differing cultural perceptions of what constitutes a malocclusion, differing perceptions of malocclusion between orthodontic specialists and general dentists, and difficulties in achieving a sufficient degree of examination consistency in use of existing malocclusion indices all lead to difficulty in making summary statements.

In view of these difficulties, probably the best available data come from the National Health Examination survey of youths aged 12–17 in the United States during the years 1966–70.[139] This survey of a representative sample of youths employed the TPI (Treatment Priority Index) of Grainger (described in Chapter 5). The results are shown in Table 6–10. They show that a higher proportion of black youths than white youths seem to have either normal occlusion or minor malocclusion. There is little difference shown between males and females among white youths; however, a notably higher proportion of black females seem to have very severe malocclusion, relative to black males. The differences between white males and females in this regard seem less marked.

Orthodontic treatment is popular and widely received in the United

Table 6–10. Percent Distribution of Youths Aged 12–17 by Orthodontic Treatment Need According to the Treatment Priority Index (TPI), United States, 1966–70*

	TPI Score	All	White Male	White Female	Black Male	Black Female
0	(Normal occlusion)	11.0%	10.2%	10.7%	15.0%	14.3%
1–3	(Minor malocclusion)	34.8	33.6	35.7	36.4	37.3
4–6	(Definite malocclusion)	25.2	26.0	25.5	23.3	18.8
7–9	(Severe malocclusion)	13.0	12.7	13.2	13.5	11.0
10+	(Very severe malocclusion)	16.0	17.5	14.9	11.8	18.6

*U.S. Public Health Service.[139] See Chapter 5 for discussion of the Treatment Priority Index.

States. However, it is not known how the amount of treatment received relates to the data shown in Table 6–10.

SUMMARY

Results of epidemiological studies show dental caries is considerably more prevalent in Western industrialized countries than in economically developing countries. This situation has obviously existed for considerable time, although in recent years there have been signs that the pattern may be shifting. There are indications of a decline in caries prevalence in the United States and some other Western industrialized countries and a sharp rise in caries prevalence, at least in urban areas, in developing countries. This rise in caries prevalence in these countries is likely to pose a major public health problem for them in the future.

Oral cancer and cleft lip and palate have remained fairly static in their prevalence, which probably will change little until acceptable prevention for these conditions can be developed. Orthodontic treatment seems to be becoming more popular in the United States, but it is not known how this occurrence is related to the prevalence of malocclusion or to occlusal dysfunction.

Periodontal disease is widespread throughout the world, and generally appears to be less severe in the Western industrialized countries, particularly among higher socioeconomic groups. However, periodontal disease still seems to be responsible for a greater degree of tooth loss than does dental caries. Treatment for periodontal disease in the United States is likely to occupy the time of dental personnel to a greater extent in the future, especially if caries prevalence declines further and if the trend toward greater life expectancy continues. Dental personnel can expect to see more and more older patients who are keeping their teeth well into old age.

References

1. Alfano, M. C. Understanding the role of diet and nutrition in dental caries. p. 6–12. (In Changing perspectives in nutrition and caries research. New York, Medcom, 1979. 52 p.)

2. American Cancer Society. 1977 cancer facts and figures. New York, The Society, 1976. 31 p.
3. Andlaw, R. J. Diet and dental caries—a review. J. Human Nutrit., 31:45–52, Feb. 1977.
4. Ånerud, Åge, Löe, Harald, Boysen, Hans, and Smith, Martyn. The natural history of periodontal disease in man: changes in gingival health and oral hygiene before 40 years of age. J. Periodont. Res., 14:526–40, Nov. 1979.
5. Bagramian, R. A., and Russell, A. L. Epidemiologic study of dental caries experience and between-meal eating patterns. J. Dent. Res., 52:342–47, Mar.–Apr. 1973.
6. Banting, D. W., Ellen, R. P., and Fillery, E. D. Prevalence of root surface caries among institutionalized older persons. Community Dent. Oral Epidemiol., 8:84–8, Apr. 1980.
7. Barmes, D. E. Features of oral health care across cultures. Internat. Dent. J., 26:353–68, Sept. 1976.
8. ———. Epidemiology of dental disease. J. Clin. Periodont., 4:80–93, Dec. 1977.
9. ———. A progress report on adult data analysis in the WHO/USPHS International Collaborative Study. Internat. Dent. J., 28:348–60, Sept. 1978.
10. Baume, L. J. Caries prevalence and caries intensity among 12,344 schoolchildren of French Polynesia. Arch. Oral Biol., 14:181–205, Feb. 1969.
11. Bay, I., and Gad, T. Arsager til ekstraktion af permanente taenderi Danmark. Tandlaegbladet, 76:103–14, Feb. 1972.
12. Beal, J. F. The dental health of five-year-old children of different ethnic origins resident in an inner Birmingham area and a nearby borough. Arch. Oral Biol., 18:305–12, Mar. 1973.
13. Bonito, A. J. The United States study of dental manpower systems in relation to oral health status: the private practice system. Final report for USPHS contract no. NO1-DH-34051. Baltimore, University Maryland Dental School, 1977. Part I (vii + 113 p.), Part II (vii + 142 p.) Part III (vii + 151 p.), Part IV (vii + 106 p.).
14. Bowen, W. H., Amsbaugh, S. M., Monell-Torrens, S., et al. A method to assess cariogenic potential of foodstuffs. Am. Dent. A. J., 100:677–81, May 1980.
15. Bryan, E. T., Howard, W. H., and Vancleave, M. L. Dental health status of school children in Tennessee. Unpublished manuscript, 1980. 7 p. typescript.
16. Burt, B. A. Influences for change in the dental health status of populations: an historical perspective. J. Pub. Health Dent., 38:272–88, Fall 1978.
17. Burt, B. A., et al. A study of dietary intake, food patterns, and dental health; analysis of data from the NHANES I survey. Final report for USPHS contract no. 223–79–2092. Ann Arbor, University Michigan, 1980. xii + 154 p. Also published as U.S. Public Health Service, National Center for Health Statistics. Diet and dental health; a study of relationships. DHHS Publ. No. (PHS) 82–1675. National Center for Health Statistics Rep. Ser. 11, No. 225. Washington, D.C., Government Printing Office, 1982. vii + 85 p.
18. Carlos, J. P., and Gittelsohn, A. M. Longitudinal studies of the natural history of caries—II. A life-table study of caries incidence in the permanent teeth. Arch. Oral Biol., 10:739–51, Sept.–Oct. 1965.
19. Chilton, N. W., and Miller, M. F. Epidemiology. p. 119–43. (In International Conference on Research in the Biology of Periodontal Disease. Chicago, University Illinois School Dentistry, 1977. xxi + 482 p.)
20. Corbett, M. E., and Moore, W. J. Distribution of dental caries in ancient British populations. IV: The 19th century. Caries Res., 10:401–14, 1976.
21. Coykendall, A. L. On the evaluation of *Streptococcus mutans* and dental caries. (In Stiles, H. M., Loesche, W. J., and O'Brien, T. C., eds. Proceedings of Microbial Aspects of Dental Caries. Spec. Suppl. Microbial Abstr., 3:703–12, 1976.)
22. Curzon, M. E., and Curzon, J. A. Dental caries in Eskimo children of the Keewatin District in the Northwest Territories. Canad. Dent. A. J., 36:342–5, Sept. 1970.
23. Cutress, T. W., et al. Adult oral health and attitudes to dentistry in New Zealand 1976. Wellington, Medical Research Council of New Zealand, 1979. x + 274 p.
24. DePaola, D. P. Human diet and dental caries: effect of diet in the early years. Paper given at the Workshop of Cariogenicity of Food, Beverages, Confections, and Chewing Gum. Chicago, American Dental Association, Sept. 15–17, 1977.
25. DePaola, P. F. First report on Boston Dental Health Survey. Report submitted to the Massachusetts Department of Public Health, 1980. 13 p. typescript.
26. Dreizen, Samuel, Mann, A. W., Spies, T. D., and Hunt, F. M. Prevalence of dental caries in malnourished children. Am. J. Dis. Child., 74:265–73, Sept. 1947.
27. Dubos, Rene. The mirage of health. New York, Doubleday, c1959. 230 p.

28. Finn, S. B., and Glass, R. B. Sugar and dental decay. World Review Nutrit. Dietetics, 22:304–26, 1975.
29. Fisher, F. J. A field survey of dental caries, periodontal disease and enamel defects in Tristan da Cunha. Brit. Dent. J., 125:447–53, Nov. 19, 1968.
30. Foster, M. K., and Hunt, A. M. A study of dental manpower systems in relation to oral health status. Part 1: Ontario. Final report for Health and Welfare grant no. 606–1334–43. Toronto, University Toronto Dentistry Faculty, 1978. iii + 508 p. + summary 44 p.
31. Garn, S. M., Rowe, N. H., and Cole, Patricia E. Husband-wife similarities in dental caries experience. J. Dent. Res., 56:186, Feb. 1977.
32. Glass, R. L. Secular changes in caries prevalence in two Massachusetts towns. Caries Res., 15:445–50, 1981.
33. Gray, P. G., Todd J. E., Slack, G. L., and Bulman, J. S. Adult dental health in England and Wales, 1968. London, Her Majesty's Stationery Office, 1970. vi + 294 p.
34. Greene, J. C. Epidemiology of congenital clefts of the lip and palate. Pub. Health Rep., 78:589–602, July 1963.
35. Greene, J. C., et al. Epidemiologic study of cleft lip and cleft palate in four states. Am. Dent. A. J., 68:387–404, Mar. 1964.
36. Gustafsson, B. E., et al. The Vipeholm dental caries study. The effect of different levels of carbohydrate intake on caries activity in 436 individuals observed for five years. Acta Odont. Scand., 11:232–364, Sept. 1954.
37. Hargreaves, J. A. Changes in diet and dental health of children living in the Scottish Island of Lewis. Caries Res., 6:355–76, 1972.
38. Harris, R. Biology of the children of Hopewood House, Bowral, Australia. 4. Observations on dental caries experience extending over five years (1957–1961). J. Dent. Res., 42:1387–99, Nov.–Dec. 1963.
39. Hartles, R. L. Carbohydrate consumption and dental caries. Am. J. Clin. Nutrit., 20:152–6, Feb. 1967.
40. Heifetz, S. B., Horowitz, H. S., and Korts, D. C. Prevalence of dental caries in white and black children in Nelson County, Virginia, a rural southern community. J. Pub. Health Dent., 36:79–87, Spring 1976.
41. Hennon, D. K., Stookey, G. K., and Muhler, J. C. Prevalence and distribution of dental caries in preschool children. Am. Dent. A. J., 79:1405–14, Dec. 1969.
42. Hughes, J. T., and Rozier, R. G. The survey of dental health in the North Carolina population; selected findings. p. 21–37. (In Bawden, J. W., and De Friese, G. H., eds. Planning for dental care on a statewide basis; the North Carolina dental manpower project. Chapel Hill, Dental Foundation North Carolina, 1981. xvii + 227 p.)
43. Hunter, P. B. V. The prevalence of dental caries in 5-year-old New Zealand children. N. Z. Dent. J., 75:154–7, July 1979.
44. Hurtarte, E. A., and Scrimshaw, N. S. Dental findings in a nutritional study of school children in five Guatemalan highland villages. J. Dent. Res., 34:390–6, June 1955.
45. Hyatt, T. P. Report of an examination made of two thousand one hundred and one high school pupils. Dent. Cosmos, 52:507–11, Apr. 1920.
46. Jackson, Douglas. Sugar and dental caries: myth and fact. London, Bouverie, 1978. 30 p.
47. Jakobsen, Jan. Recent reorganization of the Public Dental Health Service in Greenland in favor of caries prevention. Community Dent. Oral Epidemiol., 7:75–81, Apr. 1979.
48. King, N. M., Shaw, L., and Murray, J. J. Caries susceptibility of permanent first and second molars in children aged 5–15. Community Dent. Oral Epidemiol., 8:151–8, June 1980.
49. Kleemola-Kujala, Eija, and Räsänen, Leena. Dietary pattern of Finnish children with low and high caries experience. Community Dent. Oral Epidemiol., 7:199–205, Aug. 1979.
50. Klein, Henry. The family and dental disease. IV. Dental disease (DMF) experience in parents and offspring. Am. Dent. A. J., 33:735–43, June 1946.
51. Klein, H., and Palmer, C. E. Dental caries in American Indian children. Pub. Health Bul. no. 239, Washington, D.C., Government Printing Office, 1937. 54 p.
52. ———. Studies on dental caries. V. Familial resemblance in the caries experience of siblings. Pub. Health Rep., 53:1353–64, Aug. 5, 1938.
53. ———. Studies on dental caries. VII. Sex differences in dental caries experience of elementary school children. Pub. Health Rep., 53:1685–90, Sept. 23, 1938.

54. ———. Studies on dental caries. XII. Comparison of the caries susceptibility of the various morphological types of permanent teeth. J. Dent. Res., 20:203–16, June 1941.
55. ———. Community economic status and the dental problem of school children. Pub. Health Rep., 55:187–205 Feb. 2, 1940.
56. Klein, Henry, and Shimizu, Toyo. The family and dental disease. I. DMF experience among husbands and wives. Am. Dent. A. J., 32:945–55, Aug. 1945.
57. Knutson, J. W., and Klein, H. Studies on dental caries. IV. Tooth mortality in elementary school children. Pub. Health Rep., 53:1021–32, June 24, 1938.
58. Köhler, B., and Bratthall, D. Intrafamilial levels of *Streptococcus mutans* and some aspects of the bacterial transmission. Scand. J. Dent. Res., 86:35–42, 1978.
59. Köhler, L., and Holst, K. Dental health of four-year-old children. Acta Paediatr. Scand., 62:269–78, May 1973.
60. Lennon, M. A., Davies, R. M., Downer, M. C., and Hull, P. S. Tooth loss in a 19th century British population. Arch. Oral Biol., 19:511–6, July 1974.
61. Lilienthal, B., Goldsworthy, N. E., Sullivan, H. R., and Cameron, D. A. The biology of the children of Hopewood House, Bowral, N. S. W. I. Observations on dental caries extending over five years (1947–1952). Med. J. Austral., 1:878–81, June 20, 1953.
62. Löe, Harald, Theilade, Else, and Jensen, S. B. Experimental gingivitis in man. J. Periodont., 36:177–87, May–June 1965.
63. Löe, H., Ånerud, Å., Boysen, H., and Smith, M. The natural history of periodontal disease in man. Study design and baseline data. J. Periodont. Res., 13:550–62, Nov. 1978.
64. ———. The natural history of periodontal disease in man. Tooth mortality rates before 40 years of age. J. Periodont. Res., 13:563–72, Nov. 1978.
65. ———. The natural history of periodontal disease in man: the rate of periodontal destruction before 40 years of age. J. Periodont., 49:607–20, Dec. 1978.
66. Lövdal, Arne, Arnö, Arnulf, and Waerhaug, Jens. Incidence of clinical manifestation of periodontal disease in light of oral hygiene and calculus formation. Am. Dent. A. J., 56:21–33, Jan. 1958.
67. Ludwig, T. G., and Bibby, B. G. Geographic variations in the prevalence of dental caries in the United States of America. Caries Res., 3:32–43, 1969.
68. McEniery, T. M., and Davies, G. N. Brisbane dental survey 1977. A comparative study of caries experience of children in Brisbane, Australia, over a 20-year period. Community Dent. Oral Epidemiol., 7:42–50, Feb. 1979.
69. McGregor, A. B. Changing diet and its effect on caries prevalence in Ghana. Abstr. J. Dent. Res., 42:1086–7, Sept.–Oct. 1963.
70. Mackeprang, Muriel, and Hay, Sylvia. Cleft lip and palate mortality study. Cleft Palate J., 9:51–63, Jan. 1972.
71. Mackeprang, Muriel, Hay, Sylvia, and Lunde, A. S. Completeness and accuracy of reporting of malformations on birth certificates. Health Reports, DHEW, 87:43–9, Jan. 1972.
72. Mäkinen, K. K. The role of sucrose and other sugars in the development of dental caries: a review. Internat. Dent. J., 22:363–86, Sept. 1972.
73. Mandel, I. D. Dental caries. Am. Scientist, 67:680–8, Nov.–Dec. 1979.
74. Mann, A. W., Dreizen, S., Spies, T. D., and Hunt, F. M. A comparison of dental caries activity in malnourished and wellnourished patients. Am. Dent. A. J., 34:244–52, Feb. 15, 1947.
75. Mansbridge, J. N. Heredity and dental caries. J. Dent. Res., 38:337–347, Mar.–Apr. 1959.
76. Marshall Day, C. D. Nutritional deficiencies and dental caries in Northern India. Brit. Dent. J., 76:115–22, Mar. 1944.
77. Marthaler, T. M. Epidemiological and clinical dental findings in relation to intake of carbohydrates. Caries Res., 1:222–38, 1967.
78. Martinsson, T. Socio-economic investigation of school children with high and low caries frequency. III. A dietary study based on information given by the children. Odont. Revy, 23:93–113, 1972.
79. Mellanby, M. Diet and the teeth. Part III. The effect of diet on dental structure and disease in man. London, Medical Research Council, H.M.S.O., 1934. 180 p.
80. Miller, W. D. Agency of micro-organisms in decay of human teeth. Dent. Cosmos, 25:1–12, Jan. 1883.
81. Möller, I. J. Impact of oral diseases across cultures. Internat. Dent. J., 28:376–80, Sept. 1978.

82. Möller, I. J., Pindborg, J. J., and Roed-Petersen, B. The prevalence of dental caries, enamel opacities and enamel hypoplasia in Ugandans. Arch. Oral Biol., 17:9–22, Jan. 1972.
83. Möller, I. J., Poulsen, S., and Nielsen, V. O. The prevalence of dental caries in Godhavn and Scoresbysund districts, Greenland. Scand. J. Dent. Res., 80:169–80, 1972.
84. Moore, W. J., and Corbett, M. E. The distribution of dental caries in ancient British populations. I. Anglo-Saxon period. Caries Res., 5:151–68, 1971.
85. ———. The distribution of dental caries in ancient British populations. II. Iron Age, Romano-British and Mediaeval periods. Caries Res., 7:139–53, 1973.
86. ———. The distribution of dental caries in ancient British populations. III. The 17th century. Caries Res., 9:163–75, 1975.
87. ———. Dental caries experience in man; historical, anthropological and cultural diet-caries relationships, the English experience. p. 3–19. (In Rowe, N. H., ed. Proceedings of a symposium on diet, nutrition, and dental caries. Ann Arbor, University Michigan, 1978. 133 p.)
88. Newbrun, Ernest. Cariology. Baltimore, Williams and Wilkins, 1978. xv + 289 p.
89. Newbrun, E., and Frostell, G. Sugar restriction and substitution for caries prevention. Caries Res., 12(Suppl. 1):65–73, 1978.
90. Newbrun, E., Hoover, C., Mettraux, G., and Graf, H. Comparison of dietary habits and dental health of subjects with hereditary fructose intolerance and control subjects. Am. Dent. A. J., 101:619–26, Oct. 1980.
91. Nizel, A. E., and Bibby, B. G. Geographic variations in caries prevalence in soldiers. Am. Dent. A. J., 31:1619–26, Dec. 1944.
92. Pedersen, P. O. Dental disease in Europe and Greenland. Royal Soc. Health J., 91:88–91, 101. Mar.–Apr. 1971.
93. Pelton, W. J., Pennell, E. H., and Druzina, Anton. Tooth morbidity experience of adults. Am. Dent. A. J., 49:439–45, Oct. 1954.
94. Peterson, J. K. A supervised brushing trial of sodium monofluorophosphate dentrifices in a fluoridated area. Caries Res., 13:68–72, 1979.
95. Pickerill, H. P. The prevention of dental caries and oral sepsis. 3rd ed. London, Baillière, Tindall and Cox, 1923. xi + 340 p.
96. Pindborg, J. J. Epidemiological studies of oral cancer. Internat. Dent. J., 27:172–8, June 1977.
97. Poulsen, S., and Möller, I. J. The prevalence of dental caries, plaque and gingivitis in 3-year-old Danish children. Scand. J. Dent. Res., 80:94–103, 1972.
98. Ranney, R. R. Pathogenesis of periodontal disease. p. 223–300. (In International Conference on Research in the Biology of Periodontal Disease. Chicago, University Illinois School Dentistry, 1977. xxi + 482 p.)
99. Ringelberg, M. L., Matonski, G. M., and Kimball, A. W. Dental caries-experience in three generations of families. J. Pub. Health Dent., 34:174–80, Summer 1974.
100. Rogers, A. H. Evidence for the transmissibility of dental caries. Austral. Dent. J., 22:53–6, Feb. 1977.
101. Russell, A. L., and Ayers, Polly. Periodontal disease and socioeconomic status in Birmingham, Alabama. Am. J. Pub. Health, 50:206–14, Feb. 1960.
102. Russell, A. L., Leatherwood, E. C., Le Van Hien, and Van Reen, Robert. Dental caries and nutrition in South Vietnam. J. Dent. Res., 44:102–11, Jan.–Feb. 1965.
103. Russell, A. L., Leatherwood, E. C., Consolazio, C. F., and Van Reen, Robert. Periodontal disease and nutrition in South Vietnam. J. Dent. Res., 44:775–82, July–Aug. 1965.
104. Russell, A. L. International nutrition surveys: a summary of preliminary dental findings. J. Dent. Res., 42:233–44, Jan.–Feb. 1963.
105. ———. Dental caries and nutrition in Lebanon. J. Dent. Res., 45:957–63, May–June 1966.
106. ———. World epidemiology and oral health. p. 21–39. (In Kreshover, S. J., and McClure, F. J., eds. Environmental variables in oral disease. Washington, D.C., American Association Advancement Science, Publ. no. 81, 1966. xii + 311 p.)
107. ———. Epidemiology of periodontal disease. Internat. Dent. J., 17:282–96, June 1967.
108. ———. Carbohydrates as a causative factor in dental caries: epidemiological evidence. p. 635–44. (In Sipple, H. L., and McNutt, K. W. Sugars in nutrition. New York, Academic Press, 1974. xii + 768 p.)
109. Sardo Infirri, J., and Barmes, D. E. Epidemiology of oral diseases—differences in national problems. Internat. Dent. J., 29:183–90, Sept. 1979.

110. Saxén, Irma. Epidemiology of cleft lip and palate; an attempt to rule out chance correlations. Brit. J. Preven. Soc. Med., 29:103–10, June 1975.
111. ______. Etiological variables in oral clefts. Helsinki, University Helsinki, 1975. 40 p.
112. Schamschula, R. G., Keyes, P. H., and Hornabrook, K. R. W. Root surface caries in Lufa, New Guinea. I. Clinical observations. Am. Dent. A. J., 85:603–8, Sept. 1972.
113. Schamschula, R. G., Barmes, D. E., Keyes, P. H., and Gulbinat, Walter. Prevalence and interrelationships of root surface caries in Lufa, Papua New Guinea. Community Dent. Oral Epidemiol., 2:295–304, Dec. 1974.
114. Schamschula, R. G., et al.: WHO study of dental caries etiology in Papua New Guinea. Geneva, World Health Organization, offset Publ. no. 40, 1978. 199 p.
115. Schei, Olav, Waerhaug, Jens, Lövdal, Arne, and Arnö, Arnulf. Alveolar bone loss as related to oral hygiene and age. J. Periodont., 30:7–16, Jan. 1959.
116. Schlack, C. A., Restarske, J. S., and Dochterman, E. F. Dental status of 71,015 naval personnel at first examination in 1942. Am. Dent. A. J., 33:1141–6, Sept. 1, 1946.
117. Senn, W. W. Incidence of dental caries among aviation cadets. Mil. Surg., 93:461–4, Dec. 1943.
118. Shaw, J. H. Nutrition and dental caries. p. 415–567. (In National Research Council, Committee on Dental Health. Survey of the literature on dental caries. Washington, D.C., Nat. Acad. Sciences—Nat. Res. Council, Publ. 225, 1952. ix + 567 p.)
119. Sheiham, Aubrey. The epidemiology of chronic periodontal disease in Western Nigerian schoolchildren. J. Periodont. Res., 3:257–67, 1968.
120. ______. Dental cleanliness and chronic periodontal disease: studies on populations in Britain. Brit. Dent. J., 120:413–8, Nov. 1970.
121. Silness, Jan, and Löe, Harald. Periodontal disease in pregnancy. II. Correlation between oral hygiene and periodontal condition. Acta. Odont. Scand., 22:121–34, Feb. 1964.
122. Smith, C. J. Global epidemiology and aetiology of oral cancer. Internat. Dent. J., 23:82–93, Mar. 1973.
123. Sullivan, H. R., and Harris, R. The biology of the children of Hopewood House, Bowral, N.S.W. II. Observations extending over five years (1952–1956). 2. Observations on oral conditions. Austral. Dent. J., 3:311–7, Oct. 1958.
124. Takeuchi, M. Epidemiological study on dental caries in Japanese children before, during, and after World War II. Internat. Dent. J., 11:443–57, Dec. 1961.
125. Taylor, G. F., and Marshall-Day, C. D. Osteomalacia and dental caries. Brit. Dent. J., 69:316, Nov. 1940.
126. Todd, Jean E. Children's dental health in England and Wales, 1973. London, Her Majesty's Stationery Office, 1975. vi + 387 p.
127. Todd, J. E., and Whitworth, A. Adult dental health in Scotland, 1972. London, Her Majesty's Stationery Office, 1974. viii + 257 p.
128. Toverud, Guttorm. The influence of war and post-war conditions on the teeth of Norwegian school children. I. Eruption of permanent teeth and status of deciduous dentition. Milbank Mem. Fund Quar., 34:354–430, Oct. 1956.
129. ______. The influence of war and post-war conditions on the teeth of Norwegian school children. II. Caries in the permanent teeth of children aged 7–8 and 12–13 years. Milbank Mem. Fund Quar., 35:127–96, Apr. 1957.
130. ______. The influence of war and post-war conditions on the teeth of Norwegian school children. III. Discussion of food supply and dental condition in Norway and other European countries. Milbank Mem. Fund Quar., 35:373–459, Oct. 1957.
131. U. S. Public Health Service, National Center for Health Statistics. Dental visits; volume and interval since last visit; United States, 1969, by Wilder C. S. DHEW Publ. No. (HSM) 72–1066-Ser. 10–No. 76. Washington, D.C., Government Printing Office, 1972, 37 p.
132. ______. Edentulous persons, United States, 1971, by Burnham, C. E. DHEW Publ. No. (HRA) 74–1516-Ser. 10–No. 89. Washington, D.C., Government Printing Office, 1974. iv + 31 p.
133. ______. Periodontal disease in adults, United States, 1960–1962, by Kelly, J. E., and Van Kirk, L. E. PHS Publ. No. 1000–Ser. 11–No. 12. Washington, D.C., Government Printing Office, 1965. 30 p.
134. ______. Oral hygiene in adults; United States, 1960–1962, by Kelly, J. E., Van Kirk, L. E., and Garst, Caroline C. PHS Publ. No. 1000-Ser. 11-No. 16. Washington, D.C., Government Printing Office, 1966. 30 p.

135. ______. Decayed, missing, and filled teeth in adults, United States, 1960–1962, by Kelley, J. E., Van Kirk, L. E., and Garst, Caroline C. PHS Publ. No. 1000-Ser. 11-No. 23. Washington, D.C., Government Printing Office, 1967. 47 p.
136. ______. Periodontal disease and oral hygiene among children, by Kelley, J. E., and Sanchez, M. J. DHEW Publ. No. (HSM) 72–1060-Ser. 11-No. 117. Washington, D.C., Government Printing Office, 1972. iv + 28 p.
137. ______. Periodontal disease among youths 12–17 years, United States, by Sanchez, M. J. DHEW Publ. No. (HRA) 74–1623-Ser. 11-No. 141. Washington, D.C., Government Printing Office, 1974. iii + 28 p.
138. ______. Decayed, missing, and filled teeth among youths 12–17 years, United States, by Kelley, J. E., and Harvey, C. R. DHEW Publ. No. (HRA) 75–1626-Ser. 11-No. 144. Washington, D.C., Government Printing Office, 1974. iii + 34 p.
139. ______. An assessment of the occlusion of the teeth of youths 12–17 years, United States, by Kelley, J. E., and Harvey, Clair R. DHEW Publ. No. (HRA) 77–1644-Ser. 11-No. 162. Washington, D.C., Government Printing Office, 1977. vi + 65 p.
140. ______. Basic data on dental examination findings of persons 1–74 years, United States, 1971–1974, by Kelly, J. E., and Harvey, C. R. DHEW Publ. No. (PHS)79–1662-Ser. 11-No. 214. Washington, D.C., Government Printing Office, 1979. vi + 33 p.
141. ______. Facts of life and death. Washington, D.C., Government Printing Office, 1967. 33 p.
142. ______. Vital statistics of the United States, 1976. Vol. 11—Mortality, Part B. DHEW Publ. No. (PHS)79–1102. Washington, D.C., Government Printing Office, 1979. 711 p.
143. ______. Facts of life and death. DHEW Publ. No. (PHS)79–1222. Washington, D.C., Government Printing Office, 1979. iv + 47 p.
144. ______. Decayed, missing, and filled teeth among persons 1–74 years, United States 1971–1974 by Harvey, Clair R., and Kelly, J. E. DHHS Publ. No. (PHS) 81–1678–Ser. 11–No. 223. Washington, D.C., Government Printing Office, 1981. iv + 55 p.
145. Waerhaug, Jens. Epidemiology of periodontal disease: a review of literature p. 181–271. (In Ramfjord, S. P., Kerr, D. A., and Ash, M. M. eds. World workshop in periodontics. Ann Arbor, University Michigan, 1966. xv + 458 p.)
146. Wallace, J. S. The cause and prevention of decay in teeth. 2nd ed. London, Churchill, 1902. 108 p.)
147. Zacherl, W. A., and Long, D. M. Reduction in caries attack rate—non-fluoridated community. Abstr. J. Dent. Res., 58(Spec. Issue A):227, Jan. 1979.

III PREVENTION AND CONTROL OF ORAL DISEASES

CHAPTER 7

THE PREVENTION AND CONTROL OF DENTAL CARIES: FLUORIDATION

Wesley O. Young
David F. Striffler
Brian A. Burt

INTRODUCTION

In most Western civilizations, dental caries is a highly prevalent disease (see Chapter 6). As a consequence, control of dental caries is a concern of all of the people and not merely a few. Nevertheless, the fact that it is not a fatal disease imposes constraints upon the methods that may be applied in its control. The Pasteur treatment for rabies, for example, was acceptable for many years despite the definite hazard accompanying its application, because this hazard was slight compared with the much greater danger of death from untreated rabies.

An ideal control measure for dental caries, however, must be devoid of hazard to life or function. It must, of course, be effective. Its potency must be maintained for a substantial time span, preferably for the lifetime of the individual. It should take effect immediately upon application, and it should reach all of the people in the population. Its cost should fall within the means of the community, whether cost is measured in dollars or as a requirement for skilled personnel or facilities. In short, the ideal control measure for dental caries must have immediate, high, and lasting effectiveness, be innocuous, and reach all of the people at a cost in money and facilities well within the economic capabilities of the community.

Some of these requirements are met by timely and competent restorative care. Restorative care, however, is not available to many who are in need,

Some of this chapter is drawn from chapters prepared by A. L. Russell, D.D.S., M.P.H., for the second edition of this text. Dr. Russell, a distinguished epidemiologist, was formerly with the National Institute of Dental Research, U.S. Public Health Service, and later with the School of Public Health, The University of Michigan.

and can prove highly expensive for individual patients and the community (see Chapter 11). Rarely can dental caries in a community be controlled by restorative care alone.

The preventive agent that has so far proved most potent and practicable is the fluoride ion. The most effective and efficient method of bringing the benefits of fluoride to a community is by fluoridation of public water supplies, defined as the adjustment of fluoride in a public water supply to bring its concentration to an optimum level to prevent dental caries. That optimum level is around 1.0 part per million (ppm) in a temperate climate.

The discovery of the role of fluoride in drinking water is an intriguing facet of the history of dentistry. It also illustrates many aspects of the assessment of dental diseases as outlined in Chapters 5 and 6.

A CLASSIC EPIDEMIOLOGICAL STUDY

One of the most brilliant programs ever carried out in the epidemiology of chronic disease was the series of studies that led to the demonstration of the caries-inhibitory properties of fluoridated water.

It began, as is so frequently the case in scientific progress, with the study of something else. That something was a peculiar condition of dental enamel known along the Continental Divide as "Colorado Brown Stain." This condition was considered more of an oddity than a matter of importance. It was harmless enough, though it could be disfiguring in some instances. Frederick S. McKay, fresh from dental school in Philadelphia at the turn of the century, had not encountered the condition before he opened a dental office in Colorado Springs, Colorado. It was distinctly different from the commonplace blotching of enamel (idiopathic enamel opacities) found in every third to fifth person in other areas. As far as McKay knew, it was described nowhere in scientific literature. He determined to find out more, and in 1908, with the encouragement of and some financial aid from the Colorado Springs Dental Society, he began a systematic investigation.

He soon found that the condition was highly prevalent in Colorado Springs and in surrounding El Paso County but that it was to be found only in long-term residents, individuals who had been born there or who had come to the city as infants in arms. The etiological agent, then, was something in the environment that was active during the period of formation of teeth. McKay collaborated with G. V. Black, a major figure in dental history, to write the first detailed description of mottled enamel.[19]

McKay found that mottling was endemic in many other communities along the Divide and the plains to the east. It was quite apt to be found where deep artesian wells were the source of water. Within any community the persons affected had almost invariably been users of the same water supply. No other experience or way of life tended to be shared by all. The conclusion was inescapable: the agent responsible for mottling was some common constituent of the community water supplies.

Yet, a priori, this explanation was unacceptable. Repeated chemical analyses, covering all known elements found in drinking water, failed to discover anything common to all of the waters associated with mottled enamel. Nevertheless, McKay could reach no other conclusion. In communities like Andover and Britton, South Dakota, where mottling was sometimes so extreme that it was disfiguring, he began to advise mothers to obtain water for use by their children from sources other than the community supply. In Oakley, Idaho, McKay found that children living on the outskirts of the city, using water from a private spring, were free of mottling. He advised the citizens of Oakley to abandon their old supply and tap this spring for a new source. In 1925 the community voted a bond issue for mains to bring the spring water into the city—the first known instance of community action to improve dental health by an alteration in the domestic water. Children born in Oakley subsequent to the change were free of mottled enamel.[110]

In 1931, about the time that permanent teeth free of mottling were beginning to erupt in Oakley children, McKay sent several samples of suspected waters to H. V. Churchill, an Alcoa chemist who was applying new methods of spectrographic analysis to water samples. Churchill identified fluoride in each of the samples, in amounts ranging up to 14 ppm.[34] Almost simultaneously, similar findings were announced by Smith, Lantz, and Smith of the University of Arizona,[150] and by Velu and Balozet,[165] who had been studying *le darmous* (the local name given to an extreme degree of dental fluorosis) in Moroccan sheep. The causative agent was identified.

The immediate reaction of the scientific community was one of concern, because fluoride in high concentrations was known to be a protoplasmic poison. The discovery touched off a considerable number of studies to determine whether fluorides in the amounts normally found in the water supply, or elsewhere in the environment, were injurious to human health. But McKay had noted something else—something possibly beneficial—in these fluoride communities. As early as 1928 he felt confident enough to publish his opinion that the prevalence of dental caries actually was reduced in amount by the same waters that produced mottled enamel.[112]

A search of dental literature will uncover the names of many researchers and clinicians predating McKay who speculated that fluoride in tooth enamel might inhibit dental caries.[151] These people failed to develop the idea further, either because the notion seemed to be of no practical importance or because they were inhibited by the technology of their times. By contrast, McKay and a co-worker went on to explore the possibility and then to demonstrate that fluoride ingestion could be adjusted to an optimal intake without hazard to the individual, at small cost, and with a consequent sweeping reduction in the mass prevalence of dental caries. This co-worker was H. Trendley Dean of the United States Public Health Service.

McKay's studies did not end with the advent of Dean. The two men were fast friends and, on occasion, active collaborators. McKay continued to make personal contributions, notably the observation that the caries-inhibitory effect of fluoride water was still discernible in persons as old as 45 years.[111] Dean's work did not begin with the fluoride–dental caries hypothesis either. He had already shown that "mottled" enamel could be manifested in a wide range of degrees, from fine, lacy markings so faint that they could not be seen except in light of just the proper quality and intensity and coming from just the proper angle to an extreme hypoplasia in which the enamel was pitted, stained, and highly friable. He had devised a community index of fluorosis based on seven grades of severity.[40] Later, he modified this index to permit comparisons among populations on a quantitative basis and documented the prevalence of the condition for the United States as a whole[39] (see Chapter 5). These studies served as the groundwork for his later investigations of the fluoride-caries relation.

He had examined schoolchildren for fluorosis in 51 South Dakota communities in 1938.[42] There was a definite inverse relation between the prevalence of fluorosis in these areas and the prevalence of caries as reported in a survey four years earlier. Similar comparisons between Colorado and eight Wisconsin cities showed the same general pattern.[38] This was presumptive evidence that the relation was a true one. A direct test of the hypothesis was designed.

Experience gained in the study of endemic fluorosis indicated that communities to be surveyed must be chosen with great care when the presence and amount of fluoride in the domestic water was of crucial importance. Sound conclusions could be reached only in those communities with a common water supply unaltered during the lifetime of the people to be examined and with a stable fluoride level over a period long enough to establish and define the range of fluctuation.[41] These criteria were satisfied by Galesburg, Monmouth, Macomb, and Quincy–four cities in central Illinois. Galesburg and Monmouth were supplied with waters from wells 2,400 feet deep that averaged, over the course of a year, 1.8 and 1.7 ppm of the fluoride ion. Macomb and Quincy used surface waters averaging 0.2 ppm. Direct examinations were given to 319 children in Galesburg, 148 in Monmouth, 112 in Macomb, and 316 in Quincy. The children were 12 to 14 years of age, with lifetime residence in their respective cities. The prevalence of dental caries was found to be twice as high in the low as in the high fluoride cities.[43] In the words of the investigators, it was

> . . . obvious that whatever effect the waters with relatively high fluoride content (over 2.0 ppm of F) have on dental caries is largely one of academic interest; the resultant permanent disfigurement of many of the users far outweighs any advantage that might accrue from the standpoint of partial control of dental caries. On the other hand, the demonstration of such marked dental caries differences as were observed at Galesburg and Quincy made advisable a quantitative study of the influence on dental caries of waters with lower ranges of fluoride concentration. If marked inhibitory influences were operative at concentration levels as low as the minimal threshold of endemic fluorosis (1.0 ppm), the findings would be of considerable import.[44]

Accordingly, a study was made of children aged 12 to 14 years with lifetime residence in eight suburban Chicago communities with various stable fluoride levels in the domestic waters and later extended to 13 additional cities in Illinois, Colorado, Ohio, and Indiana.[44, 45] This "21 cities" study is considered an epidemiological landmark; its crucial findings are shown graphically in Figures 7–1 and 7–2. Dental caries in these children was related directly to the amount of fluoride in the water they had used from birth:

> Strikingly low dental caries prevalence was found associated with the continuous use of domestic waters whose fluoride (F) content was as low as about 1 part per million, a concentration which under the conditions prevailing in the localities studied produced only sporadic instances of the mildest forms of dental fluorosis of no practical esthetic significance.[45]

This finding in itself did not establish the cause-and-effect relation between fluoridation and reduced prevalence of caries, but it did set the stage for a test of this proposition—provided, of course, that the test could be conducted without hazard to the communities involved.[5] Assurance that this was the case was developed over years of study with people using waters with fluoride levels much higher than the proposed 1.0 ppm.

Four pioneer studies in controlled fluoridation, in which the fluoride concentration in the water supplies of the communities was brought up to 1.0 to 1.2 ppm, were begun in 1945 and 1946. One, under the direction of Dean and his associates, was carried out in Grand Rapids, Michigan.[46] The others,

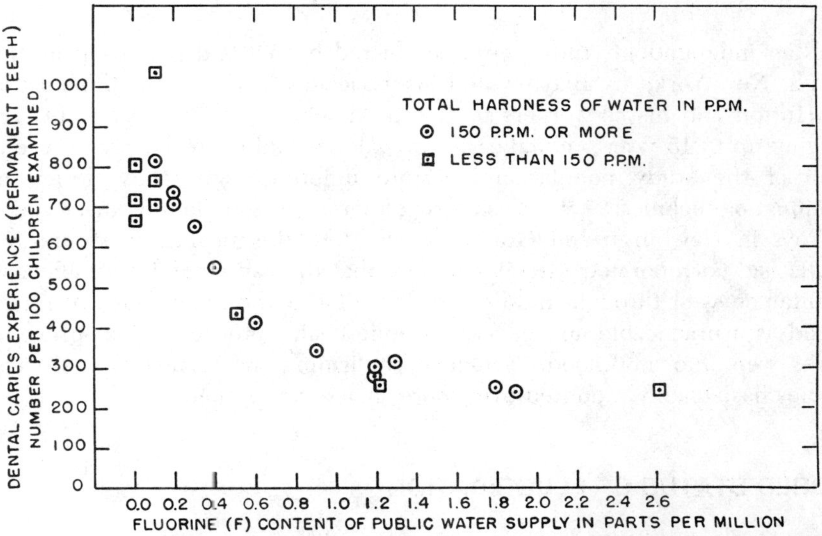

Figure 7–1. Variation in dental caries experience rates observed in 7,257 selected white schoolchildren, aged 12–14 years, in 21 cities of four states, according to fluoride concentration and hardness value of the public water supply. (From Dean, H. T., Arnold, F. A., Jr., and Elvove, Elias. Domestic water and dental caries. V. Additional studies of the relation of fluoride domestic waters to dental caries experience in 4,425 white children, aged 12 to 14 years, of 13 cities in 4 states. Pub. Health Rep., 57:1155–79, Aug. 7, 1942.)

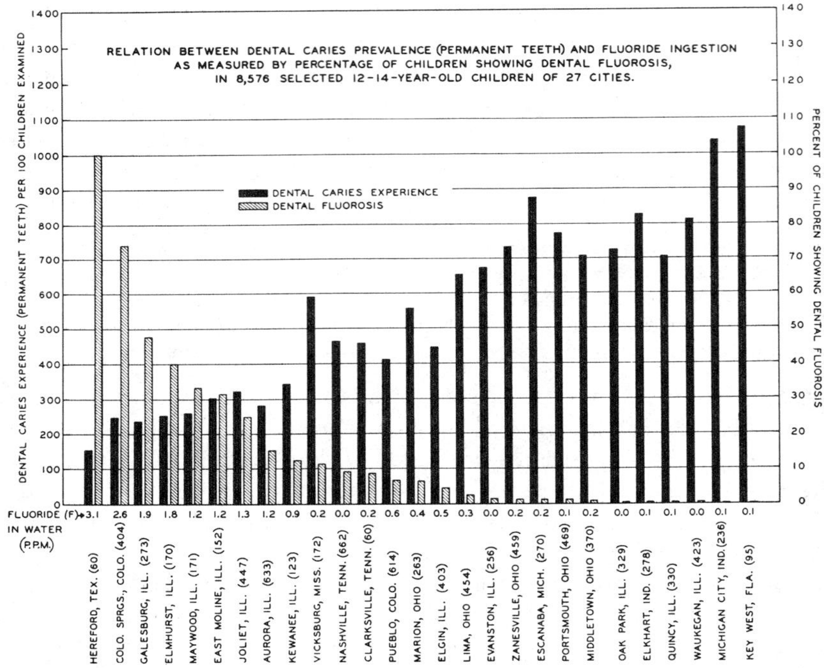

Figure 7–2. Dental caries experience of permanent teeth related to endemic dental fluorosis. (Unpublished data from the files of H. Trendley Dean.)

each an independent study, were conducted by Ast and his group in Newburgh, New York;[7] by Blayney and his associates in Evanston, Illinois;[20] and by Hutton and his co-workers in Brantford, Ontario.[87] At the end of terms ranging up to 15 years, dental caries prevalence had been sharply reduced in each of the study populations, despite differences in study design and examination technics.[4, 6, 21, 88] Disfiguring fluorosis was not found during specific surveys in Newburgh and Grand Rapids.[141] In the meantime, studies with adults had corroborated McKay's finding that the caries-inhibitory effect was maintained well through middle age.[59, 143] Fluoridation had thus been established as a practicable and effective public health procedure that prevented caries well into adulthood. Evidence confirming the results of these early studies has steadily mounted over more than a generation.

WORLD STATUS OF FLUORIDATION

Determination of the number of countries in which fluoridation is operating and the size of the population receiving fluoridated water is not easy. Many countries provide the necessary information to agencies such as the World Health Organization (WHO) or the *Fédération Dentaire Internationale* (FDI), but some of the information is vague. Data here are taken from the 1977 edition of the FDI's *Basic Fact Sheets,*[66] a compendium of summary information on dental health and dental services in member countries, supplied by the dental associations of the countries themselves.

In 1977, there were 38 countries reporting fluoridation projects reaching some 208 million people. Nations with the largest populations receiving fluoridated water were the United States, 108 million; the U.S.S.R., 38.2 million; Canada, 8.4 million; Brazil, 7.5 million; Australia, 6.4 million; Venezuela, 4.4 million; and Chile, 4.3 million. The city-states of Singapore (2.3 million) and Hong Kong (3.9 million) are totally fluoridated. Australia, Canada, Chile, Ireland, New Zealand, Panama, and the United States have one third to one half or more of their populations served by fluoridated water. At the other end of the scale, 13 of the 38 countries reported that only one city in the country was fluoridated (Singapore and Hong Kong not included).

Ireland has a mandatory fluoridation law that successfully withstood a legal challenge that went to the Irish High Court.[114] Brazil has a federal law requiring fluoridation in all communities of 50,000 people or more.[66]

There are also countries where fluoridation has made little headway; Europe particularly has seen slow progress. Moderate progress was seen in the U.S.S.R. (15 per cent of the population), Czechoslovakia, Poland, and Britain, but recent progress in some of these countries has been slow. On the other hand, there is no fluoridation at all in the Federal German Republic (West Germany), Austria, France, Italy, Denmark, and Norway. It is not banned in those countries (except perhaps Denmark, where a law on additives is interpreted to exclude fluoridation) as is sometimes claimed, but the political climate in all of them makes fluoridation a dead issue for now. Sweden, after having one experimental project for some years, repealed the legislation allowing communities to fluoridate.[28] The matter was raised again in 1981 with the appointment by the Swedish Ministry of Health and Social Affairs of a commission to study the subject anew. The commission concluded that fluoridation was safe and effective, but it recommended no change in the law on the grounds of infringement of individual rights and unknown long-term environmental effects, and because caries was declining anyway (Sweden has had school-based preventive fluoride programs for years). There was a dissenting minority opinion attached to this report recommending fluoridation, but it seems that Swedish communities will still not be allowed to fluoridate.[159]

The other main setback in Europe, as opposed to lack of progress, came in the Netherlands, where some excellent pioneering studies had led to the provision of fluoridated water for three million people. Political maneuvers resulted in the cessation of all fluoridation in 1976.[66] The background to this action has been described in *Consumer Reports.*[10]

Fluoridation in the United States

In 1982, fluoridation was estimated to be reaching some 112 million people in the United States, about half of the population.[36] Nearly 11 million of these people were receiving water naturally fluoridated at 0.7 ppm F or more; the greatest concentration of naturally fluoridated communities is found in Texas, Illinois, and New Mexico.[163] Most progress has been made in the bigger cities; the 50 percent of the total population that receives fluoridated water is reached by 13 percent of the water supplies,[101] and 42 of the 50 largest cities are now fluoridated.[36] There are over 700 communities in the United States that have been fluoridating for 25 years or more; many of the naturally fluoridated communities have been using the same water source for more than three generations. The proportion of state populations reached by fluoridation ranges from close to 100 percent in Maryland, Wisconsin, and Tennessee to 2 to 4 percent in Utah and Nevada.

A listing of all fluoridated communities in the United States is given in *Fluoridation Census 1975*, published by the U.S. Public Health Service.[162] A new edition of this work is due by early 1983.

Local, State, and Federal Government Roles in Fluoridation

The decision to fluoridate is usually made by the local community, with varying involvement of state governments. Mandatory state fluoridation laws stand in seven states: Connecticut (the first, passed in 1965), Georgia (1973), Illinois (1967), Nebraska (1973), Minnesota (1967), Ohio (1969), and South Dakota (1969). Three of these states permit exception by referendum, and two have population limits. Two of them have funding provisions for local communities. Michigan and Delaware both had passed mandatory laws in 1968, but neither now stands. Delaware is one of a group of states that require a referendum before a community can fluoridate; the other states in this group are Maine, New Hampshire, Nevada, and Utah. Weak mandatory laws, which may not be enforceable, are in place in Kentucky and Puerto Rico. It is unlikely that any more states will pass mandatory laws requiring fluoridation because the political tenor of the times does not seem to favor legislation of this nature. The mandatory state laws have been generally successful, because fluoridation is well advanced in all states that have them.

The U.S. Public Health Service, first through its Division of Dental Health and then through its Dental Disease Prevention Activity of the Centers for Disease Control in Atlanta, has provided funds and consultative expertise to promote fluoridation. Federal funds were available through the Division of Dental Health in 1965–67, and 13 states used them to begin fluoridation projects. These funds were specifically earmarked for fluoridation, while some federal contract funds had previously been used for demonstration projects.[156] The program funds in the mid-1960s disappeared as the cost of the Vietnam war increased. Again in 1978–81, the Dental Disease Prevention Activity had a budget of up to nine million dollars per year for distribution to states and communities for fluoridation. Some 765 communities, with a population of nearly 11 million, benefited directly.[65]

With the Reagan administration, these funds are now to be consolidated into block grants.[24] Federal funds may therefore still be available to states for fluoridation, but fluoridation will have to compete intrastate with other preventive health programs for its funds. States may decide themselves whether to use these preventive health block grant funds for fluoridation or not. Dentistry has an interest in ensuring that a reasonable share of these funds goes to fluoridation in each state.[157]

PHYSIOLOGY AND METABOLISM OF FLUORIDE

It was stated at the beginning of this chapter that a preventive measure for dental caries must be devoid of hazard to life or function. Fluoridation at or around 1.0 ppm meets that requirement. Dental personnel should have a reasonable knowledge of how fluoride works and what happens to it in the human body, both to be responsible promoters of the measure and to answer the questions of patients and the public who want to learn more about it.

Mechanisms of fluoride's action in preventing dental caries are described briefly in Chapter 8.

Availability

Fluorine is one of the most reactive of elements and is therefore never found naturally in its elemental form. The fluoride ion, however, is abundant in nature and occurs almost universally in soils and waters in varying concentrations. Soil samples have averaged 292 ppm F,[134] and it has been estimated that the earth's crust averages 880 ppm F.[15] Soil fluoride concentration generally increases with depth, though surface concentrations can be unusually high in volcanic areas, where the soil contains material blown out from deep in the earth. Seawater contains 1.2 to 1.4 ppm F.[153] Fresh surface waters generally have very low concentrations, 0.2 ppm F or less, whereas concentrations of up to 29.5 ppm F have been recorded in deep well waters in Arizona.[106] Fluoride's ubiquity in soil and water means that all plants and animals contain fluoride to some extent.

Given this ubiquity, it is difficult to understand how any form of life, on land or in the sea, could have evolved and survived unless it was able to cope with a continuous intake of fluoride from its environment, including feast or surge periods during which the amounts ingested would reach peaks many times higher than the average over a longer period of time. All of the evidence is fully consistent with the proposition. Species for species, the fluoride content of plants remains remarkably constant whether they are grown in soil with much or with little fluoride. There is no consistent difference in the fluoride content of the soft tissues of freshwater and saltwater fish; very little fluoride appears in cow's milk, and the amount is increased only slightly, if at all, by the addition of large amounts of fluorides to the drinking water or grain ration.[105] Negligible amounts of fluoride are stored in human soft tissues, and these concentrations do not rise with increased levels of fluoride in the individual's domestic water.[3, 149] It is clear that no serious imbalance exists between life processes and the ordinary amounts of fluoride acquired from the environment.

Studies on Fluoride and Human Health prior to 1945

There was no certainty about the upper limits of these "ordinary amounts," however, when Dean was carrying out his pioneering studies. Prior to the 1940s, studies of the effects of fluoride in humans had been concerned with massive intakes of fluoride. The most important was the landmark research with cryolite workers studied by Roholm.[137] Some of these men and women had been exposed to heavy concentrations of dust that averaged about 97 percent cryolite (a sodium-aluminum fluoride, Na_3AlF_6). Their daily absorption was estimated at 0.2 to 1.0 mg F per kilogram of body weight (for a person weighing 150 pounds, that is about 14 to 68 mgs F per day). Some workers had been employed as long as 31 years. Under these conditions a number of toxic effects were observed, principally gastric complaints and osteosclerosis. But the amounts inhaled by these workers far exceeded the amounts available from potable waters. Studies were needed to determine whether any undesirable physiological effect, beyond enamel mottling, might be produced by the relatively minute levels of the ion carried by domestic water supplies.

A series of studies in the early 1940s by McClure, a biochemist with the U.S. Public Health Service, answered some fundamental questions. First, examining medical histories of young military draftees and high school boys from many parts of the United States, he found no difference in bone fracture experience among men who had grown up with waters containing a range of fluoride concentrations, from negligible fluoride to 6.0 ppm F.[104]

A second study of equal significance demonstrated that fluoride in urine was "strikingly proportional" to the amount of fluoride in domestic water supplies ranging from 0.5 to 5.1 ppm.[107] This finding was based on determinations on urine samples from men from what were low fluoride areas at that time, such as the District of Columbia, Indianapolis, Chicago, and New Hampshire, against samples of urine from men in high fluoride areas in Texas and Illinois. In addition, no differences between these groups were found with respect to occult blood, albumin, and glucose in the urine. Further balance studies, in which young men lived in rooms controlled for varying temperatures and humidity and received varying amounts of fluoride in food and water, led to the conclusion that the elimination of absorbed fluoride via urine and perspiration is almost complete when the quantities absorbed do not exceed 4.0 to 5.0 mgs daily.[108] McClure suggested that these may be the limits of fluoride that could be ingested daily without "appreciable hazard" of bodily storage of fluoride.

But higher intakes could occur in such communities as Bartlett, Texas, where community water carried about 8.0 ppm F. Accordingly, in 1943, a U.S. Public Health Service team gave detailed physical and oral examinations to a sample of persons who had lived in Bartlett for 15 years or more. There was no indication that this fluoride exposure had had any adverse effect, other than mottling of dental enamel, upon the health or well-being of these people.[100] These and other studies on human population groups were supported by a large body of evidence obtained by direct experimentation with large animals—sheep, swine, and dairy cattle—as well as with numerous experimental laboratory animals, particularly the white rat.

This, in summary, was the state of information at the time the first fluoridation trials were begun in 1945. Research had established that:

1. The healthy human body possessed a prompt and efficient excretory mechanism for fluorides that minimized the danger of long-term accumulation.
2. Skeletal damage, the usual first sign of chronic intoxication from large doses of fluorides, could not be demonstrated in users of fluoride-bearing domestic waters.
3. Large groups of people had used waters carrying up to 8.0 ppm F for long periods of time without impairment of general health.
4. Caries-inhibitory benefits might be expected around 1.0 ppm F, a concentration too low to produce objectionable mottling.

Since that time, a great deal of research has gone into the metabolism of fluoride. This research is well summarized in the 1970 monograph of the World Health Organization, *Fluorides and Human Health*,[170] and the 1979 monograph of the American Association for the Advancement of Science, *Continuing Evaluation of the Use of Fluorides.*[91]

Absorption, Excretion, and Retention

Ingested fluoride is absorbed mainly from the upper gastrointestinal tract. About 80 percent of fluoride in food is absorbed, as is 85 to 97 percent of fluoride in water.[37] Absorption can vary, especially if calcium, magnesium, or aluminum ions are present with the fluoride. These cations will "bind" fluoride and prevent its absorption.[167] Trace amounts of fluoride leave the blood within minutes, concentrating in bone and the kidneys. Most ingested fluoride is excreted by healthy individuals in the urine,[92] with about half of it excreted in urine within 24 hours.[167]

Fluoride has an affinity for the calcified tissues, i.e., bone and developing teeth. Fluoride that is not excreted is deposited in these hard tissues, though storage is dynamic rather than inert. Bone fluoride levels range from 800 to 10,000 ppm, depending on many factors, including age and fluoride intake.[166] Fluoride levels in outer enamel layers range from 400 to 3,000 ppm and decrease rapidly with greater depth. Fluoride concentrations in soft tissue rise or fall parallel to serum levels, but because the excretion and deposition mechanisms operate so rapidly there is negligible retention of fluoride in the soft tissue fluids.[167] Some fluoride has been found in the aorta, apparently associated with calcification of that blood vessel.[149] Deposition in the placenta is also associated with islets of calcified tissue.[63] A greater proportion of ingested fluoride is excreted in older persons than in the young.[167]

Blood serum contains organic and inorganic fluoride compounds. Organic fluoride in serum appears to be independent of the fluoride concentration in drinking water.[77] Absorbed fluoride is transported by the blood serum as inorganic fluoride; it is this inorganic fluoride that is cleared quite rapidly. Most blood fluoride is organic, so that some earlier analyses of total blood fluoride relative to fluoride intake are now considered invalid.[77] In healthy adults, serum fluoride levels are around 0.02 ppm F. In persons with chronic kidney failure it can be 0.05 to 0.09 ppm.[92]

The only disease condition requiring special consideration in regard to fluoride use is chronic kidney failure. The importance of renal clearance in the body's regulatory mechanism means that when kidneys are not functioning properly, the amount of fluoride stored in the body can increase. Whereas fluoride concentration in bone increases steadily with age in all persons, these levels can become excessive in persons with long-term chronic kidney failure. Checks on serum fluoride concentration of kidney patients can help determine if the fluoride intake of the patient should be reduced. Kidney patients who receive dialysis for long periods with distilled fluoride-free water have maintained serum fluoride levels of 0.06 ppm F, whereas some dialyzed with fluoridated water have recorded levels of 0.24 ppm F. Serum fluoride levels of around 0.09 ppm F have been suggested as the upper limit before a dialyzing kidney patient should reduce fluoride intake, although evidence for this recommendation comes only from a few case studies.[92] As a precautionary measure, fluoride-free dialysate should be used for patients maintained by dialysis for long periods, though there is insufficient evidence to recommend the use of fluoride-free drinking water for all patients with renal disease.[92]

Fluoride is not the only mineral of concern in renal dialysis—iron, for example, is of greater concern. Responsible dialysis treatment centers ensure that deionized water is used as dialysate for all patients.

Sources of Fluoride Intake

Fluoride's abundance in soils and plants means that all animals and humans consume fluoride to some extent. Numerous studies have attempted to estimate the average daily intake of fluoride from all sources. The results are not entirely consistent, reflecting both the variability of the human diet and different analytical methods used when such minute amounts are being analyzed.[161] A reasonable estimate for an adult male is 1.0 to 3.0 mgs F per day from food alone, increasing to 2.0 to 5.0 mgs F per day in a fluoridated area.[153] This range, however, can easily be exceeded by particular individuals—the authors have heard the story, attributed to Professor Neil Jenkins, of a retired gentleman in Newcastle, England, whose daily intake was around 12 mgs F daily. This vigorous old gentleman was in the habit of drinking some 22 cups of tea daily (tea is rich in fluoride and Newcastle's water is fluoridated), plus imbibing up to eight pints of Newcastle Brown Ale (also made with fluoridated water) in the local pub each evening. Little of this fluoride intake was retained: urinalysis showed about 11 mgs F daily was excreted.

It has been suggested that dietary intake of fluoride may be increasing because of the amount of processed food and drink now prepared with fluoridated water. Taves[161] found no evidence to support this notion, but agreed that analytical methods were not sufficiently precise to allow valid comparisons of recent data with that of 20 years or so ago. If an increase has occurred in that period, it is likely to be less than 10 percent.[161]

Dental Fluorosis

Studies in areas fluoridated at 1.0 ppm have shown that 7 to 16 percent of children born and reared in the area exhibit mild or very mild dental fluorosis.[8, 39, 141] Actually, the use of the term "fluorosis" in this context is misleading because teeth in the mild and very mild categories are aesthetically pleasing rather than unsightly.[49] Perhaps the older term of "mild mottling" might be better here. No fluorosis rated as moderate or worse, that is with some degree of brown stain, has been reported in areas fluoridated at 1.0 ppm unless other forms of fluoride (e.g., dietary supplements) have been given as well.

Fluoride Toxicity

Claims that fluoridation is harmful rather than beneficial to human health have constantly bedeviled the progress of fluoridation. Dental personnel need to be aware that in high concentrations fluoride can be hazardous. They should be equally aware that there is a world of difference between a single intake of 5.0 grams and constant intake of 2.0 to 5.0 mgs F daily. Fluoride is thus like many other nutrients—beneficial in small amounts, toxic in high amounts.

Information on fluoride toxicity levels cannot of course be taken from controlled studies with humans. Available data are from a mix of case studies of various kinds and research on workers in certain industrial processes, such as those studied by Roholm.[137]

Ingestion of 2.5 to 5.0 grams F (5.0 to 10 grams of sodium fluoride) by an adult male results in a rather unpleasant death within two to four hours if first aid is not applied immediately. The estimated equivalent dose for a 10-kilogram child (about a one-year-old) is 535 mgs F.[82] Crippling skeletal fluorosis can eventually occur in an adult if 10 to 25 mgs F are ingested or inhaled daily for a period of 10 to 20 years. The potentially toxic effects of fluoride ingestion are summarized in Table 7–1.

If an individual is known or suspected to have taken a potentially toxic amount of fluoride, first aid consists of inducing vomiting as quickly as possible or ingesting a material to bind fluoride—milk is usually the most readily available.

Table 7–1. Degrees of Potentially Toxic Ingestion of Fluoride

Effect	Fluoride Intake, Time*
Acute fatal poisoning, adults†	2.5–5.0 grams, 2–4 hours
Acute fatal poisoning, 10 kg child†	535 mgs, 2–4 hours
Acute fatal poisoning, 3-year-old child‡	Approx. 435 mgs, approx. 3 hours
Acute fatal poisoning, adult renal dialysis patient§	Dialysate fluid 35–50 ppm F, for 3 hours
Short-term nonserious nausea in elementary schoolchildren‖	93–375 ppm F in drinking water, small amounts; symptoms within 30 minutes
Severe skeletal fluorosis†	10–25 mgs F daily, 10–20 years
Osteosclerosis, radiographic changes in human bone¶	8–20 mgs F daily, 10–20 years
Dental fluorosis¶	2–8 mgs F daily in first 8 years
Acute fatal poisoning in animals†	Approx. 50 mgs F/kg body weight
Interference with reproduction, thyroid disturbance, loss of body weight, and lameness in cattle†	40–60 ppm F in feed daily for several years

*With drinking water fluoridated at 1.0 ppm, an adult would have to drink 660 gallons in two to four hours to reach the lower limit of a fatal dose. The 10 kg child (about a one-year-old) would have to drink 115 gallons in two to four hours. Severe skeletal fluorosis could only result from drinking 2.6 to 6.6 gallons of water daily for 10 to 20 years if none of the fluoride was excreted.

†Hodge, 1979.[82]

‡Horowitz, 1977.[86]

§Morbidity and Mortality Weekly Report (MMWR), 1980.[116]

‖Hoffman et al., 1980.[83]

¶Hodge and Smith, 1965.[81]

The American Dental Association (ADA) has recommended, as a safety precaution, that fluoride materials for home use contain no more than 264 mgs F if packaged in a bulk container (tablets, mouthrinse) or up to 300 mgs F if the material is individually packaged.[2]

On the other hand, there are many instances of remarkable toleration of high quantities of fluoride without ill effects. Osteoporosis patients have received 30 to 70 mgs F per day for years under supervision, usually given with calcium so that not all the fluoride was unbound. Adverse effects are generally no worse than nausea, stomach pains, and occasional diarrhea. The greatly elevated levels of serum fluoride may be associated with some arthritic-type joint pain, but it is not certain whether these pains come from the treatment or the disease itself.[93]

While all dental personnel should be aware of these details, accidents involving fluoride since 1945 have been extremely rare.[82] It can be stated that municipal water fluoridated at 1.0 ppm, or even considerably higher, carries zero risk of any acute toxic reaction and no risk of a chronic toxic reaction apart from mottled dental enamel at higher concentrations.

FLUORIDATION AND HUMAN HEALTH

Like many nutrients, fluoride is beneficial in small amounts but toxic in large quantities, the concept of "dose-response." It has been declared an essential human nutrient by the Food and Nutrition Board of the National

Research Council, the group that provides the recommended dietary allowances for all nutrients.[121]

Few public health measures have been subjected to the degree of research on safety that fluoridation has received. Some of the studies relative to human health have been described. The Newburgh-Kingston fluoridation project, one of the "original four," included a medical component. Participating children received a complete physical examination, selected physical measurements, and laboratory and radiographic studies. Complete histories were also taken. No significant difference in general health between children in the two cities was seen at annual or final examinations. Height and weight were the same, and the onset of menstruation came at equivalent ages. No differences in bone density could be demonstrated in radiographs of the right hand, the knees, and the lumbar spine. There was essential similarity in vision and hearing tests and in findings for skeletal maturation, hemoglobin level, erythrocyte and leukocyte counts, and quantity of sugar, albumin, red blood cells, and casts in urine. On the final examination, 19 of 476 children in Newburgh (4.0 percent) and 20 of 405 children in Kingston (4.9 percent) were referred to the family physician for conditions including such minor ailments as a plantar wart or ringworm. Long-term downward trends in stillbirth and maternal and infant mortality rates continued in each of the cities. Each had about the same experience with deaths from cancer and from cardiovascular-renal disease. The overall conclusion reached was: "No differences of medical significance could be found between the two groups of children"; thus, further evidence was added to that already available on the safety of water fluoridation.[145]

Meanwhile, investigations by health departments within such states as Illinois had shown no differences in health between persons living in fluoride and nonfluoride areas For the United States as a whole no differences could be found in death rates for 1949–50 between 32 cities with established water fluoride levels of 0.7 ppm or more and 32 randomly selected nearby cities with valid histories of 0.25 ppm F or less in the domestic supply. Mortality rates were about the same for cancer, heart disease, intracranial lesions, nephritis, and cirrhosis of the liver.[78]

More recently, mortality rates for 478 cities with populations of 25,000 or more were examined for the periods 1949–50, 1959–61, and 1969–71. Data were collected on total deaths, as well as cardiovascular-renal disease deaths, heart disease deaths, and cancer deaths. The evidence indicated that fluoridation neither increased nor decreased overall mortality or mortality for the three specific causes of death studied.[146] The stimulus for this analysis came from testimony before a Congressional Committee, in 1975, by Burk and Yiamouyiannis, that fluoridation led to an increase in deaths due to cancer.[25] At the time, Dr. Yiamouyiannis was an executive of the National Health Federation, an organization backed by health-food stores and related interests and noted for its opposition to fluoridation. Dr. Burk was a former official at the National Cancer Institute of the National Institutes of Health. Their argument was based on mortality data from the 10 largest fluoridated American cities between 1950 and 1970 compared with 10 other selected nonfluoridated cities over the same period. The crude mortality data, unadjusted for age, sex, or race, showed a greater increase in cancer deaths in the fluoridated cities compared with the nonfluoridated cities over the 20-year period.

Criticism of this analysis was based on the inappropriateness of the crude mortality data, because the populations of the big cities during that 20-year period had become older and changed their ethnic composition. Yiamouyiannis and Burk repeated their work in 1977, this time with some age adjustment.[171] They claimed that their data still showed an excess of cancer deaths in the fluoridated cities, though reduced from the first report. A number of independent analyses of the same data, in both Britain and the United States, employed more detailed age-sex-race adjustments and failed to reach the same conclusions as Yiamouyiannis and Burk.[51, 62, 84, 125, 136, 155]

The alleged cancer-fluoridation link was not new at this time; similar charges had been made for years. In previous years, however, no substantive data were put forward to support the charge. Over the years, opponents have claimed that fluoridation causes just about every affliction known, but none of these charges has been substantiated with evidence of harm to humans from water fluoridated at 1.0 ppm.

One such allegation, still heard from time to time, is that fluoridation causes an increase in the congenital malformation known as Down's syndrome (mongolism). This allegation began with a series of papers by Rapaport, formerly of the University of Wisconsin, published in Paris.[128-130] Rapaport claimed to show from birth records in Wisconsin and Illinois that the incidence of mongolism was higher in fluoridated than in nonfluoridated areas. Rapaport, however, made several serious errors in his research design. These have been described by Russell.[142] The most serious error was to assume that the city of birth was the place of residence of the mother, which is clearly not the case in areas with a large rural population. In addition, Rapaport's data on fluoride content of water supplies were frequently erroneous and out-of-date. More rigorous independent studies in the United States and England have failed to show any correlation between fluoridation and Down's syndrome.[18, 61, 122]

Research on fluoride's effect on the human organism should continue because there are still some unknown factors. But bearing in mind that adults, on average, ingest 2.0 to 5.0 mgs F per day in their normal diets, that 10 to 11 million Americans (and many other peoples around the world) have been drinking naturally fluoridated water, at 1.0 ppm or more, for generations, and that over 100 million Americans have been drinking fluoride-supplemented water for years, there is a great deal of empirical evidence that suggests that fluoridation at 1.0 ppm is not harmful. Certainly it leads to no serious ill health. Allegations of various sensitivity reactions are heard, but efforts to prove cause and effect have not been successful. Western scientific method, upon which technological advances are based, cannot "prove a negative," so experiments cannot be designed to prove that fluoridation causes no harm. The occasional allegation of a sensitivity reaction should be investigated seriously, but with the passage of time the probability becomes nearer to 100 percent that fluoridation at 1.0 ppm is beneficial and produces no undesirable side effects.

Drinking Water Standards

The U.S. Environmental Protection Agency (EPA) has the responsibility for setting national standards for acceptable drinking water under the Safe Drinking Water Act (PL 93–523). Most of these standards deal with defining acceptable levels of bacterial and chemical contaminants. In the standards promulgated in 1975–76 (the National Interim Primary Drinking Water Regulations), the EPA made reference to naturally occurring fluoride above 2.0 ppm as a "contaminant," requiring removal from drinking waters. This standard was obviously well intended, with the goal of reducing dental fluorosis in affected areas, but it received a great deal of criticism. Some opponents of fluoridation misinterpreted it to say that "the EPA has said that fluoride is a contaminant." A more practical reason for opposition from public authorities was the cost of defluoridating or changing sources of drinking water. Defluoridation, the removal of excessive amounts of naturally occurring fluoride from a water supply, is a more expensive process than fluoridation. Many communities that use drinking water naturally fluoridated at more than 2.0 ppm are small and unable to bear the cost of meeting the standard. The state of South Carolina, for example, in requesting the repeal of the 2.0 ppm F "contaminant" ceiling, estimated that it would cost some $12 million to comply. Perhaps most important, few of the small communities concerned were interested in defluoridating—the degree of fluorosis they had did not concern them and they did not suffer any other ill effects, so why bother?

The Interim Primary Drinking Water Regulations of 1980[60] left the upper limit of 2.0 ppm F but included an explanatory statement that this standard did not contradict the beneficial effects of fluoride in reducing dental decay. Whether this statement really helped clarify things, especially since the rather unfortunate word "contaminant" was retained, is questionable.

With the Safe Drinking Water Act due for renewal in 1982, considerable public discussion is being held on redefining standards. Some want all reference to fluoride taken out. Others say the maximum "contaminant" level should be raised to, say, 3.0 ppm F (which would excuse about three quarters of the communities now required to defluoridate) and that the existing 2.0 ppm F maximum level be made a Secondary Standard, meaning a nonenforceable regulation—in practical terms, a guideline.

This debate illustrates the difficulty of establishing public policy in areas in which effects are not clear-cut. Should the control of fluorosis be a subject for national standards, or should these standards be confined to more "serious" matters? Should states set their own standards, or should fluorosis be left to local initiative? Is there any rationale for saying a community with 2.1 ppm F in its drinking water must defluoridate, while a community with 1.9 ppm F does not have to? Other questions arise readily. Even with the renewal of the Safe Drinking Water Act, this debate is likely to continue.

DENTAL BENEFITS OF FLUORIDATION

Fluoridation studies are numerous in the United States and in many other countries. These studies vary widely in their design and operation, but they are remarkably uniform in their results. The conclusion from this mass of information is that fluoridation reduces the prevalence of dental caries in children by 50 to 70 percent, depending on the ages studied. Over a lifetime, fluoridation has been estimated to reduce caries by about 40 percent.[90] There is little doubt that fluoridation has been an important factor in the reduction in caries prevalence in the United States, as was noted in Chapter 6.

A summary of results of the original four studies is shown in Table 7–2. After terms ranging up to 15 years of fluoridation, DMF teeth in children aged 12–14 or 13–14 years were lowered by 48, 56, 57, and 70 percent to a level of three or four DMF teeth per child. These were independent studies, utilizing different procedures. The Grand Rapids and Brantford data were based on mirror-and-explorer examinations. Mirror-and-explorer examinations were supplemented with radiographs in Newburgh, and radiographic examination was supplemented with mirror-and-explorer examinations in Evanston.

Newbrun has reviewed and analyzed several studies in other countries.[123, 124] Caries reductions in Canada, Australia, Britain, New Zealand, the Netherlands, and the German Democratic Republic (East Germany) are all in the 44 to 60 percent range. The World Health Organization (WHO) reports that similar reductions following fluoridation have been found in Brazil, Chile, Colombia, Czechoslovakia, Finland, Ireland, Japan, Switzerland, and the U.S.S.R.[169]

The first fluoridation studies were designed on the hypothesis that no caries inhibition would be seen in children born prior to the time of fluoridation. But instead in these children there was an almost immediate

Table 7–2. General Comparison of DMF Teeth per Child, and Missing Teeth per Child, at the End of the Study Term in Four Pioneer Fluoridation Communities*

Community	Year	DMF Teeth per Child	Percent Difference	Missing Teeth per Child	Percent Difference
Grand Rapids (F)	1944–45	9.58		0.84	
Ages 12–14	1959	4.26	−55.5	0.29	−65.5
Evanston (F)	1946	9.03		0.19	
Ages 12–14	1959	4.66	−48.4	0.06	−68.4
Sarnia (No F)	1959	7.46		0.75	
Brantford (F)	1959	3.23	−56.7	0.22	−70.7
Ages 12–14					
Kingston (No F)	1960	12.46		0.92	
Newburgh (F)	1960	3.73	−70.1	0.10	−89.1
Ages 13–14					

*Adapted from Ast and Fitzgerald.[6] Grand Rapids and Newburgh started fluoridation in 1945. Evanston and Brantford started fluoridation in 1946. Sarnia and Kingston are fluoride-deficient.

downward trend in mean numbers of DMF permanent teeth, demonstrable in most instances after two years of study. In younger children this effect was due almost entirely to a reduction in occlusal caries in permanent first molars that had been in eruption at the time of fluoridation. This advantage was largely lost within the next few years, though the important protection for smooth surfaces of these teeth was demonstrable eight years later.[11, 13, 144] The principal benefits were enjoyed by children who were born as the fluoridation study began or thereafter.[33, 67, 75, 85, 94]

Benefits in Adulthood

Fluoridation does not just benefit children; the cariostatic mechanism appears to provide permanent prevention rather than just a delay. In Colorado Springs, Colorado, for example (where McKay's curiosity first started things), it was possible to demonstrate that the physical characteristics of the water supply had not varied in any essential manner for 70 years prior to 1950.[143]

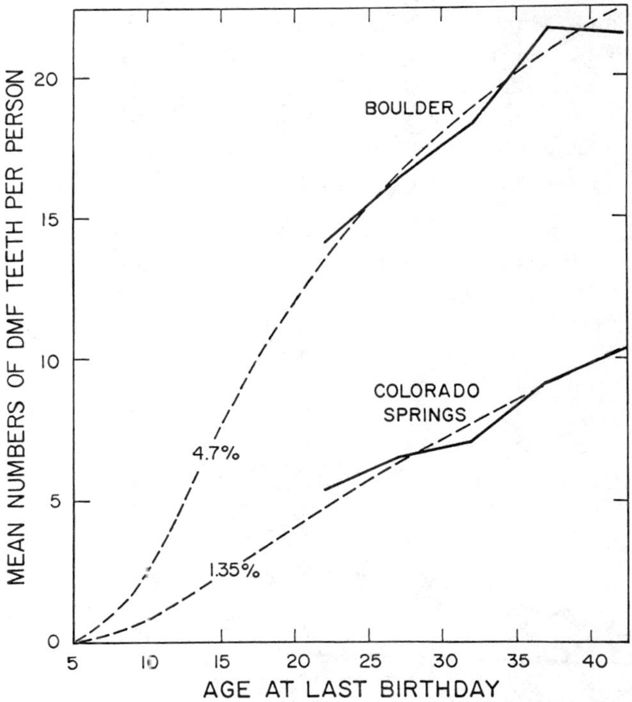

Figure 7–3. Dental caries experience of native-born residents of Colorado Springs, Colorado, with lifetime use of a fluoride-bearing water, and of Boulder, Colorado, with lifetime use of a fluoride-deficient water. The dotted lines represent estimates of the permanent tooth attack rate per year in each population. (From Russell, A. L., and Elvove, Elias. Domestic water and dental caries. VII. A study of the fluoride-dental caries relationship in an adult population. Pub. Health Rep., 66:1389–401, Oct. 26, 1951.)

Nor had there been any important fluctuation in fluoride levels for the period between 1906 and 1930, because groups of native residents aged 20–44 years in 1950 showed essentially the same degree of dental fluorosis throughout that age range. It was also possible to demonstrate that the city water of Boulder, Colorado (less than 100 miles away), had been almost fluoride-free over this same span of time. Dental caries status of lifelong residents of the two cities, aged 20–44 years, is shown in Figure 7–3. Differences in tooth mortality are shown in Figure 7–4. Throughout the age range studied, Colorado Springs natives showed about 60 percent fewer decayed, missing, and filled permanent teeth than did natives of Boulder, who had lost three or four times as many permanent teeth. The oldest Colorado Springs group (aged 40–44 years) had fewer DMF teeth per person than the youngest Boulder group (aged 20–24 years). Under these circumstances the caries-inhibitory effect, so similar to that previously demonstrated in children, persisted without apparent diminution through the age of 44 years, with no suggestion that it might be lost after that time.[139, 143] Benefits were apparent in all teeth throughout life, from the most susceptible (Table 7–3) to the least susceptible (Fig. 7–5). Similar benefits extending into adulthood were demonstrated in Aurora, Illinois, a city naturally fluoridated at 1.2 ppm.[59]

In England, Murray[119, 120] examined the effects of fluoridated water on adults up to 65 years old. He compared the dental status of adults in Hartlepool, a city with a low socioeconomic status and 1.5 to 2.0 ppm F naturally present in its water, with that of adults in York, a city with a higher socioeconomic status and 0.2 ppm F in its drinking water. At all age groups from 15 to 65, DMF values were higher in York. The proportion of adults

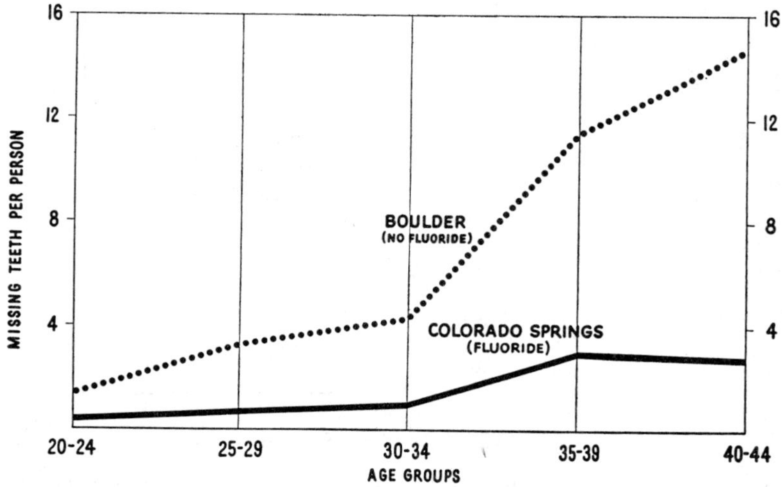

Figure 7–4. Permanent tooth mortality from all causes in adult natives of a fluoride-deficient community (Boulder, Colorado) and of a community with 2.5 ppm F in the water supply (Colorado Springs, Colorado). (From Russell, A. L., and Elvove, Elias. Domestic water and dental caries. VII. A study of the fluoride-dental caries relationship in an adult population. Pub. Health Rep., 66:1389–401, Oct. 26, 1951.)

Table 7–3. Status of Permanent First Molar Surfaces in Lifelong Residents of Boulder, Colorado (with Negligible Fluoride in the Community Water), and of Colorado Springs, Colorado (with an Average Fluoride Content of 2.5 ppm in the Community Water)*

			Average Numbers of First Molar Surfaces per Person					
				Mandibular			Maxillary	
Location	**Ages**	**Numbers Examined**	*Missing*	*Decayed or Filled*	*Present and Sound*	*Missing*	*Decayed or Filled*	*Present and Sound*
Boulder (fluoride-deficient)								
	20–24	51	1.08	3.98	4.94	1.47	3.47	5.06
	25–29	41	3.17	3.80	3.03	1.10	4.37	4.53
	30–34	29	3.28	3.90	2.82	2.41	3.21	4.38
	35–44	34	6.62	2.21	1.17	5.15	2.65	2.20
Colorado Spings (2.5 ppm F)								
	20–24	72	.42	1.80	7.78	.28	1.04	8.68
	25–29	101	.89	1.74	7.37	.64	1.28	8.08
	30–34	82	.98	2.00	7.02	.61	1.69	7.70
	35–39	75	1.86	1.62	6.52	1.40	1.56	7.04
	40–44	55	1.91	2.06	6.03	2.73	1.56	5.71

*Russell, A. L. Measures available for the prevention and control of dental caries. p. 89–125. (In Young, W. O., and Striffler, D. F. The dentist, his practice, and his community. 2nd ed. Philadelphia, Saunders, 1969. xiii + 346 p.)

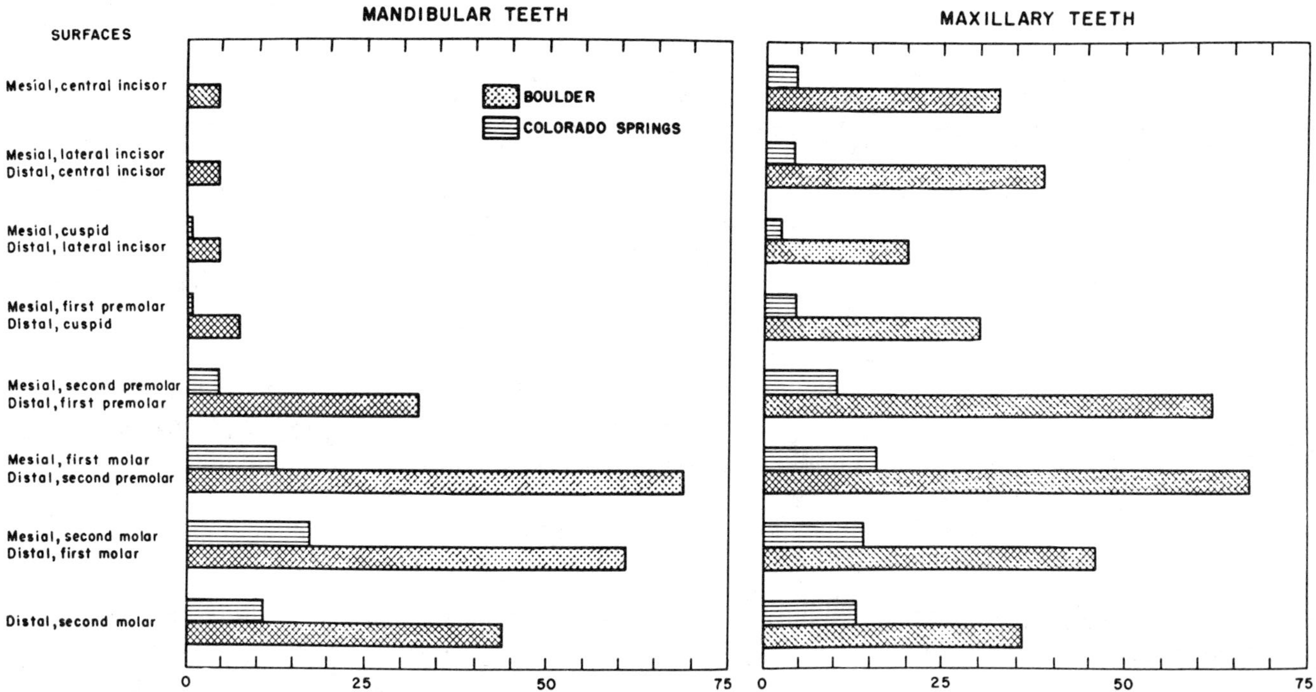

Figure 7–5. Percentages of approximal surfaces that are decayed, filled, or missing because of dental caries in adults aged 25 to 34 years in Boulder, Colorado (using a fluoride-deficient drinking water), and in Colorado Springs, Colorado (using a water with 2.5 ppm of fluoride). (From Russell, A. L. The inhibition of approximal caries in adults with lifelong fluoride exposure. J. Dent. Res., 32:138–43, Feb. 1953.)

edentulous in York was 23.6 percent; in Hartlepool, 11.7 percent. Among dentate persons, there were more teeth lost per person in York in every age group. Separated into two broad age categories, these dental data show some interesting patterns (Table 7–4). The proportion of edentulous in the 15–34 age group was eight times greater in York than in Hartlepool, but little different in the 35–65 group. Among the dentate, there were more teeth missing, on average, among York residents in both age groups. If the edentulous are more likely to be those not interested in their dental health, while dentate persons are assumed to have a greater interest in their oral welfare, it can be concluded that fluoridation has a protective effect against caries up to age 34, even among those without much interest in their oral health. After age 35, however, when periodontal disease becomes the greatest reason for tooth loss (see Chapter 6), fluoridation does little to prevent loss of teeth among this group. Among the dentate, however, Hartlepool residents retain more teeth at all ages, suggesting that with some interest in oral health the benefits of fluoridation are maintained at least to age 65.

These conclusions might be firmer if more data were available, such as on oral hygiene status, amount of periodontal disease, and utilization of services. York was the higher socioeconomic community, with a considerably more favorable dentist:population ratio. The data in Table 7–4 suggest, however, that fluoridation offers a powerful benefit even to those uninterested in dental health. Furthermore, they confirm Russell's earlier finding[140] that fluoridation has little impact on periodontal disease. (Topical fluoride therapy may be useful in plaque control for the individual patient—see Chapter 9. Existing evidence, however, does not suggest any such role for water fluoridation.)

More recently, adults in a fluoridated area were found to have considerably less root caries than adults in a nonfluoridated area.[152] This finding is important, because with an aging population that keeps more teeth longer, the prevalence of root caries is likely to increase and become a greater treatment problem than it is now. Fluoridation is likely to be a powerful influence in its control.

A medical benefit of fluoridation throughout life is likely to be its influence in controlling osteoporosis, the bone-fragility condition seen in some older persons, especially older women. Although not yet conclusive, evidence is

Table 7–4. Edentulousness and Tooth Loss among Dentate Persons, for 2,135 Adults in Hartlepool (1.5 to 2.0 ppm F) and 2,639 Adults in York (0.2 ppm F), England*

	Hartlepool		York	
Age Group	*Percent Edentulous*	*Mean Missing Teeth in Dentate*	*Percent Edentulous*	*Mean Missing Teeth in Dentate*
15–34	0.4	1.9	3.2	3.6
35–65	32.3	5.9	35.8	9.0
All	11.7	2.9	23.6	6.5

*Murray, 1971.[119, 120]

increasing that regimens of fluoride (50 to 60 mgs/day) with calcium and estrogen can prevent osteoporosis in older women.[93, 133] The role of water fluoridation in this picture may not be major but is likely to be of some benefit.

Another medical benefit may follow an intriguing report that suggests that fluoridation may be associated with reduced prevalence of Alzheimer's disease, the senility seen in some older persons and now recognized as a disease rather than a normal consequence of aging.[154] The authors suggest that the mechanism may be the affinity of fluoride to bind aluminum; the presence of aluminum ions in brain tissue has been observed in patients suffering from Alzheimer's disease.

Prenatal Benefits

Some disagreement has existed about whether fluoridation produces dental benefits in the developing fetus. One report from the Evanston fluoridation study, for example, showed that children who received fluoridated water *in utero* as well as postnatally had fewer carious lesions than those who received it only postnatally.[22] Other authorities, however, have not found this effect.[11, 85] In an exhaustive review, Driscoll[56] concluded that there was probably no prenatal benefit because (1) the most caries-susceptible teeth had not calcified before birth, and (2) the placenta acted as a partial barrier to fluoride's reaching the fetus. Driscoll, however, was unable to rule out completely the possibility of some prenatal benefit.

It is clear that fluoridation is quite safe for the developing fetus; no special precautions for expectant mothers are needed in a fluoridated area.

Effects on Different Tooth Surfaces

Fluoridation reduces the prevalence of caries in children by 50 to 70 percent overall, but it has differing effects on different tooth surfaces. Studies in New Zealand and the Netherlands have shown that the greatest benefit, approaching 90 percent, is found on buccal and lingual smooth surfaces. Proximal surfaces benefit about 55 percent; pit-and-fissure surfaces get least benefit, about 30 to 40 percent.[13, 103] Murray's study of 15-year-olds in Hartlepool and York, England, found that those in Hartlepool had a mean DMF of 4.96, whereas those in York had a mean DMF of 8.95 (44.6 percent less). But the number of carious approximal surfaces of molars was 11 times greater in York.[118]

Effects on the Primary Dentition

Fluoridation reduces caries in the primary dentition[6, 80, 97, 160] to about the same extent as is found in the permanent dentition. Caries reductions reported are in the general range of 25 to 55 percent, but different reporting methods make it difficult to specify more than that.

Partial Exposure to Fluoridation

The concentration of about 1.0 ppm F is regarded as optimum for maximum caries reduction with minimum fluorosis. Many communities, however, have water naturally fluoridated at suboptimum levels, such as 0.4 to 0.7 ppm F. Some benefits still accrue in such instances, and dental benefits are generally proportional to the fluoride concentration.[58] A decision on whether it is worth fluoridating a community whose water contains, say, 0.6 ppm F is not easily made. The cost of fluoridating may not necessarily be worth the additional dental benefits expected.

Further evidence of the benefits of partial exposure comes from three communities where fluoridation started and stopped some years later. The three communities are in Scotland, East Germany, and Wisconsin.[48, 98, 99] In each instance a decline in caries prevalence was seen in young children after fluoridation began, but this decline was not continued after fluoridation stopped.

The United States is a highly mobile society. Many people have therefore spent part of their lives in a fluoridated area and part in a nonfluoridated area. The benefit of part exposure to fluoridated water in adulthood is not known, but there is some evidence that partial exposure in childhood confers some benefit, proportional to the length of exposure. This effect was found in the interim and final reports of the Newburgh-Kingston study.[6, 8] More recently, a study of children in a nonfluoridated area found that those with some residence history in a fluoridated area had significantly better dental health than did those children resident in a nonfluoridated area all their lives.[30]

Summary of Dental Benefits from Fluoridation

Fluoridation is the most effective and efficient means of reducing dental caries on a community-wide basis.[27] It reduces caries prevalence by 50 to 60 percent in the permanent dentition among children born and reared in a fluoridated community. Caries reductions of about the same degree are seen in the primary dentition. Benefits are greatest on free smooth surfaces and anterior teeth, next best on proximal surfaces, and least on pit-and-fissure surfaces.

Whereas there is probably little dental benefit for the developing fetus, fluoridation does have lifelong dental benefits for adults—it is wrong to consider fluoridation a benefit for children only. Benefits in adult life are found in lower DMF values, greater tooth retention, and less root caries. Partial exposure to fluoridation in childhood, common in present-day United States society, provides partial benefits.

With such a vast literature on the subject, reviews can be helpful. An annotated bibliography by Campbell,[32] published in 1963, is an excellent review of research to that time. More recent reviews by Backer-Dirks[12] and Backer-Dirks, Kunzel, and Carlos[14] are recommended.

ECONOMICS OF FLUORIDATION

There are several ways of looking at the costs of fluoridation. The city manager will want to know what effect the initial installation and operating costs of fluoridation equipment will have on the city's budget, and therefore perhaps on local taxes—a subject that makes any city council nervous. Proponents of fluoridation in a community (who may well include the city manager just mentioned) want to stress the impressive cost-effectiveness of the measure. Dental practitioners, while exercising professional responsibility in supporting fluoridation, will be aware that it is likely to have some impact on their practices. (It should be mentioned that opponents of fluoridation will stress "costs" as social costs—ill health, for example.)

Water fluoridation in the United States in 1981 is said to cost about 35 cents per person per year on average.[36] In any one community the annual cost can range from 20 cents to $2.50 per person per year. Factors that influence the per capita cost are (1) the size of the community—the bigger the population to be reached, the lower the per capita cost; (2) the number of fluoride injection points required; (3) the amount and type of equipment to be used; (4) the type of fluoride chemical used, its price, plus the cost of transportation and storage; and (5) probably the expertise of water plant personnel.

City managers may well be impressed with this low per capita cost but will want to know what the initial expenditure is likely to be. This information may best come from the state health department's water supply division, because each community has its own characteristics. As a guide to likely initial expenditures, however, the data in Table 7–5 will help. These figures for five American and one British community show that whereas per capita cost is generally inversely proportional to the population to be served, expenditures on equipment and material are naturally greater in larger communities.

Fluoride compounds used in fluoridation are sodium fluoride and sodium silicofluoride, both solids, and hydrofluosilicic acid, a liquid. The availability, and hence price, of all three is highly variable and can be greatly affected by transportation costs, which will also vary greatly. If a water system has several sources of supply, separate sets of fluoridation equipment may be required for each. Where natural fluoride content is relatively high, less fluoride needs to be added, thus reducing cost of supplies to some extent. In higher temperatures, optimum concentration is lower because more water is drunk. U.S. Public Health Service recommendations on fluoride concentrations in various temperature ranges are shown in Table 7–6. These recommendations are based principally on a series of studies by Galagan and his colleagues[69-72]

Table 7–5. Estimated Annual Cost per Person of Fluoridation, in 1981 U.S. Dollars for Selected Cities in the United States and England*

City	Population	Fluoride Injection Points	Dollar Costs *Total Equipment*	Dollar Costs *Annual F Chemical*	Dollar Costs *Annual Per Capita*†
Denver, Colorado	900,000	5	$130,000	$45,000	$0.06
Macon, Georgia	120,000	2	48,200	26,800	0.26
Ann Arbor, Michigan	105,000	1	17,000‡	8,555	0.10
Watford, England	77,000	2	72,000	4,894	0.16
Mason, West Virginia	2,500	1	1,550	1,700	0.74
New Cumberland, West Virginia	1,700	2	2,890	1,070	0.80

*Data from the U.S. Public Health Service, Centers for Disease Control, Dental Disease Prevention Activity, June 1982; City of Ann Arbor Water Treatment Plant, Ann Arbor, Michigan; and Colne Valley Water Company, Watford, England.

†Amortized equipment (at 10 percent per year over 10 years) and annual chemical cost only.

‡Estimated replacement cost with volumetric feeder.

Table 7–6. Fluoride Levels Recommended for Cool and Warm Climates*

Annual Average of Maximum Daily Air Temperatures (degrees Fahrenheit)†	Recommended Control Limits (F concentrations ppm)		
	Lower	*Optimum*	*Upper*
50.0–53.7	0.9	1.2	1.7
53.8–58.3	0.8	1.1	1.5
58.4–63.8	0.8	1.0	1.3
63.9–70.6	0.7	0.9	1.2
70.7–79.2	0.7	0.8	1.0
79.3–90.5	0.6	0.7	0.8

*U.S. Public Health Service, 1962.[164]
†Based on temperature data obtained for a minimum of five years.

that measured fluoride concentrations of drinking waters, dental fluorosis, dental caries, and fluid intake in the American West—another example of using dental fluorosis as a proxy measure of optimum fluoride concentration for an area. The validity of the recommendations from the Galagan studies was later confirmed by Richards and his colleagues.[132]

Personnel costs are difficult to quantify. Maintenance of functioning equipment takes only several minutes per day of an efficient plant operator's time, in which case personnel costs are virtually negligible. The U.S. Public Health Service recommends that water plant operators receive at least one day per year of training[36] to allow them to remain efficient and up-to-date. This training may be given by health department water supply personnel or university faculty.

Reviews of fluoridation costs in other countries have been given by Kunzel[97] and Dowell.[54] An excellent manual on the engineering aspects of fluoridation is available from the U.S. Environmental Protection Agency.[16]

Savings in Treatment Costs

Costs of restorative care for children are sharply reduced by fluoridation. It was shown in one aspect of the Newburgh-Kingston study that initial dental care for six-year-old children cost 58 percent less in fluoridated Newburgh than in nonfluoridated Kingston.[9] These savings came from fewer extractions needed, fewer restorations, and a smaller proportion of complex restorations. Comparable findings came from two more recent British studies, which reported a 49 percent saving for children aged 4–5 and 54 percent for children aged 11–12.[55, 168] Yet another way of presenting cost savings in children's dental treatment came from New Zealand, where in fluoridated areas it was found that 450 school dental nurses (see Chapter 12) could carry out treatment that previously required 690 nurses.[47]

Some caveats are required, however, in interpreting findings on cost savings. Whereas children's restorative costs are certainly cut, fluoridation's effect on costs of adult dental care is less clear. Some might hypothesize that dollar savings achieved early in life are lost in later life, because greater tooth retention will increase the requirement for periodontal treatment and crowns and bridges in later years (see Chapter 11). In terms of direct expenditures only, total neglect and complete removal of remaining teeth at an early age are the cheapest forms of dental care. The greater the degree of tooth retention, the more that dental services are likely to be needed in the later years of life.[29] Of course, this argument applies to monetary expenditures only—the value of a healthy dentition throughout life will vary from one individual to another, but it is always hard to quantify.

A second caveat concerns the provision of diagnostic and preventive services to children in a fluoridated area. If many of these services are only marginally necessary, their provision will add to the cost of services without providing much in the way of benefits. With declining caries rates and the associated diminished need for restorations, diagnosis and prevention become a greater proportion of total cost of dental care. Children with an obviously low caries attack rate in a fluoridated area do not need to visit the dentist as often and require radiographs less frequently. Whether they need topical fluoride applications at all is a moot point, especially if they are using fluoride toothpaste and perhaps mouthrinsing with fluoride solutions. But if dentists continue to see such children twice a year and apply the full battery of diagnostic and preventive services each time, the potential savings of some 50 percent of the cost of treatment will be drastically reduced. This possibility had been recognized as early as 1956[172] and has since been specified in more detail.[26]

These subjects require careful study by dental personnel. They are good examples of why the preventive power of fluoridation must be seen as influencing all of dental practice and dental education, and not simply as a good way to reduce the numbers of carious lesions in children's teeth.

Some impact of fluoridation on dental practice has already been described. In a detailed study in the mid-1960s, Douglas and his colleagues[53] compared dental practices in naturally fluoridated and nonfluoridated communities in the Midwest. They found little difference in dentist:population ratios between the two and also little difference in dentists' incomes. There were differences in the types of treatment provided, and the dentists in the fluoridated areas appeared to be getting more satisfaction out of their practices. It is difficult to say how much these findings still apply in the 1980s. The dentists in the nonfluoridated areas, for example, were harried by the constant "drilling and filling" demands for children with high caries rates. With the diminished caries rates of the 1980s, that type of situation is probably a lot less common, so the "satisfaction" conclusion may have become less clear-cut.

Certainly the practice of dentistry for children has changed, as reported in an analysis of data from one pedodontic practice.[57] Of 511 patients entering the practice between 1948 and 1950 (*before* water fluoridation and other preventive programs), 86 percent needed restorative care and 41 percent required treatment of the pulp. Caries attack was so severe that four patients had to have all their primary teeth removed. Advanced carious lesions required the extraction of 24 permanent molars during the two-year period. An analysis of patients entering the practice between 1977 and 1979, *after* fluoridation, showed a dramatic change. More than 60 percent indicated no need for restorative care, and less than 10 percent required treatment of the pulp.

There is no question that dentistry is going to have to adjust to the altering disease patterns and shifting demographic profiles of society. Fluorides are major factors forcing the need for change. Whereas not all the adaptations required—in personnel requirements, dental education, specialty designations, perhaps care provision and reimbursement mechanisms—are going to be comfortable, dentistry can be proud of the constantly improving dental health of the public. The profession's role in promoting fluoridation has been an act of public service that few other professions can match.

PROMOTION OF FLUORIDATION

> Seldom has there been a measure to protect the public's health which has been so effective, so certain, and so simple. And yet, curiously enough, seldom has a program for safeguarding health evoked an outcry so vehement, so sustained, and so successful in blocking action.[126]

This 1961 statement is still true, even if the nature of the outcry has changed since then. The promotion of water fluoridation requires carefully planned leadership by practicing dental professionals—a special type of leadership with which they may not be entirely comfortable and for which little in their education and background may have prepared them. The development of water fluoridation was a product of science *but its promotion must be primarily on the basis of political action,* because the decision to fluoridate is eventually made by public officials or the electorate, not by dental professionals. Once a mayor or city council begins to be convinced of the desirability of fluoridation, the (usually unstated) question will be: "If I support the measure, will I lose votes?" The answer will reflect a political assessment.

The American Dental Association (ADA) has a clear-cut policy of support for fluoridation and has spelled out the professional responsibility of dentists and dental societies to promote the measure. The ADA recognizes that this role calls for ". . . leadership beyond the usual point."[1] But despite this policy and the endorsement of fluoridation by numerous official and voluntary health agencies and professional scientific organizations, many practicing dentists have not accepted their responsibility to promote fluoridation. A National Opinion Research Center study in the 1950s indicated, for example, that only 2 percent of the dentists questioned claimed to have participated in the organization of a fluoridation movement in their communities.[95] There is no more recent evidence to suggest that things have changed.[68] Nor is there evidence available to show that other dental professionals have done any better than their dentist co-workers in regard to promoting fluoridation. The progress that has been made in fluoridation has been due largely to the dedicated efforts of a small but hard-working group of dental professionals, both in public health and in private practice, whose enthusiasm and efforts have done much to raise the prestige of dentistry in the eyes of the other health professions as well as the public.

There is a great deal still to be learned about how to work effectively in the community to ensure a favorable public reaction to fluoridation. The information that is available comes primarily from two sources. Social scientists—from fields such as sociology, psychology, political science, and cultural anthropology, which examine various facets of the reactions of individuals singly and together in the community—have tentatively suggested some approaches. Those dental professionals, physicians, public health workers, and community leaders who have been engaged actively in fluoridation during the past decades can make suggestions based on experience and judgment.

Public Attitudes about Fluoridation

There is a reasonable body of social science literature on public attitudes about fluoridation. Much of it dates from the 1960s and may or may not be applicable in the 1980s.[68] The attraction of the issue for social scientists was often the community conflict it set off.[117]

The major point for dental professionals to remember is that most people are uninformed on the subject. A Gallup Poll in 1977 found that 51 percent of American adults did not know what fluoridation was. Of those who did know, only about 10 percent were opposed; most were either in favor or undecided.[74] These for-and-against figures can be misleading when it comes to political action, however. Many of those in favor are passively so, not necessarily willing to work actively for fluoridation (including dental professionals). Many of those opposed, however, are dedicated in their beliefs and prepared to act on them. As "single-issue" political groups have shown, a small group can clearly have its interests enacted if it is sufficiently well organized and hardworking.

Proponents of fluoridation have frequently been surprised by the vehemence and the dedication of opponents. A basic error of many health professionals trained in scientific thinking is the assumption that all persons think in rational terms and are therefore able to be convinced by scientific argument. This assumption all too often is false; the problem then arising for proponents is that they are often ill-equipped for dealing with the ensuing spirited conflicts. When attitudes other than complete approval are based on honest doubts or when they have some rational foundation, they can be identified and perhaps modified to some extent. But if opposition stems from irrational opinions, unconscious anxieties, or cultural viewpoints different from those held by the promoter, the problem is far greater.

There have been many attempts to categorize the various antifluoridationists, the rationale being that if this can be done, then individual and group opposition to fluoridation can be predicted and steps taken to counter it during promotional efforts. Unfortunately, the infinite complexities of human beliefs and behavior have resulted in a picture of antifluoridationists that is anything but clear.

A number of studies in the United States have concentrated on the attitudes of persons who vote against fluoridation on referenda. Some of these studies concluded that opponents feel a sense of deprivation or of powerlessness, an alienation from the forces that direct society, and that they hold a grudge against the people whom they see to be directing these forces. In this "antiestablishment" view, opposition to fluoride is seen by alienated persons as a means of expressing their general discontent with society at large rather than being more directly concerned with the merits of the measure itself.[76, 79, 102, 127, 148] "Alienation" has become a fashionable word and hence is in danger of losing its precise meaning, but here it means the process by which the complications, the value scales, the pace, and the pressures of life in competitive Western society act as forces that produce conscious or unconscious effects in an individual. The individual reacts, consciously or unconsciously, against these social forces in a variety of ways. It is likely that wherever social divisions are present there will be numbers of people who will use issues like fluoridation to express their vague and even unconscious desires to articulate discontent. Alienation could combine with the "antiscientific" attitude, held by some people, to promote a deep feeling of frustration.[35]

It has been suggested that an opponent of fluoridation is more likely to be an older, childless person of lower than median income and education, but a referendum can also fail in a young, high-income, and highly educated community.[147] Opposition, and certainly lack of support, can come from those who are merely doubtful or uncommitted.

The prevailing image of the profluoridationist is one of a younger married person with small children and with above-median income and education.[35, 115] But even this image is confused by the finding of support for fluoridation in all socioeconomic groups[73] and by an investigation in California, where greater opposition to fluoridation was found among nonmanual groups than among manual workers.[79] Linn[102] reviewed public attitudes on fluoridation and concluded that opposition stems from multiple causes and that the only single factor to emerge with any consistency was alienation. It is likely that alienation is still a powerful factor in public attitudes in the 1980s, though negative attitudes can also be shaped by honest concerns about ill health and long-term environmental effects.

Opposition to Fluoridation

The dichotomous nature of fluoridation ensures that there will be organized political opposition to its adoption. The first referendum on the subject was in 1950, in Stevens Point, Wisconsin. McNeil[113] has given an entertaining description of that campaign, showing how fluoridation can quickly flare up into a major political issue in a community. In recent years, opponents have exploited the climate of antiregulatory attitudes, special-interest politics, greater environmental sensitivity, and skepticism about governmental policies and officials.

Many communities that have begun fluoridation have had legal suits brought against them in an effort to stop the measure. In the short run, a few have been successful, but most have not. Successful lawsuits (successful only in the lower courts) to stop fluoridation have usually been based on the issues of personal liberty and religious beliefs.[31, 158] By 1965 there were 13 occasions in which a state supreme court had upheld the legality and constitutionality of fluoridation. Six of these decisions had been referred to the U.S. Supreme Court, which on every occasion either dismissed appeals or refused review.[135] No American court of last resort has ever ruled against fluoridation for any reason.

For many years, no American court at any level had ever ordered fluoridation to cease on the grounds that it was harmful.[17] More recently, however, two lower court judgments against fluoridation have been delivered. In November 1978 the judge in the Court of Common Pleas in Allegheny County, Commonwealth of Pennsylvania, ordered fluoridation to cease in the Westview Water Authority, a suburban area near Pittsburgh. The judge accepted the alleged link between fluoridated water and cancer, described previously. The decree further ordered that the prohibition should remain in effect until a final hearing was held or until the matter was submitted to the Pennsylvania Department of Environmental Resources. On appeal, the Commonwealth Court allowed fluoridation to continue, pending the decision of the Department of Environmental Resources. In January 1979 the Department ruled that the evidence on the alleged fluoridation-cancer link was "unpersuasive" and ordered the Water Authority to continue fluoridation (which in fact it had never ceased doing). In March 1982 the Commonwealth Court of Pennsylvania ruled that the Court of Common Pleas of Allegheny County does not have jurisdiction over actions by the State Department of Environmental Resources. Further appeals are likely.

In February 1982 a visiting judge in the Circuit Court of Alton, Illinois, ruled that the Illinois statute requiring mandatory fluoridation was unconstitutional. The decision came some 20 months after the close of a trial in April 1980. The Illinois Supreme Court, however, will allow the continued enforcement of the statute requiring fluoridation of public water systems pending the appeal of the Circuit Court order.

These two court decisions may reflect the antiregulatory attitudes of the times, but they also reflect a more sophisticated approach by those opposed to fluoridation. Most states have small "Pure Water Councils," affiliated with each other to some extent, which spring to life to oppose fluoridation when the question arises in a community. There is also a handful of "experts," Ph.D.'s, physicians, and dentists, who tend to appear anywhere in the country (or even in other countries) to support a local antifluoridation group. National opposition during the 1970s was centered in the California-based National Health Federation. With some change of executives in that organization, the opposition has now largely moved to the National Health Action Committee in Delaware, Ohio.

Local Political Action

Some communities adopt fluoridation by city council action, but referenda are common. Proponents much prefer council action because it gives them the chance of making their case before a small and interested group in an orderly fashion. If the city council has any doubt, however, whether on the issue itself or on adopting it solely by council action, it is likely to sidestep the issue and put the matter up for referendum—to "let the people decide" after a period of "public debate." Referenda, unfortunately, are usually conducted in an acrimonious and hysterical atmosphere in which the merits of the issue can become lost in personal attacks and the trading of half-truths and insults.

Knutson estimated in 1970 that over 900 referenda had been held in the United States and that over two thirds had been lost, chiefly through the political inexperience of the proponents.[96] An unknown but large number have been held since then, and the won/lost record appears to be getting no better.[23]

Dental Professionals' Role in Fluoridation Campaigns

In a political campaign it is generally recommended that dental professionals keep a reasonably low profile in a broadly based community group, *because fluoridation can only be adopted with broad community support.*

The first step is to become informed thoroughly about the technical aspects of fluoridation. Dental practitioners should first find out whether or not fluorides are present in the drinking water.* The state or local health department can provide this information as well as a description of engineering characteristics of the water system. Dental professionals should have some general understanding of the sources of water and the methods used for water treatment. In most instances, the state or local health department can provide at least tentative estimates of cost and identify any particular engineering problems that may complicate fluoridation.

At this point, it would be wise for the dental professionals to refresh their knowledge of the medical and dental studies that provide the scientific bases for fluoridation. Health departments or university faculty can be of help here.

It is important to find out what previous efforts have been made to institute fluoridation and, if so, the individuals who were involved and a history of what transpired. It is also wise to study the history of other controversial issues that may have arisen in the community in recent years

---

*As obvious as this step may seem, it has sometimes been ignored and fluoridation efforts have been initiated in communities with optimum or near optimum amounts of fluoride in the water supply. Dental professionals practicing in a fluoride area may not recognize immediately the low caries prevalence because the patients coming to the office are the very ones who need treatment—a self-selected, biased sample. Also, if they have never practiced in a nonfluoride area, they have no basis for comparison.

and to identify persons who were involved and who may be expected to form the hard core of opposition to fluoridation.

One of the most important steps is to analyze the power structure in the community and locate the individuals who are most likely to assist in bringing about favorable action. Every community is unique and there is no easy formula for identifying correctly all of the key persons and groups in any specific public issue. It is helpful, however, to try to determine the individuals who are influential because they occupy official positions in government, the various voluntary organizations that are a part of the life of the community, and those persons who, although perhaps not visibly or officially active in community groups, mold the opinion of a significant number of others.

Among those who occupy positions of responsibility, it is natural to think first of those who can take official action to institute fluoridation, such as the mayor and members of the city council or village board. For example, the mayor, simply by remaining neutral, can successfully foil a fluoridation campaign.[138] The health officer and members of the health department play important roles, as can the school administration—particularly if a parent-teacher organization is expected to be an active group. The role of other public employees, such as the superintendent of the waterworks, the town clerk, or city attorney, may not be apparent immediately. These individuals may not be in a position to initiate action directly or make major policy decisions, but they often can prevent (or facilitate) action by subtle and covert efforts. (Fluoridation may be delayed for long periods of time, for example, by dilatory tactics in purchasing equipment or ordering chemicals.)

Others, although not elected to official positions, have an important impact on community life because of what might be called "quasi-public" positions. The attitudes of the editor and staff of the local newspaper are an important consideration. Similarly, the support or opposition of a radio or television station, or of a key "personality" in their programming, can make the difference between success and failure. "Celebrities" from sports or show business can also be influential. Support of other professional groups—physicians, pharmacists, water plant engineers—is fundamental.

In addition, it has been common in fluoridation campaigns to work through existing community organizations such as parent-teacher groups, service clubs, sororities, fraternal orders, and labor unions. As valuable as these organizations are, it is important to remember that each ordinarily reaches only a small segment of the population. Characteristically, these groups often do not touch the lower socioeconomic groups in a community—the same groups that are not reached by communications through the newspapers, radio, and television. This segment of the community must be reached by face-to-face contact. To do so effectively requires the identification of individuals who are influential with certain groups but who may not be well known in the community.

If initial contacts with particular groups and influential individuals suggest that opinions are negative on the basis of incorrect or insufficient knowledge, it would be wise to slow down attempts to initiate fluoridation and change the emphasis to a low-pressure educational program with the community leaders. As previously mentioned, responsible community leaders who oppose fluoridation frequently have no strong objections to the procedure itself but rather to the symbolism of fluoridation. Strong opponents, however, are unlikely to be changed by any action and in educational efforts must be worked around.

Adoption by City Council

At such time as the organized dental professionals have reason to think that knowledge and opinions among leadership groups have become generally favorable to fluoridation, it should be possible (again through indirect and low-pressure techniques) to prevail upon one or two such leaders to introduce the subject of fluoridation through the appropriate local government channels. If the educational campaign has been effective, the proposal to fluoridate may well come spontaneously from the leadership group without additional stimulation. Alternatively, an interested community group may take the lead in having the resolution put before the council.

After the decision has been reached to place a fluoridation proposal before the governing body (but before it actually is discussed in an open meeting), the proponents have an additional educational task. They should inform members of the governing body and other key individuals about the opposition to fluoridation and the arguments that probably will be advanced against it.

It is important to solicit the aid of the mass media. Newspapers, radio, and television can turn a fluoridation issue into an unwholesome public spectacle in which the real issues may be forgotten. The question is how publicity can be kept in proportion. Experience shows that if full discussion is conducted with representatives of the mass communications media, some reporters will agree not to magnify the fluoridation issue unnecessarily and to keep coverage on as scientific a plane as possible.

Since the meeting of the governing body that will decide the fluoridation issue probably will be well attended by the opposition, it should also be well attended by those favoring the proposal.

Clearly it is not possible to spell out all the details of an educational and political campaign, since improvisation will be needed to meet local conditions. But in summary, the dental professionals should:

1. Begin by working with known official and unofficial leaders in the health and welfare areas, including members of the professional groups concerned.
2. Assess the leaders' initial knowledge of and attitudes toward fluoridation.
3. Provide needed education subtly and at a slow pace.
4. Not call attention initially to themselves as fervent fluoridation supporters nor give evidence of any plan to promote fluoridation actively.
5. Not identify themselves as the initiators or innovators of the change but leave it to another community group to take leadership.

6. Maintain a professional and nonpolitical role on the public level, avoiding the error of competing publicly with politicians in the political arena, and behave in a fashion that both lends dignity to and permits them to occupy the professional roles in which they can be most secure. Dental professionals can be more active on the private level, but their activities should be directed toward the decision-making group rather than toward the public in general.

Referenda

As described earlier, referenda are to be avoided if possible, but that seems to be getting more and more difficult to ensure. When a referendum looms, dental professionals have a leadership role to play, but it must be carefully defined because professional people can get caught in the dilemma of what is known as "conflicting role expectations."[131] What this means is that health professionals, especially dental professionals accustomed to working in the quiet of their own offices, can become acutely uncomfortable when suddenly placed in the glare of the political spotlight. It is more than just distaste for political hurly-burly. In an issue concerning health, such as fluoridation, they are expected by their colleagues and by laymen to participate as professional experts. Furthermore, the "role" of expert is the one to which they are accustomed and in which they can operate most comfortably. But once the issue of fluoridation is to be decided by referendum, it becomes an open political question. In this instance the community can expect that those supporting fluoridation will act as partisan lobbyists for an issue that has been defined by the community as controversial and political. In these campaigns the professional health workers, not surprisingly, may choose to spurn the role of a political partisan and to assume a detached professional role, refusing to engage in public debate and holding themselves aloof after giving their professional advice.

Raulet's study[131] found that the efforts of the dentists and other members of the health professions met with unfavorable reaction from the community for two different reasons. The community expected partisans in a political campaign to be motivated by their own self-interests and to conduct a propaganda campaign to further those interests. Since the health professionals supporting fluoridation were seen as political partisans, their endorsements of fluoridation and their attempts at health education (presented in their professional role) were not accepted as expert testimony. At the same time their efforts to maintain professional dignity and to avoid engaging in open controversy were interpreted as arrogance.

This study suggests that once the issue of fluoridation has become the subject of a referendum, physicians, dentists, and other health workers cannot expect to maintain the detached role of a professional expert in the health field. They must expect that their actions will be interpreted by the public as those of a partisan participant in a political debate. Referendum tactics must be structured accordingly.

Good results can follow when dental professionals act to form a citizens' committee that coordinates the campaign, often as the "Citizens for Healthy Teeth" or some such name. Interested citizens often come from PTA groups, school boards, other professions, business people, and voluntary agencies—the "doers" in a community. The resulting committee can have a rather upper-middle-class tone, so blue-collar workers, perhaps through union locals, should also be sought to join the group. To the extent possible, so should representatives of ethnic minorities and senior citizens. If active political party representatives are involved, care should be taken to see that the major political parties are represented. Fluoridation should not be a politically partisan issue; the last thing needed is to have it become so because the coordinating committee has inadvertently become identified with members of one party.

An expert in political organization and communication is invaluable as a member of the committee or as a consultant to it. In many states there are legal requirements for registration of a political action committee, and an expert can help with these details, as well as with overall strategy and specific tactics. The coordinating committee should use all appropriate methods of health education and political dissemination, including advertisements and news releases. A speakers' bureau, to provide talks to civic groups, and mass mailings are among the procedures often indicated. Leaflets and pamphlets should be printed in terminology and language understandable by the group to which they are directed. The political expert can help with reaching the large segments of the population that ordinarily do not participate in organizations and who are not influenced to a major extent by mass media. Any respectable effort to reach the uncommitted should be considered.

An important role for dental professionals is in organizing training sessions for all persons participating in the fluoridation campaign. In conducting educational efforts, dental professionals must attempt not only to be scientifically accurate but also to express the facts and concepts in simple, clear, positive terms. It will be necessary to discuss the nature of those who are opposing fluoridation and the reasons for their opposition. Extreme care should be taken that these comments are not derogatory nor of the "name-calling" variety. In addition, it is pointless to attempt to suppress opponents or to deny them an audience. First, they will find a way to express their views by one device or another. Second, efforts to suppress their presentations are likely to backfire and make the public sympathetic with their cause.

Although it is desirable for members of dental societies to remain in the background, it usually is not possible. They often will be asked to appear before public meetings and sometimes are challenged to public debates by members of the opposition. Whether or not to accept an invitation to debate a fluoridation opponent cannot be answered definitively. As described previously, behavioral science research indicates that a refusal to debate may be interpreted by the public as professional arrogance, the lack of a sense of fair play, and evidence of a dictatorial attitude. On the other hand, it must be recognized that a debate with a skillful opponent of fluoridation cannot be "won." A skilled opponent can imply, for example, that fluoridation is in the same category as dumping chemical waste, uncontrolled radiation, or acid rain, and that proponents are trying to increase both unnecessary regulation and taxes.

Importing experts from "outside" the community is a subject to be considered carefully. There are examples of where this has backfired badly and where it has succeeded—for both proponents and opponents. Decisions must be made on an individual basis.

Successful referendum campaigns have been reported in the dental literature, and strategies for dealing with fluoridation in the political arena have now been well defined. Recommended are papers by McGuire[109] and Boriskin and Fine,[23] based on successful referenda in Lansing, Michigan, and Oakland, California, to *keep* existing fluoridation, and the review by Domoto, Faine, and Rovin[52] of the successful campaign to initiate fluoridation in Seattle, Washington. Isman[89] describes a temporarily successful strategy in Portland, Oregon, while Dolinsky and others[50] have described the value of the involvement of a broad range of community organizations and agencies in a campaign. Evans and Pickles[64] take a broader look at the statewide initiative in fluoridation politics.

The common theme in these reports is that fluoridation is *politics*. It demands the use of the media, publicity, education, intensive door-to-door canvassing, telephone campaigns, getting-out-the-vote on polling day—which probably means arranging transportation for many people. Above all it means consistent hard work over a long period and starting with a solid preparation.

SUMMARY

Fluoridation is safe, effective, and inexpensive. It is by far the most efficient and effective method for reducing the prevalence of dental caries in a community. Fluoridation does not benefit just children; its role in remineralization of incipient lesions and its preventive effects on root caries make it beneficial for persons of all ages. It may help in reducing bone-fragility disease in older persons.

Fluoridation is also a subject of considerable political controversy in many places. Dental professionals can exercise their responsibilities by doing what they can to have it adopted and retained in their own communities.

References

1. American Dental Association, Council on Dental Health. Statement of American Dental Association on role of dentists and dental societies in the promotion of fluoridation. Am. Dent. A. Tr., 103:44, 1962.
2. American Dental Association, Council on Dental Therapeutics. Accepted dental therapeutics. 38th ed. Chicago, The Association, 1979. xxix + 385 p.

3. Armstrong, W. D. Mechanisms of fluoride homeostasis. Arch. Oral Biol., 4:156–9, Aug. 1961.
4. Arnold, F. A., Jr., et al. Fifteenth year of the Grand Rapids fluoridation study. Am. Dent. A. J., 65:780–5, Dec. 1962.
5. Ast, D. B. The caries-fluorine hypothesis and a suggested study to test its application. Pub. Health Rep., 58:857–79, June 4, 1943.
6. Ast, D. B., and Fitzgerald, Bernadette. Effectiveness of water fluoridation. Am. Dent. A. J., 65:581–8, Nov. 1962.
7. Ast, D. B., Finn, S. B., and McCaffrey, Isabel. The Newburgh-Kingston caries-fluorine study. I. Dental findings after three years of water fluoridation. Am. J. Pub. Health, 40:716–24, June 1950.
8. ———. The Newburgh-Kingston caries-fluorine study. XIV. Combined clinical and roentgenographic dental findings after ten years of fluoride experience. Am. Dent. A. J., 52:314–25, Mar. 1956.
9. Ast, D. B., et al. Time and cost factors to provide regular periodic dental care for children in a fluoridated and nonfluoridated area: final report. Am. Dent. A. J., 80:770–6, Apr. 1970.
10. A two-part report on fluoridation. Part 1: the cancer scare. Consumer Rep., 43:392–6, July 1978.
11. Backer-Dirks, O. The relation between the fluoridation of water and dental caries experience. Internat. Dent. J., 17:582–605, Sept. 1967.
12. ———. The benefits of water fluoridation. Caries Res., 8(Suppl. 1):2–15, 1974.
13. Backer-Dirks, O., Houwink, B., and Kwant, G. W. The result of 6½ years of artificial drinking water in the Netherlands; The Tiel-Culemborg experiment. Arch. Oral Biol., 5:284–300, Dec. 1961.
14. Backer-Dirks, O., Kunzel, W., and Carlos, J. P. Caries-preventive water fluoridation. Caries Res., 12(Suppl. 1):7–14, 1978.
15. Barth, T. F. W. The geochemical cycle of fluorine. J. Geol., 55:420–6, 1947. Chem. Abstr., 42:1536, 1948.
16. Bellack, Ervin. Fluoridation engineering manual. Washington D.C., Environmental Protection Agency, 1972 (reprinted 1974, 1980). viii + 94 p.
17. Bergen, R. P. Legal status of fluoridation. Am. Med. A. J., 211:555–6, Jan. 19, 1970.
18. Berry, W. T. C. A study of the incidence of mongolism in relation to the fluoride content of water. Am. J. Ment. Def., 62:634–6, Jan. 1958.
19. Black, G. V., and McKay, F. S. Mottled teeth—an endemic developmental imperfection of the teeth heretofore unknown in the literature of dentistry. Dent. Cosmos, 58:129–56, Feb. 1916.
20. Blayney, J. R., and Tucker, W. H. The Evanston dental caries study. J. Dent. Res., 27:279–86, June 1948.
21. Blayney, J. R., and Hill, I. N. Fluorine and dental caries. Am. Dent. A. J., 74: (special issue) 233–302, Jan. 1967.
22. ———. Evanston dental caries study. XXIV. Prenatal fluorides—value of waterborne fluorides during pregnancy. Am. Dent. A. J., 69:291–4, Sept. 1964.
23. Boriskin, J. M., and Fine, J. I. Fluoridation election victory: a case study for dentistry in effective political action. Am. Dent. A. J., 102:486–91, Apr. 1981.
24. Brandt, E. N., Jr. Block grants and the resurgence of federalism. Pub. Health Rep., 96:495–7, Nov.–Dec. 1981.
25. Burk, D., and Yiamouyiannis, J. Fluoridation and cancer. 94th Congress, first session. Congress. Record, 121:7172–6, July 21, 1975.
26. Burt, B. A. Diagnostic and preventive services in a national incremental dental plan for children. J. Pub. Health Dent., 37:31–46, Winter 1977.
27. Burt, B. A., ed. The relative efficiency of methods of caries prevention in dental public health; proceedings of a conference at The University of Michigan, June 6–8, 1978. Ann Arbor, University Michigan, 1979. 326 p.
28. Burt, B. A., and Petterson, E. O. Fluoridation: developments in Sweden. Brit. Dent. J., 133:57–9, July 18, 1972.
29. Burt, B. A., and Warner, K. E. Prevention of oral disease; its potential for containing the costs of dental care. (In Kudrle, R. T., and Meskin, L. H., eds. Opportunities for cost-containment in dentistry. Minneapolis, University Minnesota Press, in press.)
30. Burt, B. A., Loesche, W. J., and Eklund, S. A. Caries experience and *S. mutans* counts with varying exposure to fluoridated water. Abstr. J. Dent. Res., 61:225, Mar. 1982.

31. Butler, H. W. Legal aspects of fluoridating community water supplies. Am. Dent. A. J., 65:653–8, Nov. 1962.
32. Campbell, Irene R. The role of fluoride in public health: a selected bibliography. Cincinnati, Kettering Laboratory College Medicine, University Cincinnati, 1963. v + 108 p.
33. Carlos, J. P., Gittelsohn, A. M., and Waddon, Williams, Jr. Caries in deciduous teeth in relation to maternal ingestion of fluoride. Pub. Health Rep., 77:658–60, Aug. 1962.
34. Churchill, H. V. Occurrence of fluorides in some waters of the United States. J. Ind. and Eng. Chem., 23:996–8, Apr. 10, 1931.
35. Cohen, Lois K. A sociologist looks at fluoridation. Oregon Dent. J., 35:26–30, June 1966.
36. Collins, J. J., Public Health Adviser, Dental Disease Prevention Activity, Centers for Disease Control, U.S. Public Health Service, Atlanta, Ga. Personal communication, Aug. 2, 1982.
37. Cremer, H.–D., and Buttner, W. Absorption of fluorides. p. 75–91. (In World Health Organization. Fluorides and human health. Geneva, The Organization, 1970. 364 p.)
38. Dean, H. T. Endemic fluorosis and its relation to dental caries. Pub. Health Rep., 53:1443–52, Aug. 19, 1938.
39. ______. The investigation of physiological effects by the epidemiological method. p. 23–31. (In Moulton, F. R., ed. Fluorine and dental health. Washington, American Association Advancement Science, 1942. 101 p.)
40. Dean, H. T., Dixon, R. M., and Cohen, Chester. Mottled enamel in Texas. Pub. Health Rep., 50:424–42, Mar. 29, 1935.
41. Dean, H. T., and Elvove, Elias. Some epidemiological aspects of chronic endemic dental fluorosis. Am. J. Pub. Health, 26:567–75, June 1936.
42. Dean, H. T., Elvove, Elias, and Poston, R. F. Mottled enamel in South Dakota. Pub. Health Rep., 54:212–28, Feb. 10, 1939.
43. Dean, H. T., et al. Domestic water and dental caries, including certain epidemiological aspects of oral *L. acidophilus*. Pub. Health Rep., 54:862–88, May 26, 1939.
44. ______. Domestic water and dental caries. II. A study of 2,832 white children, aged 12 to 14 years, of 8 suburban Chicago communities, including *Lactobacillus acidophilus* studies of 1,761 children. Pub. Health Rep., 56:761–92, Apr. 11, 1941.
45. Dean, H. T., Arnold, F. A., Jr., and Elvove, Elias. Domestic water and dental caries. V. Additional studies of the relation of fluoride domestic waters to dental caries experience in 4,425 white children, aged 12 to 14 years, of 13 cities in 4 states. Pub. Health Rep., 57:1155–79, Aug. 7, 1942.
46. Dean, H. T., et al. Studies on mass control of dental caries through fluoridation of the public water supply. Pub. Health Rep., 65:1403–8, Oct. 27, 1950.
47. Denby, G. C., and Hollis, M. J. The effect of fluoridation on a dental public health programme. N. Z. Dent. J., 62:32–6, Jan. 1966.
48. Department of Health and Social Security (Great Britain). The fluoridation studies in the United Kingdom and the results achieved after eleven years. London, Her Majesty's Stationery Office, 1969. vii + 44 p. (p. 33–44)
49. Diefenbach, V. L., Nevitt, G. A., and Frankel, J. M. Fluoridation and the appearance of teeth. Am. Dent. A. J., 71:1129–37, Nov. 1965.
50. Dolinsky, H. B., et al. A health systems agency and a fluoridation campaign. J. Pub. Health Policy, 2:158–63, June 1981.
51. Doll, R., and Kinlen, L. Fluoridation of water and cancer mortality in the U.S.A. Lancet, 1:1300–2, June 1977.
52. Domoto, P. K., Faine, R. C., and Rovin, Sheldon. Seattle fluoridation 1973: prescription for victory. Am. Dent. A. J., 91:583–8, Sept. 1975.
53. Douglas, B. L., et al. Impact of water fluoridation on dental practice and dental manpower. Am. Dent. A. J., 84:355–67, Feb. 1972.
54. Dowell, T. B. The economics of fluoridation. Brit. Dent. J., 140:103–6, Feb. 3, 1976.
55. Downer, M. C., Blinkhorn, A. S., and Attwood, D. Effect of fluoridation on the cost of dental treatment among urban Scottish schoolchildren. Community Dent. Oral Epidemiol., 9:112–6, June 1981.
56. Driscoll, W. S. Review of clinical research on prenatal fluorides. J. Dent. Child., 48:109–17, Mar.–Apr. 1981.
57. Eichenbaum, I. W., Dunn, Naomi A., and Tinanoff, Norman. Impact of fluoridation in a private pedodontic practice: thirty years later. J. Dent. Child., 48:211–14, May–June 1981.
58. Eklund, S. A., and Striffler, D. F. Anticaries effect of various concentrations of fluoride in drinking water: evaluation of empirical evidence. Pub. Health Rep., 95:486–90, Sept.–Oct. 1980.

59. Englander, H. R., and Wallace, D. A. Effects of naturally fluoridated water on dental caries in adults. Pub. Health Rep., 77:887–93, Oct. 1962.
60. Environmental Protection Agency. Interim primary drinking water regulations. Fed. Register, 45:57332–57, Aug. 17, 1980.
61. Erickson, J. D., et al. Water fluoridation and congenital malformations: no association. Am. Dent. A. J., 93:981–4, Nov. 1976.
62. Erickson, J. D. Mortality in selected cities with fluoridated and nonfluoridated water supplies. New Engl. J. Med., 298:112–6, May 18, 1978.
63. Ericsson, Y., and Malmnas, C. Placental transfer of fluorine investigated with F^{18} in man and rabbit. Acta Obs. and Gyn. Scand., 41:144–58, 1962.
64. Evans, C. A., and Pickles, Tomm. Statewide antifluoridation initiatives: a new challenge to health workers. Am. J. Pub. Health, 68:59–62, Jan. 1978.
65. Expiring fluoridation program success despite short lifespan. ADA News, Nov. 23, 1981.
66. Fédération Dentaire Internationale. Basic fact sheets. London, The Fédération, 1977. various pagings and appendices.
67. Forrest, Jean R., and James, P. M. C. A blind study of enamel opacities and dental caries prevalence after eight years of fluoridation of water. Brit. Dent. J., 119:319–22, Oct. 5, 1965.
68. Frazier, P. Jean. Fluoridation: a review of social research. J. Pub. Health Dent., 40:214–33, Summer 1980.
69. Galagan, D. J., and Lamson, G. G., Jr. Climate and endemic dental fluorosis. Pub. Health Rep., 68:497–508, May 1953.
70. Galagan, D. J. Climate and controlled fluoridation. Am. Dent. A. J., 47:159–70, Aug. 1953.
71. Galagan, D. J., et al. Climate and fluid intake. Pub. Health Rep., 72:484–90, June 1957.
72. Galagan, D. J., and Vermillion, J. R. Determining optimum fluoride concentrations. Pub. Health Rep., 72:491–3, June 1957.
73. Gamson, W. A., and Irons, P. H. Community characteristics and fluoridation outcome. J. Soc. Issues, 17:66–74, Winter 1961.
74. General Accounting Office. Reducing tooth decay—more emphasis on fluoridation needed; a report to the Congress of the United States. Washington, D.C., Government Printing Office, 1979. v + 52 p.
75. Grainger, R. M., and Coburn, C. I. Dental caries of the first molars and the age of children when first consuming naturally fluoridated water. Canad. J. Pub. Health, 46:347–54, Sept. 1955.
76. Green, A. L. The ideology of anti-fluoridation leaders. J. Soc. Issues, 17:13–25, Dec. 1961.
77. Guy, W. S. Inorganic and organic fluoride in human blood. p. 125–47. (In Johansen, E., Taves, D. R., and Olsen, T. O., eds. Continuing evaluation of the use of fluorides. AAAS Selected Symposium no. 11. Boulder, Colo., Westview, 1979. xxviii + 321 p.)
78. Hagan, T. L., Pasternack, M., and Scholz, Grace. Waterborne fluorides and mortality. Pub. Health Rep., 69:450–4, May 1954.
79. Hahn, H. D. Fluoridation and patterns in community politics. J. Pub. Health Dent., 25:152–7, Fall 1965.
80. Hill, I. N., Blayney, J. R., and Wolf, W. The Evanston dental caries study. XVI. Reduction in dental caries attack rates in children six to eight years old. Am. Dent. A. J., 53:327–33, Sept. 1956.
81. Hodge, H. C., and Smith, F. A. Fluorine chemistry. Vol. 4 of a series, Simons, J. H., ed. New York, Academic Press, 1965. xviii + 786 p.
82. Hodge, H. C. The safety of fluoride tablets or drops. p. 253–74. (In Johansen, E., Taves, D. R., and Olsen, T. O., eds. Continuing evaluation of the use of fluorides. AAAS Selected Symposium no. 11. Boulder, Colo., Westview, 1979. xxviii + 321 p.)
83. Hoffman, R., et al. Acute fluoride poisoning in a New Mexico elementary school. Pediatrics, 65:897–900, May 1980.
84. Hoover, R. N., McKay, F. W., and Fraumeni, J. F. Fluoridated drinking water and the occurrence of cancer. J. Nat. Cancer Inst., 57:757–68, Oct. 1976.
85. Horowitz, H. S., and Heifetz, S. B. Effects of prenatal exposure to fluoridation on dental caries. Pub. Health Rep., 82:297–304, Apr. 1967.
86. Horowitz, H. S. Abusive use of fluoride. Edit. J. Pub. Health Dent., 37:106–7, Spring 1977.
87. Hutton, W. L., Linscott, B. W., and Williams, D. B. The Brantford fluorine experiment. Interim report after five years of water fluoridation. Canad. J. Pub. Health, 42:81–7, Mar. 1951.

88. ______. Final report of local studies on water fluoridation in Brantford. Canad. J. Pub. Health, 47:89–92, Mar. 1956.
89. Isman, Robert. Fluoridation: strategies for success. Am. J. Pub. Health, 71:717–21, July 1981.
90. Jackson, D., Murray, J. J., and Fairpo, C. G. Life-long benefits of fluoride in drinking water. Brit. Dent. J., 134:419–22, May 15, 1973.
91. Johansen, Erling, Taves, D. R., and Olsen, T. O., eds. Continuing evaluation of the use of fluorides. AAAS Selected Symposium no. 11. Boulder, Colo., Westview, 1979. xxviii + 321 p.
92. Johnson, W. J., Taves, D. R., and Jowsey, Jennifer. Fluoridation and bone disease in renal patients. p. 275–93. (In Johansen, E., Taves, D. R., and Olsen, T. O. Continuing evaluation of the use of fluorides, AAAS Selected Symposium no. 11. Boulder, Colo., Westview, 1979. xxviii + 321 p.)
93. Jowsey, Jennifer, Riggs, B. L., and Kelly, P. J. Fluoride in the treatment of osteoporosis. p. 111–23. (In Johansen, E., Taves, D. R., and Olsen, T. O., eds. Continuing evaluation of the use of fluorides. AAAS Symposium no. 11. Boulder, Colo., Westview, 1979. xxviii + 321 p.)
94. Katz, Simon, and Muhler, J. C. Prenatal and postnatal fluoride and dental caries experience in deciduous teeth. Am. Dent. A. J., 76:305–11, Feb. 1968.
95. Kesel, R. G. Dental practice. p. 95–238. (In Hollinshead, B. S., dir. The survey of dentistry; the final report. Washington, D.C., American Council Education, c1961. xxxiv + 603 p.)
96. Knutson, J. W. Water fluoridation after 25 years. Am. Dent. A. J., 80:765–9, Apr. 1970.
97. Kunzel, W. The cost and economic consequences of water fluoridation. Caries Res., 8(Suppl. 1):28–35, 1974.
98. ______. Effect of an interruption in water fluoridation on the caries prevalence of the primary and secondary dentition. Caries Res., 14:304–10, 1980.
99. Lemke, C. W., Doherty, J. M., and Arra, M. C. Controlled fluoridation: the dental effects of discontinuation in Antigo, Wisconsin. Am. Dent. A. J., 80:782–6, Apr. 1970.
100. Leone, N. C., et al. Medical aspects of excessive fluoride in the water supply. Pub. Health Rep., 69:925–36, Oct. 1954.
101. Leukhart, C. S. An update on water fluoridation: triumphs and challenges. Pediatr. Dent., 1:32–7, Mar. 1979.
102. Linn, E. L. An appraisal of sociological research on the public's attitudes towards fluoridation. J. Pub. Health Dent., 29:36–45, Winter 1969.
103. Ludwig, T. G. The Hastings Fluoridation Project. V. Dental effects between 1954 and 1964. N. Z. Dent. J., 61:175–9, July 1965.
104. McClure, F. J. Fluoride domestic waters and systemic effects. I. Relation to bone-fracture experience, height and weight of high school boys and young selectees of the armed forces of the United States. Pub. Health Rep., 59:1543–58, Dec. 1, 1944.
105. ______. Fluorine and other trace elements in nutrition. Am. Med. A. J., 139:711–6, Mar. 12, 1949.
106. ______. Water fluoridation; the search and the victory. Bethesda, National Institutes Health, 1970. xi + 302 p.
107. McClure, F. J., and Kinser, C. A. Fluoride domestic waters and systemic effects. II. Fluorine content of urine in relation to fluorine in drinking water. Pub. Health Rep., 59:1575–91, Dec. 8, 1944.
108. McClure, F. J., et al. Balances of fluorine ingested from various sources in food and water by five young men. Excretion of fluorine through the skin. J. Ind. Hygiene and Toxicol., 27:159–70, June 1945.
109. McGuire, Karen M. Strategies for a fluoridation campaign. Mich. Dent. A. J., 63:681–6, Oct. 1981.
110. McKay, F. S. Mottled enamel: the prevention of its further production through a change of water supply at Oakley, Idaho. Am. Dent. A. J., 20:1137–49, July 1933.
111. ______. Mass control of dental caries through the use of domestic water supplies containing fluorine. Am. J. Pub. Health., 38:828–32, June 1948.
112. ______. The relation of mottled enamel to caries. Am. Dent. A. J., 15:1429–37, Aug. 1928.
113. McNeil, D. R. The fight for fluoridation. New York, Oxford, 1957. 241 p.
114. MacNeill, Seamus. The fluoridation case in Ireland—legal and scientific evaluations. Irish Dent. A. J., 18:59–67, Mar.–Apr. 1972.

115. Mausner, Bernard, and Mausner, Judith. The anti-scientific attitude. Scient. Am., 192:35–9, Feb. 1955.
116. Morbidity and Mortality Weekly Report. Fluoride intoxication in a dialysis unit—Maryland. MMWR, 29:134–6, Mar. 28, 1980.
117. Motz, Annabelle B. The fluoridation issue as studied by social scientists. p. 347–64. (In Richards, N. D., and Cohen, Lois K., eds. Social sciences and dentistry; a critical bibliography. The Hague, Sijthoff and Fédération Dentaire Internationale, 1971. 381 p.)
118. Murray, J. J. Caries experience of 15-year-old children from fluoride and non-fluoride communities. Brit. Dent. J., 127:128–31, Aug. 5, 1969.
119. ———. Adult dental health in fluoride and non-fluoride areas. Part 1. Mean DMF values by age. Brit. Dent. J., 131:391–5, Nov. 2, 1971.
120. ———. Adult dental health in fluoride and non-fluoride areas. Part 3. Tooth mortality by age. Brit. Dent. J., 131:487–92, Dec. 7, 1971.
121. National Research Council, Food and Nutrition Board. Recommended dietary allowances. 9th ed. Washington, D.C., National Academy of Sciences, 1980. ix + 185 p. (p. 156–9)
122. Needleman, H. L., Pueschel, S. M., and Rothman, K. J. Fluoridation and the occurrence of Down's syndrome. New Engl. J. Med., 291:821–3, Oct. 17, 1974.
123. Newbrun, Ernest. Cost-effectiveness and practicality features in the systemic use of fluorides. p. 27–48. (In Burt, B. A., ed. The relative efficiency of methods of caries prevention in dental public health. Ann Arbor, University Michigan, 1979. 326 p.)
124. ———. Systemic fluorides: an overview. Canad. Dent. A. J., 46:31–7, Jan. 1980.
125. Oldham, P. D., and Newell, D. J. Fluoridation of water supplies and cancer—a possible association? Appl. Statist., 26:125–35, 1977.
126. Paul, B. D. Fluoridation and the social scientist: a review. p. 1–12. (In Paul, B. D., Gamson, W. A., and Kegeles, S. S., eds. Trigger for community conflict: the case of fluoridation. J. Soc. Issues, 17:1–84, Dec. 1961.)
127. Pinard, Maurice. Structural attachments and political support in urban politics: the case of fluoridation referendums. Am. J. Sociol., 68:513–26, Mar. 1963.
128. Rapaport, I. Contribution a l'etude du mongolisme. Role pathogenique du fluor. Bul. Acad. Nat. Med. (Paris), 140:529–31, 1956.
129. ———. Nouvelles recherches sur le mongolisme. A propos du role pathogenique du fluor. Bul. Acad. Nat. Med. (Paris), 143:367–70, 1959.
130. ———. Oligophrenie mongolienne et caries dentaires. Rev. Stomatol. (Paris), 46:207–18, 1963.
131. Raulet, H. M. The health professional and the fluoridation issue: a case of role conflict. J. Soc. Issues, 17:45–54, Dec. 1961.
132. Richards, L. F., et al. Determining optimum fluoride levels for community water supplies in relation to temperature. Am. Dent. A. J., 74:389–97, Feb. 1967.
133. Riggs, B. L., et al. Effect of the fluoride/calcium regimen on vertebral fracture occurrence in postmenopausal osteoporosis. New Engl. J. Med., 306:446–50, Feb. 25, 1982.
134. Robinson, W. O., and Edgington, G. Minor elements in plants and some accumulator plants. Soil Science, 60:15–28, 1945.
135. Roemer, R. Water fluoridation: public health responsibility and the democratic process. Am. J. Pub. Health, 55:1337–48, Sept. 1965.
136. Rogot, E., et al. Trends in urban mortality in relation to fluoridation status. Am. J. Epidemiol., 107:104–12, Feb. 1978.
137. Roholm, Kaj. Fluorine intoxication. A clinical-hygienic study with a review of the literature and some experimental investigations. London, Lewis, 1937, 364 p.
138. Rosenthal, D. B., and Crain, R. L. Executive leadership and community innovation: the fluoridation experience. Urban Affairs Quar., 1:39–57, Mar. 1966.
139. Russell, A. L. The inhibition of approximal caries in adults with lifelong fluoride exposure. J. Dent. Res., 32:138–43, Feb. 1953.
140. ———. Fluoride domestic water and periodontal disease. Am. J. Pub. Health, 47:688–94, June 1957.
141. ———. Dental fluorosis in Grand Rapids during the seventeeth year of fluoridation. Am. Dent. A. J., 65:608–12, Nov. 1962.
142. ———. Letters to Dr. Rapaport and Dr. Forrest. p. 262–5. (In Royal Commission on the fluoridation of public water supplies. Hobart, Tasmania, Government Printing Office, 1968. 268 p.)

143. Russell, A. L., and Elvove, Elias. Domestic water and dental caries. VII. A study of the fluoride-dental caries relationship in an adult population. Pub. Health Rep., 66:1389–401, Oct. 26, 1951.
144. Russell, A. L., and Hamilton, Peggy M. Dental caries in permanent first molars after eight years of fluoridation. Arch. Oral Biol., 6:50–7, July 1961.
145. Schlesinger, E. R., et al. Newburgh-Kingston caries-fluorine study. XIII. Pediatric findings after ten years. Am. Dent. A. J., 52:296–306, Mar. 1956.
146. Schneiderman, M. A. Fluoridation and health: a short review of some evidence from the United States. Bethesda, National Cancer Institute, National Institutes Health, 1979. 8 p., processed.
147. Shaw, C. T. Characteristics of supporters and rejectors of a fluoridation referendum and a guide for other community programs. Am. Dent. A. J., 78:339–41, Feb. 1969.
148. Simmel, Arnold. A signpost for research on fluoridation conflicts: the concepts of a relative deprivation. J. Soc. Issues, 17:26–36, Dec. 1961.
149. Smith, F. A., et al. The effects of the absorption of fluoride. V. The chemical determination of fluoride in human soft tissues following prolonged ingestion of fluoride at various levels. Am. Med A. Arch. Indust. Health, 21:330–2, Apr. 1960.
150. Smith, Margaret C., Lantz, Edith M., and Smith, H. V. The cause of mottled enamel, a defect of human teeth. Technical Bulletin no. 32, Tucson, University Arizona College Agriculture, 1931.
151. Sognnaes, R. F. Historical perspectives. p. 5–31. (In Johansen, E., Taves, D. R., and Olsen, T. O., eds. Continuing evaluation of the use of fluorides. AAAS Selected Symposium no. 11. Boulder, Colo., Westview, 1979. xxviii + 321 p.)
152. Stamm, J. S., and Banting, D. W. Comparison of root caries prevalence in adults with life-long residence in fluoridated and non-fluoridated communities. Abstr. J. Dent. Res., 59(Spec. Issue A) 405, Mar. 1980.
153. State of Michigan, Office of Science and Technology. Report of the Governor's Task Force on Fluorides. Lansing, Office Science and Technology, 1979. v + 81 p. (p. 26–41)
154. Still, C. N., and Kelley, Paul. On the incidence of primary degenerative dementia vs. water fluoride content in South Carolina. Neurotoxicology, 1:125–31, 1980.
155. Strassburg, M. A., and Greenland, S. Methodologic problems in evaluating the carcinogenic risk of environmental agents. J. Environ. Health, 41:214–7, Jan.–Feb. 1979.
156. Striffler, D. F., et al. Fluoridation of water supplies in small rural communities. Pub. Health Rep., 80:25–32, Jan. 1965.
157. Striffler, D. F. The switch to block grants: a challenge to state dental directors. Edit. J. Pub. Health Dent., 41:212–3, Fall 1981.
158. Strong, G. A. Liberty, religion, and fluoridation. Am. Dent. A. J., 76:1398–409, June 1968.
159. Swedish Ministry of Health and Social Affairs. The use of fluoride in dental caries prevention; summary of a report by the Swedish Fluoride Commission. Stockholm, The Ministry, 1981. 30 p. typescript.
160. Tank, Gertrude, and Storvick, C. A. Caries experience of children one to six years old in two Oregon communities (Corvallis and Albany). I. Effect of fluoride on caries experience and eruption of teeth. Am. Dent. A. J., 69:749–57, Dec. 1964.
161. Taves, D. R. Is fluoride intake in the United States changing? p. 149–57. (In Johansen, E., Taves, D. R., and Olsen, T. O., eds. Continuing evaluation of the use of fluorides. AAAS Selected Symposium no. 11. Boulder, Colo., Westview, 1979. xxviii + 321 p.)
162. U.S. Public Health Service, Centers for Disease Control. Fluoridation census 1975. Atlanta, Government Printing Office, 1977. iv + 407 p.
163. U.S. Public Health Service, Division of Dental Health. Natural fluoride content of community water supplies 1969. Washington, D.C., Government Printing Office, n.d. iii + 75 p.
164. U.S. Public Health Service. Public Health Service drinking water standards 1962. P.H.S. Publication No. 956. Washington, D.C., Government Printing Office, 1962. viii + 61 p.
165. Velu, H., and Balozet, L. Darmous (dystrophic dentaire) du mouton et solubilite du principe actif des phosphates naturels qui le provique. Bul. Soc. Path. Exot., 24:848–51, Nov. 12, 1931.
166. Weidmann, S. M., and Weatherell, J. A. Distribution in hard tissues. p. 104–28. (In World Health Organization. Fluorides and human health. Geneva, The Organization, 1970. 364 p.)
167. Whitford, G. M. Fluorides: mechanisms of action, efficiency, and safety. p. 5–18. (In

Horowitz, Alice M., and Thomas, H. B. Dental caries prevention in public health programs: proceedings of a conference, October 17–18, 1980. Bethesda, National Institutes Health, 1981. xv + 161 p.)

168. Whittle, J. G., and Downer, M. C. Dental health and treatment needs of Birmingham and Salford school children. Brit. Dent. J., 147:67–71, Aug. 7, 1979.
169. World Health Organization. Fluoridation and general health. WHO Chron., 23:505–12, Nov. 1969.
170. ———. Fluorides and human health. Geneva, The Organization, 1970. 364 p.
171. Yiamouyiannis, J., and Burk, D. Fluoridation and cancer: age-dependence of cancer mortality related to artificial fluoridation. Fluoride, 10:102–23, July 1977.
172. Young, W. O., and Pelton, W. J. Planning a dental prepayment program for children in an area of low caries prevalence. Am. Dent. A. J., 53:38–46, July 1956.

Additional Readings

Barrett, Stephen, and Rovin, Sheldon, eds. The toothrobbers; a pro-fluoridation handbook. Philadelphia, Stickley, c1980. xii + 131 p.

Brown, W. E., ed. Oral health, dentistry, and the American public; the need for an improved oral care delivery system. Norman, Okla., University Oklahoma Press, c1974. xx + 372 p.

Crain, R. L., Katz, Elihu, and Rosenthal, D. B. The politics of community conflict; the fluoridation decision. Indianapolis, Bobbs-Merrill, c1969. xix + 269 p.

Davies, G. N. Cost and benefit of fluoride in the prevention of dental caries. World Health Organization Offset Publication no. 9. Geneva, WHO, 1974. vii + 91 p.

Forrester, D. J., and Schulz, E. M., Jr., eds. International workshop on fluorides and dental caries reduction. Baltimore, University Maryland School Dentistry, 1974. 327 p.

Newbrun, Ernest. Fluorides and dental caries; contemporary concepts for practitioners and students. 2nd ed. Springfield, Ill., Thomas, 1975. xxi + 181 p.

CHAPTER 8

OTHER METHODS FOR THE PREVENTION AND CONTROL OF DENTAL CARIES

Brian A. Burt

The current accent on prevention in dental practice has been referred to as a "boom." This development may be enhanced by the growing awareness of Americans in matters of personal health and fitness, so it can be expected that public interest in the prevention of oral diseases will continue to increase.

ETIOLOGY OF CARIES

Dental caries is a highly complex disease. Because details of its etiology are provided in texts such as Newbrun's *Cariology*,[174] only a brief and necessarily simplified outline is given here.

Dental caries is an infectious, transmissible disease of bacterial origin. The causative bacteria are harbored in adherent dental plaque, and for many of these bacteria the mouth is a natural reservoir. Under specific conditions, certain of these bacteria can ferment carbohydrate to produce acid, which in turn can demineralize adjacent tooth enamel. At its earliest stages this demineralization process can be reversed; remineralization seems to be dependent upon the concentration of fluoride, calcium, and phosphorus in the plaque. If demineralization proceeds, however, clinical caries develops.

Caries is thus a disease that can only develop with the following:

1. Bacterial agents—The presence of bacteria in the dental plaque capable of producing acid as one by-product of their own metabolism.

2. A suitable substrate—The acid-producing bacteria require a suitable substrate to metabolize in the dental plaque. Carbohydrate, especially refined carbohydrate, is the most favorable substrate.

3. A susceptible host—Dental enamel (or cementum, in the case of root caries) that is susceptible to dissolution by plaque acids, and saliva that for various reasons does not buffer these acids adequately.

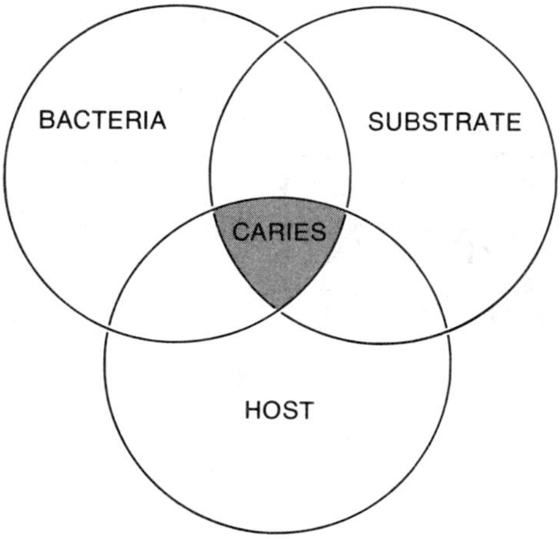

Figure 8–1. A simple ecological model to show the interaction of factors required for caries to develop. A fourth factor, time, is necessary for the clinical manifestations of the disease to become evident.

4. Time—Clinical caries only develops after repeated and undisturbed acid action has led to sufficient demineralization, which allows further bacterial invasion of the tooth and eventual permanent loss of tooth substance.

The interaction of the first three of these factors is illustrated in Figure 8–1. Time can be imagined as superimposed over the whole figure in a third dimension. Caries is thus a *multifactorial* disease (see Chapter 4); only if all four factors are present will clinical signs of caries become evident. This is a good example of "disease ecology." Prevention of caries aims to upset this ecological balance by influencing either the host enamel or cementum, the bacterial agent, or the plaque substrate.

METHODS OF PREVENTION

Dental caries is best prevented in the community by means of water fluoridation, as discussed in Chapter 7. Other effective methods for prevention and control of caries, both for the community and for individual patients, are as follows:

1. Dietary supplements of fluoride
2. Fluoridation of school water supplies
3. Topical application of fluoride compounds, both professionally applied and self-applied
4. Pit-and-fissure sealants
5. Dietary control
6. Plaque control

Research with antibiotics to date has been disappointing, though it is conceivable that the problems of nonspecificity and development of resistant organisms may be overcome in the future.[64] At present, however, antibiotics do not offer a practical means of controlling caries. Similarly, research efforts to develop a vaccine against dental caries may one day bear fruit, but there is still a long way to go. (If an effective vaccine against dental caries is ever developed and widely used, the implications for the practice of dentistry will be profound. As it is, caries prevalence in developed countries is already diminishing sufficiently [see Chapter 6] to have implications for dental practice.)

These methods are all termed "primary prevention," meaning that they are specific procedures that prevent the disease from occurring in the first place. The concept of "levels of prevention," described by Leavell and Clark,[138] is a useful one. "Secondary prevention," in this context, refers to early diagnosis and prompt and adequate treatment of disease. A dental example of secondary prevention is diagnosis and treatment of incipient carious lesions at a recall appointment. "Tertiary prevention," a term not often used, refers to rehabilitation after the defect and disability have been treated.

Restorative dental care has a place in the control of caries as secondary or tertiary prevention. The high costs of restorative care and the uneven utilization of dental services, however, make it unlikely that treatment needs to repair the damage of caries will ever be completely met, even in a wealthy country with a good supply of dentists. In developing countries, restorative care for the control of the growing problem of dental caries is practically nonexistent as an option because of shortages of resources (see Chapter 6).

Evidence for Effectiveness

The effectiveness of agents used to prevent dental caries should be based, as much as possible, on the results of well-conducted clinical trials carried out with human populations. (See Chapters 5 and 10.) The development of a preventive agent typically begins with hypotheses developed from existing knowledge or from epidemiological studies. It then proceeds through toxicological tests and animal studies. If results are promising and if the safety of the material for use in humans can be established, large-scale clinical trials in human populations are the final step. The research and development required to reach this point, however, can be long and expensive. Accordingly, some manufacturers, in an effort to recoup their investment, market products that have not received the final test of human clinical trials. But regardless of how good the theoretical basis for a preventive agent is and regardless of how promising animal and laboratory studies have been, practitioners should be discouraged from using the agent unless there is evidence of its effectiveness in humans.

Usually more than one clinical trial is required of a new agent before it can be accepted as effective, because clinical trials can occasionally produce false positive or false negative results. Moreover, results of trials may vary widely because of differences in their design, procedures used, types of personnel employed, types of examiners, age of subjects tested, and disease experience in the population from which the test subjects are drawn. Sometimes there are only subtle differences in concentration or method of application of the test material from one trial to another. If a number of clinical trials with the same material are carried out and results are all in the same direction (even if not of the same magnitude), it usually can be accepted that the regimen or agent is effective. (The requirements for a clinical trial in humans are described in Chapter 5.) For example, one of the strongest proofs of the effectiveness of water fluoridation is the extraordinary consistency of the beneficial results obtained from trials conducted in different countries by different examiners under differing conditions. That replication of evidence is in itself impressive.

The American Dental Association (ADA), through its Council on Dental Therapeutics (CDT), periodically reviews the evidence for caries-preventive agents as well as for other pharmaceutical materials used in dentistry. The findings and recommendations of the CDT are updated and published biennially in the ADA's *Accepted Dental Therapeutics*, the latest edition of which should be available in every dental office.

Choice of preventive agents and procedures, either for an individual or for groups, is based on effectiveness, acceptance, cost, and practicality. Effectiveness for different agents varies by age and by disease patterns, such as whether there is a preponderance of either fissure caries or proximal lesions. Acceptance and practicality can be based on cultural standards (e.g., toothbrushing is a normal practice in America) and individual tastes and motivation. Cost should always be a principal factor in choice of any preventive treatment.

FLUORIDES

The National Research Council of the United States[169] has declared fluoride an essential nutrient, one necessary for normal human growth as well as for dental benefits. Fluoride compounds, like many vitamins and essential minerals, are toxic if ingested in excessive amounts. Despite the familiarity with them brought about by their widespread use, they should always be applied with respect. The death of a child in New York as a result of flagrant abuse of fluoride has been reported,[98] a tragedy that emphasizes the need to follow meticulously the recommendations given in *Accepted Dental Therapeutics*.

Mode of Action of Fluoride

There are several probable ways in which fluoride works; its dental benefits most likely come from a combination of all of them.[60, 140, 193] First, fluoride reduces the solubility of dental enamel by both systemic and topical action. The traditional view has been that fluoride ingested prior to tooth eruption enhances the development of fluorapatite at the enamel surface and that this fluorapatite is resistant to the demineralizing acids that initiate the carious process. This mechanism is still thought to occur, but it is unlikely that it can fully account for the degree of reduction in caries incidence seen with various forms of fluoride therapy. Second, the topical effect of fluoride in reducing enamel solubility occurs during the repeated cycles of demineralization and remineralization in the early stages of the carious lesion,[174] when the continuous presence of a low level of fluoride in the plaque leads to a gradual establishment of a well-crystallized and more acid-resistant apatite in the enamel surface.[129, 219]

The third likely mechanism results from fluoride in the dental plaque itself, clearly a topical rather than a systemic action of fluoride. Plaque is relatively rich in fluoride. Although most of this fluoride is chemically bound to organic consitutents of plaque and is therefore not available in free ionic form, it nevertheless seems to inhibit glycolysis, the process by which sugar is metabolized by bacteria to produce acid. There is also some evidence that the bound fluoride inhibits the production of extracellular polysaccharide by cariogenic bacteria, a necessary process for plaque adherence to smooth enamel surfaces. The relatively small amount of fluoride that is not bound in dental plaque is available to react with enamel under specific conditions, as already described.[60]

As a further possible mechanism, there is evidence that fluoride may have specific bactericidal action on cariogenic bacteria in the plaque,[147] especially in higher concentrations and at low pH.

Fluorides have their most pronounced benefits on the smooth enamel surfaces, followed by proximal surfaces, with the least benefits in the pits and fissures.[18, 96, 149] Although one study found pronounced benefits in occlusal surfaces following the application of an amine fluoride gel over five consecutive days,[206] this procedure is not practical in most instances.

Dietary Supplements of Fluoride

The object of dietary supplementation of fluoride is to mimic the action of water fluoridation. Dietary supplements are widely used around the world, in the form of tablets, lozenges, drops, liquids, and fluoride-vitamin preparations for pediatric use. Fluoridated salt is available in a number of countries. There has been some small-scale experimentation with fluoridated milk, but the variable consumption patterns of milk and concerns over distribution make fluoridated milk an impractical preventive measure.[214]

Most fluoride tablets contain 1.0 mg of fluoride, although tablets with 0.5 or 0.25 mg are also available for use by younger children. Fluoride tablets were orginally in a "pill" form to be swallowed; more recently, some tablets are being made as lozenges, meant to be sucked a minute or two before swallowing, in order to get both topical and systemic effects. Tablets contain either neutral sodium fluoride (NaF) or acidulated phosphate fluoride (APF). There appears to be little difference between neutral NaF and APF in terms of effectiveness, although the APF tablets are rather more expensive.

A number of studies in the United States, Europe, and Australia show that fluoride tablets taken daily can result in a 50 to 80 percent reduction in caries in the primary teeth when taken as prescribed. Best results are found when supplementation is begun before two years of age and continued for at least three to four years.[28] Reductions of about the same magnitude have been recorded for the permanent dentition,[28] with the greatest reduction—around 80 percent—occurring in one study conducted in the Boston area.[2] It is likely, however, that the groups studied in this and similar studies[157] are selected groups who show above-average motivation and adherence to prescribed dental health behavior. Driscoll's study in North Carolina, conducted in rural schools with children who chewed an APF tablet once or twice each school day, provided results that are perhaps more to be expected in average populations. After six years, Driscoll reported reductions of 29 percent, based on approximately two fewer DMF surfaces per child compared with controls.[53] There were no additional benefits from chewing and ingesting two rather than one tablet per day. Benefits of a slightly lower magnitude were found to persist a year and a half after the supervised school-based program ceased[51] and were still detectable four years after the program ended.[52]

The fluoride-vitamin preparations, often prescribed by pediatricians for young infants, appear to have effects similar to those of other fluoride supplements.[91] The addition of vitamins does not appear to increase or decrease the effectiveness of fluoride. Dental practitioners should be aware that a physician's prescription of vitamins for an infant is often terminated at a young age. If a child dependent on the fluoride-vitamins for intake of fluoride does have the prescriptions terminated before the recommended age for fluoride supplementation, additional supplementation of fluoride will be necessary.

The current recommendations of the ADA and the American Academy of Pediatrics (AAP) on fluoride supplementation are shown in Table 8–1. They are based on the age of the child and the concentration of fluoride in the water supply. For children under two years of age, both organizations now recommend 0.25 mg per day, although the AAP formerly recommended 0.5 mg per day.[6] The revised AAP schedule now agrees with that of the ADA.[5] Although the difference between 0.5 mg and 0.25 mg per day may seem minor, when ingested consistently it could be sufficient to lead to very mild

Table 8–1. Dosage Levels of Supplemental Fluoride Recommended by the American Dental Association and the American Academy of Pediatrics, by Age and Concentration of Fluoride in Water*

	Concentration of Fluoride in Water (in ppm)		
Age	*<0.3*	*0.3–0.7*	*>0.7*
0–2 years	0.25 mg†	0.00 mg	0.00 mg
2–3 years	0.50 mg	0.25 mg	0.00 mg
3–13 years‡	1.00 mg	0.50 mg	0.00 mg

*American Dental Association, Council on Dental Therapeutics.[9]

†Adjusted allowance in total milligrams of fluoride per day.

‡The American Academy of Pediatrics recommends 16, rather than 13, as the termination age.[5]

dental fluorosis in an infant whose teeth are still developing. In the Boston-area study, in which an 80 percent reduction in caries in the permanent dentition was recorded, a considerable number of the children ingesting 0.5 mg of fluoride daily in infancy exhibited very mild dental fluorosis.[2] Case histories of dental fluorosis from oversupplementation in infancy have also been recorded.[44] A 1980 survey found that a number of well-meaning physicians in fluoridated areas were prescribing fluoride supplements inappropriately,[158] thus inadvertently increasing the risk of dental fluorosis. Infants are usually seen by a physician before they attend a dentist, so local dental societies should ensure that physicians in their area are prescribing in accordance with the regimen shown in Table 8–1.

There is no reason to prescribe fluoride supplements for an expectant mother on the basis that the fluoride will aid the developing teeth of the infant. The U.S. Food and Drug Administration ruled in 1966 that the evidence did not support the advertising of claims that administration of fluorides prenatally would increase the caries resistance of offspring and accordingly banned such advertisements.[224] Although the placenta may not act as a barrier to fluoride in the manner once thought,[218] there is insufficient evidence to support the prenatal administration of fluoride for the purpose of increasing the resistance to caries of the offspring.[9] This statement does not reject the possibility of prenatal benefits; it simply means that the evidence is lacking. While some spectacular claims to the contrary have been made,[74, 75] these claims appear to based on questionable research design. The whole intriguing question of the efficacy of prenatal fluorides was examined in a symposium at the 1980 Annual Meeting of the ADA, subsequently reported in the *Journal of Dentistry for Children.*[103]

The decision of whether or not to prescribe fluoride supplements for an infant depends largely on the other dietary intake of fluoride the infant is receiving, including that from water.[54, 55] Very little fluoride is found in mother's milk, so that a child who is being *totally* breast-fed, with no additional water given between feedings, can have fluoride supplements prescribed with confidence. This recommendation applies whether or not the child resides in a fluoridated area, because either way the child will be receiving little fluoride. If the child is being partly breast-fed and partly formula-fed, more caution by the practitioner in prescribing fluoride is in order. A number of infant formulas and baby foods were found in the past to contain relatively high concentrations of fluoride,[55, 221] though major American manufacturers of these products have since taken steps to correct this problem. If the child resides in a fluoridated area, supplementation should not be carried out if the child is receiving any tap water. When there is doubt, caution on the part of the practitioner seems to be the best policy.

In summary, practitioners should know the fluoride content of the water in their communities and follow the ADA recommendations for fluoride supplementation. For breast-fed infants, good judgment and moderate caution should dictate what course of action is taken.

Fluoridated Salt

The addition of fluoride to salt is considered the most efficient way of bringing the benefits of systemic fluoride to populations in many developing countries where there is no piped water. Fluoridated salt was first used in Switzerland in 1955; the mountainous nature of that country prevented many communities from having municipal water supplies. The reduction in caries incidence in communities using fluoridated salt consistently paralleled that found in communities having water fluoridation, and public acceptance of the fluoridated salt in Switzerland has been good.[161]

The early studies used salt fluoridated to 90 parts per million (ppm). In 1970, this concentration was increased to 250 ppm (250 mg per kg of salt). Estimates of the ideal concentration of fluoride in salt have been made from studies of urinary excretion of fluoride. Data suggest that 250 ppm now appears to be the most suitable concentration.

The effects of fluoridated salt have also been studied in Colombia, Spain, and Hungary, with results generally similar to those found in Switzerland.[161] Salt fluoridation may become more common, especially in developing countries. Given the mass distribution of food in the United States and Canada, along with the frequent occurrence of natural fluoride, salt would not appear to be a suitable vehicle for fluoride in those countries.

Fluoridation of School Water Supplies

An alternative to community water fluoridation is the fluoridation of a school's drinking water. This procedure has been shown to reduce dental caries among schoolchildren by about 40 percent.[87, 107] It is most applicable in rural schools where fluoridation of community waters is not feasible. Relative to community water fluoridation, the disadvantages of this method are that children do not receive the benefits until they begin school and that they consume the water only when school is in session. In order to compensate for this belated and abbreviated exposure, the school water is usually fluoridated at 4.5 times the optimum concentration recommended for community fluoridation in the same geographical area. School water fluoridation has been introduced in 13 states in the United States; it was established in approximately 450 schools by 1981. North Carolina and Kentucky have particularly large programs. It is not known if the procedure is used in countries outside the United States.

The fluoridation equipment in the school is usually monitored by an employee of the school system who has been properly trained, usually by personnel from the state's health department. Only one mishap with school water fluoridation has been reported,[92] fortunately without lasting ill-effects. Safety guidelines set by the Centers for Disease Control (U.S. Public Health Service, Atlanta) in association with the Environmental Protection Agency[25] minimize the potential for mishaps. States can publish their own standards from these guidelines; Kentucky is an example of one state that has done so.[213]

Fluorides Applied Topically

Dental personnel should be familiar with the composition of the fluoride compounds used in the dental office or prescribed for home use. Table 8-2 provides general guidance in regard to quantities and concentrations of the most frequently used fluoride compounds applied topically.

Professionally Applied Fluorides

Early work with topical fluorides began even before the first additions of fluoride to community water supplies and led to the procedure known as the "Knutson technic."[132] This technic involves the use of a 2.0 percent solution of NaF given in a series of four applications over a period of several days, following an initial prophylaxis. The technic is recommended for children aged 3, 7, 10, and 13 to coincide with the eruption of new teeth. Reductions of caries on the order of 40 percent have been reported with this technic.[35]

The principal disadvantage of the Knutson technic was the necessity of applying the solution on four separate occasions at each of the four ages. In the 1950s, the annual application of stannous fluoride (SnF_2) at a concentration of 8.0 percent was reported to give beneficial results similar to those achieved with NaF. The SnF_2 had the advantage that it only had to be applied once

Table 8–2. Concentration and Quantity of Fluoride in Commonly Used Topical Fluoride Compounds*

Compound	Concentration (ppm)	Quantity
Topically applied by dental personnel:		
2.00% NaF—Knutson technic	9,050	45.0 mg in 5 ml†
1.23% APF solution, gel or prophylaxis paste	12,300	62.0 mg in 5 gm
8.00% SnF_2 solution	19,363	97.0 mg in 5 ml
Mouthrinses:		
0.20% NaF—weekly	905	9.0 mg in 10 ml‡
0.05% NaF—daily	226	2.0 mg in 10 ml
0.10% SnF_2—daily	242	2.0 mg in 10 ml
APF rinse (0.1% fluoride)—weekly	1,000	10.0 mg in 10 ml
APF rinse (0.022% fluoride)—daily	200	2.0 mg in 10 ml
		1.0 mg in 5 ml of oral rinse supplement ("rinse and swallow")
Dentifrices:		
0.76% Sodium monofluorophosphate	1,000	1.0 mg per gm§
0.40% SnF_2‖	966	1.0 mg per gm
0.243% NaF	1,105	1.1 mg per gm

*Some figures rounded.
†A topical application or prophylaxis uses about 5 ml or 5 gm of material.
‡Amounts of 5 and 10 ml are used in supervised mouthrinsing.
§An average load of toothpaste on the brush is about 1 gm.
‖No longer marketed in the United States.

annually. It also had the disadvantage, however, of being relatively unstable and hence had to be mixed prior to each application. In addition, some staining problems were reported, and the material had an unpleasant taste.[35] Better results have been reported with semiannual applications of SnF_2,[35] and the material is now available in a stable formulation.

Since the early 1960s, APF has probably become the most widely used topical fluoride for professional application. The material has a pH of about 3.0 and was developed following experimental work that showed that the uptake of fluoride by enamel was greater in an acid environment.[35] It has been tested in several concentrations, the most common being 1.23 percent of fluoride, usually present as NaF, in orthophosphoric acid. APF has been successfully tested in both solution and gel form, but the gel is by far the most widely used today. Its advantages are that it is convenient to handle; can be applied from a tray, which requires less time than the constant application of a solution;[36] and is readily stored. The material is nonirritating and nonstaining, will tolerate the addition of flavorings, and is acceptable to patients.[100]

Professionally applied topical fluorides were developed on the basis that the fluoride would react with enamel to form a fluorapatite; a prophylaxis was thus considered mandatory before the application of the fluoride. Subsequently, however, the value of the prophylaxis prior to a professional application of fluoride came to be questioned,[220] in light of the development of alternative theories of fluoride action described earlier. If clinical research shows that a prophylaxis is not necessary, there will be a considerable saving of time, and hence cost, in the professional application of topical fluorides. For the present, the professionally applied fluoride procedures are considered less cost-effective than the variety of self-applied measures used in public health programs,[90] though the former clearly have a role with selected patients in the private office.

Fluoride-containing prophylaxis pastes are widely used in dentistry; the reasoning behind their development was that the prophylaxis and the professional fluoride application could be carried out at one time. Results from clinical trials using the professionally applied prophylaxis pastes, however, have been inconsistent.[46, 180] While routine use of fluoride-containing prophylaxis pastes is recommended in dental practice, it is not used as a substitute for a professional application of topical fluoride.[9]

Self-Applied Fluorides

Some fluoride compounds may be applied by the individual rather than by a dental professional. Because such procedures lead to benefits of much the same magnitude as those received from professionally applied fluorides, they are obviously more cost-effective in a public health program. At the individual level, self-applied fluorides can be used to complement the professional treatment received from the dentist or hygienist.

Individualized Gel-Tray Application. A study by Englander and his colleagues[58] in Cheektowaga, New York, produced impressive reductions in dental caries among schoolchildren aged 11–14. Their procedure was to fabricate individualized trays for each child; the children then held these trays with a neutral NaF or APF gel in place for six minutes each school day over a period of two school years. Dental hygienists supervised the procedure.

With such intensive application it is not surprising that results were good, but the procedure is expensive and is not currently used in public health programs because of its limited cost-effectiveness. This study did demonstrate, however, the benefits of intensive fluoride therapy to individual patients who are especially susceptible to caries.

Supervised Brushing with Fluoride Solutions, Prophylaxis Pastes, and Gels. Public health programs of supervised brushing have been employed in Norway and Sweden in the past. The brushing material generally used was a neutral NaF solution with between 0.5 and 1.0 percent of fluoride, brushed on under supervision once every two months during the school year.[222] While several evaluations in Scandinavia and elsewhere showed the procedure to be moderately beneficial,[150] rinsing with fluoride solutions has been found to be more effective.[29] As a result, the supervised brushing procedure is now being superseded by rinsing programs in Scandinavian school-based programs.[190]

Supervised brushing programs using 9.0 percent SnF_2 with a zirconium silicate abrasive have been popular in some areas of the United States. These annual or biannual "brush-ins" sometimes attracted a lot of publicity and large group participation. Results of studies to evaluate this procedure, however, have given equivocal results in terms of dental benefits. Gish and colleagues[71] in Indiana recorded a 37 percent reduction in caries among children aged 6–14 over a three-year period, and Muhler and associates[167] reported substantial benefits in the Virgin Islands after one year. But other studies in the United States and Canada showed little benefit.[65, 78, 110] Questionable dental benefits and relatively high costs, in addition to the development of other more cost-effective methods of self-application of fluoride, are the chief reasons why "brush-ins" are not recommended today. Moreover, the stannous fluoride-zirconium silicate material is no longer manufactured in the United States.

Studies to test the efficacy of supervised brushing with APF prophylaxis paste two to four times per year also demonstrated little benefit from the procedure.[148, 162, 163, 223] The procedure was reported as being unpopular with participants. Better results have been attained from programs of supervised brushing with APF solutions[43] and APF gels when used frequently[160] or when preceded by a self-applied brushing with a nonfluoride prophylaxis paste.[108] Not all studies with these materials, however, have yielded positive results.[84]

The concept of supervised brushing has been widely tested with a variety of fluoride materials and frequencies of application, but results do not fit into a clear-cut pattern. In addition, fluoride mouthrinsing has emerged as a more cost-effective procedure for public health programs.[90]

Brushing with fluoride-containing prophylaxis pastes or gels has little application to the individual patient under the care of a dentist or hygienist. These materials are not the same as fluoride dentifrices.

Fluoride Mouthrinses. The idea of mouthrinsing with dilute solutions of fluoride is not new.[27, 231] A number of different formulations have been widely tested and are being widely used.[94, 97] Both NaF and APF rinses have been extensively tested; others tested to a lesser extent include SnF_2, ammonium fluoride, and amine fluoride. Fluoride mouthrinses are suitable for use both in public programs and by individual patients at home.

Materials most often recommended for use are NaF in either 0.2 percent concentration used weekly or 0.05 percent fluoride used daily.[9, 97] Use of the 0.2 percent NaF on a weekly basis appears to be most suitable for school-based public programs.[94] By 1981 about 8 to 10 million children in the United States were enrolled in programs using this technic. Daily rinsing appears to confer only slightly greater benefits than weekly rinsing,[56, 89] and the slight differences noted do not compensate for the greater practicality and lower cost of weekly rinsing in a school-based program. For the individual patient, however, daily use is probably more appropriate as part of the daily oral hygiene routine. Dentists can either prescribe a material for home use or patients can purchase 0.05 percent NaF or 0.1 percent SnF_2 mouthrinse over the counter in drug stores and supermarkets. Two over-the-counter fluoride mouthrinses have been accepted by the ADA—*Fluorigard* (0.05 percent NaF) and *Stancare* (0.1 percent SnF_2).[9]

A considerable number of studies show that use of recommended NaF mouthrinses results in reductions in caries on the order of 35 percent.[31, 47, 97, 106, 189, 195] There has been one report indicating similar benefits to be derived from 0.025 percent NaF daily,[68] Positive benefits have also been reported in the primary dentition.[188] Comprehensive reviews of the numerous studies on fluoride mouthrinses have been provided by Torell and Ericsson[222] and Birkeland and Torell.[31]

Several studies using APF rinse, 1.23 percent fluoride at pH 4.0, have indicated reductions on the order of 20 to 30 percent.[31] APF "rinse-and-swallow" rinse, available by prescription, has also been shown to be beneficial.[1] The "rinse-and-swallow" approach provides both systemic and topical benefits. A limited number of tests with SnF_2 rinse, 0.1 percent, have shown positive caries reductions.[151, 182] One of these studies resulted in reductions of 33 to 43 percent in caries incidence in a fluoridated area, thus indicating that benefits additional to those derived from fluoridated water can be achieved.[182] Other fluoride compounds have been tested for rinsing such as ammonium fluoride[47] and amine fluoride.[185] These tests did not produce results superior to those obtained with neutral NaF.

Rinsing with neutral NaF, rather than with other fluoride compounds, either on the weekly or on the daily regimen is recommended for several reasons:[97] (1) more studies showing the benefits of neutral NaF rinsing have been carried out; (2) NaF solution can be readily made up at schools, whereas other solutions are best formulated in a commercial laboratory (this factor alone considerably reduces the cost of the program); and (3) NaF solutions do not have the objectionable taste of SnF_2 or the acid taste of APF solutions.

There is evidence that the benefits from long-term use of fluoride mouthrinsing programs are impressive. In Sweden, for example, 10 years of rinsing produced benefits in children similar to those obtained from ingestion of fluoridated water for the same period.[30] However, it is not known to what extent the benefits of mouthrinsing are retained, whereas the benefits from fluoridated water extend into adulthood (see Chapter 7).

In summary, mouthrinsing with fluoride is a recommended procedure at a public health or individual level. It is of particular value for caries-susceptible patients, but it is a useful prophylactic measure for all. It is cheap, simple, and beneficial. A number of prescribed and over-the-counter mouthrinses have been classified as efficacious by the ADA,[9] and an excellent reference paper on the use of fluoride mouthrinses has been given by Ripa.[187]

Fluoride Dentifrices. Because toothbrushing is an established practice in most Western societies, a variety of preventive and therapeutic agents (both known and hypothetical) have been added to dentifrices over the years. Early efforts to produce therapeutic dentifrices included the addition of ammonia,[83, 128] antibiotics,[64] chlorophyll, and other additives with "anti-enzyme action."[9] None of these additives, however, proved to be beneficial.

To date, fluoride is the only additive to a dentifrice known to be of benefit in the prevention of caries. Use of a fluoride toothpaste seems to provide some added benefits even in fluoridated areas[142, 159, 227] and is also a successful adjunct to other forms of fluoride therapy.[112] Dentifrices without active ingredients—that is, those that contain abrasive and flavoring agents only and are thus intended for oral hygiene and cosmetic benefits—have no anticaries action by themselves. The earliest attempts to add fluoride to dentifrice were unsuccessful because of the use of incompatible abrasives (particularly calcium-based abrasives), many of which bound the fluoride, making it unavailable. The first successful clinical trials using a fluoride additive, however, had a SnF_2/calcium pyrophosphate formulation.[166] The beneficial results reported were replicated in a number of other studies,[104, 120, 126, 165, 210] which reported reductions of dental caries in the range of 15 to 30 percent.

Subsequent studies using fluorides of various types with different abrasives have generally produced moderate caries reductions of around 15 to 30 percent. These include SnF_2 with insoluble metaphosphate abrasive,[34, 171, 211, 212] sodium monofluorophosphate in several different concentrations and with several different abrasive systems,[11, 61, 67, 73, 114, 121, 142, 154, 164, 170, 179, 217] SnF_2 in a hydrated silica gel formulation,[66] and amine fluoride.[159, 185]

Dentifrices with NaF as an additive were disappointing in their early tests,[109] again probably because of binding of the fluoride by other constituents of the toothpaste.[9] Subsequently, however, several dentifrices with NaF as the active ingredient have been successfully tested in both Europe[57, 67, 134, 227] and North America.[24, 184, 234]

By 1979, the ADA had accepted four dentifrices that used sodium monofluorophosphate 0.76 percent *(Aquafresh, Colgate with MFP, Macleans, Aim)* and two with SnF_2 0.4 percent as the active ingredient (*Crest* and *Aim*).

Subsequently, *Advanced Formula Crest* with 0.243 percent NaF was accepted in late 1980, as was *Aim* with sodium monofluorophosphate.* Some 80 percent of toothpastes sold in the United States are now ADA-accepted fluoride-containing toothpastes,[202] though there are numerous other fluoride-containing dentifrices widely available, as any perusal of the shelves in a drugstore or supermarket will reveal. Many of these other brands have not been tested clinically, although now that the initial problems with incompatible abrasive systems have been overcome most toothpastes containing fluoride are probably beneficial. Practitioners are well-advised, however, to recommend brands accepted by the ADA. Brushing with fluoride dentifrices is a recommended procedure for everybody with teeth.

Fluoride Varnishes. A fluoride varnish is not intended to be as permanent as a fissure sealant; rather it is a vehicle for holding fluoride in close contact with the tooth for a period of time. Studies in Sweden have suggested that the fluoride varnish is effective in reducing caries,[93, 133] though a similar study in England did not give nearly as good results.[168]

Although accepted in Sweden and other countries, fluoride varnishes are not available in the United States.

Combined Use of Fluorides

Most studies of the effect of fluoride on prevention of dental caries have been with individual procedures, but the growing awareness that fluoride acts in several different ways[60, 140, 193] has led to interest in the multiple use of fluorides. For example, there appears to be sound rationale for combining the less frequent use of concentrated fluorides (especially those with a low pH), to promote deposition of fluoride in enamel and to inhibit bacterial growth, with the frequent use of more dilute fluoride to promote remineralization.[48] Even before the multiple action of fluoride was understood, the U.S. Navy was using its "three agent" program—SnF_2 in a prophylaxis paste, in an aqueous solution, and in a dentifrice.[203] Additional benefits to children in fluoridated areas have been demonstrated with the use of dentifrices,[229] mouthrinses, and gel-tray technics,[88, 182] and with intensive self-application of fluoride in custom-made trays[59] as well as in a comprehensive program of preventive and restorative care.[22] Benefits derived from an annual professional application of SnF_2 in a fluoridated area are less clear.[105] Multiple fluoride therapy, whether in fluoridated or nonfluoridated areas, is especially beneficial for caries-susceptible patients. For example, Dreizen and colleagues[49] reported excellent results in preventing caries among patients who received radiation treatment for oral cancer, a treatment that leads to dysfunction of the salivary glands. The loss of the salivary buffer makes these patients highly susceptible to caries. Such therapy includes topical applications of fluoride, daily fluoride

---

*Both *Crest* and *Aim* had previously been accepted by the ADA with 0.4 percent stannous fluoride. By 1981, however, no dentifrices with stannous fluoride were being marketed in the United States.

rinsing, and use of a fluoride-containing dentifrice. In the public health field, additional programs of fluoride application in fluoridated areas, while effective, may not always be cost-effective. In nonfluoridated areas, multiple types of fluoride therapy have been shown to be effective in public health programs.[112]

For the individual patient in a fluoridated area who has little caries problem, professional applications may be of dubious additional value. If the patient is already brushing with a fluoride-containing dentifrice and rinsing daily with a fluoride solution at home, the protection obtained should be adequate and at minimum expense to the patient. More caries-susceptible patients, even in a fluoridated area, may benefit from additional fluoride therapy such as professional applications of fluoride gel in the dental office.

PIT–AND–FISSURE SEALANTS

It has been long recognized that fissured occlusal surfaces are the most vulnerable to caries.[116] In one United States community, over 90 percent of lesions in first permanent molars of children up to age 11 were occlusal lesions or occlusal with palatal/lingual extensions.[77] Occlusal surfaces are also those least protected by fluorides.[18, 113] The rationale for use of a physical barrier to caries in newly erupted occlusal surfaces is therefore sound. Indeed, Hyatt's suggestion[116] of the "prophylactic odontotomy" in 1923 has probably led to the present concept of the "preventive restoration," an approach to caries control perhaps seen more often than it should be.[119] (It is interesting to note that Hyatt's suggestion was not universally accepted even before the days of modern sealants.[130])

By the mid-1960s cyanoacrylates had been used as pit-and-fissure sealant materials with some success,[45] but production of these materials was not continued.[209] A new material at the time, based on bisphenol-A glycidyl methacrylate (bis-GMA) was highly successful in a feasibility trial[38] and remains the basis of materials now in use.

Although not all trials with pit-and-fissure sealants have been successful, there is sufficient evidence to show that sealants are efficacious in the prevention of caries when used correctly.[186, 209] Results of these studies have shown that meticulous attention to application technic is essential, for even slight moisture contamination will result in failure of the sealant to bond to the tooth surface. Acid etching is essential prior to the application of the sealant. Some manufacturers supply a 50 percent phosphoric acid for this purpose, though good results have also been achieved with a 30 percent unbuffered solution.[191, 208] Etching allows "tags" of sealant to penetrate the enamel, enhancing retention.[208, 209] In one extensive study in Kalispell, Montana (the longest study of fissure sealants yet reported), 40 percent of all the sealant was fully retained five years after a single application of bis-GMA sealant.[111] The retention rate was twice as high on mandibular teeth as it was on maxillary teeth, a result attributable to differences in tooth morphology and accessibility.[209] In the Kalispell study, there was a 90 percent reduction in dental caries on teeth where the sealant was completely retained. On teeth where the sealant was partially retained, there was an 83 percent reduction, but only a 13 percent reduction where the sealant was completely missing.

Public health studies have shown that auxiliaries can apply sealant as successfully as dentists;[139] the technic, though simple, demands meticulous application. There may also be value in sealing early carious lesions, rather than merely just sound surfaces.[82] Sealants have been successfully used in combination with other fluoride therapies.[22] Indeed, because fluoride works least effectively on occlusal surfaces, sealants complement fluoride as part of preventive therapy for many individuals.

The ADA recognizes seven pit-and-fissure sealants as being fully acceptable. These are *NuvaSeal P.A.* (meaning pre-activated), *Nuvacote, Delton, Delton (tinted), Kerr, Concise* white sealant, and *Oralin.*[8] No doubt this list will change with some frequency. *Delton* has been shown to be somewhat more effective than *NuvaSeal* in comparative studies, although both were beneficial in preventing caries when employed in the same study.[33]

Application of pit-and-fissure sealant is an expensive professionally applied procedure, so practitioners should be selective in their choice of patients to receive it. Fissure sealants are most effectively applied on newly erupted molars and premolars, because if the sealing is delayed long after eruption only caries-resistant teeth are likely to be sealed, with no benefit to the patient.[181] The cost-effectiveness of pit-and-fissure sealants in public health use is uncertain,[20, 101] though it should improve as less demanding technics and materials are developed that would lead to improved retention rates and reduced time needed for their application.

DIETARY CONTROL OF CARIES

It was stated in Chapter 6 that there is little reason to conclude that inadequate nutrition, whether during tooth development or subsequently, will lead to dental caries. While further research is needed on the consequences of introducing a developmentally malnourished patient to a highly cariogenic diet, little developmental malnourishment is found today in the United States or other Western societies. Despite this evidence, the suggestion that caries can be controlled by nutritional counseling has become fashionable in some dental circles in the United States, though some of the more fanciful approaches have been criticized.[228] Of course, the general nutritional status of a patient is rightly the concern of the attending dentist who as an ethical health professional is concerned with the patient's total health. But even in those instances where nutritional counseling is required, dental professionals should not delude themselves that such counseling is likely to improve the caries status of the patient concerned. (As stated in Chapter 6, the terms "diet" and "nutrition" ought not to be used interchangeably. "Diet" is simply food and drink taken into the mouth, regardless of what happens to them. "Nutrition" is more than just ingestion and includes digestion, absorption, and assimilation.)

If the carious process is accelerated by the presence of sugars in the mouth, caries should be inhibited if sugars are not present in the mouth. The evidence for relating sugar consumption to dental caries in population groups was given in Chapter 6. Additional evidence for the etiological role of sugary diets is their use in inducing caries in experimental animals over many years,[175] as well as in initiating caries in humans under controlled experimental conditions.[226] The studies of Bunting[37] and Jay[122] at The University of Michigan in the mid-1930s repeatedly showed that there was a greater prevalence of caries in children with high-sugar diets than in those with low-sugar diets. These studies led to the development of Jay's program for control of dental caries by dietary means,[123, 124] to be discussed later in this section.

Consumption of Sugar

The material generically known as sugar is a disaccharide, sucrose, which is the most common variety of sugar consumed by humans.[204] Sucrose is added to a wide variety of processed foods; purchasers of supermarket staples such as canned soups, salad dressings, and processed meats will notice how frequently sugar is high on the list of ingredients. Sucrose consumption in the United States peaked in the 1920s at a little over 120 pounds per head per year and has tended to decline since then.[12] This trend does not mean that the American sweet taste is diminishing, because other sugars, especially those in corn syrup, are being increasingly used in processed foods. Corn syrup contains predominantly fructose and other monosaccharides, and is a cheaper sweetener than ssucrose. Table 8–3 shows the consumption of the various sweeteners in the United States from 1970 to 1982. It can be seen that while sucrose consumption is declining, it still is the predominant sugar consumed. Corn syrup consumption is increasing, and the consumption of all caloric sweeteners combined is still stable.

In addition to the partial switch from sucrose to corn syrup in processed food, two other major changes have taken place in the consumption pattern of sugars and other carbohydrates since the early twentieth century:

Table 8–3. Per Capita Consumption of Various Sweeteners, United States, 1970–82*

	Consumption (lbs/capita/year)			
Year	*Sucrose*	*Corn Syrup*	*All Caloric Sweeteners*†	*Noncaloric Sweeteners*‡
1970	101.8	19.3	122.6	5.8
1972	102.8	21.3	125.6	5.1
1974	96.5	25.3	123.0	5.9
1976	94.6	30.1	126.1	6.1
1978	93.1	34.3	128.7	6.9
1980	84.9	41.1	127.4	7.1
1982	73.8	48.2	123.3	8.2

*U. S. Department of Agriculture, personal communication, June 16, 1983.
†Includes sucrose, corn syrup, honey, and special syrups.
‡In sugar equivalents, chiefly saccharin.

1. The proportion of calories obtained from carbohydrate foods has swung from a preponderance obtained from starches (bread, potatoes, whole grain cereals) to one obtained from sugars.[225]

2. Use of sugar has changed from discretionary use (i.e., by way of the sugar bowl on the table) to its consumption by way of processed foods, the so-called hidden sugar. At present, 75 percent of all sugars consumed come from processed foods.[40] The ubiquity of this hidden sugar makes it difficult for people to reduce sugar consumption significantly without substantial change in dietary practices.

There is little doubt in the dental world today that the relation between sugar and caries is one of cause and effect.[41] Because there appear to be only minor differences between sucrose and various monosaccharides in terms of cariogenic potential,[135] many think there is little to be gained, in terms of caries reduction, by substituting fructose or dextrose for sucrose in food processing.[176] The question of relative cariogenicity of sucrose and fructose in human diets, however, has not been completely resolved.[156] Similarly, there is apparently no important difference in cariogenicity between refined sugar and brown sugar or between refined sugar and "natural" sugars such as honey. Sucrose is the "arch-criminal" of dental caries mainly because so much more of it is consumed relative to other sugars.[172]

The food item that has probably received most attention in recent years concerning sugar content is presweetened breakfast cereal. The issue of whether or not there should be some control of the advertising of these products on television programs geared primarily to children was the center of considerable public discussion in the late 1970s. Many breakfast cereals *do* contain a high concentration of sugar, as shown in Table 8–4. Several field studies have attempted to determine if presweetened cereals by themselves add to the caries experience of children, but the results have thus far been inconclusive.[63, 72, 194] Animal studies with presweetened breakfast cereals generally show a more direct relation between sugar content of the cereal and caries experience,[152] but the diets of laboratory animals can be rigidly controlled in a way that human diets cannot. Regardless of how cariogenic any one food is, it is difficult to demonstrate its cariogenicity in humans if only because of the heterogenicity of human foods and eating habits. The inconclusive results of human studies with presweetened breakfast cereals are therefore not surprising.

Food manufacturers are adding more sugar to more foods because they say the public likes it and it increases the marketability of their products.[173] If a suitable substitute for sugar in food processing could be found, it is likely that many manufacturers would use it, if marketability were not impaired. But there are two barriers to the development of suitable sugar substitutes. One is that sugar has such a variety of desirable characteristics from the food manufacturer's point of view that it is difficult to replace; as well as having a sweet taste, sugar adds body, luster, and texture to a food product, promotes the emulsification of fats, and acts as a preservative. While corn syrup is being increasingly used as a sweetener in place of sucrose in processed foods for

Table 8–4. The Concentration of Sucrose and Other Sugars in Selected Breakfast Cereals, United States, 1980*

Cereal	Concentration of Sugar (percent of dry weight)
Kellogg's Sugar Smacks	56
Kellogg's Apple Jacks	53
Post Super Sugar Crisp	49
Kellogg's Frosted Rice	46
Kellogg's Cocoa Krispies	46
Kellogg's Froot Loops	46
Kellogg's Sugar Frosted Flakes	46
Quaker Fruity Pebbles	46
Quaker Cookie Crisp	46
Quaker 100% Natural	32
Nabisco Honey Bran	25
Post Granola	25
Quaker Life	18
Kellogg's All Bran	18
Kellogg's Rice Krispies	11
Kellogg's Product 19	11
Nabisco Rice Chex	7
Nabisco Corn Chex	7
Nabisco Shredded Wheat	3.5

*From manufacturers' information on the box.

economic reasons, the other desirable qualities of sucrose have to come from food additives.

A second reason for the slow development of sugar substitutes in the United States concerns legal considerations. There are tedious and expensive hurdles to be jumped in convincing government regulatory agencies that new sugar substitutes, or other food additives for that matter, are sufficiently safe to be marketed. An excellent discussion on these and related issues is found in Newbrun's book, *Cariology.*[174]

Some sugar substitutes, such as the noncaloric saccharin, are in common use in the United States and elsewhere. Aspartame, a dipeptide composed of two naturally occurring amino acids became available in the United States in 1982. Other substitutes are the sugar alcohols, mannitol and sorbitol, used in many sugarless chewing gums. These sugar alcohols have an advantage over sucrose (in terms of cariogenesis) because they do not lower the pH of the dental plaque to a point at which enamel demineralization occurs, though they can be fermented by cariogenic bacteria, particularly *Streptococcus mutans.*[174] The preventive value of partial substitution of sucrose by sorbitol and mannitol in the diet remains uncertain, though it is presumed to convey some benefit.

At present the most promising of several potential sugar substitutes is the sugar alcohol xylitol. In a series of studies in the Finnish city of Turku,[198, 199] a volunteer group of adults made virtually complete substitution of sucrose in their diet by xylitol, a change made possible with the cooperation of food manufacturers for the two years of the study. A second group consumed fructose instead of sucrose, and a third group consumed the usual sucrose-containing diet. By necessity, this study deviated from an ideal clinical trial in that the participants were self-selected and were aware of their group assignment. Still, the magnitude of the differences in new caries experience between the groups was impressive. Over the two-year period there were practically no new carious lesions in the xylitol group, while there were more than seven in the group eating the normal (sucrose) diet and four new lesions in the fructose group. Lesions in the adult test subjects (average age 27.5) were almost all on smooth surfaces. The quantity of plaque formed in the xylitol group was also significantly lower.[201] In a separate study in Turku,[200] subjects consumed an average of four sticks a day of chewing gum containing xylitol, in addition to a normal diet. Control group subjects consumed the same amount of chewing gum containing sucrose in addition to the usual diet. After a year the test group subjects had 0.3 new DMF carious surfaces compared with nearly four surfaces in the sucrose group.

Xylitol cannot be metabolized by cariogenic microorganisms and in addition does not reduce the pH of plaque.[137] As a consequence, the replacement of sucrose by xylitol in the dental plaque is thought to "starve" the cariogenic microorganisms, thus sharply reducing their numbers. This apparent *anti*cariogenic effect, in addition to the *non*cariogenic attributes of xylitol, suggests that even its partial substitution for sucrose is likely to be more effective in caries control than is the present partial substitution of sucrose by mannitol and sorbitol.[156, 200]

At present, xylitol is not available in the United States. It did appear for a short time as an ingredient in Wrigley's *Orbit* chewing gum, but was later withdrawn by the company after an animal study suggested that xylitol might be carcinogenic. Because xylitol does imitate some of the other desirable properties of sugar, it could be attractive for food manufacturers to use in place of sucrose once the question of its safety becomes settled enough to meet the rigid criteria of the United States government.

Determinants of Cariogenicity of the Diet

Sugar Content

Sugar is probably not the only food item that leads to caries but it is by far the most potent one. Sugar is a cariogenic food because cariogenic organisms, notably *S. mutans*, metabolize it readily to produce extracellular polysaccharides. Acid production, and hence a lowered pH of the plaque, is a consequence of this metabolism. The extracellular polysaccharides increase the retentiveness (on smooth surfaces) and the bulk of the plaque. One of the unique properties of *S. mutans* is that it is aciduric, meaning that it can thrive in an acid environment, so that as the acid production continues, the organism continues to multiply and grow.[146] In pits and fissures, other acid-producing organisms as well as *S. mutans* probably initiate caries.

Starches in due course can be broken down in the oral cavity and metabolized by cariogenic bacteria, but this process occurs much more slowly than the metabolism of sugar. For that reason starchy foods, such as bread and potatoes, do not appear to be particularly conducive to caries. On the other hand, after sugar is taken into the oral cavity, the pH of plaque drops rapidly.[125, 155, 215]

An almost complete abstinence from sucrose leads to extremely low levels of dental caries, as seen in persons suffering from the rare disease of hereditary fructose intolerance.[177] (Hereditary fructose intolerance is a metabolic disorder that requires lifetime restraint in eating sugar.) By contrast, epidemiological studies show that there is little relation between total quantities of sucrose in the normal diet and caries levels.[39] These findings suggest that there is a "threshold" level for sucrose consumption and that once this threshold is exceeded, additional amounts of sucrose per se may not have all that much effect. Of course, additional consumption can also mean additional *frequency* of consumption, which is a different story.

Physical Form of the Diet

The sugar ingested in the diet is considered to be more damaging if it is in a physically sticky form; the sugar in chewy toffees is likely to be more cariogenic than the same amount of sugar in a soft drink. The importance of physical form of the food has been demonstrated in animal studies and was also confirmed in human subjects in the Vipeholm study.[79]

It was discussed in Chapter 6 that beliefs in the anticariogenic properties of "detersive foods" have little substance. The value of nonsticky fibrous foods such as apples, carrots, and celery, long endorsed by dental health education, may be indirect—presumably a carrot is better than candy as an after-school snack. But nothing is sacred any more, for even the apple has been shown to lower plaque pH soon after ingestion.[70] The influence of this finding on caries initiation and progression is unknown, and may be of little importance—acidogenesis is but one factor in cariogenesis, and it is even possible that the inherent acidity of the apple influenced the readings obtained.

Frequency of Consumption of Sugary Foods

One of the effects of sugar ingestion is that within a few minutes the pH of the dental plaque can drop to a point low enough to demineralize enamel, thus initiating the caries process. This drop in pH, followed by gradual recovery over the following half hour if no further food is eaten, was first described by Stephan[215] in 1940; the curve described by plotting pH against time is known as the "Stephan Curve." If sugary foods are eaten frequently—for instance, at half-hour intervals—the dental plaque is kept at a low acid pH because the frequent infusions of sugar reactivate the plaque. In such instances, the acidity of the plaque of a person who is frequently eating candy throughout the day, for example, may be kept below the critical pH level for demineralization (5.2 to 5.5) for a considerable period. On the other hand, the person who eats sugary food only once or twice during the day will lower the pH of the plaque for a much shorter period. The technology for measuring plaque pH is much more sophisticated today than it was in Stephan's time, but his original work has been confirmed by more precise measurements.[118]

Again, animal studies have generally shown that caries rates are closely allied to frequency of snacking. In epidemiological studies, data from the National Health and Nutrition Examination Survey (NHANES) of the United States in 1971–74 showed a strong correlation between the reported frequency of ingestion of sugary snacks and DMF values for all age groups in a representative sample of the United States population.[39] This finding confirmed other studies with human populations,[79, 230] though some conflicting results have also been reported in this area.[21] Difficulties in obtaining reliable dietary information, as well as the inherent difficulty of relating recent dietary history to lifetime caries experience, probably account for this lack of universality. On balance, however, the frequency of eating sugar-containing foods, especially between meals, is an important correlate of caries.

Ingestion with Meals or between Meals

This point is somewhat related to frequency, although the rationale is slightly different. Saliva flow increases during a meal. If a sugar-containing food is eaten with a meal rather than by itself, the extra buffering capacity of the increased saliva flow helps to prevent the pH level of the plaque from dropping to a critically low level, and the pH level that is reached quickly returns to normal.[174] In the NHANES survey there was a strong relation between the reported consumption of sugar between meals and DMF values, but practically none between total consumption of sugar (which would include that eaten with meals) and DMF values.[39]

Are There Protective Factors in Foods?

It has been suggested that the low caries prevalence in ancient civilizations came partly from protective factors in the coarse and unrefined nature of the diet consumed, factors presumably lost in modern food processing. One modern food with reported protective factors is cheese; there is evidence to show that finishing a meal with cheese reduces the acidity of plaque[196] and therefore presumably its cariogenicity. Apart from fluoride, certain other trace elements in the diet such as molybdenum have been associated with low prevalence of caries,[197] and others such as selenium have been associated with a high prevalence of caries.[80] These trace elements may well be involved in a manner as yet not understood, but at this time this information has no practical implications for caries control.

Among the various food additives intended to reduce the carious attack, the addition of phosphates has probably received most attention. In numerous animal studies phosphates have been shown to reduce caries when added to the diet, but studies among humans have been disappointing.[125, 141] The reductions in caries have been too small to be of any significance and the phosphate materials tend to have an unpleasant taste and thus are not readily accepted. The approach may be sufficiently promising, however, to warrant continued research.

For the present, there are no known "caries-fighting" food additives. The presumed anticariogenic property of cheese makes good newspaper copy, but because consumption of between-meal snacks is of more consequence than what is eaten with meals, it seems to have little practical significance.

Control of Caries by Dietary Means

The dietary control regimen of Jay[123, 124] is sound and effective. However, Jay's regimen demands almost total abstinence from all forms of carbohydrate for a short period, with a gradual return to limited carbohydrate intake. Such dietary change demands too high a degree of motivation from most patients[23] and could only be successfully applied by those whom Chambers[42] refers to as "susceptible to prevention." Drastic reduction of all forms of carbohydrate might also be unwise because it could result in excessive intake of fat, which could have greater consequences to general health.[136] Dental caries needs to be kept in perspective. The select Committee on Nutrition and Human Needs of the United States Senate, in its dietary guidelines for the United States, has recommended that the population as a whole should eat more carbohydrate, not less.[225] The recommendation emphasizes, however, consumption of more *unrefined* carbohydrate (e.g., fruit, potatoes, and rice) and considerably less *refined* carbohydrate. In light of current knowledge, the approach of Jay and his colleagues can be modified to highlight selective reduction of refined carbohydrates, since general advice to "reduce sugar consumption" is of little value to the average dental patient. Many may have no idea how much they are consuming, and in any case it is hard to comply with such advice given the ubiquity of sugar in the modern diet. Advice to patients should be aimed at the reduction of sugary foods eaten frequently between meals.

Not all patients need to change their dietary habits. Given the decline in caries prevalence described in Chapter 6, large numbers of dental patients will present with few carious lesions. For such persons, it would seem to be taking things out of perspective to recommend a major change in lifestyle in order to prevent a small amount of disease. Individuals who are more susceptible to caries, on the other hand, may benefit considerably. Dietary counseling in the dental office may be more efficient if it is concentrated on susceptible patients rather than directed to all patients. Technics for dietary counseling have been described in several textbooks.[178, 183]

On a community basis, dental health education should concentrate on making known the fact that sugary snacks between meals are damaging to teeth. Realistically, not many members of the public can be expected to respond to this message. It goes against the culture of current society, especially for those in the caries-prone teenage years, when 22 to 45 percent of the day's nutrient intake can come from between-meal snacks.[115] Nevertheless, individuals should at least receive the facts. How well they act upon this knowledge is another problem altogether and dealt with elsewhere in this book (see Chapter 15).

An interesting approach to public education is taken in Switzerland. Food products there may be labeled "Zahnschonend" (safe for teeth) if they do not lower the pH of interdental plaque below 5.7 for up to 30 minutes after consumption.[117] Tests are carried out telemetrically with the plaque electrode. "Zahnschonend" products are usually sweetened with xylitol (nonacidogenic) or the more slowly fermenting sorbitol, mannitol, maltitol, or *Lycasin* (a starch derivative). Fructose does not pass the test. The impact of this program on the dental health of the Swiss people has not been determined.

In the United States, the ADA has a national task force attempting to reduce the availability of cariogenic foods in schools.[207] There is evidence to show that the nonavailability of sugary foods on school premises leads to lower DMF scores among the children at the school.[62, 192] As mentioned earlier, the dental profession has also supported efforts to obtain federal control on the number and types of advertisements for highly sugared foods on television programs directed primarily at young children.[99] Even if these well-intentioned efforts are ultimately successful, it is difficult to predict the subsequent impact on caries. In the same vein, the research efforts to determine the cariogenicity of individual foods[32] may be misdirected, because foods are not usually eaten in isolation, though they are usually tested that way. Even if a valid rank order of cariogenic foods can be developed, this does not necessarily mean that individuals referring to it are reducing the cariogenicity of their diets. If snacking on one highly cariogenic food is avoided in favor of repeated snacking on an apparently less cariogenic food, the patient may still not be better off.

In summary, dietary control of caries for the individual can still be based on a modification of the precepts enunciated by Jay many years ago. In particular, consumption of sugary snacks between meals should be controlled, especially by caries-susceptible patients. The strategies for achieving this end will vary from patient to patient. Development of less cariogenic diets on a community basis will be advanced if suitable sugar substitutes become widely used in food processing. Xylitol appears to be the most promising alternative, though others are being developed.[205] While much has yet to be learned about cariogenic diets and the precise relation between foods eaten and the development of dental caries, sufficient knowledge exists to enable dental personnel to offer sound advice and guidance to patients who need it.

PLAQUE CONTROL

Because the bacterial agents causing dental caries are in the dental plaque, caries is theoretically preventable by regular and careful oral hygiene procedures to remove that plaque. The old adage is that "a clean tooth never decays." Caries control by oral hygiene is based on the "nonspecific plaque hypothesis," which implies that all bacteria in plaque are of equal cariogenicity and should therefore be removed.[146] Efforts to relate individual oral hygiene status to a lower incidence of caries have been disappointing,[10] however, though hardly surprising in view of the multifactorial causes of caries. Although some relation between the level of plaque scores and the development of caries among adults has been reported,[127] the prevailing thinking among researchers is that poor motivation and improper technic have been responsible for the inability of instructional programs aimed at improving oral hygiene status to have much effect on the initiation or progression of caries.[26, 86, 216]

The problems in application of oral hygiene procedures to prevent dental caries are two. The first is to persuade people to practice the procedures at the desired intensity and with the necessary day-in-day-out consistency.[95] The second is to have the necessary mechanical procedures performed well enough to remove the plaque from caries-susceptible areas, even in well-motivated individuals.[153] Among children, the success of a professionally administered flossing program in preventing caries has been reported,[232] but other studies using dental floss have reported failure.[4, 76, 95] The wisdom of teaching young children to floss is questioned by many dental professionals who fear that some children may do more harm than good to developing dental structures.

In this prevailing atmosphere of skepticism about the caries-preventive benefits of oral hygiene practices, new interest has been sparked by a remarkable series of studies from the Swedish researchers Lindhe and Axelsson. Their studies in the Swedish city of Karlstad have indicated that caries incidence in children can be virtually eliminated by meticulous plaque removal carried out by trained dental auxiliaries at frequent intervals.[15, 16, 17, 143] These intervals were two weeks in younger children, while in older children spectacular results were maintained when the time between cleanings was extended to eight weeks after an initial two years at two-week intervals.[144]

The procedures involved in the professional cleaning of children's teeth as described by Axelsson and Lindhe[15] are as follows:

1. Detailed initial explanations of oral disease etiology and purpose of treatment by the dentist or auxiliary carrying out the treatment. Involvement of the family is considered integral to the program's success.

2. Identification of plaque in patient's mouth by disclosing tablet, then demonstration of correct toothbrushing technic for removing the stain. Patient uses dental floss under supervision. These oral hygiene instructions are repeated throughout the course of treatment as necessary.

3. Rubber cup cleaning of accessible surfaces and engine-mounted pointed bristle used for cleaning fissures in occlusal surfaces. A fluoride-containing prophylactic paste is used for these procedures.

4. Interdental cleaning, again by dentist or auxiliary providing the treatment, with dental floss and reciprocating interproximal tips. Again, the fluoridated prophylactic paste is forced interdentally and kept in close contact with the proximal surfaces by the floss and the tips.

Benefits from this technic come from (1) plaque removal, (2) intensive use of topical fluoride paste, and (3) dental health education and oral hygiene practices at home. To test the effect of oral hygiene alone, nonfluoridated prophylaxis paste and dentifrice were used in one subgroup in Karlstad. Results showed no difference in caries increment over one year[16] when compared with the group using fluoridated paste and dentifrice, leading to the conclusion that oral hygiene measures alone produced the benefits.

The reported reduction of caries incidence in the Karlstad studies is remarkable. For example, seventh-grade children, aged 13–14, averaged only 0.17 new decayed and filled permanent tooth surfaces (DFS) over two years, whereas controls averaged 8.15 DFS—a 98 percent reduction.[15] Reductions of this order demand that the "Lindhe-Axelsson approach" be examined seriously.

There have been several attempts to replicate these results.[3, 13, 19, 81] Results from these studies, although good, are not nearly as impressive as those recorded in Karlstad. Badersten and her group, for example, studied children aged 10–12 in Malmo, Sweden.[19] They used the same prophylactic procedures as Lindhe and Axelsson on a monthly basis, even supplemented with 0.2 percent NaF rinse at the end of each cleaning session. Test group children in one year registered 3.4 DF surfaces compared to the control group's 4.5 DFS, an unremarkable 24 percent reduction. Another study with children aged 10–11 in Linkoping, Sweden, moved the concept into much larger groups.[81] The 51 percent reduction achieved over three years was impressive, but the test group still averaged 6.3 DFS in that time. Agerbaek and others,[3] applying a modified version of Lindhe and Axelsson's approach (mechanical procedures alone without the dental health education and parental involvement), achieved a 70 percent reduction in seven-year-old children in the first year, but only 33 percent in the second year. Test group children averaged 1.83 DF surfaces over the two years.

These studies suggest that the virtual elimination of caries by professional plaque removal is possible, but that it demands the heroic efforts and extraordinary enthusiasm, some might say evangelism, that Lindhe and Axelsson brought to their work.[3, 19] This approach also requires dental equipment on-site at schools (or workplace for adults) and up to three hours of dental treatment per year,[81] and therefore seems a likely preventive option only in those countries that have established school or industrial dental services. Its application in a public health context is virtually out of the question in the United States and many other countries on a cost-effectiveness basis alone.

Lindhe and Axelsson's studies have shed fresh light on the role of oral hygiene in preventing caries—perhaps a clean tooth really does not decay. Neither practitioners nor public health administrators, however, should expect the usual routine personal oral hygiene measures to prevent all caries. As an adjunct to fluoride therapy, regular professional cleaning might be applicable for highly motivated caries-susceptible patients in practices where the dentist or hygienist has the right degree of charisma.

References

1. Aasenden, R., DePaola, P. F., and Brudevold, F. Effects of daily rinsing and ingestion of fluoride solutions upon dental caries and enamel fluoride. Arch. Oral Biol., 17:1705–14, Dec. 1972.
2. Aasenden, R., and Peebles, T. C. Effects of fluoride supplementation from birth on deciduous and permanent teeth. Arch. Oral Biol., 19:321–6, Apr. 1974.
3. Agerbaek, N., et al. Effect of professional toothcleaning every third week on gingivitis and dental caries in children. Community Dent. Oral Epidemiol., 6:40–1, Jan. 1978.
4. Ainamo, J., and Parviainen, K. Occurrence of plaque, gingivitis and caries as related to self-reported frequency of toothbrushing in fluoride areas in Finland. Community Dent. Oral Epidemiol , 7:142–6, June 1979.
5. American Academy of Pediatrics, Committee on Nutrition. Fluoride supplementation: revised dosage schedule. Pediatrics, 63:150–2, Jan. 1979.
6. ______. Fluoride as a nutrient. Pediatrics, 49:456–9, Mar. 1972.
7. American Dental Association, Council on Dental Materials and Devices. List of certified dental material and devices, revised to Jan. 1, 1979. Am. Dent. A. J., 98:272–83, Feb. 1979.
8. American Dental Association, Council on Dental Materials, Instruments, and Equipment. J. W. Stanford, Secretary. Personal communication, June 17, 1981.
9. American Dental Association, Council on Dental Therapeutics. Accepted dental therapeutics. 38th ed. Chicago, The Association, 1979. xxix + 385 p.
10. Andlaw, R. J. Oral hygiene and dental caries—a review. Internat. Dent. J., 28:1–6, Mar. 1978.
11. Andlaw, R. J., and Tucker, G. I. A dentifrice containing 0.8 percent sodium monofluorophosphate in an aluminum oxide trihydrate base. A 3-year clinical trial. Brit. Dent. J., 138:426–32, June 3, 1975.
12. Antar, M. A., Ohlson, M. A., and Hodges, R. E. Changes in retail market food supplies in the United States in the last seventy years in relation to the incidence of coronary heart disease, with special reference to dietary carbohydrates and essential fatty acids. Am. J. Clin. Nutrit., 14:169–78, Mar. 1964.
13. Ashley, F. P., and Sainsbury, R. H. The effect of a school-based plaque control programme on caries and gingivitis. Brit. Dent. J., 150:41–5, Jan. 20, 1981.
14. Association recognizes OTC fluoride rinses. ADA News, 11:1, July 7–14, 1980.
15. Axelsson, P., and Lindhe, J. The effect of a preventive programme on dental plaque, gingivitis and caries in school children. Results after one and two years. J. Clin. Periodont., 1:126–38, 1974.
16. ______. Effect of fluoride on gingivitis and dental caries in a preventive program based on plaque control. Community Dent. Oral Epidemiol., 3:156–60, Aug. 1975.
17. Axelsson, P., Lindhe, J., and Waseby, J. The effect of various plaque control measures on gingivitis and caries in schoolchildren. Community Dent. Oral Epidemiol., 4:232–9, Nov. 1976.
18. Backer-Dirks, O., Houwink, B., and Kwant, G. W. The results of 6½ years of artificial drinking water in the Netherlands; the Tiel–Culemborg experiment. Arch. Oral Biol., 5:284–300, Dec. 1961.
19. Badersten, A., Egelberg, J., and Koch, G. Effect of monthly prophylaxis on caries and gingivitis in schoolchildren. Community Dent. Oral Epidemiol., 3:1–4, Feb. 1975.
20. Bagramian, R. A. Oral hygiene procedures and pit and fissure sealants. p. 123–51. (In Burt, B. A., ed. The relative efficiency of methods of caries prevention in dental public health. Proceedings of a workshop at The University of Michigan, June 5–8, 1978. Ann Arbor, University Michigan, 1979. 326 p.)
21. Bagramian, R. A., and Russell, A. L. Epidemiologic study of dental caries experience and between-meal eating patterns. J. Dent. Res., 52:342–7, Mar.–Apr. 1973.
22. Bagramian, R. A., Srivastava, S., and Graves, R. C. Effectiveness of combined preventive methods on erupting teeth in children in a fluoridated community. Community Dent. Oral Epidemiol., 7:246–51, Oct. 1979.
23. Becks, H. The physical consistency of food and refined carbohydrate restrictions—their effect on caries. J. Dent. Res., 27:405–12, June 1948.
24. Beiswanger, B. B., Gish, C. W., and Mallatt, M. E. Effect of a sodium fluoride-silica

abrasive dentifrice upon caries. Abstr. J. Dent. Res., Abstr. no. 1072, 60(Spec. Issue A):577, Mar. 1981.
25. Bellack, E. School water supply fluoridation. Environmental Protection Agency publication no. EPA-430/9–75–004. Washington, D.C., Government Printing Office, 1972. 18 p.
26. Bibby, B. G. Do we tell the truth about preventing caries? J. Dent. Child., 33:269–79, Sept. 1966.
27. Bibby, B. G., et al. Preliminary reports on the effect of dental caries of the use of sodium fluoride in a prophylactic cleaning mixture and in a mouthwash. J. Dent. Res., 25:207–11, Aug. 1946.
28. Binder, K., Driscoll, W. S., and Schutzmannsky, G. Caries-preventive fluoride tablet programs. Caries Res., 12(Suppl. 1):22–30, 1978.
29. Birkeland, J. M., and Jorkjend, L. Effect of mouthrinsing and toothbrushing with fluoride solutions on caries among Norwegian schoolchildren. Community Dent. Oral Epidemiol., 3:201–7, Sept. 1975.
30. Birkeland, J. M., Broch, L., and Jorkjend, L. Benefits and prognoses following 10 years of a fluoride mouthrinsing program. Scand. J. Dent. Res., 85:31–7, Jan. 1977.
31. Birkeland, J. M., and Torell, P. Caries-preventive fluoride mouthrinses. Caries Res., 12(suppl. 1):38–51, 1978.
32. Bowen, W. H., et al. A method to assess cariogenic potential of foodstuffs. Am. Dent. A. J., 100:677–81, May 1980.
33. Brooks, J. D., et al. A comparative study of two pit and fissure sealants: three-year results in Augusta, Ga. Am. Dent. A. J., 99:42–6, July 1979.
34. Brudevold, F., and Chilton, N. W. Comparative study of a fluoride dentifrice containing soluble phosphate and a calcium-free abrasive: second-year report. Am. Dent. A. J., 72:889–94, Apr. 1966.
35. Brudevold, F., and Naujoks, R. Caries-preventive fluoride treatment for the individual. Caries Res., 12(suppl. 1):52–64, 1978.
36. Bryan, E. T., and Williams, J. E. The cariostatic effectiveness of a phosphate-fluoride gel administered annually to school children; final results. J. Pub. Health Dent., 30:13–6, Winter 1970.
37. Bunting, R. W. Diet and dental caries. Am. Dent. A. J., 22:114–22, Jan. 1935.
38. Buonocore, M. G. Caries prevention in pits and fissures sealed with an adhesive resin polymerized by ultraviolet light; a two-year study of a single adhesive application. Am. Dent. A. J., 82:1090–3, May 1971.
39. Burt, B. A., and Eklund, S. A. Sugar consumption and dental caries: some epidemiological patterns in the United States. p. 171–80. (In Hefferen, J. J., Ayer, W. A., and Koehler, H. M., eds. Foods, nutrition and dental health; volume 3 of a series. Park Forest South, Ill., Pathotox, 1981. vii + 265 p.)
40. Cantor, S. M. Patterns of use. p. 19–29. (In National Academy of Sciences. Sweeteners: issues and uncertainties. Academy forum, fourth of a series. Washington, D.C., The Academy, 1975. vii + 260 p.)
41. Carlos, J. P. Sugar and dental caries: research study in humans. Evidence submitted to the Federal Trade Commission, Washington, D.C., Nov. 20, 1978. 14 p. typescript.
42. Chambers, D. W. Susceptibility to preventive dental treatment. J. Pub. Health Dent., 33:82–90, Spring 1973.
43. Conchie, J. M., McCombie, F., and Hole, L. W. Three years of supervised toothbrushing with a fluoride-phosphate solution. J. Pub. Health Dent., 29:11–9, Winter 1969.
44. Corpron, R. E., and Burt, B. A. Fluorosis from supplementation with fluoride tablets: a case report. Mich. Dent. A. J., 60:615–8, Dec. 1978.
45. Cueto, E. L., and Buonocore, M. G. Sealing of pits and fissures with an adhesive resin: its use in caries prevention. Am. Dent. A. J., 75:121–8, July 1967.
46. DePaola, P. F., and Mellberg, J. R. Caries experience and fluoride uptake in children receiving semiannual prophylaxes with an acidulated phosphate fluoride paste. Am. Dent. A. J., 87:155–9, July 1973.
47. DePaola, P. F., et al. Effect of high-concentration ammonium and sodium fluoride rinses in dental caries in schoolchildren. Community Dent. Oral Epidemiol., 5:7–14, Jan. 1977.
48. DePaola, P. F., et al. The anticaries effect of single and combined topical fluoride systems in schoolchildren. Arch. Oral Biol., 25:649–53, 1980.
49. Dreizen, S., et al. Prevention of xerostomia-related dental caries in irradiated dental patients. J. Dent. Res., 56:99–104, Feb. 1977.

50. Driscoll, W. S. Review of clinical research on prenatal fluorides. J. Dent. Child., 48:109–17, Mar.–Apr. 1981.
51. Driscoll, W. S., Heifetz, S. B., and Brunelle, J. A. Treatment and posttreatment effects of chewable fluoride tablets on dental caries: findings after 7½ years. Am. Dent. A. J., 99:817–21, Nov. 1979.
52. ———. Caries preventive effects of fluoride tablets in school children four years after discontinuation of treatments. Am. Dent. A. J., 103:878–81, Dec. 1981.
53. Driscoll, W. S., Heifetz, S. B., and Korts, D. C. Effects of chewable fluoride tablets on dental caries in schoolchildren: results after six years of use. Am. Dent. A. J., 97:820–4, Nov. 1978.
54. Driscoll, W. S., and Horowitz, H. S. A discussion of optimal dosage for dietary fluoride supplementation. Am. Dent. A. J., 96:1050–3, June 1978.
55. ———. Dosage recommendations for dietary fluoride supplements. Am. J. Dis. Child., 133:583–4, July 1979.
56. Driscoll, W. S., et al. Caries-preventive effects of daily and weekly fluoride mouthrinsing in an optimally fluoridated community: findings after eighteen months. J. Pediatr. Dent., 3:316–20, Dec. 1981.
57. Edlund, K., and Koch, G. Effect on caries of daily supervised toothbrushing with sodium monofluorophosphate and sodium fluoride dentifrices after 3 years. Scand. J. Dent. Res., 85:41–5, Jan. 1977.
58. Englander, H. R., Keyes, P. H., and Gestwicki, M. Clinical anticaries effect of repeated topical fluoride applications by mouthpieces. Am. Dent. A. J., 75:639–44, Sept. 1967.
59. Englander, H. R., et al. Incremental rates of dental caries after repeated topical sodium fluoride applications in children with lifelong consumption of fluoridated water. Am. Dent. A. J., 82:354–8, Feb. 1971.
60. Ericsson, S. Y. Cariostatic mechanism of actions of fluorides: clinical observation. Caries Res., 11(Suppl. 1):2–23, 1977.
61. Fanning, E. A., Gotjamanos, T., and Vowles, N. J. The use of fluoride dentifrices in the control of dental caries: methodology and results of a clinical trial. Austral. Dent. J., 13:201–6, June 1968.
62. ———. Dental caries in children related to availability of sweets at school canteens. Med. J. Austral., 1:1131–2, May 31, 1969.
63. Finn, S. B., and Jamison, H. C. The relative effects of three dietary supplements on dental caries. J. Dent. Child., 47:33–7, Mar.–Apr. 1980.
64. Fitzgerald, R. J. The potential of antibiotics as caries-control agents. Am. Dent. A. J., 87:1006–9, Oct. 1973.
65. Fleming, W. J., Burgess, R. C., and Lewis, D. W. Effects on caries of self-application of a zirconium silicate paste containing 9% stannous fluoride. Community Dent. Oral Epidemiol., 4:142–8, July 1976.
66. Fogels, H. R., et al The relative caries-inhibiting effects of a stannous fluoride dentifrice in a silica gel base. Am. Dent. A. J., 99:456–9, Sept. 1979.
67. Forsman, B. Studies on the effect of dentifrices with low fluoride content. Community Dent. Oral Epidemiol., 2:166–75, 1974.
68. ———. The caries preventing effect of mouthrinsing with 0.025 percent sodium fluoride solution in Swedish children. Community Dent. Oral Epidemiol., 2:58–65, 1974.
69. Frankl, A. N., and Alman, J. E. Report of a three-year clinical trial comparing a toothpaste containing sodium monofluorophosphate with two marketed products. J. Oral Therap. Pharmacol., 4:443–50, May 1968.
70. Geddes, D. A., et al. Apples, salted peanuts and plaque pH. Brit. Dent. J., 142:317–9, May 17, 1977.
71. Gish, C. W., et al. Self-application of fluoride as a community preventive measure: rationale, procedures, and three-year results. Am. Dent. A. J., 90:388–97, Feb. 1975.
72. Glass, R. L., and Fleisch, S. Diet and dental caries: dental caries incidence and the consumption of ready-to-eat cereals. Am. Dent. A. J., 88:807–13, Apr. 1974.
73. Glass, R. L., and Shiere, F. R. A clinical trial of a calcium carbonate base dentifrice containing 0.76% sodium monofluorophosphate. Caries Res., 12:284–9, 1978.
74. Glenn, F. B. Immunity conveyed by a fluoride supplement during pregnancy. J. Dent. Child., 44:39–43, Sept.–Oct. 1977.
75. ———. Immunity conveyed by sodium-fluoride supplement during pregnancy: Part II. J. Dent. Child., 46:17–24, Jan.–Feb. 1979.
76. Granath, L. E., et al. Intraindividual effect of daily supervised flossing on caries in schoolchildren. Community Dent. Oral Epidemiol., 7:147–50, June 1979.

77. Graves, R. C., and Burt, B. A. The pattern of the carious attack in children as a consideration in the use of fissure sealants. J. Preven. Dent., 2:28–32, May–June 1975.
78. Gunz, G. M. The effect of self-applied fluoride paste. J. Pub. Health Dent., 31:177–81, Summer 1971.
79. Gustafsson, B. E., et al. The Vipeholm dental caries study. The effect of different levels of carbohydrate intake on caries activity in 436 individuals observed for five years. Acta Odont. Scand., 11:232–364, Sept. 1954.
80. Hadjimarkos, D. M. Selenium: a caries-enhancing trace element. Caries Res., 3:14–22, 1969.
81. Hamp, S.-E., et al. Effect of a field program based on systematic plaque control on caries and gingivitis in schoolchildren after 3 years. Community Dent. Oral Epidemiol., 6:17–23, Jan. 1978.
82. Handelman, S. L., Washburn, F., and Wopperer, P. Two-year report of sealant effect on bacteria in dental caries. Am. Dent. A. J., 93:967–70, Nov. 1976.
83. Hawes, R. R., and Bibby, B. G. Evaluation of a dentifrice containing carbamide and urease. Am. Dent. A. J., 46:280–6, Mar. 1953.
84. Heifetz, S. B., Horowitz, H. S., and Driscoll, W. S. Two-year evaluation of a self-administered procedure for the topical application of acidulated phosphate-fluoride; final report. J. Pub. Health Dent., 30:7–12, Winter 1970.
85. Heifetz, S. B., and Suomi, J. D. The control of dental caries and periodontal disease; a fundamental approach. J. Pub. Health Dent., 33:2–6, Winter 1973.
86. Heifetz, S. B., et al. Programs for the mass control of plaque; an appraisal. J. Pub. Health Dent., 33:91–5, Spring 1973.
87. Heifetz, S. B., Horowitz, H. S., and Driscoll, W. S. Effect of school water fluoridation on dental caries: results in Seagrove, N.C., after eight years. Am. Dent. A. J., 97:193–6, Aug. 1978.
88. Heifetz, S. B., et al. Combined anticariogenic effect of fluoride gel-trays and fluoride mouthrinsing in an optimally fluoridated community. Clin. Preven. Dent., 6:21–8, Jan.–Feb. 1979.
89. Heifetz, S. B., Meyers, R., and Kingman, A. A comparison of the anticaries effectiveness of daily and weekly rinsing with sodium fluoride solutions: findings after two years. J. Pediatr. Dent., 3:17–20, 1980.
90. Heifetz, S. B. Cost-effectiveness of topically-applied fluorides. p. 69–104. (In Burt, B. A., ed. The relative efficiency of methods of caries prevention in dental public health. Proceedings of a workshop at The University of Michigan, June 5–8, 1978. Ann Arbor, University Michigan, 1979. 326 p.)
91. Hennon, D. K., Stookey, G. K., and Muhler, J. C. The clinical anticariogenic effectiveness of supplementary fluoride-vitamin preparations—results at the end of four years. J. Dent. Child., 34:439–42, Nov. 1967.
92. Hoffman, R., et al. Acute fluoride poisoning in a New Mexico elementary school. Pediatrics, 65:897–900, May 1980.
93. Holm, A. K. Effect of fluoride varnish (Duraphat) in preschool children. Community Dent. Oral Epidemiol., 7:241–5, Oct 1979.
94. Horowitz, A. M., and Horowitz, H. S. School-based fluoride programs: a critique. J. Preven. Dent., 6:89–96, Apr. 1980.
95. Horowitz, A. M., et al. Effects of supervised daily dental plaque removal by children after 3 years. Community Dent. Oral Epidemiol., 8:171–6, Aug. 1980.
96. Horowitz, H. S. Fluoride: research on clinical and public health applications. Am. Dent. A. J., 87:1013–8, Oct. 1973.
97. ———. The prevention of dental caries by mouthrinsing with solutions of neutral sodium fluoride. Internat. Dent. J., 23:585–90, Dec. 1973.
98. ———. Abusive use of fluoride. Edit. J. Pub. Health Dent., 37:106–7, Spring 1977.
99. ———. The arch criminal is still at large. Edit. J. Pub. Health Dent., 37:301–4, Fall 1977.
100. ———. Review of topical applications; fluorides and fissure sealants. Canad. Dent. A. J., 46:38–42, Jan. 1980.
101. ———. Pit and fissure sealants in private practice and public health programmes: analysis of cost-effectiveness. Internat. Dent. J., 30:117–26, June 1980.
102. ———. The future for self-applied fluorides. J. Pub. Health Dent., 41:255–9, Fall 1981.
103. ———, moderator. Perspectives on the use of prenatal fluorides: a symposium. Presented at the annual session of the American Dental Association, New Orleans, La., Oct. 1980. Published in J. Dent. Child., 48:102–33, Mar.–Apr. 1981.

104. Horowitz, H. S., et al. Evaluation of a stannous fluoride dentifrice for use in dental public health programs. I. Basic findings. Am. Dent. A. J., 72:408–22, Feb. 1966.
105. Horowitz, H. S., and Heifetz, S. B. Evaluation of topical applications of stannous fluoride to teeth of children born and reared in a fluoridated community; final report. J. Dent. Child., 36:65–71, Sept.–Oct. 1969.
106. Horowitz, H. S., Creighton, W. E., and McClendon, B. J. The effect on human dental caries of weekly oral rinsing with a sodium fluoride mouthwash; a final report. Arch. Oral. Biol., 16:609–16, May 1971.
107. Horowitz, H. S., Heifetz, S. B., and Law, F. E. Effect of school water fluoridation on dental caries: final results in Elk Lake, Pa., after 12 years. Am. Dent. A. J., 84:832–8, Apr. 1972.
108. Horowitz, H. S., et al. Evaluation of self-administered prophylaxis and supervised toothbrushing with acidulated phosphate fluoride. Caries. Res., 8:39–51, 1974.
109. Horowitz, H. S., and Heifetz, S. B. Clinical tests of dentifrices. Pharmacol. Therapeut. Dent., 2:235–44, 1975.
110. Horowitz, H. S., and Bixler, D. The effect of self-applied SnF_4–$ZrSiO_4$ prophylactic paste on dental caries: Santa Clara County, California. Am. Dent. A. J., 92:369–73, Feb. 1976.
111. Horowitz, H. S., Heifetz, S. B., and Poulsen, S. Retention and effectiveness of a single application of an adhesive sealant in preventing occlusal caries, final report after five years of study in Kalispell, Montana. Am. Dent. A. J., 95:1133–9, Dec. 1977.
112. Horowitz, H. S., et al. A program of self-administered fluorides in a rural school system. Community Dent. Oral Epidemiol., 8:177–83, Aug. 1980.
113. Houwink, B., Backer-Dirks, O., and Kwant, G. W. A nine-year study of topical application with stannous fluoride in identical twins and the caries experience five years after ending the applications. Caries Res., 8:27–38, 1974.
114. Howat, A. P., Holloway, P. J., and Davies, T. G. H. Caries prevention by daily supervised use of MFP gel dentifrice; report of a 3-year clinical trial. Brit. Dent. J., 145:233–5, Oct. 1978.
115. Howe, S. M., and Vaden, A. G. Factors differentiating participants and nonparticipants of the National School Lunch Program. I. Nutrient intake of high school students. Am. Dietetic A. J., 76:451–8, 1980.
116. Hyatt, T. P. Prophylactic odontotomy. Dent. Cosmos, 65:234–41, Mar. 1923.
117. Imfeld, T., and Muhlemann, H. R. Evaluation of sugar substitutes in preventive cariology. J. Preven. Dent. 4:8–14, Mar.–Apr. 1977.
118. ———. Cariogenicity and acidogenicity of food, confectionery, and beverages. Pharmacol. Therapeut. Dent., 3:53–68, 1978.
119. Jackson, D. Caries experience in English children and young adults during the years 1947–1972. Brit. Dent. J., 137:91–8. Aug. 6, 1974.
120. James, P. M. C., and Anderson, R. J. Clinical testing of a stannous fluoride-calcium pyrophosphate dentifrice in Buckinghamshire school children. Brit. Dent. J., 123:33–9, July 4, 1967.
121. James, P. M. C., et al. A 3-year clinical trial of the effect on dental caries of a dentifrice containing 2% sodium monofluorophosphate. Community Dent. Oral Epidemiol., 5:67–72, Mar. 1977.
122. Jay, P. Lactobacillus acidophilus and dental caries. Am. J. Pub. Health, 28:759–61, June 1938.
123. ———. The reduction of oral Lactobacillus acidophilus counts by the periodic restriction of carbohydrate. Am. J. Orthodont. Oral Surg., 33:162–84, Mar. 1947.
124. Jay, P., Beeuwkes, A. M., and Husbands, J. Dietary program for the control of dental caries. Ann Arbor, Overbeck, c1965. 30 p.
125. Jenkins, G. N. Current concepts concerning the development of dental caries. Internat. Dent. J., 22:350–62, Sept. 1972.
126. Jordan, W. A., and Peterson, J. K. Caries inhibiting value of a dentifrice containing stannous fluoride: final report of a two-year study. Am. Dent. A. J., 58:42–4, Jan. 1959.
127. Kennon, S., et al. The relationship between plaque scores and the development of caries in adult dentition. Clin. Preven. Dent., 1:26–31, Mar.–Apr. 1979.
128. Kesel, R. G. The effectiveness of dentifrices, mouthwashes, and ammonia-urea compounds in the control of dental caries. p. 88–102. (In Easlick, K. A., ed. Dental caries. St. Louis, Mosby, 1948. 234 p.)
129. Kidd, E. A., et al. Influence of fluoride in surface enamel and degree of dental fluorosis on caries development in vitro. Caries Res., 14:196–202, 1980.

130. Klein, H., and Palmer, C. E. "Therapeutic odontotomy" and "preventive dentistry." Am. Dent. A. J., 27:1054–5, July 1940.
131. Knutson, J. W. Sodium fluoride solutions: technique for application to the teeth. Am. Dent. A. J., 36:37–9, Jan. 1948.
132. Knutson, J. W., and Armstrong, W. D. Effect of topically applied sodium fluoride on dental caries experience. Pub. Health Rep., 58:1701–15, Nov. 19, 1943.
133. Koch, G., Petersson, L. G., and Ryden, H. Effect of fluoride varnish (Duraphat) treatment every six months compared with weekly mouthrinses with 0.2 percent NaF solution on dental caries. Swed. Dent. J., 3:39–44, 1979.
134. Koch, G., and Lindhe, J. The state of the gingivae and the caries increment in schoolchildren during and after withdrawal of various prophylactic measures. p. 271–81. (In McHugh, W. D., ed. Dental plaque. London, Livingstone, 1970. 298 p.)
135. Koulourides, T., et al. Cariogenicity of nine sugars tested with an intraoral device in man. Caries Res., 10:427–41, 1976.
136. Kreitzman, S. Human diet and dental caries. Paper given at the Workshop on Cariogenicity of Foods, Beverages, Confections and Chewing Gum, American Dental Association, Sept. 15–17, 1977.
137. Larmas, M., Makinen, K. K., and Scheinin, A. Turku sugar studies. VIII. Principal microbiological findings. Acta Odont. Scand., 34:285–328, 1976.
138. Leavell, H. R., and Clark, E. G. Preventive medicine for the doctor in his community; an epidemiologic approach. 3rd ed. New York, McGraw-Hill, 1965. xvi + 684 p.
139. Leske, G. S., Pollard, S., and Cons, N. The effectiveness of dental hygienist teams in applying a pit and fissure sealant. J. Preven. Dent., 3:33–6, Mar.–Apr. 1976.
140. Levine, R. S. The action of fluoride in caries prevention; a review of current concepts. Brit. Dent. J., 140:9–14, Jan. 6, 1976.
141. Lilienthal, B. Phosphates and dental caries. Monographs in Oral Science, Vol. 6. Basel, Karger, 1977. 107 p.
142. Lind, O. P., et al. Anticaries effect of a 2% Na_2PO_3 F-dentifrice in a Danish fluoride area. Community Dent. Oral Epidemiol., 4:7–14, Jan. 1976.
143. Lindhe, J., and Axelsson, P. The effect of proper oral hygiene and topical fluoride application on caries and gingivitis in Swedish schoolchildren. Community Dent. Oral Epidemiol., 1:9–16, 1973.
144. Lindhe, J., Axelsson, P., and Tollskog, G. The effect of proper oral hygiene on gingivitis and dental caries in schoolchildren. Community Dent. Oral Epidemiol., 3:150–5, Aug. 1975.
145. Lobene, R. R. Chemotherapeutics for the prevention of dental plaque. J. Preven. Dent., 3:32–8, Jul.–Aug. 1976.
146. Loesche, W. J. Chemotherapy of dental plaque infections. Oral Sci. Rev., 9:63–107, 1976.
147. ———. Topical fluorides as an antibacterial agent. J. Preven. Dent., 4:21–6, Jan.–Feb. 1977.
148. Long, J. G. Self-applied fluoride paste: effect on dental caries. J. Pub. Health Dent., 32:161–4, Summer 1972.
149. Ludwig, T. G. The Hastings fluoridation project. V. Dental effects between 1954 and 1964. N. Z. Dent. J., 61:175–9, July 1965.
150. McConchie, J. M. The potential benefits of "brush-in" programmes as regards prevention of dental caries, dental health education and public relations. p. 259–304. (In Forrester, D. J., and Schulz, E. M., Jr., eds. International workshop on fluorides and dental caries reductions. Baltimore, University Maryland, 1974. 327 p.)
151. McConchie, J. M., et al. Caries-preventive effect of two concentrations of stannous fluoride mouthrinse. Community Dent. Oral Epidemiol., 5:278–83, Nov. 1977.
152. McDonald, J. L., Jr., and Stookey, G. K. Animal studies concerning the cariogenicity of dry breakfast cereals. J. Dent. Res., 56:1001–6, Aug. 1977.
153. McGuire, M. K., et al. Evaluation of an oral disease control program administered to a clinic population at a suburban dental school. J. Periodont., 51:607–13, Oct. 1980.
154. Mainwaring, P. J., and Naylor, M. N. A three-year clinical study to determine the separate and combined caries-inhibiting effects of sodium monofluorophosphate toothpaste and an acidulated phosphate-fluoride gel. Caries Res., 4:202–12, 1978.
155. Makinen, K. K. The role of sucrose and other sugars in the development of dental caries: a review. Internat. Dent. J., 22:363–86, Sept. 1972.
156. Makinen, K. K. Xylitol and oral health. Adv. Food Res., 25:137–58, 1979.
157. Margolis, F. J., et al. Fluoride: ten-year prospective study of deciduous and permanent dentition. Am. J. Dis. Child., 130:794–800, July 1975.

158. Margolis, F. J., et al. Fluoride supplements for children: a survey of physicians' prescription practices. Am. J Dis. Child., 134:865–8, Sept. 1980.
159. Marthaler, T. M. Caries inhibition by an amine fluoride dentifrice: results after 6 years in children with low caries activitiy. Helv. Odont. Acta, 18:35–44, Apr. 1974.
160. Marthaler, T. M., Konig, K. G., and Muhlemann, H. R. The effect of a fluoride gel used for supervised brushing 15 or 30 times per year. Helv. Odont. Acta, 14:67–77, Oct. 1970.
161. Marthaler, T. M., et al. Caries-preventive salt fluoridation. Caries Res., 12:15–21, 1978.
162. Mellberg, J. R., Nicholson, C. R., and Trubman, A. The acquisition of fluoride by tooth enamel in vivo from self-applied APF gel and prophylaxis paste. Caries Res., 7:173–8, 1973.
163. Mellberg, J. R., Peterson, J. K., and Nicholson, C. R. Fluoride uptake and caries inhibition from self-application of an acidulated phosphate-fluoride prophylaxis paste. Caries Res., 8:52–60, 1974.
164. Møller, I. J., Hoist, J. J., and Sorensen, E. Caries reducing effect of a sodium monofluorophosphate dentifrice. Brit. Dent. J., 124:209–13, Mar. 5, 1968.
165. Muhler, J. C. Effect of a stannous fluoride dentifrice on caries reduction in children during a three-year study period. Am. Dent. A. J., 64:216–24, Feb. 1962.
166. Muhler, J. C., et al. Comparison between the anticariogenic effects of dentifrices containing stannous fluoride and sodium fluoride. Am. Dent. A. J., 51:556–9, Nov. 1955.
167. Muhler, J. C., et al. The clinical evaluation of patient-administered SnF_2-$ZrSiO_4$ prophylactic paste in children. I. Results after one year in the Virgin Islands. Am. Dent. A. J., 81:142–5, July 1970.
168. Murray, J. J., Winter, G. B., and Hurst, C. P. Duraphat fluoride varnish: a 2-year clinical trial in 5-year-old children. Brit. Dent. J., 143:11–7, July 5, 1977.
169. National Research Council, Food and Nutrition Board. Recommended dietary allowances. 8th ed. Washington, D.C., National Academy Sciences, 1974. v + 128 p. (p. 98–9)
170. Naylor, M. N., and Glass, R. L. A 3-year clinical trial of calcium carbonate dentifrice containing calcium glycerophosphate and sodium monofluorophosphate. Caries Res., 13:39–46, 1979.
171. Naylor, M. N., and Emslie, R. D. Clinical testing of stannous fluoride and sodium monofluorophosphate dentifrices in London school children. Brit. Dent. J., 123:17–23, July 4, 1967.
172. Newbrun, E. Sucrose, the arch criminal of dental caries. Odont. Rev., 18:373–86, 1967.
173. ———. The role of food manufacturers in the dietary control of caries. Am. Soc. Preven. Dent., 4:33–44, Sept.–Oct. 1974.
174. ———. Cariology. Baltimore, Williams and Wilkins, 1978. xv + 298 p.
175. ———. Dietary carbohydrates: their role in cariogenicity. Med. Clin. N. Am., 63:1069–86, Sept. 1979.
176. Newbrun, E., and Frostell, G. Sugar restriction and substitution for caries prevention. Caries Res., 12(suppl. 1):65–73, 1978.
177. Newbrun, E., et al. Comparison of dietary habits and dental health of subjects with hereditary fructose intolerance and control subjects. Am. Dent. A. J., 101:619–26, Oct. 1980.
178. Nizel, A. E. Nutrition in preventive dentistry: science and practice. 2nd ed. Philadelphia, Saunders, 1981. xi + 611 p. (p. 417–52)
179. Peterson, J. K. A supervised brushing trial of sodium monofluorophosphate dentifrices in a fluoridated area. Caries Res., 13:68–72, 1979.
180. Peterson, J. K., et al. Effectiveness of an acidulated phosphate fluoride-pumice prophylactic paste: a two-year report. J. Dent. Res., 48:346–50, May–June 1969.
181. Poulsen, S., et al. Evaluation of a pit-and-fissure sealant program in a public dental health service after 2 years. Community Dent. Oral Epidemiol., 7:154–7, June 1979.
182. Radike, A. W., et al. Clinical evaluation of stannous fluoride as an anticaries mouthrinse. Am. Dent. A. J., 86:404–8, Feb. 1973.
183. Randolph, P. M., and Dennison, C. I. Diet, nutrition, and dentistry. St. Louis, Mosby, 1981. xi + 358 p (p. 139–67)
184. Reed, M. W. Clinical evaluation of three concentrations of sodium fluoride in dentifrices. Am. Dent. A. J., 87:1401–3, Dec. 1973.
185. Ringelberg, M. L., et al. The caries-preventive effect of amine fluorides and inorganic fluorides in a mouthrinse or dentifrice after 30 months of use. Am. Dent. A. J., 98:202–8, Feb. 1979.

186. Ripa, L. W. Occlusal sealants: rationale and review of clinical trials. Internat. Dent. J., 30:127–39, June 1980.
187. ———. Fluoride rinsing: what dentists should know. Am. Dent. A. J., 102:477–81, Apr. 1981.
188. Ripa, L. W., and Leske, G. S. Two years' effect on the primary dentition of mouthrinsing with a 0.2% neutral NaF solution. Community Dent. Oral Epidemiol., 7:151–3, June 1979.
189. Ripa, L. W., Levinson, A., and Leske, G. S. Supervised weekly rinsing with a 0.2% neutral NaF solution; results from a demonstration program after three school years. Am. Dent. A. J., 100:544–6, Apr. 1980.
190. Rise, J., and Haugejorden, O. Monitoring and evaluation of results of community fluoride programs in Norway during the 1960s and 1970s. Community Dent. Oral Epidemiol., 8:79–83, Apr. 1980.
191. Rock, W. P. Fissure sealants: further results of clinical trials. Brit. Dent. J., 136:317–21, Apr. 16, 1974.
192. Roder, D. M. The association between dental caries and the availability of sweets in South Australian school canteens. Austral. Dent. J., 18:174–82, June 1973.
193. Rølla, G. Effects of fluoride on initiation of plaque formation. Caries Res. 11(Suppl. 1):243–61, 1977.
194. Rowe, N. H., Anderson, R. H., and Wanninger, L. A. Effects of ready-to-eat breakfast cereals on dental caries experience in adolescent children: a three-year study. J. Dent. Res., 53:33–6, Jan–Feb. 1974.
195. Rugg-Gunn, A. J., Holloway, P. J., and Davies, T. G. H. Caries prevention by daily fluoride mouthrinsing. Brit. Dent. J., 135:353–60, Oct. 16, 1973.
196. Rugg-Gunn, A. J., et al. The effect of different meal patterns upon plaque pH in human subjects. Brit. Dent. J., 139:351–6, Nov. 4, 1975.
197. Schamschula, R. G., et al. WHO study of dental caries etiology in Papua, New Guinea. WHO Offset Publ. No. 40. Geneva, WHO, 1978. 199 p.
198. Scheinin, A., Makinen, K. K., and Ylitalo, K. Turku sugar studies. I. An intermediate report on the effect of sucrose, fructose and xylitol diets on the caries incidence in man. Acta Odont. Scand., 32:383–412, 1974.
199. ———. Turku sugar studies. V. Final report on the effect of sucrose, fructose, and xylitol diets on the caries incidence in man. Acta Odont. Scand., 34:179–216, 1976.
200. Scheinin, A., et al. Turku sugar studies. XVIII. Incidence of dental caries in relation to 1-year consumption of xylitol chewing gum. Acta Odont. Scand., 33:269–78, 1975.
201. Scheinin, A., and Makinen, K. K. Turku sugar studies; an overview. Acta Odont. Scand., 34:405–8, 1976.
202. Scholle, R. H. Will the manufacturer of the best fluoride dentifrice please stand. Edit. Am. Dent. A. J., 102:958, June 1981.
203. Scola, F. P. Self-preparation stannous fluoride prophylactic technique in preventive dentistry: report after two years. Am. Dent. A. J., 81:1369–72, Dec. 1970.
204. Shannon, I. L. Sucrose—the tooth's mortal enemy; fluoride—the tooth's best friend. J. Dent. Child., 44:133–6, July 1976.
205. Shaw, J. H. Sweeteners—an overview. Dent. Abstr., 26:172–5, Apr. 1981.
206. Shern, R. J., et al. Clinical study of amine fluoride gel and acidulated phosphate fluoride gel. Community Dent. Oral Epidemiol., 4:133–6, July 1976.
207. Shory, N. L. Report of the ADA national task force on the prohibition of confection sales in schools. p. 233–8. (In Hefferen, J. J., Ayer, W. A., and Koehler, H. M., eds. Foods, nutrition and dental health: volume 3 of a series. Park Forest South, Ill., Pathotox, 1981. vii + 265 p.)
208. Silverstone, L. M. Fissure sealants; laboratory studies. Caries Res., 8:2–26, 1974.
209. ———. Operative measures for caries prevention. Caries Res., 12(Suppl. 1):103–12, 1978.
210. Slack, G. L., et al. Clinical testing of a stannous fluoride-calcium pyrophosphate dentifrice in Essex school girls. Brit. Dent. J., 123:26–32, July 4, 1967.
211. Slack, G. L., et al. Clinical testing of stannous fluoride-insoluble metaphosphate dentifrice in Kent school girls. Brit. Dent. J., 123:9–16, July 4, 1967.
212. Slack, G. L., Bulman, J. S., and Osborn, J. F. Clinical testing of fluoride and non-fluoride containing dentifrices in Hounslow school children. Brit. Dent. J., 130:154–8, Feb. 16, 1971.
213. Sprouse, L. W., and Brooks, J. A manual for rural school fluoridation. DHEW Publ. no. (HSA) 76–15029. Washington, D.C., Government Printing Office, 1976. 83 p.

214. Stamm, J. W. Milk fluoridation as a public health measure. Canad. Dent. A. J., 38:446–8, Dec. 1972.
215. Stephan, R. M. Changes in hydrogen-ion concentration on tooth surfaces and in carious lesions. Am. Dent. A. J., 27:718–23, May 1940.
216. Sutcliffe, P. A longitudinal clinical study of oral cleanliness and dental caries in school children. Arch. Oral Biol., 18:765–70, July 1973.
217. Thomas, A., and Jamison, H. Effect of combination of two cariostatic agents on caries of children: two-year clinical study of supervised brushing in children's homes. Acad. Med. N. J. Bul., 14:241–6, Dec. 1968.
218. Thylstrup, A. Distribution of dental fluorosis in the primary dentition. Community Dent. Oral Epidemiol., 6:329–37, Nov. 1978.
219. Thylstrup, A., et al. Enamel changes and dental caries in 7-year-old children given fluoride tablets from shortly after birth. Caries Res., 13:265–76, 1979.
220. Tinanoff, N., Wei, S. H. Y., and Parkins, F. M. Effect of a pumice prophylaxis on fluoride uptake in tooth enamel. Am. Dent. A. J., 88:134–9, Feb. 1974.
221. Tinanoff, N., and Mueller, B. Fluoride content in milk and formula for infants. J. Dent. Child., 45:53–5, Jan.–Feb. 1978.
222. Torell, P., and Ericsson, Y. The potential benefits to be derived from fluoride mouth rinses. p. 113–66. (In Forrester, D. J., and Schultz, E. M., eds. International workshop on fluorides and dental caries reductions. Baltimore, University Maryland, 1974. 327 p.)
223. Trubman, A., and Crellin, J. A. Effect on dental caries of self-application of acidulated phosphate fluoride paste and gel. Am. Dent. A. J., 86:153–7, Jan. 1973.
224. U. S. Department of Health, Education, and Welfare, Food and Drug Administration. Oral prenatal drugs containing fluorides for human use. Fed. Register, 31:13537, Oct. 20, 1966.
225. U. S. Senate, Select Committee on Nutrition and Human Needs. Dietary goals for the United States. 2nd ed. Washington, D.C., Government Printing Office, 1977. xii + 83 p.
226. von der Fehr, F. R., Löe, H., and Theilade, E. Experimental caries in man. Caries Res., 4:131–48, 1970.
227. von der Fehr, F. R., and Møller, I. J. Caries-preventive fluoride dentifrices. Caries Res., 12:(Suppl. 1)31–7, 1978.
228. Voss, A. C. A dietitian's view of nutrition crusaders. Ohio Dent. J., 53:33–8, Sept. 1979.
229. Wei, S. H. The potential benefits to be derived from topical fluorides in fluoridated communities. p. 178–240. (In Forrester, D. J., and Schultz, E. M., eds. International workshop on fluorides and dental caries reductions. Baltimore, University Maryland, 1974. 327 p.)
230. Weiss, R. L., and Trithart, A. H. Between-meal eating habits and dental caries experience in pre-school children. Am. J. Pub. Health, 50:1097–1104, Aug. 1960.
231. Weisz, W. S. The reduction of dental caries through use of a sodium fluoride mouthwash. Am. Dent. A. J. 60:438–56, Apr. 1960.
232. Wright, G. Z., Banting, D. W., and Feasby, W. H. The Dorchester dental flossing study; final report. Clin. Preven. Dent., 1:23–6, May–June 1979.
233. Zacherl, W. A. Clinical evaluation of neutral sodium fluoride, stannous fluoride, sodium monofluorophosphate and acidulated fluoride-phosphate dentifrices. Canad. Dent. A. J., 38:35–8, Jan. 1972.
234. ______. Clinical evaluation of a sodium fluoride-silica abrasive dentifrice. Abstr. J. Dent. Res., Abstr. no. 1071, 60(Spec. Issue A):577, Mar. 1981.

CHAPTER 9

PREVENTION AND CONTROL OF PERIODONTAL DISEASE AND OTHER ORAL DISEASES AND ANOMALIES

Brian A. Burt

Periodontal disease is described in Chapter 6 as a highly prevalent global disease. Its presence and severity are most directly related to age and to the lack of good oral hygiene. Because periodontal disease is the major cause of tooth loss in adults, its prevention and control are fundamental steps toward improved oral health in most communities.

Unfortunately, there is no parallel to water fluoridation for the prevention of periodontal disease; its prevention and control are based on removal of plaque at regular intervals. While plaque removal can be carried out by a dental professional to a considerable extent, effective plaque control demands at least a reasonable effort by the person concerned. While partial control of caries can thus be achieved at the community level without purposeful individual action, *no control of periodontal disease is possible without conscious action on the part of the individual.* The individual's interest, awareness, and the elusive concept of motivation are thus all-important. In those many instances in which primary prevention cannot be achieved, the same approaches and procedures can be used to control further progress of the disease, thus leaving the patient with a functioning, if not completely disease-free, dentition.

Dentists and hygienists play a major role in controlling periodontal disease both by their own treatment efforts and by educating patients to carry out the necessary self-care procedures. Education of patients, and even more so the public, can be a frustrating task at times, but the successes achieved in patient education can also be among the most rewarding aspects of dental practice.

ETIOLOGY OF PERIODONTAL DISEASE

The etiology of periodontal disease is still not completely understood, although enough is known for effective preventive measures to be undertaken.

Some two hours after cleaning, a structureless pellicle derived from saliva forms on the tooth surface.[22] Plaque, "a soft concentrated mass consisting mainly of a large variety of bacteria held together in an intermicrobial substance,"[117] then forms on the pellicle. Plaque has also been defined as:

> . . . a soft, concentrated mass consisting mainly of a large variety of bacteria together with a certain amount of cellular debris which develops within a short time of refraining from tooth brushing. . . . It is not removed by rinsing with water. . . .[28]

These definitions, though useful and widely quoted, may be oversimplified because the amount of plaque as well as its microbial and biochemical composition varies with the site of formation, the duration of accumulation, the composition of the diet, and other factors yet to be determined.[22]

After plaque has been completely removed, it re-forms slowly on the tooth surface for about three days and then increases rapidly to reach a maximum bulk after seven days.[116] Plaque forms more readily if fermentable carbohydrates are present in the diet,[24] though it can still form to some extent in their absence. Plaque forms naturally in the human mouth, and its causative role in initiating periodontal disease has been demonstrated many times since the early experimental gingivitis studies in humans.[78]

The term *periodontal disease* is used in this chapter to refer generically to the spectrum of periodontal conditions, from gingivitis to the destructive loss of attachment and bony support. Some use the expression in the plural form (periodontal diseases), although this matter still needs clarification, as will be discussed. *Gingivitis* refers to a reversible inflammatory condition of the papilla and the gingival margin, whereas *destructive periodontal disease*, or *periodontitis*, is used to describe chronic progression of the inflammatory condition into pocket formation, loss of attachment, and eventually loss of bony support. Where acute necrotizing ulcerative gingivitis (ANUG) and juvenile periodontitis (formerly called periodontosis) are being specifically referred to, those terms are specifically used.

Ranney[97] defines gingivitis-periodontitis as:

> Inflammation, beginning in the gingiva, which may extend into subjacent periodontal structures, producing loss of attachment of the periodontal structures from the tooth. The condition can be subdivided clinically into gingivitis and periodontitis on the basis of loss of attachment progressing apical to the cementoenamel junction (the original, most coronal extent of connective tissue attachment and most apical extent of epithelial attachment). This division confines all pathologic changes in gingivitis to the gingiva only; in periodontitis, additional alterations occur in one or more of the other periodontal tissues (cementum, periodontal ligament, alveolar bone). Gingivitis and periodontitis are grouped together by this definition, since current evidence is insufficient to suggest different etiologies, periodontitis seeming to be an extension of the same processes operative in gingivitis. Future evidence may warrant reconsideration of this position.

Periodontal disease is caused by bacteria present in dental plaque.[108] Few bacteria can be isolated from around healthy gingival tissue,[108, 117] though with gingivitis there is a considerable increase in the numbers and complexity of bacteria. Plaque forming in the gingival sulcus, called *subgingival plaque*, has a considerably different bacterial structure from that found in *supragingival plaque*.[117] Studies of experimental gingivitis in subjects with previously excellent oral hygiene have shown that when all oral hygiene procedures are stopped for a period of 21 days, the plaque collects rapidly (as described previously), but seems to reach a maximum mass after seven days. Over time, however, undisturbed plaque from the gingival margin shows a change in its bacterial character, shifting from one dominated by bacteria of the *Streptococcus* genus to one dominated by *Actinomyces*[84, 114] without a measurable change in mass. This information suggests that gingival inflammation may come from proportional changes in bacteria rather than just an increase in plaque mass and lends further support to the "specific plaque hypothesis" of Loesche.[83] This concept of bacterial specificity also suggests that what is generically called periodontal disease may be a group of diseases with similar clinical profiles but with different etiologies and clinical courses.[90] This view seems to contrast with that given by Ranney in his definition of gingivitis-periodontitis, in which periodontitis is seen as an extension of gingivitis. It is clear that considerably more research is needed to clarify the nature of the disease or diseases.

THE NATURAL HISTORY OF PERIODONTAL DISEASE

The natural history of periodontal disease has received surprisingly little attention, probably because of the long-term chronic nature of the condition. Studies in this field, among others, were conducted by Löe and his associates in Norway and Sri Lanka.[6, 80, 81, 82] Briefly, the studies have shown that with excellent oral hygiene status maintained by the individual over a long period of time, the loss of attachment is negligible and excellent periodontal health is maintained. Whereas some loss of attachment with increasing age is probably physiological, it appears that as long as excellent oral hygiene status is maintained, the loss can be of clinically insignificant proportions, at least up to 40 years of age. On the other hand, in those individuals whose oral hygiene status is poor, loss of attachment can be substantial and rapid and can lead to tooth loss even before 40 years of age. Undisturbed plaque accumulations lead to destructive periodontal disease and ultimately to tooth loss in any population.[15] Studies on populations over 40 years of age have not yet been reported.

Among different individuals, the same degree of plaque accumulation will lead to different degrees of inflammatory gingival response. This difference is to be expected, given the nature of individual variation to agents of disease (discussed in Chapter 5). With periodontal disease, this individual variation has stimulated considerable research into host resistance factors—the "immune response" of the individual.[60] At present, the immune response to the challenge of periodontal disease is too poorly understood to have any practical application, although in time it may be a basis for better prevention of the condition.

Chronic periodontal disease is highly prevalent and constitutes a major public health problem (see Chapter 6). There are other more acute forms of periodontal disease that are seen much less commonly, and they will be described here briefly. They are mentioned to emphasize the point that their treatment and control are based on the same fundamental principle that governs prevention and treatment of the far more frequent chronic periodontal disease—regular and consistent plaque removal.

Acute Necrotizing Ulcerative Gingivitis

Acute Necrotizing Ulcerative Gingivitis (ANUG) is an acute form of periodontal disease, characterized by rapid development and usually by pain. ANUG is defined by Ranney[97] as:

> A disease involving necrosis and ulceration of the surface of the gingiva, with underlying inflammation; it usually begins in the col area, resulting in the clinically pathognomonic "punched-out" papilla, and is characterized by a relative proliferation of fusiforms and spirochetes, including invasion of gingival tissue by the organisms.

In Western populations, this disease is predominantly seen in teenagers and young adults; occurrence may be higher in developing nations. It is probably not communicable, though it may occur in people living under similar conditions in barracks or dormitories. Individual cases, however, are not unusual. It can be accompanied by extreme malaise with elevated temperature and has been associated with emotional or psychic stress. Its precise etiology is unclear. Once the pain and acute symptoms have been brought under control, treatment and further prevention proceed as those for chronic periodontal disease.

Juvenile Periodontitis

The condition of juvenile periodontitis, formerly called periodontosis, is characterized by the clinical picture of severe destructive periodontal disease, but it characteristically occurs in young individuals. Usually there are no obvious signs of accompanying gingival inflammation, and the disease can occur in persons whose oral hygiene appears to be reasonably good. Ranney[97] defines the condition as:

> . . . severe loss of attachment and destruction of bone adjacent to permanent first molars and/or incisors in children, adolescents or young adults.

Studies by Waerhaug[121, 122] indicate that the disease is characterized by extremely rapid apical migration of subgingival plaque. Apparently the transformation of supragingival plaque to subgingival plaque occurs sooner in persons with juvenile periodontitis than in those without it, and the subsequent apical migration of the subgingival plaque, once established, is extremely rapid. In addition, the tissue response to small amounts of subgingival plaque is highly exaggerated—hence the observation of earlier years, when the disease was referred to as periodontosis, that it occurred in the absence of plaque. It is now accepted that plaque is the causative agent, though very small amounts of plaque are sufficient to induce severe disease. When compared with clinically normal sites, subgingival plaque in juvenile periodontitis contains increased proportions of gram-negative anaerobic rods, as well as many other organisms that are difficult to classify.[91]

Waerhaug[122] found that patients with the condition responded well to total plaque control, but the plaque control had to be virtually total. Established pockets were removed surgically in Waehaug's regimen and subgingival plaque was removed professionally at each three-month recall. Patients were instructed in the thorough oral hygiene procedures that they needed to carry out themselves. Those who responded well to these procedures kept the disease under control. Those who responded incompletely did not and the disease progressed. Waerhaug stresses that early diagnosis, which is not necessarily easy, is essential to successful treatment of the condition.

Why do these individuals respond in such an exaggerated fashion to what may be a relatively small disease challenge? One suggestion is that they suffer from a selective cell-mediated immunodeficiency and therefore have poor host resistance to the disease challenge.[59] Again, there is at present no practical application of this suggestion, although studies of such individuals may help advance knowledge of the individual immune response.

Once the condition of juvenile periodontitis has been correctly diagnosed, treatment and control procedures are no different from those for patients with chronic destructive periodontal disease—just more intensive.

APPROACHES TO PREVENTION AND CONTROL OF PERIODONTAL DISEASE

Primary prevention of periodontal disease, in practical terms, is difficult to separate from secondary prevention and control of the disease at a low level of gingivitis. Even treatment of established disease, once any necessary surgery has been carried out, follows procedures similar to those used in primary prevention.

There is little evidence for any preventive benefits to be achieved by changes in diet or nutrition,[68, 111] although the role of diet and nutrition should continue to be explored.[4] No magic mouthrinses have yet been developed,[13] even though chemotherapeutic rinses (to be discussed later in this chapter) are used to some extent in other countries. None, however, is currently available for use in the United States. Rinsing with water removes loose debris, but not dental plaque.[62] Chewing fibrous foods does not remove dental plaque,[65, 86] and no toothpaste is yet available with the property of preventing calculus from forming.[112] In short, mechanical plaque removal remains the basis for prevention and control of periodontal disease.[74, 75, 120]

Primary prevention of periodontal disease requires consistent, thorough removal of plaque on a lifetime basis. The rationale is to remove plaque before it matures to the point at which gingivitis begins. Some people are capable of maintaining adequate oral hygiene status largely by their own efforts, but many people are not. The dental professional will consistently see some level of gingivitis in these patients and may become frustrated in the effort to eliminate the gingivitis entirely. With these patients, the dental professional's approach should be to maintain the gingivitis at as low a level as possible, but to be prepared to settle for some disease rather than none. Expectations of idealistic dentists and hygienists can often be unrealistically high. It should be remembered that the ultimate aim of dental care is to maintain a functioning dentition rather than to achieve the complete absence of disease. As long as a moderate level of gingivitis can be stabilized and loss of periodontal support prevented, the patient will maintain a functioning dentition.

For practical prevention and control of the disease, both in population groups and in the individual patient, Löe[75] made a fundamental point when he stated that the crucial transition phase of the progression of the disease is when supragingival plaque becomes subgingival. So long as plaque accumulation remains supragingival, where plaque formation begins,[117] it can be controlled by simple mechanical means, most of which are carried out by the individual patient. Once plaque becomes subgingival, the individual patient cannot control the disease by self-care and professional intervention is necessary.

Plaque control methods for prevention and control of periodontal disease consist of (1) mechanical plaque removal by the individual, (2) mechanical plaque removal by the dental professional, and (3) chemotherapeutic methods of plaque control.

Mechanical Plaque Removal by the Individual

Self-care by the individual is the key to periodontal health. Unless the individual is able to maintain at least a reasonable level of oral cleanliness throughout life by regular and consistent home care, the benefits of treatment by dental professionals will be limited.[107] Individual effort means mechanical plaque removal with the toothbrush and aids like dental floss, the interproximal brush, and wood points. Natural self-cleansing mechanisms are inadequate to remove plaque,[71] as are the traditional toothcleaning practices such as the "chewing stick," used in some cultures as an oral hygiene mechanism.[106] When used under supervision, however, the chewing stick may be as efficient as a toothbrush in populations accustomed to it.[93] The implication is that in countries where the chewing stick is a normal cultural practice, efforts to improve the efficiency and regularity of its use may help to control periodontal disease.

Given the fundamental nature of individual oral hygiene practices in the promotion of oral health, it is surprising how little is known about basic things such as the best type of toothbrush to use and how often to brush. Research studies that have been conducted in these areas have often been run for only short periods and with atypical populations, such as dental or dental hygiene students. Long-term effects and the projection of results to the general population are thus difficult to assess.

Frequency of Toothbrushing. The best available information indicates that a thorough oral cleansing should be carried out at 24- to 48-hour intervals.[54, 58] When one considers the time needed for plaque to mature, the old adage of brushing after every meal, which was usually impractical anyway, seems unnecessary. Thorough cleaning at 24-hour intervals is a routine that probably best fits in with most people's daily schedules and is one that is compatible with gingival health. This appears to be a practical regimen for dentists and hygienists to recommend for their patients.

Type of Toothbrush. Little research has been carried out on the best type of toothbrush; what evidence there is suggests that it really does not matter much.[47, 111] Children clearly should use a smaller brush, and the dentist and hygienist may want to recommend different sizes and degrees of softness depending on each patient's manual dexterity, enthusiasm, and oral health. But these recommendations are based on common sense rather than on firm evidence.

The comparative effectiveness of manual and power-driven toothbrushes has been relatively well studied.[7, 26] Again, it appears that both are equally effective if used properly. Differences between individuals are probably greater than differences between the brushes. Power brushes may be particularly useful for handicapped persons or others with low manual dexterity.

Toothbrushing Methods. A variety of toothbrushing methods, some requiring a lot of manual gymnastics, have been described in the dental literature; proponents of one method or another have traditionally been vehement in the defense of their method's efficacy. Research, however, indicates that there appears to be little inherent difference between methods in the ability to remove dental plaque.[37, 42, 46, 100, 101, 104, 105] From these research studies, limited though some of them are, the scrub method emerges as the simplest method available and one that is no less effective than any other. It requires minimal manual dexterity and patient concentration. Because dental professionals must aim for the best possible results within practical limits in educating their patients, the scrub method seems best for most persons. For some individuals receiving treatment for advanced disease, a special method may be needed, assuming they are able to manage it.

Dental Floss. A lot of dental health education materials extol the efficacy of dental floss — "brush and floss" now tends to replace the exhortation to just "brush." There is still little evidence, however, to show that flossing, as practiced by the individual, adds much to the efficiency of brushing,[46, 100, 105] nor are the limited research studies able to find a difference between waxed and unwaxed floss in cleaning efficacy.[16, 33, 53] Floss is probably helpful for many individuals with hard-to-clean contact areas, but the patient does need thorough training in its use. Patient interest needs to be assessed as well, because flossing adds to the time taken for the daily oral hygiene routine. Because the proportion of the mouth brushed by young persons aged 5–22 ranged only from 25 to 67 percent in one study,[103] anything to aid the efficiency of brushing needs to be judiciously chosen.

Patient Motivation. The individual practice of regular, thorough, and consistent oral hygiene procedures depends largely on the interest and enthusiasm of the individual patient. Some individuals may have this enthusiasm already; in others, it may need to be developed. This is no easy task, as is discussed in Chapter 15. Oral hygiene practices must fit into the lifestyle of each individual, and lifestyle changes are difficult to achieve by exhortation alone.[45]

There is no easy answer to the "motivational" problem. Carefully thought-out and well-organized "motivational programs" in groups such as schoolchildren have produced little benefit in the United States.[44, 47] Supervised daily toothbrushing with schoolchildren in Sweden did produce a reduction in gingivitis for the duration of the program,[62] but the improvement disappeared when the supervision ended.[64] Effects of individual chairside instruction, according to some investigators, have been minor,[115, 125] thus raising doubts about what "motivational programs" really do. Melsen and Agerbaek,[89] for example, found that motivational programs only succeeded in reinforcing existing favorable attitudes and not in altering negative ones.

A great deal needs to be learned about methods of altering individual behavior. For dental professionals who try to induce individual patients to improve their daily oral hygiene performance, success may depend as much upon a personal and common sense approach by the dentist or hygienist as upon anything else. Patients need to know the facts about periodontal disease, and all regimens and procedures taught to them should have a clear rationale. Some patients will respond better than others. Some will just need information, because they already are motivated; but other patients, regardless of the information given and the time spent, may show little progress in improving their oral hygiene. Objective measurement of progress by use of an index of periodontal disease and dental plaque (see Chapter 5) is necessary, because subjective impressions of progress can be misleading. Reinforcement of simple messages and constant encouragement of the individual's efforts seem to be important factors. Oral health professionals must work within the limitations of the individual patient — not to mention their own limitations.

Public health education programs intended to produce mass improvement in oral hygiene have had little measurable effect in the past.[40, 44, 71] The amount of time given to this form of education in public health programs should perhaps be reduced to a minimum, especially since more effective primary prevention procedures can be carried out. (For a discussion of dental health education, see Chapter 15.)

Mechanical Plaque Removal by Professionals

Periodontal disease can be successfully controlled when dentists and dental hygienists carry out regular and thorough plaque removal for their patients, but the frequency and thoroughness required are considerable. Success also depends on a concomitant high level of personal oral hygiene efforts practiced by the patient. The benefits of professional plaque removal have been shown in studies of children and adults who were in reasonable periodontal health to begin with, as well as in studies of adults receiving treatment for advanced disease.

Karlstad Studies. Among children, spectacular success at preventing gingivitis has been reported by the Axelsson-Lindhe group in their studies at Karlstad, Sweden.[8, 9, 11, 67] In their studies with children aged 7–14, this group provided the intensive prophylactic procedures listed on p. 225–226.[8] They include explanation of the disease etiology and treatment; identification of plaque; cleaning of accessible and occlusal surfaces; and interdental cleaning. These procedures were applied by professionals *every two weeks for two years.* In the third year, the time between these "professional cleanings," as the Karlstad researchers refer to them, was extended to four weeks for the 7–11 year olds and to eight weeks for the 13–14 year olds. The continuing good results with this reduced frequency of cleaning was attributed to the background effects of the first two years.[67] These researchers are firm in their contention that professional cleanings five to eight times per year are not enough to control gingivitis. If they are right, that might explain the mixed results from other similar studies in which the frequency of application, and perhaps the intensity of the procedures, varied.

Badersten and colleagues[12] achieved significant reduction in gingivitis in children from a working class area of Malmo, Sweden, who had prophylaxes applied 10 times per year, though their results with caries prevention were not as good (see Chapter 8). Results comparable to those from Karlstad, however, were achieved in a Norwegian study that was intended to replicate the Karlstad program; substantial reductions in caries and gingivitis were achieved in this intensive two-year project with schoolchildren.[55] A study in Denmark[1] achieved considerable reduction in gingivitis among 7-year-old children who received a professional cleaning every two weeks over a year, but the gingivitis got worse when the frequency of cleaning was reduced to once every three weeks for the second year. In the United States, prophylaxes twice per year in children aged 10–11 produced neither beneficial reductions in gingivitis nor improvements in oral hygiene levels.[99]

Prophylactic Treatment of Adults. Qualified success from routine prophylaxes (with a less intensive cleaning procedure than that used in the Karlstad regimen) in adults was reported in Norway by Lovdal and colleagues in 1961.[87] For five years, factory workers received a prophylaxis plus oral hygiene instruction at 6-month intervals and at 3-month intervals for more severely affected individuals. The greatest benefits were gained by persons whose oral hygiene status was best to begin with, and least success was achieved among those with initially poor oral hygiene. This difference in results could have been because the persons with initially better oral hygiene (the "better motivated" persons) practiced more rigorous self-care during the period of the study. In Axelsson and Lindhe's study of adults[10] in Karlstad, the professional cleanings were carried out every two months for the first two years, and every three months for the third year. In line with the philosophy of these researchers, intensive oral hygiene instruction for self-care accompanied the professional cleanings. The success reported in this study was clouded by some questions regarding group allocation procedures of the research design.

In the United States, the study of Suomi and associates[110] with office workers in California showed that a professional prophylaxis plus intensive oral hygiene instruction every two to four months reduced levels of plaque and gingivitis relative to a control group and greatly slowed the rate of loss of attachment. In a separate study of young men, Suomi and colleagues[113] found a tendency toward improved gingival health accompanying greater frequency of prophylaxes, though differences resulting from prophylaxes at 12-month, 6-month, and 4-month intervals were not pronounced. The Air Force study of Lightner and co-workers[61] found that beneficial results were proportional to the frequency of the prophylactic treatment received. The best results in this study came from the group that received four prophylaxes per year plus oral hygiene instruction at each appointment.

Defective Restorations. Where overhangs from restorations extend into the gingival crevice, plaque control is virtually impossible. One Swedish study found that 75 per cent of interproximal fillings had some subgingival defect and found also that loss of periodontal attachment was related directly to the size of the overhang.[18] Existing overhangs and other restorative defects should be removed in prophylactic treatment. Initial placement of interproximal restorations is one area in which control of caries and control of periodontal disease are involved at the same time.

Treatment of Established Periodontal Disease. The long-term studies of the effects of treatment of established chronic periodontal disease, carried out by Ramfjord and colleagues at The University of Michigan,[56, 96] suggest that extensive surgery does not seem to be the most favorable treatment for all patients with established disease. Relatively light surgical intervention (the modified Widman flap procedure) along with subgingival curettage and oral hygiene measures promoted the greatest levels of clinical attachment. Similar results came from a study in Minnesota.[95] In that study, as in the Michigan studies, the value of the light surgery plus scaling and root planing was greatest when the initial disease was more severe. With less severe disease, scaling and root planing alone gave better results. Excellent results from meticulous oral hygiene regimens following periodontal surgery have come from studies in Sweden that included patients in whom periodontal disease was far advanced.[66, 92, 102]

These studies have all demonstrated the value of continued plaque removal in the treatment of chronic periodontal disease, though there are some uncertainties over how stringent this plaque removal must be for successful posttreatment maintenance.

Professional Plus Personal Care. These studies just described indicate that professional plaque removal has an important role in the prevention and control of periodontal disease, though it must be reemphasized that the best results were obtained when excellent personal oral hygiene status was maintained by the individual. The evidence suggests that a thorough professional prophylaxis at 2- to 4-month intervals (longer in some patients), combined with a high level of daily individual oral hygiene practiced at home, is enough to maintain periodontal health in the periodontally healthy adult. In other words, these procedures are sufficient to prevent the destructive periodontal disease that leads to tooth loss. The needed frequency of the prophylaxis will vary from patient to patient, but it is becoming increasingly clear that the traditional twice-a-year or annual prophylaxis may not be enough, especially in the middle-to-later years of life.

Many persons, however, are unable to meet the necessary self-care standards, and host resistance to the periodontal challenge of mature plaque may sometimes be low. For such patients, dental professionals should probably consider carrying out the professional plaque removal procedures more frequently. In either instance, a high level of individual motivation is needed. In addition, frequent professional plaque removal can also be expensive unless carried out by auxiliaries.[23]

Plaque Removal by Chemotherapeutic Methods

The inability of many persons to remove their own dental plaque consistently results from insufficient knowledge, poor mechanical dexterity, or lack of motivation. The idea of a chemical method of plaque removal, a "magic" mouthrinse or tablet that does it all, is therefore highly attractive. Such a periodontal panacea may be developed one day, but it has not appeared yet. Research over many years, however, has uncovered some partially successful products that can be of use in specific circumstances. Further development in this area can be expected, and there is reason to be hopeful.[3]

Antibiotics have been tested with some success, but their use is impractical on a long-term basis, chiefly because of the potential for development of resistant organisms.[2, 34,70, 74] Metronidazole currently shows some promise.[84] Various enzymes, especially dextranase, intended to prevent the adhesion of plaque by interfering with bacterial metabolism have been successfully tested in animals, but have been disappointing in human studies.[70] Given the complexity of dental plaque, if enzymes are ever to be effective as routine antiplaque agents, it seems likely that a combination of enzymes will be needed.

Chlorhexidine and Alexidine

Two antiseptic agents received considerable research attention during the 1970s and have shown sufficient promise to be used selectively in dental practice in Europe. Chlorhexidine gluconate, used as a mouthrinse (10 ml, 0.2 percent concentration once or twice daily) or topical application (1.0 to 2.0 percent concentration used daily) or in a dentifrice (0.4 to 1.0 percent concentration), has been successful in reducing supragingival plaque in a number of studies.[2, 73] Alexidine dihydrochloride mouthrinse (10 to 15 ml, 0.035 to 0.05 percent concentration) has yielded similar results, though the success of either compound is not unqualified.

The early short-term studies conducted by Löe and colleagues indicated that chlorhexidine rinses inhibited the formation of plaque almost completely.[27, 76, 77] These studies led to Löe's enthusiastic endorsement of chlorhexidine in 1973.[72, 73] However, the studies were conducted with periodontally healthy dental students who ceased all oral hygiene procedures at the beginning of the studies, so the applicability of these results to the public is doubtful. Results of short-term studies by other researchers using chlorhexidine in gel and dentifrice form were less clear-cut and revealed more undesirable side effects than the results of the Löe group.[14, 31, 35] Staining of teeth and restorations was a persistent problem.[35] Even when short-term results were good, some researchers had reservations about long-term effects.[21, 41]

Short-term studies with alexidine provided results similar to those found with chlorhexidine. Reductions in plaque and gingivitis were recorded,[25, 29, 69, 109, 123] but some were of little clinical significance.[25, 109] Mild staining was also reported in all of these studies.

Results of long-term studies confirmed the reservations about the routine use of chlorhexidine. One two-year study found no changes in plaque and gingivitis levels among test subjects, although again the initial oral hygiene status in the dental student subjects of the study was excellent, possibly masking any beneficial effects of the chlorhexidine.[52] Löe and associates showed reduced levels of plaque and gingivitis in a two-year study (also with dental and medical students), although one anomalous finding was that calculus deposition increased in the test group.[79] One possible explanation is that the chlorhexidine kills plaque bacteria but does not remove the plaque.[2] The reduced vitality of the plaque then enhances its subsequent mineralization. It is also interesting to note that in the Karlstad studies chlorhexidine gel was found ineffective in plaque control.[11]

By the end of the 1970s, reservations about chlorhexidine were widely accepted, although they were not so great as to negate its use completely. On the one hand, its selective bactericidal effect against *Streptococcus mutans*[126] may lead to its use in controlling severe cases of caries. It also seems to be free of toxic reactions.[36] But on the other hand, its side effect of staining and the possibility of development of resistant organisms were enough to cause Löe to modify the earlier endorsement; on several occasions, he warned against the indiscriminate use of chlorhexidine.[74, 75] In addition, chlorhexidine does not affect subgingival plaque,[2] which suggests that any preventive use it may have must come after mechanical cleansing.

Chlorhexidine is used in the Scandinavian countries as an antiseptic rinse before oral surgery, to improve plaque control up to three to four weeks after periodontal surgery, and as an oral hygiene aid for patients with immobilized jaws recovering from fractures.[2] This limited and selective application relegates chlorhexidine to the role of a useful adjunct to mechanical cleansing in those countries where it is available.

Chlorhexidine and alexidine are not available for intraoral use in the United States, and neither is recognized in *Accepted Dental Therapeutics*.[5]

Fluoride

The chemotherapeutic agent that holds perhaps the most promise and presents the fewest problems is one in common use now: fluoride. The multiple action of fluoride in caries control was discussed in Chapter 8. Fluoride reduces acid production in plaque by inhibiting the enzyme enolase, essential for the degradation of sugars to lactic acid.[51] There is also evidence that fluoride reduces plaque bulk.[17, 119] Stannous fluoride has been suggested as a useful adjunct to plaque control after periodontal surgery in the United States.[119] One American study that assessed the effect of amine fluoride in reducing plaque and gingivitis was inconclusive,[98] but the subject seems worthy of further research.

Control of Periodontal Disease in the Community

Periodontal disease is controlled by the regular, consistent, and thorough removal of plaque. Current evidence is that regular dental attendance for professional prophylaxes, together with a high level of individual plaque removal by toothbrushing and other mechanical cleansing aids every 24 to 48 hours, is enough to maintain an adequate level of periodontal health for life in most persons. In special instances, such as those persons with juvenile periodontitis, professional intervention is necessary, but the principles of prevention and control of the disease are the same. Until a chemotherapeutic antiplaque agent suitable for widespread public use is developed, or until antimicrobial therapy can be directed against specific pathogens, dentistry's efforts must be aimed at mechanical plaque removal.

Individual patients need to combine professional plaque removal with a program of self-care, the extent of which depends upon each patient's interest, mechanical capability, and ability to attend and pay for treatment. Dental professionals need to train individual patients in methods of plaque control and need to use whatever legitimate persuasive tactics work to raise the patient's level of motivation.

In the community, public education programs should be continuous and stress the need for personal oral hygiene measures and regular dental visits. Even though these programs have generally not been successful in the past and face formidable obstacles to success, those members of the public who rarely visit the dentist still need to know why plaque control is in their own best interest. Patients who are in the habit of making annual dental visits need to be convinced that more regular prophylactic visits are necessary if periodontal health is not to deteriorate. By the same token, dentists and hygienists themselves need to be convinced of the necessity for thorough prophylaxes for their adult patients at regular intervals. Widespread acceptance of this philosophy could have profound implications for dental education and the provision of care, as well as leading to improved periodontal health in the community.

CONTROL OF OTHER CONDITIONS

Oral Cancer

There is no direct primary prevention for oral cancer. Avoidance of the risk factors listed in Chapter 6 (alcohol and tobacco are the most obvious ones) makes sense, even though a cause-and-effect relation between these factors and oral cancer has not definitely been established.

Secondary prevention or control consists of treatment following early detection. All dentists and hygienists should be on the lookout for the early signs of soft tissue changes in their patients, because the probability of successful treatment is greatest when the disease is diagnosed early. Patients presenting with those risk factors described in Chapter 6 require especially close attention. A biopsy should be carried out when there is any doubt about a lesion, and the results interpreted by a qualified pathologist. Dentists should be sufficiently practiced at biopsy procedures to carry them out confidently and competently.

In those instances in which a dentist feels a biopsy cannot be carried out, exfoliative cytology—a histological examination of surface cells scraped from a suspected lesion with a tongue blade—may be performed. Unfortunately, the accuracy of oral exfoliative cytology is highly variable, and the procedure is especially weak in detecting premalignant lesions.[19] Both false positive and false negative readings are common. The variety of clinical and histological appearances found in oral cancer casts doubt on the validity of diagnoses made from microscopic examination of surface cells alone.[57] Because final diagnosis must eventually be based on the results of a biopsy examination,[19, 57] oral exfoliative cytology is rarely indicated.

Mass screening for oral cancer is costly. Many thousands of persons must be screened in order to find very few potential lesions. Screening of special high-risk population groups, however, such as those in nursing homes or homeless people, is justified from time to time both as case-finding and as educational experiences.

Oral Clefts

Cleft lip and palate also cannot be prevented in the usual sense. A complex, polygenic mode of inheritance is involved with cleft palate, and there are also thought to be interactions of multiple genetic and environmental factors.[39] Genetic counseling, defined as the communication process that deals with the human problems associated with occurrence, or risk of occurrence, of a genetic disorder in a family,[38] can therefore be of help to prospective parents. The chance of occurrence of clefts increases considerably if there is a history of clefts in the family; risk tables have been tabulated[20] to specify the degree of risk in various patterns of family history. Genetic counseling is usually provided at the hospitals of large medical colleges.

Publicly funded programs for the treatment of this condition are generally available in other countries and in most states of the United States through the state crippled children services (CCS). Treatment of cleft palate is lengthy, complicated, and highly expensive. It requires a team approach, with oral surgeons, plastic surgeons, orthodontists, speech pathologists, and sometimes other specialists needed for successful habilitation. Such "teams" sometimes function as true teams, with careful coordination of the various specialties. On the other hand, they frequently seem to function haphazardly, though good treatment can still result. Local dental societies and dental public health authorities should be aware of the resources available in or near their communities for genetic counseling, team-treatment, and funding for treatment of this most distressing condition.

Malocclusion

While malocclusions of genetic origin cannot be prevented, those resulting from premature loss of primary teeth or the subsequent loss of permanent teeth can be. Indeed, one important aim of the prevention of dental caries in younger patients is to prevent the crowding, overeruption, and other orthodontic complications that can result from premature tooth loss.

Dental Fluorosis

Dental fluorosis is prevented by restricting the intake of fluorides by children to optimum levels during the preeruptive period of enamel formation. Dental fluorosis most commonly occurs in the permanent dentition, but has also been reported in the primary teeth.[94, 118] Although fluorosis in primary teeth is uncommon, it is now thought that the placenta does not prevent fluoride from reaching the fetus to the degree it was once thought.[118] Except in areas of very high, naturally occurring fluoride content in water, however, this information seems to be of no practical importance in preventing fluorosis.[30] Most fluorosis follows excessive ingestion of fluoride in infancy rather than in utero.

Removal of excess fluoride from a community water supply is generally more difficult and more costly than adding fluoride to fluoride-deficient water. Defluoridation programs have been successfully carried out, however, in communities such as Bartlett, Texas,[49, 50] where too much fluoride was naturally present in the water. The numbers of communities in the United States with a gross excess of naturally occurring fluoride in the drinking water may diminish in time, because the current regulations of the Environmental Protection Agency under the Safe Drinking Water Act require that excessive fluoride be removed[32] (see Chapter 7). These same regulations, it should be pointed out, also state that fluoride in the optimum concentration is beneficial to dental health.

One avoidable reason for fluorosis is the inappropriate prescription of fluoride supplements by well-meaning physicians and dentists for their patients living in fluoridated areas. A national survey in 1979 found that up to 19 percent of prescribing physicians in fluoridated areas prescribed fluoride supplements for children up to one year of age,[88] clearly an inappropriate thing to do. Dental professionals must therefore ensure that physicians in their community are prescribing fluoride supplements in accordance with the schedule recommended by the American Dental Association and the American Academy of Pediatrics (see Table 8–1).

Another entirely preventable source of unsightly enamel staining is the ingestion of tetracycline by the infant or expectant mother during the period of enamel calcification.[43, 124] Again, dental professionals in a community can use their influence to ensure that their medical and other health colleagues are aware of this possibility and the options that can be used to avoid it.

It should be noted that fluoride ingestion and tetracyclines are not the only, or even the most frequent, causes of opacities in dental enamel. Many of the conditions classified as *amelogenesis imperfecta*, and possibly some of those conditions referred to as idiopathic enamel opacities, are hereditary in nature and therefore not preventable by any present means.

Of course, as dental professionals well know, there are many other oral diseases that could have been listed here under the broad heading of "other oral diseases and anomalies." From time to time certain diseases and anomalies tend to be in vogue or seem to be more prevalent, at least as reported by the professional press or the popular media. Recently, oral herpes has been receiving considerable attention. Unfortunately, not much factual scientific information on its epidemiology, prevention, or control is yet available.

References

1. Agerbaek, Nina, et al Effect of professional toothcleansing every third week on gingivitis and dental caries in children. Community Dent. Oral Epidemiol., 6:40–1, Jan. 1978.
2. Ainamo, J. Control of plaque by chemical agents. J. Clin. Periodont., 4:23–35, Dec. 1977.
3. ______ . Bacterial control—state of the art. J. Dent. Res., 59(Spec. Issue D, part II):2137–43, Dec. 1980.
4. Alfano, M. C. Prospects for improving the prevention of inflammatory periodontal disease. J. Preven. Dent., 5:26–8, Jan.–Feb. 1978.
5. American Dental Association, Council on Dental Therapeutics. Accepted dental therapeutics. 38th ed. Chicago, The Association, 1979. xxix + 385 p.
6. Ånerud, Åge, et al. The natural history of periodontal disease in man; changes in gingival

health and oral hygiene before 40 years of age. J. Periodont. Res., 14:526–40, Nov. 1979.
7. Ash, M. M., Rainey, B. L., and Smith, W. A. Evaluation of manual and motor driven toothbrushes. Am. Dent. A. J., 69:321–5, Sept. 1964.
8. Axelsson, P., and Lindhe, J. The effect of a preventive programme on dental plaque, gingivitis and caries in school children. Results after one and two years. J. Clin. Periodont., 1:126–38, 1974.
9. ______ . Effect of fluoride on gingivitis and dental caries in a preventive program based on plaque control. Community Dent. Oral Epidemiol., 3:159–60, Aug. 1975.
10. ______ . Effect of controlled oral hygiene procedures on caries and periodontal disease in adults. J. Clin. Periodont., 5:133–51, May 1978.
11. Axelsson, Per, Lindhe, Jan, and Waseby, Jan. The effect of various plaque control measures on gingivitis and caries in schoolchildren. Community Dent. Oral Epidemiol., 4:232–9, Nov. 1976.
12. Badersten, A., Egelberg, J., and Koch, G. Effect of monthly prophylaxis on caries and gingivitis in schoolchildren. Community Dent. Oral Epidemiol., 3:1–4, Feb. 1975.
13. Bagramian, R. A. Oral hygiene procedures and pit and fissure sealants. p. 123–51. (In Burt, B. A., ed. The relative efficiency of methods of caries prevention in dental public health. Proceedings of a workshop at The University of Michigan, June 5–8, 1978. Ann Arbor, University Michigan, 1979. 326 p.)
14. Bassiouny, M. A., and Grant, A. A. The tooth-brush application of chlorhexidine. Brit. Dent. J., 139:323–7, Oct. 21, 1975.
15. Becker, W., Berg, L., and Becker, B. E. Untreated periodontal disease. A longitudinal study. J. Periodont., 50:234–44, May 1979.
16. Bergenholtz, A., and Brithon, J. Plaque removal by dental floss or toothpicks. An intraindividual comparative study. J. Clin. Periodontol., 7:516–24, Dec. 1980.
17. Birkeland, J. M. Effect of fluoride on the amount of dental plaque in children. Scand. J. Dent. Res., 80:82–4, 1972.
18. Björn, A. L., Björn, H., and Grkovic, B. Marginal fit of restorations and its relation to periodontal bone level. Odont. Revy, 20:311–21, 1969.
19. Blozis, G. G. The value of exfoliative cytology in the diagnosis of oral cancer. Internat. Dent. J., 22:481–8, Dec. 1972.
20. Bonaiti-Pellie, C., and Smith, C. Risk tables for genetic counselling in some common congenital malformations. J. Med. Genetics, 11:374–7, Dec. 1974.
21. Bosman, C. W., and Powell, R. N. The reversal of localized experimental gingivitis. A comparison between mechanical tooth-brushing procedures and a 0.2 percent chlorhexidine mouth rinse. J. Clin. Periodont., 4:161–72, Aug. 1977.
22. Bowen, W. H. Nature of plaque. Oral Sciences Rev., 9:3–21, 1976.
23. Burt, B. A., and Warner, K. E. Prevention of oral disease; its potential for containing the costs of dental care. (In Kudrle, R. T., and Meskin, L. H., eds. Opportunities for cost-containment in dentistry. Minneapolis, University Minnesota Press. In press.)
24. Carlsson, Jan, and Egelberg, Jan. Effect of diet on early plaque formation in man. Odont. Revy, 16:112–25, 1965.
25. Carlson, H. C., Porter, K., and Alms, T. H. The effect of an alexidine mouthwash on dental plaque and gingivitis. J. Periodont., 48:216–8, Apr. 1977.
26. Conroy, C. W. Comparison of automatic and hand toothbrushes: cleaning effectiveness. Am. Dent. A. J., 70:921–9, Apr. 1965.
27. Davies, R. M., et al. The effect of topical application of chlorhexidine on the bacterial colonization of the teeth and gingiva. J. Periodont. Res., 5:96–101, 1970.
28. Dawes, C., Jenkins, G. N., and Tonge, C. H. The nomenclature of the integuments of the enamel surface of teeth. Brit. Dent. J., 115:65–8, July 16, 1963.
29. Deasy, M. J., et al. Inhibitory effects of an alexidine mouthrinse on dental plaque formation. Clin. Preven. Dent., 1:6–9, Mar.–Apr. 1979.
30. Driscoll, W. S. Review of clinical research on prenatal fluorides. J. Dent. Child., 48:109–17, Mar.–Apr. 1981.
31. Emilson, C. G., and Fornell, J. Effect of toothbrushing with chlorhexidine gel on salivary microflora, oral hygiene, and caries. Scand. J. Dent. Res., 84:308–19, 1976.
32. Environmental Protection Agency. Interim primary drinking water regulations. Fed. Register, 45:57332–57, Aug. 27, 1980.
33. Finkelstein, Paul, and Grossman, Eli. The effectiveness of dental floss in reducing gingival inflammation. J. Dent. Res., 58:1034–9, Mar. 1979.

34. Fitzgerald, R. J. The potential of antibodies as caries-control agents. Am. Dent. A. J., 87:1006–9, Oct. 1973.
35. Fløtra, L., et al. Side effects of chlorhexidine mouth-washes. Scand. J. Dent. Res., 79:119–25, 1971.
36. Foulkes, D. M. Some toxicological observations on chlorhexidine. J. Periodont. Res., 8(Suppl. 12):55–7, 1973.
37. Frandsen, A. M., et al. A comparison of the effectiveness of the Charters' scrub and roll methods of toothbrushing in removing plaque. Scand. J. Dent. Res., 80:267–71, 1972.
38. Fraser, F. C. Genetic counseling. Am. J. Human Genetics, 26:636–59, Sept. 1974.
39. Fraser, G. R., and Mayo, O., eds. Textbook of human genetics. Oxford, Blackwell, 1975. 524 p.
40. Frazier, P. Jean. A new look at dental health education in community programs. Dent. Hyg., 52:176–86, Apr. 1978.
41. Gjermo, P., and Rølla, G. The plaque-inhibiting effect of chlorhexidine-containing dentifrices. Scand. J. Dent. Res., 79:126–32, 1971.
42. Hansen, F., and Gjermo, P. The plaque-removing effect of four toothbrushing methods. Scand. J. Dent. Res., 79:502–6, 1971.
43. Harcourt, J. K., Johnson, N. W., and Storey, E. In vivo incorporation of tetracycline in the teeth of man. Arch. Oral Biol., 7:431–7, July–Aug. 1962.
44. Heifetz, S. B., et al. Programs for the mass control of plaque; an appraisal. J. Pub. Health Dent., 33:91–5, Spring 1973.
45. Heifetz, S. B., and Suomi, J. D. The control of dental caries and periodontal disease; a fundamental approach. J. Pub. Health Dent., 33:2–6, Winter 1973.
46. Hill, H. C., Levi. P. A., and Glickman, I. The effects of waxed and unwaxed dental floss on interdental plaque accumulation and interdental gingival health. J. Periodont., 44:411–3, July–Dec. 1973.
47. Horowitz, Alice. Oral hygiene measures. Canad. Dent. A. J., 46:43–6, Jan. 1980.
48. Horowitz, Alice M., et al. Effects of supervised daily dental plaque removal by children after 3 years. Community Dent. Oral Epidemiol., 8:171–6, Aug. 1980.
49. Horowitz, H. S., Heifetz, S. B., and Driscoll, W. S. Partial defluoridation of a community water supply and dental fluorosis. Health Services Rep., 87:451–5, May 1972.
50. Horowitz, H. S., and Heifetz, S. B. The effect of partial defluoridation of a water supply on dental fluorosis—final results in Bartlett, Texas, after 17 years. Am. J. Pub. Health, 62:767–9, June 1972.
51. Jenkins, G. N., Edgar, W. M., and Ferguson, D. B. The distribution and metabolic effects of human plaque fluorine. Arch. Oral Biol., 14:105–19, Jan. 1969.
52. Johansen, J. R., Gjermo, P., and Eriksen, H. M. Effect of 2 years use of chlorhexidine-containing dentifrices on plaque, gingivitis, and caries. Scand. J. Dent. Res., 83:288–92, Sept. 1975.
53. Keller, S. E., and Manson-Hing, L. R. Clearance studies of proximal tooth surfaces. Part II. In vivo removal of interproximal plaque. Ala. J. Med. Sci., 6:266–74, July 1969.
54. Kelner, R. M., et al. Gingival inflammation as related to frequency of plaque removal. J. Periodont., 45:303–7, June 1974.
55. Kjaerheim, Vibeke, von der Fehr, F. R., and Poulsen, Sven. Two-year study on the effect of professional toothcleaning on schoolchildren in Oppergård, Norway. Community Dent. Oral Epidemiol., 8:401–6, Dec. 1980.
56. Knowles, J. W., et al. Results of periodontal treatment related to pocket depth and attachment level—eight years. J. Periodont., 50:225–33, May 1979.
57. Kramer, I. R. H. Carcinoma-in-situ of the oral mucosa. Internat. Dent. J., 23:94–9, Mar. 1973.
58. Lang, N. P., Cumming, B. R., and Löe, H. Toothbrushing frequency as it relates to plaque development and gingival health. J. Periodont., 44:396–405, July 1973.
59. Lehner, Thomas, et al. Immunological aspects of juvenile periodontitis (periodontosis). J. Periodont. Res. 9:261–72, 1974.
60. Lehner, Thomas. Immunological aspects of dental caries and periodontal disease. Brit. Med. Bul., 31:125–30, May 1975.
61. Lightner, L. M., et al. Preventive periodontic treatment procedures: results over 46 months. J. Periodont., 42:555–61, Sept. 1971.
62. Lindhe, Jan, and Koch, Goran. The effect of supervised oral hygiene on the gingiva of children. Progression and inhibition of gingivitis. J. Periodont. Res., 1:260–7, 1966.
63. Lindhe, Jan, Koch, Goran, and Mansson, Ulla. The effect of supervised oral hygiene on the gingiva of children. Effect of mouth rinsings. J. Periodont. Res., 1:268–75, 1966.

64. Lindhe, Jan, and Koch, Goran. The effect of supervised oral hygiene on the gingiva of children. Lack of prolonged effect of supervision. J. Periodont. Res., 2:215–20, 1967.
65. Lindhe, Jan, and Wicén, P. O. The effects on the gingivae of chewing fibrous foods. J. Periodont. Res., 4:193–201, 1969.
66. Lindhe, Jan, and Nyman, S. The effect of plaque control and surgical pocket elimination on the establishment and maintenance of periodontal health. A longitudinal study of periodontal therapy in cases of advanced disease. J. Clin. Periodont., 2:67–79, Apr. 1975.
67. Lindhe, Jan, Axelsson, P., and Tollskog, G. The effect of proper oral hygiene on gingivitis and dental caries in schoolchildren. Community Dent. Oral Epidemiol., 3:150–5, Aug. 1975.
68. Listgarten, M. A. Prevention of periodontal disease in the future. p. 61–7. (In Prevention of major dental disorders. Proceedings of a symposium held at Marabou, Sundbyberg, Sweden, June 16, 1979. 89 p.)
69. Lobene, R. R., and Soparkar, P. M. The effect of an alexidine mouthwash on plaque and gingivitis. Am. Dent. A. J., 87:848–51, Oct. 1973.
70. Lobene, R. R. Chemotherapeutics for the prevention of dental plaque. J. Preven. Dent., 3:32–8, July–Aug. 1976.
71. Löe, Harald. A review of the prevention and control of plaque. p. 259–70. (In McHugh, W. D., ed. Dental plaque. Edinburg, Livingstone, 1970. 298 p.)
72. ——— . Plaque control in periodontal disease. Am. Dent. A. J., 87:1034–6, Oct. 1973.
73. ——— . Does chlorhexidine have a place in the prophylaxis of dental diseases. J. Periodont. Res., 8(Suppl. 12):93–9, 1973.
74. ——— . Mechanical and chemical control of dental plaque. p. 32–6. (In Prevention of major dental disorders. Proceedings of a symposium held at Marabou, Sundbyberg, Sweden, June 16, 1979. 89 p.)
75. ——— . Principles and progress in the prevention of periodontal diseases. p. 255–68. (In Lehner, T., and Cimasouri, G., eds. The borderland between caries and periodontal disease. II. New York, Grune and Stratton, 1980. 288 p.)
76. Löe, H., and Rindom-Schiott, C. The effect of suppression of the oral microflora upon the development of dental plaque and gingivitis. p. 247–55. (In McHugh, W. D., ed. Dental plaque. Edinburgh, Livingston, 1970. 298 p.)
77. ——— . The effects of mouthrinses and topical application of chlorhexidine on the development of dental plaque and gingivitis in man. J. Periodont. Res., 5:79–83, 1970.
78. Löe, H., Theilade, Else, and Jensen, S. B. Experimental gingivitis in man. J. Periodont., 36:177–87, May–June 1965.
79. Löe, H., et al. Two years oral use of chlorhexidine in man. I. General design and clinical effects. J. Periodont. Res., 11:135–44, June 1976.
80. Löe, H., et al. The natural history of periodontal disease in man. Study design and baseline data. J. Periodont. Res., 13:550–62, Nov. 1978.
81. ——— . The natural history of periodontal disease in man. Tooth mortality rates before 40 years of age. J. Periodont Res., 13:563–72, Nov. 1978.
82. ——— . The natural history of periodontal disease in man; the rate of periodontal destruction before 40 years of age. J. Periodont., 49:607–20, Dec. 1978.
83. Loesche, W. J. Chemotherapy of dental plaque infections. Oral Sciences Rev., 9:65–107, 1976.
84. Loesche, W. J., and Syed, S. A. Bacteriology of human experimental gingivitis: effect of plaque and gingivitis score. Infect. Immun., 21:830–9, Sept. 1978.
85. ——— . Anaerobic nature of certain periodontal infections. p. 225–33. (In Proceedings of the International Symposium on Anaerobes, Tokyo, Japan, June 22, 1980. Tokyo, Nippon Merck Bamyu, 1980. 248 p.)
86. Longhurst, P., and Berman, D. S. Apples and gingival health; report of a feasibility study. Brit. Dent. J., 134:475–9, June 5, 1973.
87. Lovdal, A., Arno, A., Schei, O., and Waerhaug, J. Combined effect of subgingival scaling and controlled oral hygiene on the incidence of gingivitis. Acta Odont. Scand., 19:537–55, Dec. 1961.
88. Margolis, F. J., et al. Fluoride supplements for children; a survey of physicians' prescription practices. Am. J. Dis. Child., 134:865–8, Sept. 1980.
89. Melsen, Birté, and Agerbaek, Nina. Effect of an instructional motivation program on oral health in Danish adolescents after 1 and 2 years. Community Dent. Oral Epidemiol., 8:72–8, Apr. 1980.

90. Newman, M. G., et al. Studies of the microbiology of periodontosis. J. Periodont., 47:373–9, July 1976.
91. Newman, M. G., and Socransky, S. S. Predominant cultivable microbiota in periodontosis. J. Periodont. Res., 12:120–8, Mar. 1977.
92. Nyman, Sture, Rosling, Bengt, and Lindhe, Jan. Effect of professional tooth cleaning on healing after periodontal surgery. J. Clin. Periodont., 2:80–6, Apr. 1975.
93. Olsson, B. Efficiency of traditional chewing sticks in oral hygiene programs among Ethiopian schoolchildren. Community Dent. Oral Epidemiol., 6:105–9, May 1978.
94. ———. Dental findings in high-fluoride areas in Ethiopia. Community Dent. Oral Epidemiol., 7:51–6, Feb. 1979.
95. Pihlstrom, B. L., Ortiz-Campos, C., and McHugh, R. B. A randomized four-year study of periodontal therapy. J. Periodont., 52:227–42, May 1981.
96. Ramfjord, S. P., et al. Longitudinal study of periodontal therapy. J. Periodont., 44:66–77, Feb. 1973.
97. Ranney, R. R. Pathogenesis of periodontal disease. p. 223–300. (In International Conference on Research in the Biology of Periodontal Disease. Chicago, University Illinois School Dentistry, 1977. xxi + 482 p.)
98. Ringelberg, M. L., and Webster, D. B. Effects of an amine fluoride mouthrinse and dentifrice on the gingival health and the extent of plaque of school children. J. Periodont., 48:350–3, June 1977.
99. Ripa, L. W., Berenie, J. T., and Leske, G. S. The effect of professionally administered bi-annual prophylaxes on the oral hygiene, gingival health and caries scores of school children. Two-year study. J. Preven. Dent., 3:22–6, Jan.–Feb. 1976.
100. Robinson, Emerson. A comparative evaluation of the scrub and Bass methods of toothbrushing with flossing as an adjunct. Am. J. Pub. Health, 66:1078–81, Nov. 1976.
101. Rodda, J. C. A comparison of four methods of toothbrushing. N.Z. Dent. J., 64:162–7, July 1968.
102. Rosling, Bengt, Nyman, Sture, and Lindhe, Jan. The effect of systematic plaque control on bone regeneration in infrabony pockets. J. Clin. Periodont., 3:38–53, 1976.
103. Rugg-Gunn, A. J., and MacGregor, I. D. M. A survey of toothbrushing behavior in children and young adults. J. Periodont. Res., 13:382–9, July 1978.
104. Sangnes, G., Zachrisson, B., and Gjermo, P. Effectiveness of vertical and horizontal brushing techniques in plaque removal. J. Dent. Child., 39:94–7, Mar.–Apr. 1972.
105. Schmid, M. O., Balmelli, O. P., and Saxer, U. P. Plaque removing effect of toothbrush, dental floss, and a toothpick. J. Clin. Periodont., 3:157–65, Aug. 1976.
106. Sheiham, Aubrey. The epidemiology of chronic periodontal disease in Western Nigerian schoolchildren. J. Periodont. Res., 3:257–67, 1968.
107. ———. Prevention and control of periodontal disease. p. 309–67. (In International Conference on Research in the Biology of Periodontal Disease. Chicago, University Illinois School Dentistry, 1977. xxi + 482 p.)
108. Socransky, S. S. Microbiology of periodontal disease—present status and future considerations. J. Periodont., 48:497–504, Sept. 1977.
109. Spolsky, V. W., Bhatia, H. L., Forsythe, A., and Levin, B. S. The effect of an antimicrobial mouthwash on dental plaque and gingivitis in young adults. J. Periodont., 46:685–90, Nov. 1975.
110. Suomi, J. D., et al. The effect of controlled oral hygiene procedures on the progression of periodontal disease in adults. Results after third and final year. J. Periodont., 42:152–60, Mar. 1971.
111. Suomi, J. D. Prevention and control of periodontal disease. Am. Dent. A. J., 83:1271–87, Dec. 1971.
112. Suomi, J. D., et al. A clinical trial of a calculus-inhibitory dentifrice. J. Periodont., 45:139–45, Mar. 1974.
113. Suomi, J. D., et al. Study of the effect of different prophylaxis frequencies on the periodontium of young adult males. J. Periodont., 44:406–10, July 1973.
114. Syed, S. A., and Loesche, W. J. Bacteriology of human experimental gingivitis: effect of plaque age. Infect. Immun., 21:821–9, Sept. 1978.
115. Tan, H. H., and Saxton, C. A. Effect of a single dental health care instruction and prophylaxis on gingivitis. Community Dent. Oral Epidemiol., 6:172–5, July 1978.
116. Theilade, E., et al. Experimental gingivitis in man. II. A longitudinal clinical and bacteriological investigation. J. Periodont. Res., 1:1–13, 1966.

117. Theilade, Else, and Theilade, Jorgen. Role of plaque in the etiology of periodontal disease and caries. Oral Sciences Rev., 9:23–63, 1976.
118. Thylstrup, A. Distribution of dental fluorosis in the primary dentition. Community Dent. Oral Epidemiol., 6:329–37, Nov. 1978.
119. Tinanoff, Norman, and Weeks, D. B. Current status of SnF_2 as an antiplaque agent. Pediatr. Dent., 1:199–204, Sept. 1979.
120. Waerhaug, Jens. Current basis for prevention of periodontal disease. Internat. Dent. J., 17:267–81, June 1967.
121. ———. Subgingival plaque and loss of attachment in periodontosis as observed in autopsy material. J. Periodont., 47:636–42, Nov. 1976.
122. ———. Plaque control in the treatment of juvenile periodontitis. J. Clin. Periodont., 4:29–40, Feb. 1977.
123. Weatherford, T. W., Finn, S. B., and Jamison, H. C. Effects of an alexidine mouthwash on dental plaque and gingivitis in humans over a six-month period. Am. Dent. A. J., 94:528–36, Mar. 1977.
124. Witkop, C. J., Jr., and Wolf, R. O. Hypoplasia and intrinsic staining of enamel associated with tetracycline therapy. Am. Med. A. J., 185:1008–11, Sept 28, 1963.
125. Zaki, H. A., and Bandt, C. L. The effective use of a self-teaching oral hygiene manual. J. Periodont., 45:491–5, July 1974.
126. Zickert, I., Emilson, C. G., and Krasse, B. Effect on caries activity in school children by measures against S. *mutans*. J. Dent. Res., 58(Spec. Issue A): 427, Abstr. No. 1345, Jan. 1979.

IV THE EVALUATION OF SCIENTIFIC INFORMATION

CHAPTER **10**

THE EVALUATION OF SCIENTIFIC INFORMATION

Herschel S. Horowitz

INTRODUCTION

Students and practitioners of dentistry and dental public health must read many scientific reports to develop fundamental knowledge in their fields and to keep abreast of new developments. Equally important, they must be able to evaluate the quality and validity of these reports, which may influence their attitudes, actions, or practices. Readers need to know certain elemental facts about a study in order to appraise the strengths of any report of scientific research. The contents of this chapter should help readers to evaluate scientific information critically and demonstrate that a paper is not necessarily valid merely because it has been published.

Reports of inferior research are frequently quoted or used as documentation. It is sometimes difficult to detect poor research, but readers will be misled less frequently if they watch for gross errors in design, inadequate samples, improper use of statistical methods, failure to carry out procedural details, inaccuracies in reported data, unwarranted conclusions, and inappropriate or out-of-context quotes from references. In addition, the ability to discern valid research should help students and practitioners improve the quality of their own reports.

This chapter will not cover statistical formulas or procedures for computing statistical tests. That type of information may be found in statistical texts, some of which are listed at the end of this chapter. Rather, the aim of the chapter is to examine some factors that should help discriminating readers interpret, understand, and evaluate scientific literature. Relevant examples to illustrate major points will be provided, but all aspects of evaluation that deserve scrutiny cannot be reviewed because a list of possible shortcomings and items to check would be nearly endless. The few concepts of statistics discussed in this chapter have been chosen to illustrate the bases of statistical reasoning.

Many people go through two stages in evaluating the contents of scientific reports. Initially, readers tend to accept the veracity of reports unquestioningly. Later, after having been misled a few times, they become increasingly skeptical. Readers must be careful, however, not to become excessively critical, or they may remain uninformed of scientific developments. The purpose of developing skill in evaluation is to avoid the extremes of blind acceptance and blanket distrust of scientific reports.

Purposes of Scientific Information

The primary purpose of scientific literature is to communicate new information or ideas. Research on health-related issues is conducted for a variety of reasons. Studies may be done to satisfy the scientific curiosity or instincts of investigators. Others are done to convince general practitioners, specialists, or other investigators of the validity of a therapeutic hypothesis. Sometimes research is undertaken because an agency or institution requires the information to help establish policy. Studies are also conducted for a variety of audiences, for example, fellow researchers, health officials, or the public. The credibility of a report may hinge on the experience and sophistication of the intended audience.

Types of Scientific Information

One characteristic of a study, in contrast to an editorial or a case history, is that it reaches conclusions without taint of personal biases. *Bias* is an unconscious preference or inclination that inhibits impartial judgment. The distinction between bias and *prejudice* (a prejudgment or a preconceived opinion formed without knowledge or examination of the facts) rests on the unconsciousness of bias. In the context of conducting research, bias is any process at any stage of a study that tends to produce results or conclusions that differ systematically from the truth. Bias usually stems from inadequate study design, honest but systematic errors of observation, undue optimism, or insufficient evidence. Good studies attempt to remove these and other sources of bias.

In therapeutic or preventive research, proof of clinical effectiveness must be based on controlled human studies or trials that compare one or more test regimens with some other established procedure or with no intervention. Anecdotes and case reports do not constitute research, although they may offer clues to the answers of research problems. Many popular but ineffective forms of treatment and prevention have been enthusiastically adopted in the past on the basis of an unverified supposition of their value. On the other hand, there have been instances in which the curiosity or impressions of a clinician have led to important knowledge. One has only to think of McKay's curiosity about Colorado Brown Stain, which led to the subsequent studies of fluorosis, dental caries, and community fluoridation, to appreciate the potential importance of reports of personal observations. (See Chapter 7.) It must be stressed, however, that these case reports are not research.

The term *statistics* has two meanings in connection with health research; the following definitions are representative of its different contexts. Used as a plural noun, statistics—such as those encompassing the incidence or prevalence of a disease—denote compilations of figures that describe a phenomenon. When used as a singular noun, statistics is a body of methods or technics used for making decisions about the relation, stability, or completeness of collected information.

A clinical trial is a prospective research project that involves human subjects. It is designed to evaluate how well a particular regimen will work under given conditions and to provide a scientifically sound judgment of its worthiness for adoption (or retention) in accepted biomedical practice.

Statistical Planning

Thirty years ago, few researchers probably understood the rationale for the statistical technics that they commonly used. Although the sophistication of researchers has undoubtedly improved since then, so has the complexity and sophistication of statistical thought and methods. For this and other reasons, a statistician should be an integral partner in the planning and operation of a research project, as well as a participant in the tabulation, analysis, and reporting of collected data. A collaborating statistician should have experience relevant to the type of investigation that is being planned, be willing to become intimately involved with the project, and be available to give help whenever needed.

Merely turning collected data over to a statistician for processing, tabulation, and analysis is not advisable. At that stage, there is little a statistician can do to correct a poor design, improper sample sizes, or the use of inappropriate indexes. It is not reasonable to expect that statistical analysis will validate the findings of the study and somehow rectify any errors or distortions in logic. Statisticians can only assume that errors and distortions do not exist and analyze the data as presented. Although everyone may be content, both the investigator and the statistician may be deluded by spurious results obtained from inappropriate statistical analyses of bad data.

The reader of scientific literature, of course, has no way of knowing whether appropriate statistical planning has taken place. It is reassuring, however, if a statistician known to be familiar with the type of data presented in a particular report is a coauthor. This fact usually denotes that the statistician has been intimately involved in planning the research, collecting and analyzing the data, and preparing the report for publication.

Protocols for Scientific Studies

Every study should follow a written protocol or formal plan for the research. The reader of scientific reports does not have the advantage of seeing this protocol, but if the research has been funded as a contract or grant from a responsible agency, such as the National Institute of Dental Research, the reader may be assured that the protocol most likely received a thorough scientific review.

A good protocol should contain at least the major elements of the following 12 sections:

1. *Background and problem*—defining precisely the research problem, the reasons for undertaking the research, and a review of pertinent literature.
2. *Objectives or hypotheses to be tested.*
3. *Data and information to be collected*—listing and describing each item needed to accomplish the objectives or to test the hypotheses.
4. *Population to be studied*—including its selection, source, size, method of sampling, and allocation to groups.
5. *Experimental or survey procedures*—describing details of the study design and including a description of the responsibilities of all study personnel.
6. *Data-collection methods*—including definitions and criteria for each item of collected data, examples of all data collection forms to be used, and a list of all necessary supplies, equipment, and instruments.
7. *Data-analysis plans*—including details for summarization, a format for the tables that will be used, and the basic statistical tests to be performed.
8. *Reporting*—including plans for authorship and for presentations and publication of interim and final reports.
9. *A justification for staff, facilities, equipment, and supplies*—including the need for consultants.
10. *Budget*—including estimates for salaries of study personnel and consultants, travel, equipment, supplies, printing, and publication.
11. *Time schedule*—including planning, obtaining study subjects, data collection and analysis, and report writing.
12. *Human subjects clearance*—including letters that go to prospective participants and plans for their distribution and retrieval.

Preparing a good protocol should not be considered an onerous task. Those who have prepared or contributed to the preparation of protocols for studies can attest to their value in formulating thoughts about a study, aiding in its design, anticipating problems with the project, planning the analysis of data, and preparing a final report for publication. In fact, a good protocol usually simplifies the preparation of a final report because the major elements of a protocol are often integral parts of the report.

COMPONENTS OF A SCIENTIFIC REPORT

When reading a scientific report, readers should evaluate how well the various sections of the report have been prepared, beginning with the title.

Title

The title of a paper should be concise and clearly stated, yet describe its content as fully as possible. The title is important not only for catching the attention of potential readers and letting them know whether they are likely to be interested in the paper's contents but also for permitting various indexing services and libraries to put it in suitable categories for subsequent retrieval of information. The inclusion of key words in the title is therefore important.

Abstract (or Summary)

A good abstract of a scientific report permits readers to identify quickly the basic contents of the paper and thus ascertain its relevance to their interests. The abstract frequently determines whether an entire paper is read or even scanned; therefore, it should be prepared with care. An abstract should (1) state the main objectives and scope of the investigation, (2) describe briefly the methods used, (3) summarize the findings, and (4) state the main conclusions. Abstracts should not contain information or conclusions not stated in the body of the report. They should be straightforward, objective, and factual and should not contain opinions or speculation.

Introduction

The introduction or background section of a report should clearly state the reasons for conducting a survey or study. Readers of scientific reports should ask themselves if there is a need for the research undertaken in a particular study; that is, does the research have relevance to the needs of society in general or of the dental health community in particular?

Review of the Literature

Pertinent literature that summarizes current information about the problem under investigation should be reviewed thoroughly but concisely. The authors of the report should independently review the literature and not rely on or modify the review of another report. The current status of research pertinent to the particular study should also be summarized. Some reports indiscriminately and inappropriately refer to the work of other researchers. Writers of good scientific reports should not quote only those statements from the literature that support a particular point of view while ignoring other statements that cast doubt on the viewpoint. Nor should they quote statements or conclusions out of context to give the impression that the original reporters meant something other than they intended. Cited articles should be pertinent to the report and should not be used merely to accumulate respected names in the bibliography or to show that the author is well read.

Effective, critical appraisal of a report hinges on a reader's initial understanding of its aims or objectives. Therefore, these objectives should be stated clearly and precisely. They should be specific and capable of being measured. If the research is primarily descriptive, this fact should be stated. If the research is primarily explanatory, the hypotheses to be tested should be stated. If possible, the objectives should be stated as a *null hypothesis*, meaning that the procedures used in the study did not affect the nature of the observations or the results achieved. The objectives of a study may be to dispute a null hypothesis and then to accept an alternative hypothesis that may be the basis for doing the study. A reader should be wary, however, of a report that tries to prove an alternative hypothesis before developing an adequate reason for rejecting the null hypothesis.

Materials and Methods

The materials and methods used in a survey or study should be presented in detail. Treatments given to each group of subjects should be clearly described. Descriptions of the criteria used to determine whether a disease or condition was present or absent should be specific. The variables measured should be carefully delineated. The measurements should be straightforward and as free as possible from subjective interpretation. Sufficient details should be given so that a competent worker could repeat the investigation.

There are essentially four types or scales of measurement that may be applied in clinical research: nominal, ordinal, interval, and ratio. (See Chapter 5, p. 87.) Because the use of appropriate measurement scales is critical in conducting good scientific research, important aspects of each type are discussed.

Nominal Measurements. Those scales that group subjects into mutually exclusive, separate classes so that all those in a single class are equivalent with respect to some attribute are called nominal measurements. One example of a nominal measurement is to group males and females separately and assign the numbers 0 and 1 to the groups, respectively. The assignment of children to various Angle classifications of occlusion is another example of nominal measurement. Since nominal measurements consist of names or numbers assigned to categories, performing mathematical tests on them is obviously inappropriate, although it may be appropriate to determine statistically whether the observed frequencies in each class differ from the expected frequencies.

Ordinal Measurements. Those scales in which increasing or decreasing numbers denote a greater or smaller presence of an attribute or property are called ordinal measurements. Although the values can be ranked or ordered, the intervals between rankings or categories are not necessarily equal. The scale of hardness of minerals is an ordinal scale. An example in dentistry is the categorization of oral hygiene status as excellent, good, fair, or poor, with the assignment of the numbers 4, 3, 2, or 1 to these categories, respectively. It is inappropriate to state, for example, that mouths with an "excellent" oral hygiene status are four times more clean than those scored as "poor." One knows only that if the subjects were categorized correctly, persons with an "excellent" status (4) have cleaner mouths than those with a "good" status (3), and so on. Study populations may be compared on the basis of distributional patterns of ordinal data. In many reports, however, ordinal data are added, subtracted, multiplied, or otherwise compared. Although nothing prohibits one from making these comparisons, they may be misleading about the amounts of the property in question. The reader of reports in which mathematical exercises are performed on ordinal measurements should ask: "Do the results of these measurements really have any meaning? Does it matter that a group had a mean score of 3.4 initially and after some sort of intervention a decreased mean score of 2.9?" When these values are derived from an ordinal scale, the observed numerical change may be meaningless.

Interval Measurements. Those scales in which differences in the amount of a characteristic may be distinguished but, in addition, all differences among categories are of equal magnitude are called interval measurements. Temperature is an example of an interval scale. The difference between 60° and 70° Fahrenheit is the same as that between 30° and 40°F. The zero point of an interval scale is an arbitrary one. Zero degrees Fahrenheit is not an absolute value with no temperature; it has been arbitrarily chosen. Eighty degrees Fahrenheit is not twice as warm as 40°F. The numbering of years is also an interval scale. The amount of time existing between the years 1776 and 1800 is the same as between 1900 and 1924. Overjet is measured on an interval scale, with an end-to-end bite arbitrarily designated as a zero overjet.

Ratio Scales. Ratio scales differ from interval scales only in that the zero point is not arbitrary but indicates an absence of the property measured. Height and weight are both examples of ratio scales of measurement. Zero weight is no weight at all, and a 300-pound person weighs twice as much as a 150-pound person. The DMF surface increment is a ratio scale.

Another matter of concern to readers of scientific reports is whether the responses chosen by the investigators are appropriate to measure the effectiveness of treatments. The ultimate goal of a clinical trial is to treat or prevent disease in a test population. Well-designed studies should show, for example, how much dental caries was prevented by a certain regimen or the degree to which an educational campaign has improved the prevention of gingivitis. Studies that merely measure the fluoride concentration of outer enamel after a fluoride regimen or determine whether the subjects' knowledge of oral health matters has increased or whether their plaque scores have been reduced do not answer the ultimate questions about reduced incidence, prevalence, or intensity of disease. Indirect variables may or may not be highly correlated with therapeutic effectiveness, but even if they are, they do not answer the questions of reduced disease. Although there is nothing wrong with seeking answers to ancillary questions, readers should make certain that the writers have not made excessive claims for disease prevention.

Sample Selection

The study population reported upon in a scientific paper should be clearly defined. If the studied group is a sample from a larger population, that population as well as the procedures that were used to draw the sample should be concisely described.

Readers of scientific reports should ask themselves whether the sample chosen for a study is representative of a larger population than the group from which the data are actually collected. If not, the writers should not generalize or extrapolate their findings by concluding that their successful regimen will also be effective among other groups. For example, a dietary regimen that effectively reduces the incidence of dental caries in a group of institutionalized children, whose lifestyle is well controlled, may not be effective among noninstitutionalized children. A method of plaque removal tested among dental hygiene students, who probably already have relatively healthy gingival tissues and above average oral hygiene skills and knowledge, may produce results entirely different from those that might be achieved among persons in the same age range in the general population. If the writer has ignored the question of whether the nature of the sample has affected the results, the reader must decide whether the findings are only narrowly applicable or may be generalized.

Readers of a scientific report should examine closely how participants were selected for inclusion in the study. Were some potential subjects excluded from participation? If so, are the reasons for exclusion reasonable, such as having too few sound teeth remaining for evaluation, the presence of orthodontic bands, or advanced periodontal disease? Or are the exclusions likely to bias the findings and preclude the application of the findings to a larger population?

There are many examples of ways that study populations can be biased. For example, subjects in a study of periodontal disease may be patients who have sought treatment for the disease. They may have uncomfortable symptoms or some anxiety because they know others with a similar condition. Perhaps they have presented themselves because of monetary or other incentives or for the opportunity for a checkup. Sometimes subjects are solicited by direct or mailed questionnaires or by a public call for volunteers through the media. Investigators may tend to exclude submitted questionnaires that are messy or not filled out properly, or may reject volunteers who are unattractive or unkempt or who have disagreeable personalities. These self-selections by the subjects and the exclusions by the investigators may bias the sample. It should be obvious that the selection process may influence results.

Assignment of Subjects to Study Groups

Whenever possible, subjects should be randomly assigned to groups. A haphazard or systematic assignment may produce groups with different characteristics that could affect the variable under study. Knowing the method used to assign participants randomly to groups and having some idea of how well the method was followed will help readers of scientific reports determine how much credence the conclusions of a study warrant.

Readers should try to ascertain whether participating subjects were assigned to study groups in a fair and equitable way. The principal aim of allocating subjects to test and control groups is to achieve groups that are, as far as possible, equivalent in all respects relevant to the condition being measured. If the groups are truly comparable at the beginning, any group differences in the variable under study observed at the end of the investigation may be attributed to the treatment given to each group, after ruling out the possibility that the differences are chance occurrences.

Ideally, every participant should have had an equal chance of being chosen for the control or test groups. The method of group assignment should allow no systematic bias that would tend to favor one of the groups at the start of the investigation. *Simple random assignment* of subjects to groups is one of the best ways to make groups comparable with respect to known and unknown factors that might influence the outcome of a clinical trial. If in a study of dental caries prevention there are factors that may influence future caries experience—such as race, sex, or previous caries experience—the investigators may have used *stratification* or *blocking* procedures based on those factors in conjunction with random assignment. In other words, prior to random assignment to groups, participants with common characteristics are blocked (grouped) into various strata. For example, one block might comprise black males 10 to 12 years of age who have four to seven DMF surfaces. Within each block, subjects are then allocated to test and control groups by a random procedure. Blocking allows a heterogeneous population to be grouped into strata, each of which is homogeneous within limits. Blocking on appropriate variables followed by random assignment improves the chance that groups are comparable at the start, which is less likely to occur if only simple random procedures are used for assignment of subjects. No method will ensure that all study groups are exactly equal in all respects. Methods of randomization, however, do increase the likelihood that variation among groups will differ only by a minor extent, which is usually predictable and measurable.

The investigators should not assign subjects to groups in any way that completely avoids randomization. Using a control group chosen by any method other than randomization requires the assumption that either the control and test groups are identical in all important variables except the one under study or that the investigator can compensate for all relevant differences. This assumption is seldom warranted. An extreme example emphasizes the point. To evaluate the use of a fluoride dentifrice to prevent dental caries, it is obvious that the fluoride dentifrice should not be assigned to a group of dental students and the control dentifrice to a group of factory workers of the same ages. Other biases may be more subtle, but they must be detected and then eliminated or controlled. Some examples of group assignment that can cause serious problems in interpretation and that should be avoided when possible are the following:

1. For altruistic reasons, assigning all subjects with rampant caries to the study group likely to benefit the most.

2. Assigning subjects for whom consent has not been obtained to a control group and assigning subjects with consent to a test group.

3. Using all subjects at one school as controls for comparison with test subjects at another school.

4. In a study of periodontal disease, using patients of one periodontist as subjects to receive one regimen of treatment and patients of another periodontist to receive a different regimen.

5. Attempting to make groups comparable by consciously placing subjects in a group on the basis of factors thought to influence future disease or status of health.

6. Allowing subjects to select their own group assignment.

These and other questionable methods of assignment of subjects to groups are likely to influence the outcome of the study.

Writers of reports of clinical trials should give the reasons why potential candidates did not choose to participate and the number of refusals. This information may offer clues to the reasonableness of the study procedures and perhaps may help define how far the findings may be extrapolated to the general population.

Sample Characteristics

The ages of a study population should be appropriate to the particular study. For example, it may be futile to attempt to measure the effect of a caries-preventive regimen on the primary teeth of children ages 8–11. By those ages, many primary teeth have already exfoliated and, in a caries-prone population, many if not most of the remaining susceptible tooth surfaces have already become carious. Similarly, selection of a sample of eight-year-old children for the evaluation of a pit-and-fissure sealant is a poor decision. At age eight, many or most caries-susceptible pit-and-fissure surfaces of first permanent molars have already decayed, while premolars and second molars have not yet erupted. The determination of the numbers of decayed, missing, and filled permanent teeth in a group of subjects from 40 to 60 years old may be misleading because many of them have probably lost teeth from periodontal disease. A survey of occlusal relations among children with a mixed dentition is another example of a poor age selection, as is a study of loss of periodontal attachment in young adults. These examples emphasize that readers should ask themselves whether reported findings may be accepted as valid or whether the study was compromised in advance by selection of a study sample inappropriate to demonstrate the intended purpose of the research.

In surveys that compare one population with another, the populations must be truly comparable with respect to key characteristics related to the variable under study. For example, in the late 1970s, some opponents of community fluoridation claimed that death rates from cancer in 10 cities in the United States with fluoridated water were increasing compared with those in 10 cities supplied with nonfluoridated water. Their conclusions were based on crude mortality rates determined by dividing total deaths by the total population. No such conclusions can be derived from crude mortality rates because deaths from cancer vary grossly with age and to a lesser extent with sex, ethnic group, and race. When the data were independently analyzed to adjust for differences in the communities by age, sex, and race, the supposed relation completely disappeared. In other words, differences in these demographic characteristics between the two groups of communities accounted entirely for the observed differences in the crude death rates from cancer; no effect of fluoride could be discerned. Readers of scientific reports must carefully peruse reports for possible biases resulting from data that are not suitably adjusted or standardized.

Sample Size

The size of a sample is another important factor for scrutiny. The number of persons needed for a clinical trial may be determined in advance if the magnitude of new disease and the expected variation among subjects can be estimated from a pilot study or from similar data reported in the literature. When large differences between test and control groups are expected, the samples can be smaller than when small differences are expected. Selecting samples of correct size is essential if statements about the value of a regimen are to be made with assurance at the end of an investigation. Samples must be large enough so that differences among groups thought to be clinically meaningful can be shown to be statistically significant at the 5 percent, or the 0.05, level of probability ($p < 0.05$). This simply means that the risk of accepting a difference between groups when a true difference does not exist is only 5 in 100. In this case, the 5 percent chance of falsely accepting that a regimen is effective is termed a *Type I error* and α is the probability of making a Type I error. To offer greater assurance that a measured difference is real, investigators may set the α level at 1 percent or $p = 0.01$. If the sample of participants is too small, it is also possible to conclude mistakenly that a treatment has no effect when in fact a true effect exists. This latter mistake is known as *Type II error*, with the probability of making a Type II error expressed as β.

Investigators usually have given most attention to avoiding Type I errors. They have recently paid renewed attention, however, to Type II errors, principally because concern has developed that many studies with negative findings were designed with too few subjects to be able to reasonably detect a positive result even if it existed. The selection of a small α level does not protect investigators from the possibility of failing to identify an effective agent or regimen. An effective regimen should not be overlooked or rejected because the chance of detecting that effect is small. This chance of detecting a specific true effect, if it exists, is denoted as the *power* of the test and is defined as

1-β. In essence, if the findings from a study are negative (the null hypothesis is accepted), the β error or, conversely, the power of the test gives an indication of how confident one can be that the findings are truly negative. The goal in considering power when calculating sample sizes is to enhance the chances of finding real and important effects if they exist.

The power of a test becomes critically important in multigroup studies in which more than one effective treatment is being evaluated. Such a study might compare different concentrations and frequencies of using fluoride mouthrinses (all of which are likely to be effective) among groups whose differences in caries increments are likely to be slight. If the investigators judge that differences as small as 15 percent among groups are clinically meaningful and wish to demonstrate that differences this small are statistically significant, the number of subjects per group must be extremely large. Otherwise, with smaller groups, the scientists may falsely conclude that the regimens were equivalent because they failed to demonstrate statistical significance, when in fact the chance of demonstrating such significance, or the power of the test, was small—for example, less than 50 percent.

The preceding discussion does not mean that the way to overcome problems of sample size is to make study groups as large as possible in all investigations. *If the sample is large enough, a trivial difference between two study groups may be statistically significant but clinically unimportant.* Too often, studies have been reported in which clinically unimportant differences between groups are found to be statistically significant because an excessively large population for study had been recruited. It is important to avoid the conclusion that therapeutic significance exists because statistical significance has been determined. The sample size for each study must be determined individually, depending upon the number of groups, the nature and acceptability of the regimens used in each group, the expected variation in responses among participants, and the anticipated magnitude of the differences among groups. As previously mentioned, a statistician should participate in the determination of sample sizes.

In multigroup studies, the investigators should report the power (1-β) of the investigation. They should describe the statistical test used and state, for example, that there was an 80 percent chance (1-β) of correctly rejecting the null hypothesis at the 5 percent level (α), if a true difference of 15 percent among groups existed.

Control Groups and Alternative Designs

An essential component of clinical trials is the *control group*, a collection of subjects who provide responses with which the effects of test regimens may be compared. The use of controls is basic to scientific inquiry. Controls may consist of subjects who receive no treatment or a placebo (negative controls), or subjects who receive an established treatment with which a new treatment is being compared or who are given the same treatment but at a different frequency or dosage (positive controls). For example, if a new mouthrinse for the prevention of dental caries were compared with a dilute saltwater solution, the group of children using the salt water would constitute a negative control group. If the new rinse were compared with a 0.2 percent sodium fluoride rinse, the group using the sodium fluoride rinse would be a positive control group. Some studies are designed with both negative and positive control groups.

Studies with negative control groups are most useful and appropriate when the value of a new regimen is unknown or uncertain. Comparison with a negative control group is the only way to ascertain the actual magnitude of protection afforded by a new regimen. In the last few years, negative control groups have been used less often because of ethical concerns about precluding some volunteer participants from receiving beneficial treatments. Without a negative control group, however, little can be determined about the actual magnitude of the benefit of any of the treatments in the study. Even after completion of the study, there may still be uncertainty about whether any of the treatments has been effective.

One design used with increasing frequency in recent years to circumvent the problem of withholding treatments from study participants is the establishment of a baseline of existing conditions among persons at the study site. These findings at the start of the investigation serve as a basis for future comparison. The treatment regimens are then started and results of examinations conducted after various time intervals are compared with the baseline findings. This *retrospective design* employs no untreated controls, and one of its weaknesses is that natural changes that may occur with time in the condition under investigation cannot be measured. Moreover, with this design, shifts may occur in the application of diagnostic criteria at different examinations that cannot be measured or controlled. Readers of a report of a study designed this way should be aware of its weaknesses because it does not permit firm conclusions of cause and effect to be drawn. The ethical advantages of this design in some studies, however, may outweigh its weaknesses. It is undoubtedly preferable to obtaining controls from reports in the literature. In fact, the value of many of the most thoroughly accepted medical drugs, including morphine, digitalis, aspirin, insulin, penicillin, and the corticosteroids, was established in studies without concurrent comparisons. Most research on the cariostatic effects of consuming fluoridated water has also employed this retrospective design. Invariably, these studies have shown that dental benefits increase with length of consumption of the water. Although other factors in a community may have influenced dental health for better or worse during the evaluations, the influence of the consumption of fluoridated water has been so profound and the findings so consistently repeated that the conclusion of its benefits is inescapable.

Observations and Treatments

A report should specify what disease is being studied and state the specific diagnostic criteria that were used to determine whether it was present or absent. For example, to state merely that a study concerned patients with periodontal disease is inadequate because the composition of such a group of patients is open to a spectrum of interpretation among investigators. Reliability of measurements and of diagnosis is critical to the accuracy of data. A good index should have *specificity*—it should not measure an attribute in too many people who do not have the attribute. Moreover, it should have *sensitivity* so that it does not miss the attribute in people who have it. If the investigators used a well-established index, such as the DMF index for dental caries or Russell's Periodontal Index (see Chapter 5), either as originally described or as reported in the readily available proceedings of a workshop, it is not necessary to repeat the details. For example, if criteria for dental caries are the same as those described at the American Dental Association's 1968 Conference on the Clinical Testing of Cariostatic Agents, a statement to that effect is sufficient. If modifications of method or in criteria have been made, or if a new index has been applied, however, details are essential. If a new index is used, discriminating readers should ask themselves whether the index is *valid*; that is, does it measure what it purports to measure? The results of adequate pretests of the new index made to prove its validity should be presented.

Reports should contain a clear description of the questionnaires applied or treatments given and how they were given or supervised. Readers should not have to assume what was done to whom, when, where, and how.

The observations should be made by as few examiners as possible in order to reduce interexaminer variations in measurement, and the investigators should note how well different examiners agreed on measurements and how consistently each examiner repeated the same measurements at different times. In other words, a complete report will include assessments of *intraexaminer* and *interexaminer variability*, that is, measures of reliability and reproducibility. Merely stating that such assessments were done is not enough; at least a summary of the findings of those assessments should be included. Readers should be suspicious of results devoid of any measures of reproducibility and reliability, particularly when the study contains subjective elements in the diagnosis, observation, or assessment of outcome.

Critical readers should ascertain whether examinations of subjects were made in random order. The examiner should not have examined first all subjects in one group and then all subjects in another group. Intermixing subjects from different groups during examination prevents unconscious shifts in the application of diagnostic criteria by the examiners from disproportionately affecting the findings for any particular group.

Blindness

"Blindness" is another major bias-reducing technic that should be used in clinical trials. Like randomization, methods of achieving blindness help readers judge the adequacy of a trial's objectivity. The study protocol should ensure that the examiners make their measurements without knowing to which group any subject is assigned *(blind examinations)*. Whenever possible, a study should be designed in a *double-blind* manner; that is, not only should the examiners be uninformed of the group assignment of subjects but the subjects themselves also should be unaware of the groups to which they belong. A design in which subjects cannot tell which treatment they are receiving neutralizes any possible *placebo effect* a new treatment may have. This design is often important because many subjects say they feel better when given a sham treatment (placebo effect). Of course, "blinding" subjects to their assigned regimen is impossible if the regimens in different groups are obviously dissimilar or if an untreated control group is used. When a placebo is used as a control, however, it should be as similar as possible in taste, odor, color, and physical appearance to the agent under investigation. It should vary only by not containing the active ingredient. One of the most critical elements of a study plan is that the examiners should be unaware of the group assignment of any participant in order to prevent their prejudices or biases from influencing the results. Another precaution that should always be taken is to make sure the results of earlier examinations are not available to the examiners at the time of subsequent examinations so that previous findings cannot affect current diagnoses.

The use of a double-blind technic, however, does not compensate for poorly trained examiners nor for the selection of poorly designed indexes, scales, or criteria. If indexes have unspecified elements, if scales of measurement are unclear, or if precise criteria are not provided for using the indexes and scales, the findings will be suspect despite a double-blind technic. Readers of scientific reports should not accept irreproducible results merely because they were made blindly.

Readers also should be attentive to possible ways in which the blindness may be compromised. For example, if a test agent stains oral tissues, as is the case with chlorhexidine or concentrated stannous fluoride preparations, true blindness may be impossible to achieve.

If several conditions—such as the status of periodontal tissues, the presence of plaque, and the amount of dental caries—are recorded in a study, a different examiner should apply each index rather than allowing one examiner to make multiple measurements. When a different examiner is used for each assessment, one measurement is less likely to be influenced by the findings detected from another, possibly related measurement. For example, because most investigators would probably contend that gingivitis is related to the presence of plaque, they may have a tendency to observe more gingival disease in subjects with poor oral hygiene status than in subjects with good oral hygiene status.

Readers should look for other aspects of blindness. If a paper reports a study in which preventive procedures have been professionally applied, it should state that those professionals did not know which agents were active and which was the placebo. This knowledge may unconsciously have affected the relative care with which the procedures were given. The same concern applies to supervisors of self-applied treatments; if at all possible, supervisory personnel should be unaware of the contents of any of the agents. All agents used in a study, therefore, should have coded labels. Studies in which examiners, participants, and personnel giving or supervising treatments do not know which agents are being used in a particular group may be designated *triple-blind* studies. When conditions permit, this method should be followed.

Cross-Over Designs

A *cross-over design* is occasionally used in some studies in which subjects serve as their own controls. Each subject receives an active treatment for a specific time and no treatment or a placebo during a control period. Cross-over designs are unsuitable for studies of dental caries prevention because the period required for cavities to develop is too long. These designs may be useful, however, in studies of mouthrinses that may prevent the formation of plaque or benefit gingival tissues. The principal advantage of a cross-over design is that it avoids differences in prognosis and variations in response among participating subjects. Readers must assume in studies with this design that these characteristics have remained the same in each subject during the entire trial. This design is not appropriate for regimens that have a carry-over effect because the effects of the treatment phase could influence responses during the nontreatment phase. If there is the possibility of a carry-over effect, the investigators should include a sufficiently long interval between phases to permit any retained effects to dissipate. Cross-over designs are also inappropriate in studies of test regimens that may produce a permanent effect or cure, of test agents that may be retained at the site of action for prolonged periods, or of conditions that may naturally undergo a rapid change in prevalence, incidence, or morbidity.

Clinical studies should continue long enough to compare accurately the effectiveness of two or more treatments. Early trends sometimes prove later to have been wrong or initial effects may not be sustained. Publication of early findings of a study that stops prematurely may leave a legacy of misleading results.

The Presentation of Data

Findings in a scientific report should be presented clearly, objectively, and in sufficient detail to enable a reader to assess them independently. The reported data must be able to withstand careful scrutiny. Tables and graphs should be easy to interpret and contain enough information to be understood on their own but not so much information that they discourage a reader. Data should be representative rather than exhaustive or repetitive. Important findings require proper documentation. For example, it is not sufficient for a report to state simply that females fared better than males on a test regimen without showing numerical values or summary statistics that permit readers to judge the validity of such a statement.

Table 10–1. Mean Incremental DMF Surface Scores after 12 and 24 Months of Fluoride Mouthrinsing for Children in Grade 6 Present for All Examinations, According to Group, Portland, Oregon, 1971

Study Group	No. of Children	Mean DMFS Increment	Difference (%)	p*
After 12 months				
Control	210	1.46(0.27)†		
Test	198	1.05(0.24)	28.1	0.12
After 24 months				
Control	210	2.92(0.40)		
Test	198	1.65(0.28)	43.5	0.01

*Two-tailed t-test.
†Figures in parentheses are standard errors of the means.

Measures of central tendency—such as means, medians, or modes—should be given, along with measures of dispersion. Standard deviations and ranges are common measures of dispersion. Columns and rows of figures should add up to their totals. Percentages of mutually exclusive categories should add up to 100 percent, and numbers in tables and figures should correspond with those in the text. Tables and graphs should be titled completely but concisely. Readers should be able to understand the information in tables and graphs without referring to the text.

The data in each table should be organized to facilitate comparisons and show relations and trends. The heading of each vertical column should accurately describe the information contained in the column, and each side identifier should indicate the nature of the data in the corresponding horizontal row. Table 10–1 is a simple table that shows findings of a study on the caries-preventive effects of fluoride mouthrinsing.

Graphic presentations are particularly suitable for complicated sets of data or for portraying interesting relations among findings. Figure 10–1 shows a graphic representation of mean gingivitis scores measured in male and female participants in a three-year study of supervised daily dental plaque removal in school. The accompanying text should not merely repeat the information in tables or graphs but rather should summarize the material and point out interesting trends or relations among findings.

In a scientific report, reasons for loss of subjects during a trial should be explained. If attrition of subjects is greater in one group than in others, the reasons should be discussed. Data should demonstrate the comparability of groups, both for subjects who began the investigation and for those who participated throughout. For example, initial DMF surface scores should be given for all children who begin a study (to indicate initial comparability) and for those who complete three years of the study (to indicate whether remaining subjects are similar to all original participants).

When data have been collected over a lengthy period, readers should check the logic or consistency of findings. For example, because dental caries

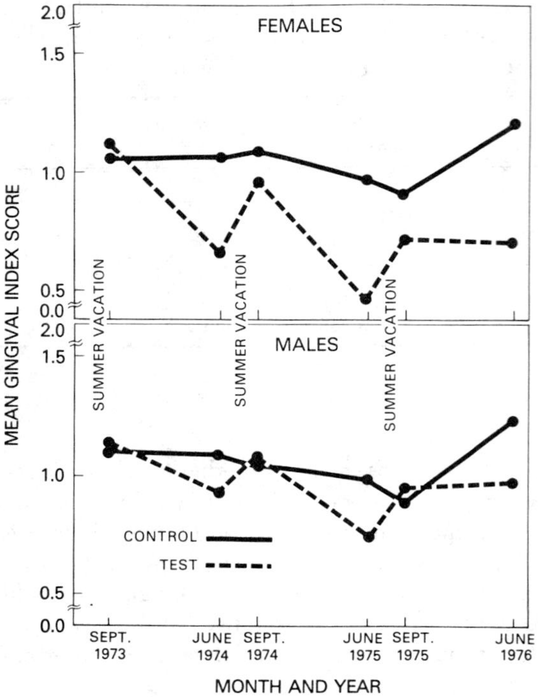

Figure 10–1. Mean gingivitis scores for females and males at each examination, East Hampton, Connecticut, September 1973 to June 1976.

in permanent teeth of children tends to develop fairly linearly between the ages of 6 and 17, the annual increment of DMF surfaces reported in studies lasting for three years or longer should increase in a fairly straight line. Gross deviations from this pattern may denote inadequate training of examiners or changes in diagnostic criteria.

The Analysis of Data

Answers to scientific problems come from carefully framed questions and properly collected data, not from esoteric or abundant analyses. Data analysis is not a process for generating information but an aid to the presentation and interpretation of findings. Methods of statistical analysis are simply tools of scientific study, much like a microscope, or like an ion probe for recording fluoride concentrations. Statistical analysis consists of applying the mathematics of chance to forecasting with various degrees of assurance the likely occurrence of an observed event or effect. To learn whether an observed effect is real, its *variability*, or how it fluctuates within the sample, must be determined. If the effect clearly exceeds the fluctuation, it is probably real or statistically significant. If the effect is relatively small in comparison with the fluctuation or variability among observations, it is likely not to be real or could have occurred by chance with a greater than acceptable degree of probability.

Readers of scientific reports should ask themselves whether the design of a study or the methods of observation warrant a statistical analysis of the results. A major defect in design or an extreme bias in the method of observation may preclude a valid analysis of the data. Any set of numbers may be subjected to statistical analysis, but the question is whether there is sufficient justification for making the computations necessary for drawing inferences.

Limitations of space preclude an extensive discussion of inappropriate statistical methods, but the following are some common errors:

1. The application of tests of statistical inference to biased data.
2. The performance of certain statistical tests on ordinal data.
3. The performance of t-tests or other *parametric* tests on dimensional data with highly skewed (nonnormal) distributions or on small groups with unequal variances.
4. The use of a series of t-tests in multiple comparisons without an adjustment for the fact that the chance of finding statistical significance increases as the number of tests performed increases.
5. The conclusion of no effect or nonsignificance in an inappropriately small sample or when the Type II error is not determined.
6. The conclusion that a trivial difference is important just because a test shows it is statistically significant.
7. The conclusion that scores of one measured variable are the cause of variation in another variable, even when a test produces a statistically significant *correlation coefficient* (r). The correlation of two variables may be large and significant, but one cannot legitimately claim causation.

In some published articles, an apparent inverse relation exists between the amount and complexity of the statistical analysis and the soundness of the investigation. Data that fail to yield a significant result when subjected to simple tests but do so after a refined or complex analysis should be scrutinized critically. It is possible that statistical significance resulted from analyzing transformed data or more information by complex methods, but the significance may reflect differences that have no practical importance. For example, if an overall evaluation of a cariostatic agent shows no general benefits, subanalyses of the data should not be done to the point at which conclusions might be drawn that the agent is effective on distal surfaces of maxillary second premolars and mesial surfaces of mandibular lateral incisors and nowhere else. Such conclusions have no practical value and are likely to be spurious. If enough analyses are made, some will produce "significant findings" by chance alone.

The practice of presenting results only as percentage reductions may also be misleading. In the interpretation of proportional caries scores, it is essential to pay equal attention to the numerator and denominator of the scores. For example, if the mean increment of new carious surfaces in the control group of a clinical trial is only 0.5 per child and if in the test group the corresponding value is 0.25 per child, this difference represents a percentage reduction of 50 percent. However, there has only been a saving of 0.25 carious surfaces per child. When one evaluates percentage reductions, one must, therefore, look critically at the absolute differences involved.

It needs to be emphasized further that readers of scientific reports should be wary of poorly conceived or carelessly conducted studies that provide "statistically significant" findings. Statistical significance denotes nothing about the biological or clinical meaning of a difference in numbers or values. Readers are deluded who think that the value or meaning of a study is authenticated merely because the results are statistically significant.

Perhaps it is most important for readers (and investigators) to distinguish between *statistical significance* and *clinical significance*. The former is a mathematical expression of the degree of confidence that an observed difference between groups represents a real difference, that a zero response would not occur if the study were repeated, and that the difference is not merely due to chance. In contrast, clinical significance is a judgment made by the researcher or reader that differences in response to intervention observed between groups are important for health. Clinical significance is a subjective determination based upon clinical experience and an understanding of the characteristics of the disease or condition being measured. It is an estimate of the practical value of the differences between a test group and a control group. Many considerations determine judgments about clinical significance. A common one is *cost-effectiveness*, or the relative cost of achieving a certain protection or effect. For example, a regimen that costs $0.50 per year per child to achieve a reduced incidence of one-half DMF surface per year may be considered cost-effective, whereas another regimen that costs $40.00 per year per child to prevent one DMF surface per year may not.

The proper use of various statistical tests, such as t-tests and F ratios, requires that dimensional data have a *normal distribution*. Many of the data collected in biomedical research are not normally distributed and thus the assumptions that are made of normality are frequently violated. Fortunately, many parametric tests used to analyze dental findings are fairly robust and may be applied legitimately when the number of observations is large even though the data are not normally distributed. There are also parametric tests based on other than normal distributions of data. Moreover, many statistical tests for analyzing data are available that are not based on assumptions of any particular distribution of data; these are called distribution-free or *nonparametric tests*.

Data that are not normally distributed are occasionally normalized by using logarithms, square roots, or other transformations of the original data in order to perform statistical tests legitimately. The scientific logic and justification for these transformations are uncertain. For example, what does it really mean to say that the cube root of some measured variable is significantly lower in one group than in another?

Many reports fail to state the statistical methods used to analyze the data. Readers should be told specifically which statistical test was used, whether it was one- or two-tailed, and what the value of the statistic and the actual probability (p) value are, rather than just be given an expression of statistical significance such as $p < 0.05$. *Two-tailed statistical tests* are generally used when there is uncertainty whether one regimen is better than another. If previous information exists that one regimen is better than another, a *one-tailed statistical test* should be used to evaluate the first regimen's superiority. A decision on whether one- or two-tailed tests are appropriate should be made during the planning phase of a study and not after the fact.

A *p value* is the probability of obtaining by chance alone a difference as large as the one observed in a trial if the null hypothesis of no effect is true. Results of analyses that yield a p value of 0.05 or less are generally thought to be significant; p values below 0.01 are highly significant. These are arbitrary demarcations. The outcome of a p-value calculation should not unduly influence decisions about the worth of a regimen. There may be an unfortunate tendency to disregard or discount the findings of a well-designed, scientifically important experiment if the findings come close but fail to achieve statistical significance.

Biologically important decisions are rarely made on the basis of a single trial or experiment. The tendency to dichotomize the results of a study into a "yes" (statistically significant, or $p < 0.05$) or "no" (not statistically significant, or $p > 0.05$) may be counterproductive and misleading; p values of, for example, 0.06 and 0.04 should not lead to definitive opposite conclusions but to closely similar ones. At the least, the analysis of a study should not necessarily be limited to a statistical approach. A more descriptive or informative analysis for quantifying data may be appropriate. Such an analysis may take the form of calculating a *confidence interval.* Although a confidence interval calculated from the data of a study may include a zero difference among groups, the interval may also range far into territory that indicates a beneficial effect of treatment. It may not be correct to classify as negative those findings that produce a confidence interval that includes zero within its boundaries but also a value indicating a strong treatment effect. Traditional significance testing focuses all interest to one precise point—the lower boundary of a confidence interval.

Conditions measured in a study may be *correlated;* that is, there may be a causal, complementary, parallel, or reciprocal association between two or more measured variables. An example is a positive relation that has repeatedly been shown between dental plaque scores and gingivitis. A *correlation coefficient* is a measure of the interdependence of two random variables that may range in value from -1 to $+1$, indicating perfect negative correlation and perfect positive correlation, respectively. The correlation coefficient is expressed as r. The amount of variation in one variable explained by another variable is determined by squaring r, and is expressed by r^2. Thus, a correlation coefficient of $+0.30$, which may be statistically significant, explains only 9 percent of the variation between two variables; 91 percent of the variation is left unexplained. Moreover, a correlation estimate *cannot* prove that one factor is the cause of another; the relation between the factors may be casual or fortuitous.

Multiple correlation (regression) analyses permit computation of the maximum total effect of combinations of independent factors on the variation of a dependent variable. These analyses determine the influence of these factors in decreasing order of their influence on the dependent variable. For example, a regression analysis may indicate that periodontal disease in an examined population may be explained in decreasing order by age, dental plaque scores, oral hygiene practices, sex, education, and income, and in total, may explain 38 percent of the variation in scores.

Discussion

The primary purpose of a discussion of results is to show the relations among the findings that have been observed. One common error found in many reports is that the discussion largely repeats the results. Instead, the discussion should present the principal elements, relations, and generalizations shown by the results. It should also point out any exceptions, inconsistencies, and lack of correlation among the findings, and should raise unsettled issues. The discussion also should include the researchers' critical assessments of their own work. This part of a report should also show how the results of the investigation agree or contrast with previously published articles or accepted precepts. Speculation about the implications or applications of the report's findings belongs in the discussion section as well. In short, the discussion gives writers an opportunity to give their opinions and ideas about the study.

Conclusions

Most reports should contain from one to several clearly stated conclusions that are based on the collected data and their analyses. Moreover, the conclusions should be relevant to the original questions posed by the investigators and should state whether each postulated null hypothesis is accepted or rejected. Of course, the conclusions should agree with the results of the statistical analysis. Readers should ask themselves whether the concluding statements generalize beyond the limits warranted from the population that has been studied. The conclusions should make biologic sense and be of practical importance. The reporters should state whether their findings and the existing body of scientific information on the same subject suggest a need for additional research. Readers should ask whether the conclusions will lead them to change their thinking, attitudes, practices, or recommendations.

References

Scientific reports as well as review articles should contain *references* that support statements made in the text. References mostly document statements made in the background review and the discussion of a report's findings. They should direct the reader to other sources for additional information. The citation of references, therefore, must be given in sufficient detail so that they can be located and checked readily. Original sources of information rather than secondary attributions should be cited in references in order to reduce chances of compounding previously made errors in documentation. A *bibliography* is either a list of works of a specific writer or, in the context of a scientific report, a list of sources of information in print on the subject of the report. Sometimes a bibliography at the end of a review is titled "Suggested Reading." Items in a bibliography should be pertinent to the subject of the paper; irrelevant items written by well-known researchers should not be included. Moreover, all the pertinent literature should be cited in references and bibliographies, and not merely those papers that support the writer's premise or findings. Readers should be wary of reports that rely heavily on personal communications in the list of references and of review articles that inordinately cite the writer's own work and that omit important references to work on the subject of the paper.

ETHICAL CONSIDERATIONS OF STUDIES WITH HUMAN SUBJECTS

During the past several years, concern has increased about ethical considerations in the conduct of biomedical research with human beings. Although many ethical considerations of research with humans may not properly belong in a chapter on the evaluation of scientific information, others do. For this reason, some discussion on several aspects of the ethics of biomedical research is provided here.

In ethical studies, the questions being asked can be answered validly, while the rights and welfare of participants remain fully protected. It is unethical to conduct a bad scientific experiment with humans. Subjects should not be asked to assume risks of possible injury, discomfort, or inconveniences in clinical studies when not enough subjects have been included for valid results; too many subjects have been recruited to establish a clinically significant point; or improperly designed random or double-blind procedures have been employed. Deficiencies in design cannot be compensated for or corrected. A poorly designed or conceived study is unethical by definition and should never have been done. Thus, the design of clinical research has broad ethical implications that deserve attention when readers evaluate scientific literature.

Studies using human subjects must follow scientific principles that provide a sound rationale for the research. Justification for the research should depend on findings obtained from laboratory studies or other clinical studies or on a thorough knowledge of pertinent scientific literature. Nearly all research institutions have now established permanent committees to review their proposed research with human subjects. Review committees must be competent to review proposed studies scientifically and to determine their acceptability in terms of local law, standards of professional conduct, and community practice.

The rights and welfare of participants in research projects must be adequately protected. Any predictable risks to subjects must be outweighed by the benefits they are likely to receive or by the importance to the public of the knowledge that will be gained. The interests of science or society must be balanced by concern for the participants' interests. Therefore, reports should contain a brief description of how subjects were recruited and informed about the study.

Informed Consent

The informed consent of patients or subjects who take part in a study must be obtained by adequate and fair methods, only after the study has been fully explained and, as far as can be ascertained, fully understood. Participation must be truly voluntary and must not be coerced in any way. Prospective subjects must be assured that individual findings will be held confidentially. Reasonable risks and benefits should be explained and put in perspective, and permission should be given for a subject to withdraw from the study at any time without prejudice.

For research on preventive methods, it is particularly important, when a placebo will be used, that subjects be informed of the likelihood of their receiving the ineffective treatment. For research other than for treatment or prevention, for example, behavioral or social research, the aspect of confidentiality of information concerning beliefs, practices, or habits of participants assumes preeminence.

Ethical considerations frequently conflict with the pursuit of scientific rigor in the design of clinical trials. When subjects are randomly assigned to groups, those in the control group will be deprived of effective treatment or prevention if the intervention is effective. Yet if no untreated or placebo-treated control group is used, it may be uncertain whether a tested regimen has been effective. Moreover, if a control group is not included in the design of a study in which two effective regimens are compared, the subjects in one of the two groups risk receiving the less effective regimen. If one of the two regimens is thought by the investigators or by a consensus of the scientific community to be more effective than the other, from an ethical standpoint, all subjects should be assigned to the group designated to receive that treatment. Unless subjects are randomly assigned to all groups, however, the trial will yield invalid scientific results. Because of the present conflicting demands of ethics and scientific rigor, the likelihood is increased that trials with scientifically compromised designs will yield inconclusive results. Good experimental design is the essential element of ethical research in humans. It is unethical to put persons needlessly at risk, however small, in experiments that cannot produce any meaningful results.

Three basic questions must be asked when a proposed study is being designed: (1) Should there be a negative control group? (2) Should the subjects be randomly assigned to groups? (3) Is it ethically acceptable to randomize subjects to groups? From a scientific standpoint, the answer to the second and third questions is routinely yes, but persons in the community with different backgrounds are likely to give different answers to these questions. There may be no uniformly right answers acceptable to all. Readers of scientific reports should think about these considerations, although at the time of reading a scientific report, an ethical judgment of the study's design may be after the fact.

REVIEWS

Other than reports of clinical studies, scientific literature includes reviews of information or state-of-knowledge articles on particular subjects. The proliferation of scientific information in the last 10 to 20 years has caused most health personnel and researchers to narrow the range of topics about which they can keep abreast. Few are able to read and absorb the contents of all scientific reports on a host of subjects. Reviews of a particular topic are usually written by experts who have firsthand knowledge of the subject and who also digest and evaluate scattered bits of information on the subject and condense them into coherent and comprehensible packages for practitioners and other scientists.

The importance of review articles for the advancement of science and the practice of a profession should not be underrated. There is a chronic shortage of people capable of writing authoritative reviews. To collect the available literature on any subject and turn it into a single, relatively unbiased, comprehensive, and yet digestible work requires much time, knowledge, and writing skill.

THE RETRIEVAL OF SCIENTIFIC INFORMATION

The amount of scientific literature is growing at an explosive rate. Several journals that contain important dental information, such as *Community Dentistry and Oral Epidemiology*, the *Journal of Preventive Dentistry*, and *Pediatric Dentistry*, have commenced publication within the last 10 years. Faced with an ever-growing body of dental literature, dental professionals must limit their reading, because of financial or time restrictions, to an increasingly smaller proportion of available publications.

A major problem in dealing with the literature of an expanding field is the storage and retrieval of information. New and economical computer technics for classifying and retrieving this information—such as the MEDLINE and MEDLARS systems of the National Library of Medicine—have simplified the problem. Even so, the person making a literature search with these systems is often overwhelmed by the large quantity of marginal literature that is automatically retrieved for apparent relevance when a request is made. Computerized literature retrieval systems have the shortcoming of being only as good as the information about a paper entered into the system. If a paper has been improperly coded for the system, reference to it will not occur when a request by key words is made. The axiom "garbage in—garbage out" (the acronym of which is GIGO) applies. Although it would seem to be desirable to eliminate questionable entries from these retrieval systems, to do so would prevent the attractive possibility of finding a previously unrecognized but pertinent report that was published in an unconventional forum.

The *Index Medicus* and the *Index to Dental Literature* are invaluable sources of scientific references. Several years ago, the latter increased its usefulness by expanding its coverage of periodical literature.

TYPES OF JOURNALS

Some journals, such as the *Journal of Dental Research, Community Dentistry and Oral Epidemiology,* and *Caries Research,* devote their contents almost exclusively to research. Usually the articles published in these journals are scrutinized carefully by referees before they are published. Journal *referees* are experts to whom the editor of a journal refers a submitted article for an opinion of its acceptability for publication. The referees are frequently, but not necessarily, members of the editorial board of the journal. A good editor will maintain a cadre of referees with expertise in different specialties. It is important for an editor to send an article to those referees best qualified to review a particular article. Each article should be sent to two or three referees who editors hope will concur on a recommendation for publication. Sometimes an editor will send a submitted article to two referees and use a third one only if the original two disagree on their recommendation for publication.

Other journals, such as the *Journal of Public Health Dentistry,* the *Journal of the American Dental Association,* and the *Journal of Periodontology,* are published for a large professional group of general practitioners or specialists. They contain research articles and reviews, but also articles of wide interest to professionals within their respective fields. These journals, too, are usually rigorously refereed and edited.

A final type of journal is hard to categorize but may be called a "throwaway," commercial, or trade journal, such as *Dental Survey, Dental Management,* or *Dental Products.* Although these publications contain articles, they rarely if ever are submitted to referees or undergo vigorous editing. It is safe to say that major research is not published in these magazines, although an occasional helpful article may be found.

A published paper may influence dental practice, community programs, and future research by scientists. The editorial board of a journal and its referees thus have an important ethical responsibility to ensure that papers appearing in their journal are scientifically sound.

Journals should not reject statistically valid papers because the findings are negative. Negative findings may seem unexciting, but they often may be just as important to health planning as positive findings. Investigators and editors have a responsibility to publish reports with negative findings if they are based on sound research.

To keep informed of scientific developments, professionals should concentrate on the core journals in their fields of interest. Probably no more than six to eight journals contain the most useful articles in each discipline. Regular perusal of such a well-chosen set of journals is probably the most effective way to maintain a reasonable level of current awareness and knowledge. Indexes to the literature and literature retrieval systems may then be used for special purposes. The reader can supplement a basic set of journals by reading review articles and the proceedings of workshops and conferences. It is also helpful to peruse compilations of abstracts such as *Dental Abstracts* and special issues of the *Journal of Dental Research* that contain abstracts of papers presented at annual sessions of the International Association for Dental Research and its component divisions. The principal value of abstracts of already published reports is to inform readers about the overall findings of a study and to help them keep up-to-date on research developments. Readers who require details of a study should seek the original publication, especially if they are writing a paper; an abstract should not be used as a reference if a full publication of the article exists. Investigator-prepared abstracts of oral presentations may have to be used as citations until a corresponding paper has been published. Upon request, investigators will usually supply complete manuscripts of papers they have presented at meetings. The manuscript invariably contains details not found in the abstract.

The status of a journal as a continuing source of scientific information can be preserved only if the editors set high standards for the articles they accept and maintain those standards by conscientious editing and refereeing policies. Reputable journals employ a peer review system to control quality. Although this system is subject to error, bias, and disagreement between reviewers and occasionally among reviewers, writers, and editors, it is better than any other known system for evaluating reports for publication.

Many papers rejected by core scientific journals may eventually be published elsewhere, but this fact does not justify relaxing the standards of editorial boards that maintain journals of high scientific quality. Writers choose journals to publish their reports for relevance to their research and for quality—the same criteria that should be used by the readers of particular journals.

EVALUATION OF WRITERS OF SCIENTIFIC REPORTS

The scientific reputation of the writer of a report is often helpful in predicting the quality of the report even before it is read. The work of writers who have a reputation for being knowledgeable about their subjects, who are recognized as having a scientific attitude toward research, and who have previously demonstrated their ability to conduct and report careful, accurate research is likely to be valid. Of course, the novice reader of scientific literature may not be familiar with the reputations of many researchers, or an article may be the work of a relatively new investigator. There are nevertheless clues to the likely quality of a report. The affiliations of the writers, where they work, what resources are available to them (such as libraries, consultants, and necessary equipment), their colleagues and co-workers, and the source of financial support for the research are all guides to assessing the expected quality of an article.

STYLE OF SCIENTIFIC WRITING

Most scientific information is communicated in writing that describes phenomena and concepts. The way in which these phenomena and concepts are expressed in language is *style,* which necessitates putting proper words in proper places.

The best scientific writing is organized, precise, clear, and brief. Unfortunately, many scientists conclude that in order to be taken seriously, they must write as "scientifically" as possible, using jargon instead of plain language. Those who defend the use of scientific idioms claim that they are briefer and more exact than ordinary language. Some scientists may unconsciously take delight that their jargon seemingly makes their field incomprehensible to outsiders and assume that use of it makes them experts in their field. Perhaps psychiatry and sociology have contributed most heavily to jargon because many of their words, picked up by other professionals and the public, no longer have a precise meaning. Consider such terms as *ambivalent, phobia, subconscious, underachiever,* and *depressed socioeconomic area.*

Science is built with stones of facts, and style determines the architecture by which those facts are expressed. The goal of good scientific writing is to communicate scientific facts and thoughts in an honest and clear way. Students should realize that they do not know what they mean until they can say what they mean plainly so that others will understand them. They should apply this standard to the scientific reports that they read as well as to their own work.

CHECKLIST FOR EVALUATING SCIENTIFIC INFORMATION

As a form of summary on evaluating scientific information, the following criteria for scoring project reports submitted by candidates for certification by the American Board of Dental Public Health are offered. These criteria were recently revised and accepted by members of the Board at their 1981 annual meeting and should serve as a good checklist for assessing the quality of scientific papers in dentistry.

1. Relevance of Project to Dental Public Health or Candidate's Agency
   a. Was the project timely?

b. Did the project provide new information, confirm findings of other reports, or was it needlessly repetitive?
c. Is it likely that application of information from the project will improve the oral health of the public or be useful to the practice of dental public health?
d. Is the project likely to lead to additional research or other projects?
e. Were the findings published or was the report suitably distributed?

2. Identification and Planned Approach to Problem (Design)
   a. Did the project clearly and concisely define or identify a specific hypothesis, problem, or need?
   b. Did the project contain a logical and realistic approach to testing a hypothesis, solving a problem, or meeting a need?
   c. Is the overall design of the project logical?
   d. Were the objectives of the project realistic and were they likely to be attained in the allotted time with the staff, facilities, materials, and finances available?
   e. Were the collected data specified, described, or defined, and were they related directly to the objectives of the project?
   f. Did the candidate seek appropriate technical assistance and consultation?
   g. Were responsibilities of participating project personnel clearly defined or outlined?
   h. Were the number and qualifications of project personnel adequate for the project?
   i. Is there evidence that the candidate understood the assumptions made in designing the project?
   j. Was the study designed with adequate concern for ethical considerations?
3. Adequacy and Pertinency of Review of Literature
   a. Does the report contain a comprehensive review of the current literature pertinent to the project?
   b. Is there evidence that the candidate understood the contents of the reviewed literature?
   c. Is there evidence that the candidate understood the significance of the work done by others?
   d. Have important background references or findings by others been omitted?
   e. Are there inappropriate references?
4. Adequacy of Procedures Used (Methods)
   a. Was an appropriate sample of the population used and was it suitably drawn?
   b. Were experimental procedures specified and described sufficiently, and were they likely to be valid, sensitive, repeatable, and reliable?
   c. Did the test procedures have a suitable control?
   d. Were appropriate methods of measurement used?
   e. If project personnel were trained, were the training methods described adequately?

   f. If new methods of measurement were used, were they adequately pretested?
   g. Were the procedures used described in sufficient detail to evaluate the work or to permit repeating the project?
   h. Were the data collected in an organized way suitable for analysis?
   i. Was bias reasonably controlled?
   j. Was the candidate successful in following the planned procedures for the project?
   k. Were the methods adequate for obtaining informed consent of participants?
5. Data Analysis and Discussion of Findings
   a. Are the findings presented clearly and are tables and graphs easy to understand?
   b. Were the statistical tests used appropriate for the collected data?
   c. Does a spot check of calculations show that they are accurate?
   d. Do the data provide answers to the questions that led to the design and execution of the project?
   e. Do the data seem to be overanalyzed?
   f. Are superfluous data presented?
   g. Is all of the discussion relevant to the findings?
   h. Were some findings overemphasized or excessively discussed and other findings underemphasized or ignored?
6. Summary and Conclusions
   a. Does the summary synthesize the project's most salient procedures and findings?
   b. Do the data support the conclusions?
   c. Are the conclusions valid?
7. Clarity of Writing and Overall Style of Report and Abstract
   a. Is the report clear, concise, and orderly?
   b. Has excessive jargon been used?
   c. Does the abstract comprise an understandable summary of the project?
   d. Are the style, grammar, spelling, and general composition of the report satisfactory?
8. Recognition of Problems and Suggested Changes if Project Were Repeated
   a. Is there evidence that the candidate is aware of weaknesses in the design or execution of the project that could have been eliminated?
   b. Would the suggested changes likely improve the project if it were repeated?
   c. Does the candidate refuse to recognize any deficiencies in the project or the report?

CONCLUDING COMMENTS

This chapter, it is hoped, should help readers to make logical and orderly analyses of scientific information. Without publication, a work barely exists and is ineffectual. Nevertheless, results should not be published if the work is trivial, faulty, poorly designed, unethical, biased, inappropriately analyzed, poorly controlled, or unsupported by adequate data. Even if results are published, they do not automatically achieve credibility. A critical appraisal of published reports is obligatory for health professionals, who are expected to implement current preventive and therapeutic methods and make valid recommendations to patients and communities. The ability to appraise reports properly will also help potential referees of journal articles and reviewers of papers and abstracts for scientific meetings.

If you, the reader, find fault with a study, ask yourself if you can think of a better way to have done it. You may come to realize that the study, although somewhat imperfect as conducted, cannot feasibly be improved, and that the investigators, having struggled with the decision to do an imperfect study or none at all, preferred the former alternative.

Suggested Reading

Altman, D. G. Statistics and ethics in medical research—misuse of statistics is unethical. Brit. Med. J., 281:1182–4, Nov. 1, 1980.

______. Statistics and ethics in medical research. VIII—improving the quality of statistics in medical journals. Brit. Med. J., 282:44–7, Jan. 3, 1981.

American Dental Association. Proceedings of the Conference on the Clinical Testing of Cariostatic Agents. Chicago, The Association, 1972. viii + 117 p.

Brown, B. W., Jr. Statistical controversies in the design of clinical trials—some personal views. Controlled Clin. Trials, 1:13–27, May 1980.

Byar, D. P., et al. Randomized clinical trials. New Engl. J. Med., 295:74–80, July 8, 1976.

Chambers, T. C., et al. A method for assessing the quality of a randomized control trial. Controlled Clin. Trials, 2:31–49, Jan. 1981.

Ciampi, A., and Till, J. E. Null results in clinical trials: the need for a decision-theory approach. Brit. J. Cancer, 41:618–29, Apr. 1980.

Colton, Theodore. Critical reading of the medical literature. p. 315–23. (In Colton, T., ed. Statistics in medicine. Boston, Little, Brown, 1974. xii + 372 p.)

Council of Biology Editors style manual—a guide for authors, editors, and publishers in the biological sciences. 4th ed. Arlington, American Institute Biological Sciences, 1978. xvii + 265 p.

Day, R. A. How to write and publish a scientific paper. Philadelphia, Institute Scientific Information Press, 1979. xi + 160 p.

Easlick, K. A., ed. Communicating in dentistry. Springfield, Ill., Thomas, 1974. ix + 228 p.

Haack, D. G. Statistical literacy: a guide to interpretation. N. Scituate, Mass., Duxbury Press, 1979. xii + 323 p.

Horowitz, H. S. Overview of ethical issues in clinical studies. J. Pub. Health Dent., 38:35–43, Winter 1978.

Horowitz, H. S., et al., eds. Principal requirements for controlled clinical trials of caries preventive agents and procedures. Internat. Dent. J., 23:505–16, Sept. 1973.

Huff, Darrell. How to lie with statistics. New York, Norton, 1954. 142 p.

Jenny, Joanna, ed. Ethical and legal considerations in dental caries research involving human subjects. Proceedings of a conference at the University of Iowa, Iowa City, Iowa, May 7–9, 1979. J. Dent. Res., 59: Spec. Issue C, July 1980.

Mosteller, Frederick, Gilbert, J. P., and McPeek, Bucknam. Reporting standards and research strategies for controlled trials—agenda for the editor. Controlled Clin. Trials, 1:37–58, May 1980.

O'Mullane, D. M. Efficiency in clinical trials of caries preventive agents and methods. Community Dent. Oral Epidemiol., 4:190–4, Sept. 1976.

Osborn, John. Statistical principles in the analysis of dental data. p. 221–44. (In Slack, G. L., and Burt, B. A., eds. Dental public health; an introduction to community dentistry. 2nd ed. Bristol, England, Wright, 1981. ix + 343 p.)

Prineas, R. J. Common problems in clinical trials. Med. J. Austral., 2:425–36, Aug. 21, 1971.

Rennie, Drummond. The ethics of medical publication. Med. J. Austral., 2:409–12, Oct. 20, 1979.

Rhein, R. W., Jr. Placebo—deception or potent therapy? Med. World News, 21:39–47, Feb. 4, 1980.

Russell, A. L. The interpretation of data and the evaluation of scientific literature. p. 63–72. (In Young, W. O., and Striffler, D. F. The dentist, his practice, and his community. 2nd ed. Philadelphia, Saunders, 1969. xvi + 346 p.)

Sackett, D. L. Bias in analytic research. J. Chron. Dis., 32:51–63, 1979.

Smart, J. V. Elements of medical statistics. 2nd ed. London, Staples Press, 1970. 176 p.

Tanur, Judith M., et al., eds. Statistics: a guide to the unknown. San Francisco, Holden-Day, 1970. xxiii + 430 p.

Ziman, J. M. The proliferation of scientific literature; a natural process. Science, 208:369–71, Apr. 25, 1980.

V MEETING THE DEMAND FOR DENTAL CARE

CHAPTER **11**

DENTAL TREATMENT NEED, DEMAND, AND UTILIZATION

David F. Striffler

INTRODUCTION

After most dental personnel have gained a little practical experience, they determine treatment needs almost without thinking about it. They look into a patient's mouth and immediately think, "Aha! A Class II amalgam ought to do nicely there. That missing lower first molar will have to be replaced by a fixed bridge, and this patient should have a couple of preventive educational sessions with the dental hygienist. He's got to learn to keep his mouth in better shape." The musing continues: "We'll see after the hygienist gets through cleaning up the mouth and instructing the patient just what periodontal therapy will be necessary." Thus, it seems clear to most dental professionals that the determination of the treatment needs and the course of therapy to be followed is a *professional* determination. Rarely is professional integrity or judgment questioned about whether the recommended treatment is best for a particular patient. It is usually only when cost enters into the equation that the dental professionals have to back off and consider what the patient can afford and what still might be an acceptable treatment procedure even if a compromise. Nevertheless, most dental professionals assume that the determination of what dental treatment is needed is their professional dental responsibility.

Contrary views, however, are beginning to be expressed by the public, giving voice to what previously may have been silent questions concerning the need for the particular treatment recommended by the dental professional, whether it is needed right now, and whether there isn't a less expensive expedient.

Regardless of whether one views the issue as a dental professional or as a patient or potential patient, serious question is being given to just exactly what constitutes appropriate, adequate, effective, and efficient dental treatment. Inherent in that questioning is whether or not a treatment need truly exists in the first place. The entire concept of accountability is now being applied across the board and not just for small businessmen, large faceless corporations, "that government in Washington," or the bureaucrats at the state capitol; health professionals now are being challenged, and challenged seriously. As evidence, one only needs to turn to the spate of consumer books and directories concerned with how to go about purchasing health care, including dental care. In answer to this flurry of consumer directories, the American Dental Association has responded to a call from the House of Delegates to prepare its own guidelines to assist dental groups that are developing directories of their own or assisting community groups in developing them. The ADA also has developed its own consumer's guide.[8]

Over 10 years ago the second edition of this textbook[55] detailed need and demand rather simply and indeed even used as an illustration a diagram (see Fig. 11–1) from an earlier version of this text[10] published two decades before. The concept of absolute need was defined as the need actually existing in a person's mouth. Detectable need was defined as that which the dentist could detect. It was also pointed out that no examination procedure could be expected to uncover all pathological conditions present. Therefore, it was recognized that there will be a difference between detectable and absolute need.

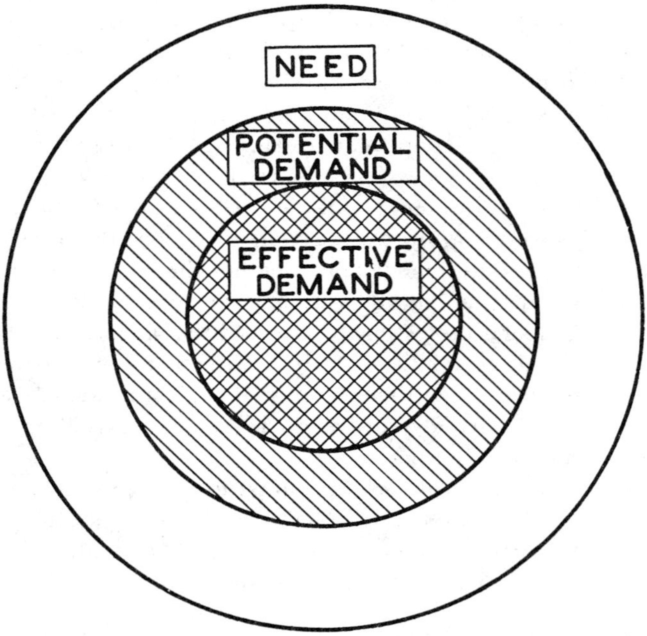

Figure 11–1. Dental treatment needs and the demand for care. (From Dollar, M. L., and Kulstad, Hugo. The economic aspects of the dental health problem. p. 24–34. [In Pelton, W. J., and Wisan, J. M., eds. Dentistry in public health. Philadelphia, Saunders, 1949. xi + 261 p.])

It is conceivable, of course, that some of the need detected by the dental professional might not truly be a need in anyone's eyes but the professional's and perhaps a few others of a similar persuasion. For example, European dentists visiting this country are sometimes surprised at the acceptance of orthodontic intervention for what they consider only slight deviations from "normal." (It might be noted that possibly no two dentists can agree on what is normal occlusion.) The dentists from abroad wonder at the number of youngsters they see with complete-mouth banding and headgears, apparently the result of cultural pressures both from within the professional culture and from the culture of affluence. So perhaps around that outer concentric circle in Figure 11–1 there should be another outer circle drawn and labeled as culturally determined need.

Overtreatment and Undertreatment

As previously mentioned, earlier editions of this book took it for granted that the definition of what constituted need was that which was detectable by professional dental personnel, primarily the dentist. Only in recent years have the concepts of overtreatment or undertreatment even been mentioned in dental circles. But because of a number of developments such as (1) the perception that there is an oversupply of dentists and dental hygienists; (2) the likelihood or actuality that new payment methods, such as capitation and prepayment, will play a much larger role in the financing of dental care; and (3) the imminence or realities of peer review and quality assurance, preauthorization, and posttreatment reviews; the concepts of overtreatment and undertreatment cannot be avoided and must be discussed.

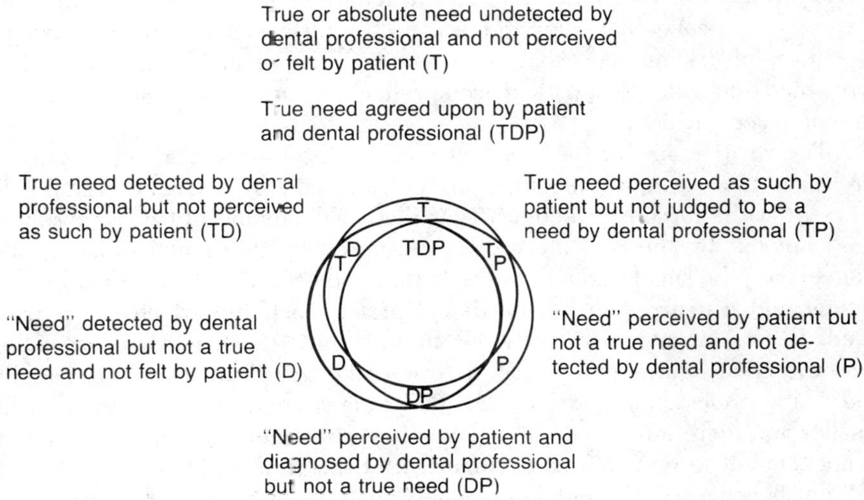

Figure 11–2. Overtreatment, appropriate treatment, and undertreatment.

In Figure 11–2 the three intersecting circles represent, first, absolute or true need as the slightly elevated center circle (T); second, the dental professional's diagnosed or declared need as the circle to the left (D); and third, the patient's perception of the patient's own needs as the circle to the right (P). The largest area in the center, that which is contained by the intersection of all three circles (TDP), is the absolute need or true need that has been detected by the dental professional and that also is felt by the patient. In this largest area, overtreatment or undertreatment is not a problem. The crescent area farthest to the left (D) represents overtreatment; that is, dental needs declared to exist by the dental professional but not true needs and not perceived by the patient. Overtreatment could be an honest error in diagnosis, or it could be the result of a deliberate recommendation for a dental service that really was not required. The inner crescent area on the left (TD) also represents need that is a professionally determined true need, but one that is not felt by the patient and one that could result in undertreatment if the patient refused the recommended treatment.

The crescent or partial circle to the far right (P) is need felt by the patient but not a true need. For example, the patient might wish to have a porcelain jacket crown placed, when in the best professional judgment a porcelain jacket crown is not indicated and no pathosis exists. Nevertheless the patient might persist and the treatment might be performed. In this instance it would be patient-induced overtreatment.

The crescent to the right (TP) just inside the outer crescent would be true need felt and perceived by the patient but not recognized as such by the dental professional. This type of need again could be an honest disagreement between patient and dental professional because the patient, for example, felt some sensitivity that the dental professional tended to discount but that later proved to be a carious lesion. Undertreatment could also occur if a prepayment plan was so constituted that dental professionals were encouraged to provide services fully covered by the plan and to ignore or put off services not fully covered or not covered at all in the plan. In this instance that type of "service" is a form of "skimming" (that is, "skimming the cream"), and not being concerned about the total patient, comprehensive care, or whether or not the patient is seen again.

The relative size of the areas covered by the intersections of the three circles in the accompanying figure is not assigned by accident. The small segment at the top designated as "T" is that small amount of true or absolute need not felt by the patient and not diagnosed by the dental professional. Conversely, the small segment at the bottom labeled "DP" is need felt by the patient and concurred in by the dental professional, but which is not true need. In this instance overtreatment could result. It is felt that most of the time the great bulk of dental need is true need agreed upon by both patient and dental professional and that the other instances of disagreement are much smaller and more infrequent. The issue of overtreatment and undertreatment is not thought to be particularly important at this time and one hopes that it will not become so. All dental personnel should be aware of it, however, and be on guard for errors of commission and omission.

Overtreatment has been of concern in medicine and in surgery particularly. A strong association exists between the number of surgeons and the number of surgical procedures carried out, just as there is a strong correlation between the number of hospital beds available and the number of days spent in a hospital per person. And there is a somewhat apocryphal story of the period when physicians went on strike and the death rate dropped.

Defining Need, Demand, and Utilization

It still appears true that the unqualified desire for dental care may be defined as "potential demand," whereas the desire plus the ability to obtain dental service may be defined as "effective demand." There are other terms that economists and others use such as "felt need" (which perhaps could be equated with "potential demand") and "utilization." From an economist's viewpoint, "utilization" probably should be used instead of "effective demand." Obviously if people are effectively demanding care, that means they are getting it and thus are utilizing dental services.

Some economists[48] maintain that utilization should refer to the number of individuals that utilize (make use of) dental services. Thus, an increase in utilization literally means that a larger number of individuals utilize dental services as measured in numbers of individuals—not quantities of services. The related concept of "utilization rate" simply refers to the proportion of a population that utilizes dental services over a specified period of time.

The contrasting concept of "demand" is referred to as an economic term most commonly expressed as a quantity of goods or services that will be purchased for a given price. The quantity of demand normally increases when prices fall and decreases when prices rise. The demand concept of economic theory does not include any reference to the number of people who are buying the quantities that are demanded at the given price. The literature seldom makes a distinction between utilization and demand and often uses the concepts interchangeably. All too often, the number of visits per person per year is the most commonly reported measure of "utilization," yet it gives neither the number of people using the services nor the quantities and prices of services purchased.

*The Viewpoint of Economists**

Of course, the familiar "supply and demand" are two of the most commonly used terms by economists. When discussing dental care, economists use these and similar terms that dental professionals perhaps do not like to hear applied to them and their services: marketplace, vendor or provider, sales, monopoly or oligopoly, customers, stock of dentists, and care delivery.

*Much of the balance of this section dealing with economic theory and Figures 11–3 through 11–8 are based on material originally drafted by Stephen Eklund, D.D.S., M.H.S.A., Dr.P.H.

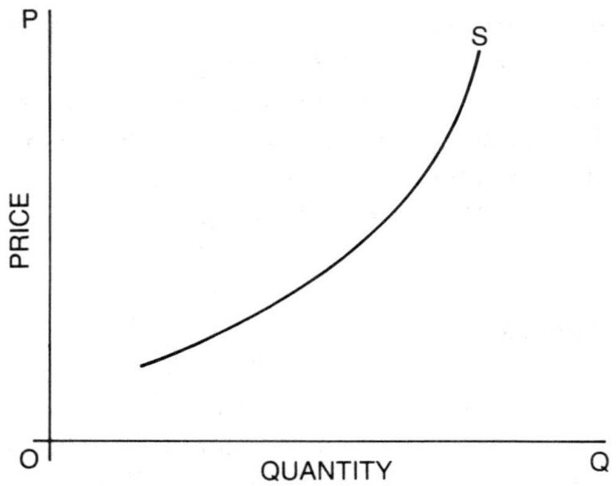

Figure 11–3. Hypothetical supply curve.

Supply is defined as the quantity of a service that will be provided at a given price (Fig. 11–3). Under most circumstances, the higher the price, the larger the quantity that suppliers are willing to make available. Demand is the quantity of a service that a consumer (patient) will buy at a given price (Fig. 11–4). For most goods and services, the lower the price, the larger the quantity that consumers are willing to buy. Explicit in both of these definitions is the concept that the quantities supplied and demanded will change as prices change.

Two other important terms, which should be distinguished from supply and demand, are need and wants. Need, according to dental professionals, is a *professionally defined* quantity of care that is required to achieve or maintain health optimal for a particular patient. Wants are the quantity of care individuals themselves feel that they need. Felt need is often used as a synonym for wants. As these needs and wants have been defined, they do not necessarily coincide. Since neither theoretically is affected by price, they may be and usually are quite different from supply or demand, at least in dental health care.

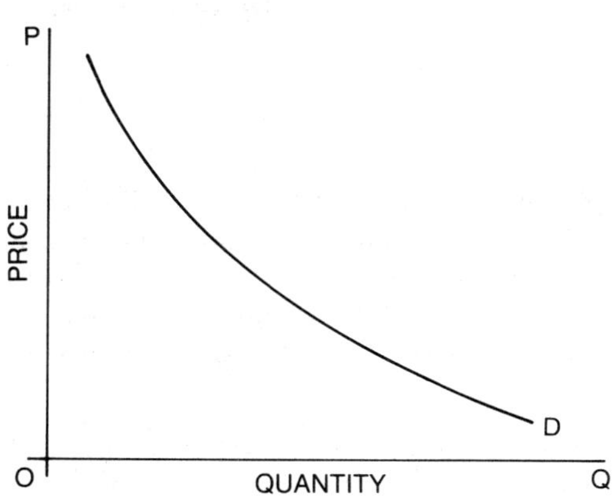

Figure 11–4. Hypothetical demand curve.

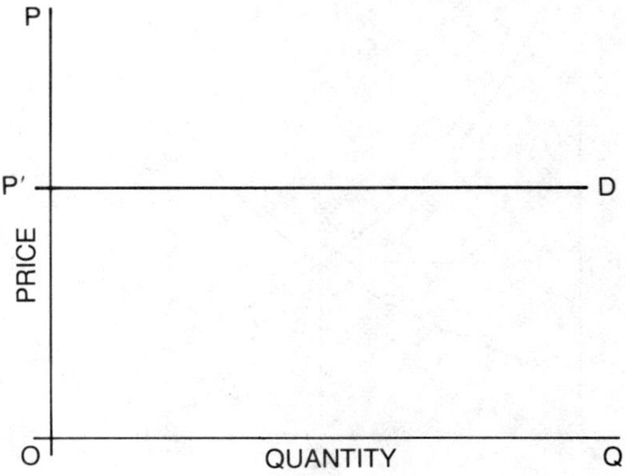

Figure 11–5. A perfectly elastic demand curve. Perfect elasticity means that demand at P′ is infinite and that above P′ it is zero.

Perfect Competition

Medical and dental care are often discussed in terms of "free enterprise" or "perfect competition."* There are four basic requirements for perfect competition.[30] First, the product of one seller must be the same as the product of any other seller. In other words, a silver amalgam restoration or a complete denture from one dentist would have to be identical to the same service from another dentist.

Second, each buyer (patient) or seller (dentist) must represent so small a part of the total market that he or she cannot individually affect the price. This requirement means that the demand curve that any dentist would face would be horizontal (Fig. 11–5). The dentist would find demand for a given service to be infinite up to and including the prevailing fee (P′) for a given service. If an individual dentist charged a higher fee, no one would purchase care from that dentist.

The third requirement of perfect competition is that all resources are completely mobile. This requirement means that the supply of professional personnel must be easy to increase or decrease. There would be no barrier to entry into the professions, such as a shortage of training positions, licensing examinations, or restrictions on the delegation of duties to auxiliary personnel.

Fourth, perfect competition would require that all people involved, both dental professionals and patients, have complete information about prices (fees), needs, all alternative treatments, and all possible outcomes. If all of the requirements for perfect competition were met, the supply and demand curves (Figs. 11–3 and 11–4) would combine to define an equilibrium price (P′) and quantity (Q′) as shown graphically in Figure 11–6. This equilibrium is the point at which the available supply is exhausted and all who are willing to pay the price have been able to buy the quantity they desire. (Note, however, that while this equilibrium balances supply and demand, it says nothing about need [professionally defined] or wants [consumer defined]).

*For further elaboration of the "free enterprise" concept, see Chapter 13.

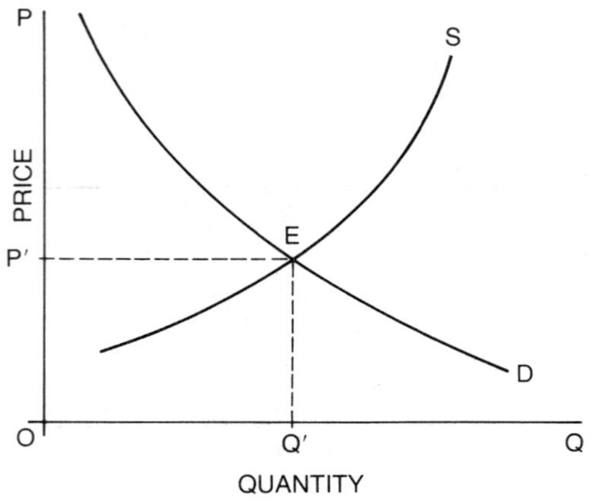

Figure 11–6. Equilibrium (E) of demand and supply.

It should be obvious that no market, including the market for dental care, is perfectly competitive. Obviously there are numerous ways in which the dental care market and health care in general do not meet the definition of a perfectly competitive market.

Deviations of Medical and Dental Care from Perfect Competition

The health care market possesses some characteristics that distinguish it from the perfect competition model. Among these characteristics is the fact that many of the consumer demands on the individual level are irregular and unpredictable. The individual consumer (patient) usually can only guess about his or her future needs (and for an individual patient, a dental professional doesn't have a much better guess). Perfect knowledge of needs and alternative treatment is thus rarely met in the instances of both medical and dental care. Both professions historically have also had limitations on advertising (and until recently rather severe limitations), which have further restricted the flow of knowledge.

Another characteristic, which may be viewed as an extension of the problem of limited information available to or on the part of the patient, is the phenomenon of provider-originated demand. Once the patient has decided to make the initial contact with the provider, the provider plays a major role in determining which specific services will be consumed. Once in the dental operatory, patients rarely are given the chance to choose among possible alternative treatments or to choose how much of a given treatment is appropriate unless they insist.

Further similarities between medicine and dentistry are found in the nature of the supply of care. In both medicine and dentistry there are limitations to the entry of practitioners because of educational and licensing requirements. There are also limitations on the use of auxiliary personnel.

No moral judgment is necessarily implied concerning these deviations from perfect competition. Because of these deviations, however, the balance of supply and demand (equilibrium) that is the result of a perfectly competitive market may not be achieved.

Differences between Medicine and Dentistry

Although there are many similarities between medicine and dentistry, there are also important differences. One of the most important of these differences is that whereas medical care is sometimes mandated for survival, survival is rarely the concern of dentistry—although the quality of life is. This difference translates into differences in the effects of personal income and price on the use of services. Given a combination of low income and high fees for care, dental care is more likely to be neglected than is medical care. Furthermore, as incomes increase or fees go down, the use of dental services will increase at a faster rate than the use of medical services (Figs. 11–7 and 11–8). Thus, the dental market is more responsive to changing economic conditions than the medical market. These phenomena have special significance in light of the growth of prepayment for dental care, and bring to the forefront the question of how much is "enough" dental care. Because the use of dental services is likely to increase as the apparent out-of-pocket price of a service drops, patients covered by prepayment will use services that they would not use if they had to pay part or all of services directly out-of-pocket themselves. To illustrate, if patients were offered a $15 service at no charge, they would more likely use that service more often than if they had to pay out-of-pocket for it. In addition, if they were offered $15 in cash or the $15 service, they would on occasion take the cash instead of the service. In other words, the $15 service is sometimes not worth $15 in the minds of patients.

An additional dilemma may arise with prepayment, because when the plan covers the fee for the service, dental providers do not directly affect the

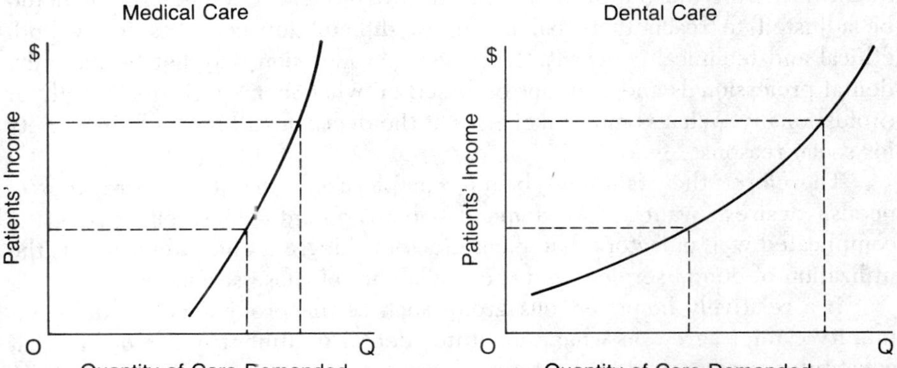

Figure 11–7. Income-to-quantity relation for medical and dental care demand. (Quantity axes are not to scale.)

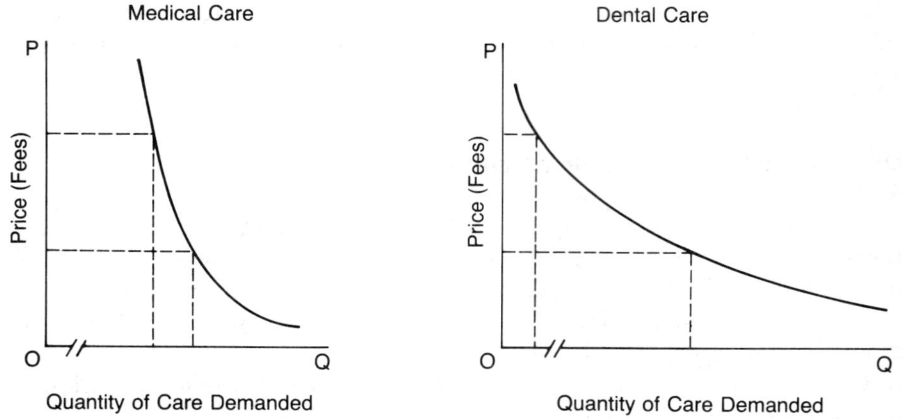

Figure 11–8. Price-to-quantity relation for medical and dental care demand. (Quantity axes are not to scale.)

covered patient when they raise their fees. The fee may become higher than the patient would ordinarily pay, but because a third party is covering the fee, the patient will continue to consume the service. Such fee increases may also have a profound effect on the patients who are not covered by prepayment. Because many patients do not see dental services as mandatory, patients not covered by prepayment may seek fewer of these services as fees increase (see demand curve, Fig. 11–4).

Although far from complete, the preceding discussion has pointed out that the deviations of the dental care market from perfect competition, the likely influence of prepayment on utilization, and the differences between demand, need, and wants all combine to make a single definition of the "right" or "proper" amount of dental care impossible. The quantity of care that dental professionals say people need, the quantity of care that patients feel they need, and the quantity of care that the market will provide, given its imperfections, are all likely to be different. Deciding which among these quantities is the most appropriate one to provide and how the system should be adjusted to reach that goal is a most difficult job complicated by both ethical and technical concerns. Moreover, the decision may not be made by dental professionals and may not be based on what seems right technically or professionally. What is more likely is that the decision will be made by society for social reasons.

Therefore, the statement bears reemphasizing that the entire area of needs, desires, wants, and demands—both potential and effective—is a complicated web of factors that affect in various degrees and interrelations the utilization of dental services and the availability of those services.

If a relatively homogeneous group such as the professional dental community cannot agree on what constitutes dental treatment needs or on what constitutes recommended treatment, one can see that introducing patients into the decision-making process will create additional confusion. And, in their stead, if patients are not the direct out-of-pocket purchasers of the care, the third-party payers are introduced into the equation to include their definitions and perceptions of need, and the treatment available to satisfy that need; then one can see that that complicated web begins to get even more tangled. The potential patient, for example, could well perceive a dental need that he or she has (or his or her child may have) and yet see no way that that need could be reasonably met. For example, a low- or even moderate-income parent might just plain feel that there is no way his or her child is going to get to the dental office—much as he or she feels the child should get there. The care may not be readily available or accessible, or there may not seem to be any conceivable way to pay for it. Given a felt need, a remedy might be rejected because the cost of that remedy is too high, not necessarily in dollars, but in pain, inconvenience, or a temporary poor appearance. If the potential patient believes that the cure is worse than the disease, even if the need for treatment is recognized, the treatment may not be realized.

Associated with this perceived need may be a complete unwillingness or reluctance to give voice to that perceived need, because of either a sense of futility or shame or some other reason. Unless scientifically oriented survey researchers actually go out and probe and measure and listen, potential demand may be greatly underestimated regardless of whether that potential demand is related to any scientific professional determination of treatment need according to generally accepted standards.

One can begin to see that the professional assessment of treatment needs and the patients' assessments of their own needs are closely related to eventual utilization. A host of interrelated factors (to be considered in more detail in the balance of this chapter) all bear upon treatment needs, demands, and utilization of dental services. It would seem, therefore, that the dental professional, if one is to make any kind of sense of these factors, will have to become knowledgeable about them and their interactions.

TREATMENT NEEDS

Epidemiological Estimation of Treatment Needs

In Section II, The Assessment of the Problem of Oral Diseases, two chapters, 5 and 6, were necessary to list the methods for assessing oral diseases and describing the distribution of oral disease patterns in population groups. One might assume that if one can assess, determine, and describe the level of disease patterns in groups of people, one ought to be able to project the *treatment* needs based upon that assessment of disease pattern. In some respects, it might even seem easy that if one can measure "decayed, missing, and filled teeth" (DMF), one certainly ought to be able to state that decayed teeth ought to be filled, that missing teeth for the most part should be replaced, and that filled teeth (other than for a periodic checkup to see that they are in good condition) probably are "okay," at least as far as dental caries goes. Not so; it is a quantum leap from an epidemiological survey of a group for purposes of describing the disease and in what patterns it occurs in that group to the determination of what the adequate estimates for treatment needs in that group might be—for example, for third-party prepayment plans for actuarial purposes. Perhaps one day sufficient experience and the availability of electronic data processing will provide procedures that will allow projections of treatment need based on prior experience with large population groups and their patterns of disease occurrence. So far those projections have not been made.[28]

North Carolina Study

An entire book[3] was devoted to reporting the dental conditions and predictions of the dental situation in North Carolina, the dental status of North Carolinians, and the needed dental personnel. One chapter in the book discussed the prediction of treatment needs from epidemiological data. That chapter[28] was only about one and one-half pages in length and concluded by saying, in part, "This problem of using epidemiological data to develop treatment needs estimates exists as the major 'missing link' in the information required for dental manpower planning." Nevertheless, Chapter 10[44] of that book took 50 pages to estimate the need for dental care and dental health manpower in North Carolina.

The researchers used data from the North Carolina Dental Disease Prevalence Survey, from NHANES I (discussed elsewhere in this chapter), and from a variety of other sources to make their estimates. They felt that their analyses permitted them at least to judge that:

1. Even though the condition of edentulism is widespread and many persons are in need of full or partial dentures, North Carolina dentists are meeting the demand, and most (i.e., 95 percent) of the need, for this kind of care.
2. Demand for restorative care appropriate to the treatment of dental caries is much lower than the epidemiological data on need would indicate as desirable. North Carolina general dentists are able to treat in one year about 30 percent of the existing buildup of decay among the State's population as well as the annual occurrence of new decay. Thus there does not appear to be a need for additional dentists to provide for restorative dental care.
3. Periodontal disease is a widespread dental health problem in North Carolina that has not been given appropriate attention and emphasis by the general public and deserves further attention from the dental profession. Given the current volume of periodontal dental services provided by North Carolina dentists, the prevalence of periodontal disease in the State represents an accumulation of untreated disease over several decades. General dentists could easily treat the newly occurring periodontal disease and some of the untreated backlog. Periodontists in North Carolina are treating 14 percent of the advanced periodontal disease. This figure represents the effective demand, as opposed to the total need for, advanced periodontal therapy. But the real problem is one of stimulating a greater level of public awareness

of the severity of the disease and a pattern of seeking care at an earlier period in the course of the disease.
4. The demand for preventive dental care services (including periodic examinations, prophylaxes, and fluoride treatments) is approximately 15 to 20 percent of the recommended standard of care.

It must be emphasized that the researchers stated that this analysis was ". . . a very subjective process necessarily based on many assumptions."

Of course, a couple of epidemiological indices perhaps are misnamed and are not epidemiological indices (except as they deal with the epidemiology of health services). They are the TPI or Treatment Priority Index of Grainger,[17] which relates to malocclusion, and the HLD or Handicapping Labio-lingual Deviation index of Draker,[12] which also deals with orthodontic treatment needs. For the most part, however, epidemiological indices of dental disease almost by definition will provide little help in determining treatment needs. Also, most clinicians would be uncomfortable relying upon what they perceive as rapidly applied indices to large groups of people in a short period of time in a kind of screening process for purposes of determining specific treatment needs. The indices were not designed to do so nor, as indicated previously, should they be used for that purpose.

Mass Inspections

It is perhaps appropriate here to discuss the apparently fallacious reasoning behind mass dental inspections and screenings in the schools for purposes of "finding out whether Jane or Johnny has a 'cavity' and needs to go to the dentist." This rapid type of mass inspection—frequently given under the poorest of conditions, often in the auditorium or gymnasium or on the stage while a basketball game is going on nearby—is in no way to be confused with scientific epidemiological surveys conducted for describing the distribution of diseases within large populations. At worst, they simply tell the child or the child's parent that the cavity that was looked at last year is bigger this year, or they get the screening dental professional in a conflict with the private dentist. At best, they may serve as a form of triage to sort out the students badly in need of care and get them to the dentist. (And they probably knew they needed to go before the screening.)

Estimating Treatment Needs

Spencer[46] presented four different approaches to obtaining estimates of need for dental care. He first defined "normative need," which is the requirement for care as determined by expert opinion; "perceived need," which is the requirement for care as determined by the patient or the public; "demand for health care," which arises out of attempts by members of the public to seek attention for their perceived needs; and, finally, "utilization," which is the actual attendance by members of the public at health care facilities to receive care. Need for dental care may be divided into three parts: diagnostic needs; preventive needs; and disease-, disability-, or dysfunction-oriented needs. Whereas such a division is somewhat arbitrary, it does indicate that need is more than just palliative or reparative treatment for disease states. It is conceded that the estimation of diagnostic and preventive needs cannot be addressed because a critical approach to their estimation is presently lacking. The estimation of need for dental care that arises from diseases, disabilities, or dysfunction may be labeled as initial backlog or incremental needs. The four different approaches to estimating need are differentiated by the basic sources of data: (1) surveys of dental status, (2) surveys of need for dental care, (3) analyses of service or treatment records, and (4) the best judgment of dental practitioners. The surveys, of course, constitute the epidemiological approach, which has already been mentioned as having its limitations.

Spencer, while recognizing the limitations of the survey or epidemiological approach, does point out that Bulman and colleagues[4] were able to generate estimates of restorative and exodontic needs in their study of demand and need for dental care in England from the charting of dental caries through the DMFT index. In further analyses of attempts to translate epidemiological indices into treatment needs, one might conclude in general that the field epidemiologist tends to underestimate the treatment needs at least in comparison to the clinician. Epidemiologists have long been taught: "When in doubt, don't count it." Clinicians when in doubt tend to go ahead in a cautious approach and restore or treat the problem. In Spencer's analysis of surveys of need for dental care per se, he concluded that the chief problem was that the criteria are not well developed and that internationally no set of criteria is currently recommended.

Spencer judged—and correctly so—that the records from dental health programs that operate on any semblance of an organized basis have not been used sufficiently in planning or evaluation. The retrospective review of records that are sufficiently comprehensive and comprehensible to permit the extraction of useful information from them is likely the most worthwhile way to estimate future needs. The work of Bader and colleagues[2] in Appalachia is a good example.

A major problem with the data from these groups is that they are rarely comparable between groups; that is, one cannot compare one group with another, because their definitions of terms and their records are not standardized. Another shortcoming, of course, is that these groups are far from representative of the population of the United States, and thus one cannot necessarily generalize from those groups to larger or other populations. At best, the findings from those groups can only be reported. Another major qualification is that the people in these groups are indeed people who *do* go to dentists at least occasionally and do not necessarily reflect the people who *do not* usually go to dentists.

The potential of third-party dental insurance carriers who could make available summaries of service records in the form of profiles of patient need for dental care has not been realized. The problems in obtaining such data from third-party carriers are discussed later in this chapter.

Surveys of Dental Status and Dental Needs

One can nevertheless use epidemiological data, especially those obtained from the National Health Survey of the U.S. Public Health Service (USPHS). The National Center for Health Statistics (NCHS) is an agency of the USPHS established in 1956 by an Act of Congress with the mandate for monitoring the health status of the American people. The NCHS carries out this function in several ways, one of which is to survey and interview representative samples of the population in a number of health areas, including dentistry. Dental surveys, as part of the National Health Survey, were carried out with adults in 1960–62, children aged 6–11 in 1963–65, and youths aged 12–17 in 1966–70. The addition of a diet/nutrition survey to the health examination survey resulted in the first National Health and Nutrition Examination Survey (NHANES I) in 1971–74.

Data from these surveys can be used to gain some idea of dental disease and dental disease conditions and at least two types of dental treatment already rendered—restorations and extractions (at least as estimated from the "M" and "F" components of the DMF index). Of course, the sheer magnitude of the amount of dental disease, dental conditions requiring treatment, and estimates of treatment already rendered is staggering. This continuous survey has already been cited frequently in Chapter 6. Data from these continuing surveys are displayed in Figures 6–4, 6–5, 6–6, 6–10, and 6–11. The surveys (references 131–140 of Chapter 6) are carried out on a regular basis and have had dental advisers and a dental component. They have most frequently examined DMF rates, periodontal disease rates, malocclusion, oral cancer, and interview reports from samples of the populations surveyed concerning their dentist-going behavior. These surveys have been carried on now for two decades, and patterns are beginning to emerge for various demographic variables such as age group, sex, ethnic group, and geographic area of the country.

National Health and Nutrition Examination Survey I (NHANES I)

A summary of the important findings to date as they apply to *dental treatment needs* from the dental examinations of the first National Health and Nutrition Examination Survey (NHANES I) is reported here.[50] The findings are based on examinations by 10 dentists during the years 1971–74 for approximately 20,000 people between the ages of 1 and 74. The 20,000 people who were examined were part of a carefully planned probability sample of the civilian noninstitutionalized population within the coterminous United States, at 65 survey locations. A dental examination was given to the entire sample. The dental examiners attempted to derive their findings as carefully and as uniformly as possible by following a written set of objective standards that had been carefully prepared in an attempt to reduce examiner variability. The dental examiners, using their best clinical judgment, estimated the kind and amount of dental treatment "required" by every person examined. In so

Table 11–1. Percent of Persons Aged 1–74 Years with Specific Dental Treatment Needs, by Age and Sex, with Standard Errors, United States, 1971–74*

Specific Dental Treatment Needed	Total	1–5 Years	6–11 Years	12–17 Years	18–44 Years	45–64 Years	65–74 Years	Total	1–5 Years	6–11 Years	12–17 Years	18–44 Years	45–64 Years	65–74 Years
Both Sexes	*Percent*							*Standard Error*						
General (at least one of the following)	64.1	16.6	63.5	67.5	72.7	67.5	61.0	1.31	1.05	2.15	1.71	1.44	2.14	2.02
Removal of debris and calculus	19.1	2.4	28.2	27.5	22.4	13.5	8.4	1.34	0.61	2.82	2.32	1.51	1.34	1.06
Gingivitis treatment	8.9	0.0	1.9	13.4	13.8	6.9	3.5	0.67	0.01	0.33	1.18	1.05	0.77	0.67
Periodontal disease treatment	10.1	0.0	0.1	2.0	12.2	19.3	15.4	0.42	0.02	0.09	0.43	0.73	1.18	0.92
Severe malocclusion treatment	2.0	0.1	6.4	7.1	0.9	—	—	0.18	0.07	0.89	0.75	0.19	—	—
Decay treatment—permanent and primary teeth	41.1	16.1	52.7	53.6	49.3	30.1	17.9	1.12	1.03	2.14	1.53	1.55	1.50	0.77
Extractions, any reason	4.8	0.1	0.4	0.6	5.8	8.4	9.8	0.31	0.07	0.21	0.15	0.54	0.76	0.73
Fixed bridges and/or partials	16.0	—	0.1	5.8	25.3	23.3	9.5	0.93	—	0.11	0.81	1.35	1.91	0.97
Repair denture or bridge	2.7	—	—	0.0	1.9	6.7	7.7	0.25	—	—	0.02	0.22	0.80	0.74
Construct full denture	6.6	—	0.0	0.1	4.2	15.6	24.8	0.34	—	0.01	0.08	0.41	1.08	1.44
Male														
General (at least one of the following)	67.5	17.1	66.5	68.4	76.9	72.3	68.2	1.36	1.41	2.60	2.02	1.67	2.33	2.15
Removal of debris and calculus	20.8	2.2	30.6	25.8	24.9	15.7	9.7	1.47	0.56	3.08	2.40	1.76	1.58	1.15
Gingivitis treatment	10.6	0.0	2.1	17.1	16.4	7.6	3.5	0.87	0.02	0.62	1.86	1.37	1.14	0.62
Periodontal disease treatment	11.8	—	0.2	2.1	14.5	22.9	19.6	0.52	—	0.17	0.56	1.02	1.55	1.57
Severe malocclusion treatment	2.3	—	6.4	7.9	1.2	—	—	0.24	—	1.06	1.15	0.32	—	—
Decay treatment—permanent and primary teeth	43.7	16.7	55.2	52.2	52.4	33.7	21.3	1.26	1.42	2.68	1.76	1.94	2.12	1.20
Extractions, any reason	5.3	0.2	0.5	0.5	6.2	9.8	12.2	0.40	0.13	0.28	0.24	0.69	1.15	1.01
Fixed bridges and/or partials	15.4	—	0.3	5.2	24.0	23.4	9.8	1.03	—	0.21	0.89	1.67	2.29	1.18
Repair denture or bridge	2.5	—	—	—	1.7	6.3	7.8	0.26	—	—	—	0.34	0.89	0.96
Construct full denture	6.7	—	—	—	4.0	16.2	29.1	0.47	—	0.02	—	0.59	1.51	1.93
Female														
General (at least one of the following)	61.0	16.1	60.5	66.4	68.9	63.1	55.5	1.42	1.30	2.59	2.42	1.53	2.70	2.23
Removal of debris and calculus	17.6	2.7	25.8	29.3	20.1	11.4	7.5	1.33	0.85	3.06	2.77	1.49	1.64	1.34
Gingivitis treatment	7.4	—	1.7	9.6	11.5	6.2	3.5	0.57	—	0.44	1.42	0.94	0.78	0.86
Periodontal treatment	8.6	0.0	0.1	1.9	10.1	16.0	12.1	0.49	0.04	0.05	0.47	0.70	1.47	0.98
Severe malocclusion treatment	1.8	0.2	6.4	6.2	0.7	—	—	0.21	0.14	1.15	0.90	0.14	—	—
Decay treatment—permanent and primary teeth	38.7	15.5	50.1	55.0	46.4	26.9	15.2	1.19	1.33	2.55	2.05	1.62	1.72	1.14
Extractions, any reason	4.4	—	0.4	0.6	5.5	7.1	8.0	0.34	—	0.24	0.27	0.54	0.82	0.93
Fixed bridges and/or partials	16.7	—	0.0	6.3	26.5	23.2	7.5	0.93	—	0.03	1.13	1.26	2.01	1.03
Repair denture or bridge	3.0	—	—	0.0	2.1	7.1	7.7	0.32	—	—	0.04	0.26	1.07	0.93
Construct full denture	6.6	—	—	0.2	4.4	15.0	21.6	0.40	—	—	0.17	0.42	1.29	1.56

*U.S. Public Health Service.[50]

doing, the status of oral hygiene and periodontal disease, the amount and adequacy of past dental care, and responses to questions at the beginning of the examination about chewing and eating difficulties were taken into consideration. The treatment recommendations could range anywhere from a simple procedure of placing a restoration in one surface of a tooth to extraction of all remaining teeth and denture construction.

Unfortunately, additional information that was elicited by interview questionnaire about the interviewees' self-perceived needs for dental care has not yet been analyzed. It would be most fascinating to correlate those self-perceived needs with what the examiners reported that they actually found, especially in consideration of Figure 11–2.

A brief summary indicates that almost 15 percent of the adult population aged 18–74 had lost all of their permanent teeth and an additional almost 10 percent had lost all of their upper or lower teeth. More women than men had two edentulous arches and more had only one edentulous arch. For more detailed information on decayed, missing, and filled teeth, periodontal disease status, and oral hygiene status, see Chapter 6, The Epidemiology of Oral Diseases.

As estimated by the examiners, almost 65 percent of the population "required" dental treatment of one type or another. More males than females needed at least one type of dental service, 67.5 percent versus 61 percent (see Table 11–1). Over 40 percent of the people needed at least one filling, with a range of a low of 16 percent for children aged 1–5 to a high of about 53 percent of children aged 6–17. Table 11–2 shows the average number per person of one-surface and two-surface restorations and restorations involving three surfaces or more that were needed by those who needed at least one filling. About one out of every 20 people needed to have at least one tooth extracted. The average number of teeth that needed to be extracted because of decay rose only slightly with increasing age, but as one might expect, the number needed to be extracted because of periodontal diseases and other reasons (usually prosthetic considerations) rose sharply with age.

Of course one can quibble about whether the 10 dentists who did the examinations for this survey would agree with 10 dentists from other parts of the country or graduates of other dental schools, or wonder if they were using different methods or standards. Nevertheless, these data are the best available on a nationwide probability sample, and they do give an indication of the treatment needs of a cross section of the population in 1971–74.

National Institute of Dental Research's Nationwide Survey of Schoolchildren

The most recent nationwide survey[52] carried out in a scientific fashion studied the dental caries prevalence of United States schoolchildren 5–17 years of age in 1979 and 1980. This study was conducted by the National Caries Program of the National Institute of Dental Research (NIDR). It was carried out using a national sample and with calibrated examiners. A summary of the key findings reports that the estimated caries prevalence in permanent teeth

Table 11–2. Average Number of 1-, 2-, and 3-Surface Fillings Needed to Restore the Permanent Teeth of Those Persons Aged 1–74 Years Who Need at Least One Filling, by Race, Sex, and Age, with Standard Errors, United States, 1971–74*

Sex and Age	1-Surface Fillings Total†	1-Surface White	1-Surface Black	2-Surface Fillings Total†	2-Surface White	2-Surface Black	3-Surface Fillings Total†	3-Surface White	3-Surface Black
				Average Number of Fillings					
Both Sexes									
All ages, 1–74 years	1.8	1.7	2.2	0.6	0.6	0.8	0.3	0.4	0.3
1–5 years	0.9	0.5	1.3	0.6	0.9	0.3	—	—	—
6–11 years	1.6	1.6	1.6	0.5	0.5	0.5	0.1	0.1	0.1
12–17 years	2.5	2.4	2.8	0.6	0.6	0.8	0.2	0.2	0.3
18–44 years	1.9	1.8	2.6	0.7	0.6	1.0	0.4	0.4	0.4
45–64 years	1.1	1.1	1.1	0.5	0.5	0.6	0.4	0.5	0.2
65–74 years	0.7	0.7	0.7	0.4	0.4	0.3	0.3	0.3	0.1
Male									
All ages, 1–74 years	1.8	1.7	2.2	0.6	0.6	0.8	0.3	0.4	0.3
1–5 years	0.6	0.5	1.0	0.8	1.0	—	—	—	—
6–11 years	1.5	1.5	1.6	0.5	0.5	0.6	0.1	0.1	0.0
12–17 years	2.4	2.3	2.7	0.6	0.5	1.0	0.2	0.2	0.3
18–44 years	1.9	1.8	2.6	0.7	0.6	1.0	0.4	0.4	0.4
45–64 years	1.1	1.1	1.0	0.6	0.6	0.6	0.4	0.5	0.1
65–74 years	0.6	0.7	0.7	0.5	0.6	0.2	0.3	0.3	0.2
Female									
All ages, 1–74 years	1.8	1.7	2.2	0.6	0.5	0.9	0.4	0.4	0.3
1–5 years	1.4	1.0	1.4	0.4	—	0.4	—	—	—
6–11 years	1.6	1.6	1.6	0.4	0.4	0.4	0.1	0.1	0.2
12–17 years	2.5	2.5	2.8	0.6	0.6	0.7	0.2	0.2	0.2
18–44 years	1.9	1.8	2.5	0.7	0.6	1.1	0.4	0.4	0.4
45–64 years	1.1	1.1	1.2	0.5	0.4	0.6	0.4	0.5	0.2
65–74 years	0.7	0.7	0.6	0.3	0.3	0.5	0.3	0.3	0.1

				Standard Error					
Both Sexes									
All ages, 1–74 years	0.06	0.06	0.10	0.02	0.02	0.06	0.02	0.02	0.03
1–5 years	0.38	0.42	0.39	0.40	0.82	0.34	—	—	—
6–11 years	0.07	0.09	0.13	0.04	0.05	0.11	0.02	0.02	0.05
12–17 years	0.09	0.10	0.18	0.05	0.05	0.11	0.02	0.03	0.05
18–44 years	0.08	0.08	0.15	0.03	0.03	0.10	0.02	0.03	0.06
45–64 years	0.08	0.08	0.15	0.05	0.05	0.09	0.05	0.06	0.04
65–74 years	0.06	0.07	0.11	0.06	0.07	0.06	0.03	0.04	0.04
Male									
All ages, 1–74 years	0.06	0.07	0.13	0.03	0.03	0.09	0.02	0.02	0.04
1–5 years	0.38	0.43	0.71	0.62	0.87	—	—	—	—
6–11 years	0.09	0.10	0.18	0.07	0.09	0.13	0.03	0.04	0.01
12–17 years	0.09	0.11	0.19	0.06	0.06	0.15	0.03	0.03	0.09
18–44 years	0.10	0.11	0.25	0.04	0.04	0.14	0.03	0.03	0.09
45–64 years	0.11	0.11	0.20	0.08	0.09	0.11	0.05	0.06	0.03
65–74 years	0.07	0.09	0.15	0.11	0.14	0.05	0.05	0.06	0.07
Female									
All ages, 1–74	0.06	0.07	0.13	0.03	0.02	0.07	0.02	0.03	0.04
1–5 years	0.47	0.71	0.61	0.36	—	0.39	—	—	—
6–11 years	0.10	0.12	0.19	0.07	0.07	0.15	0.02	0.02	0.10
12–17 years	0.14	0.15	0.35	0.06	0.06	0.12	0.02	0.03	0.05
18–44 years	0.07	0.07	0.16	0.03	0.03	0.11	0.03	0.03	0.06
45–64 years	0.09	0.09	0.19	0.05	0.05	0.14	0.06	0.07	0.09
65–74 years	0.08	0.09	0.17	0.05	0.05	0.12	0.06	0.07	0.04

*U.S. Public Health Service.[50]

†Includes data for other races, which are not shown separately.

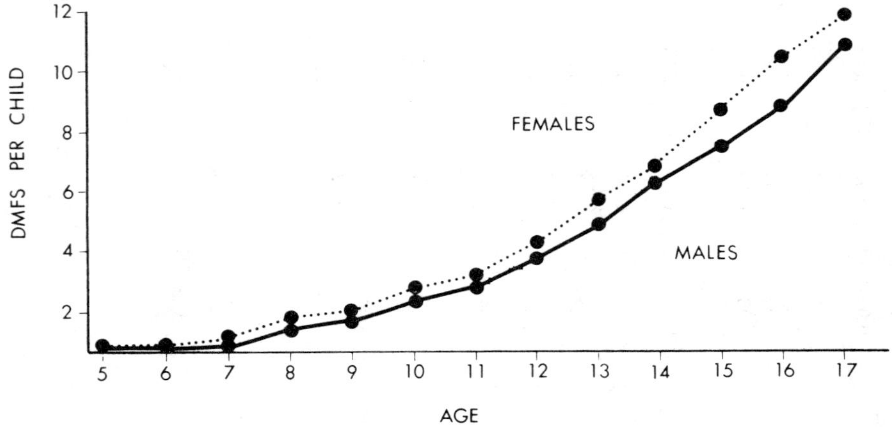

Figure 11–9. Age and sex specific prevalence of dental caries in permanent teeth for United States, 1979–1980. (From U.S. Public Health Service, National Institutes of Health, National Institute of Dental Research, National Caries Program. The prevalence of dental caries in United States children, 1979–1980; the national dental caries prevalence survey. NIH Publ. No. 82–2245. Washington, D.C., Government Printing Office, 1981. iv + 159 p.)

for some 45.3 million schoolchildren aged 5–17 in the United States was 4.77 decayed, missing, or filled tooth surfaces (DMFS) per child and some 2.91 DMF teeth. Over half of the disease was found in occlusal surfaces. By the age of 12 the children had an average of 4 DMF surfaces and by the age of 17 each child had over 11 DMF surfaces.

Again, females were found to have slightly higher caries prevalence (see Fig. 11–9), which bore out the findings of previous surveys. Some 16.7 million schoolchildren aged 5–9 were estimated to have an average of 5.31 decayed or filled primary surfaces (dfs) and 2.55 df primary teeth per child, with the children aged 5 having on average over 4 df surfaces—all in the primary dentition.

Significant was the finding that almost 17 million—over 36 percent of the some 45 million children represented in the study—were estimated to be completely caries free. At the other extreme, some 3.5 million children—almost 8 percent—had 9 or more DMF permanent teeth (see Fig. 11–10).

White children had slightly more caries experience (4.89 DMFS per child) than children of other races (4.15 DMFS per child).

The scientists analyzing the data from this survey attempted to estimate the amount of unmet need for restorative dental care by examining the components of the DMFS index, made up of D, M, and F, respectively. They found that in this survey almost 17 percent of the DMF surfaces were classified as decayed and unfilled (D), whereas over 75 percent had been restored by dental treatment (F). Only about 7 percent of permanent tooth surfaces had been extracted because of caries (M). Their judgment was that evidently the level of restorative dental care among schoolchildren in the United States is rather high, but they did not say what the basis of comparison was.

The analysts proceeded then to compare their findings from this NIDR

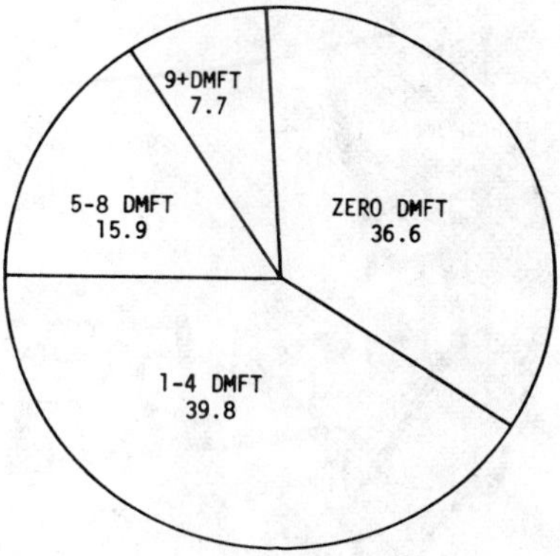

Figure 11–10. Percent distribution of United States children according to DMFT status, 1979–1980. (From U.S. Public Health Service, National Institutes of Health, National Institute of Dental Research, National Caries Program. The prevalence of dental caries in United States children, 1979–1980; the national dental caries prevalence survey. NIH Publ. No. 82–2245. Washington, D.C., Government Printing Office, 1981. iv + 159 p.)

national prevalence survey of dental caries in children with the data reported by the NHANES I for 1971–74.[50] The findings are shown in Table 11–3. Although they recognized that the data for the two surveys cannot be compared exactly, the surveys they reported were sufficiently similar in design, they felt, to warrant attempting some comparisons of the changes in caries prevalence during the interval of approximately eight years. They concluded that caries prevalence (see Table 11–3) underwent a substantial decrease during this time period for each age studied, although they added the disclaimer that ". . . quantitative statements about the magnitude of this decrease cannot be confidently made from these data."

Table 11–3. Mean DMFS for United States Children Aged 5–17 from the 1971–73 National Center for Health Statistics Survey and the 1979–80 National Institute of Dental Research Survey*

	NCHS† 1971–73		**NIDR 1979–80**	
Age	*Number in Thousands‡*	*Mean DMFS*	*Number in Thousands‡*	*Mean DMFS*
5	1,068	0.15	1,055	0.11
6	2,825	0.41	2,750	0.20
7	3,704	0.69	3,525	0.58
8	3,661	1.86	3,453	1.25
9	4,036	3.59	3,420	1.90
10	4,378	4.14	3,515	2.60
11	4,088	4.58	3,479	3.00
12	4,116	6.36	3,601	4.18
13	4,153	8.67	3,822	5.41
14	4,046	9.60	4,063	6.53
15	4,256	11.67	4,171	8.07
16	4,164	15.12	4,195	9.58
17	3,898	16.90	4,267	11.04
All Ages	48,393	7.06	45,315	4.77

*U.S. Public Health Service.[52]

†Decayed, missing, and filled surfaces among children. National Health Survey, 1971–1974. NHANES I special dental tape, National Center for Health Statistics, June 1978. Unpublished.

‡Sample weighted to represent total U.S. children.

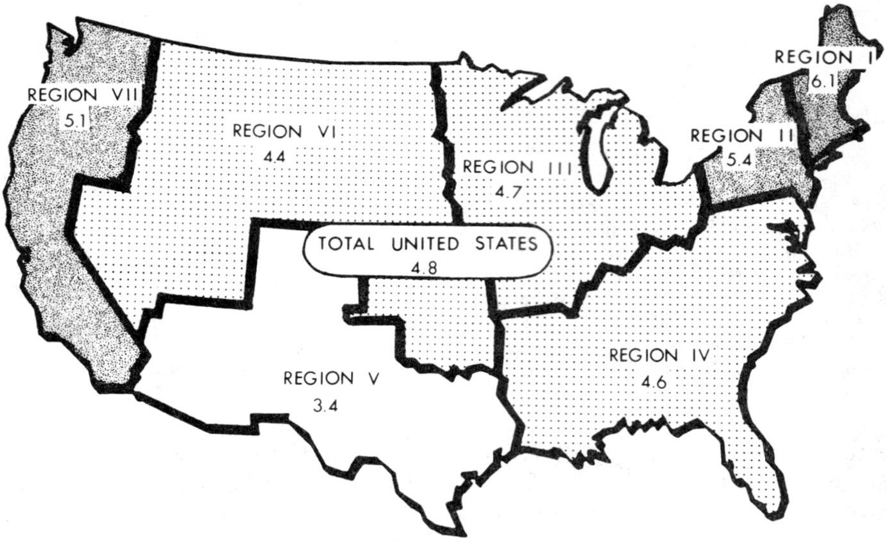

Figure 11–11. Mean DMFS for United States children by geographic region, 1979–1980. (From U.S. Public Health Service, National Institutes of Health, National Institute of Dental Research, National Caries Program. The prevalence of dental caries in United States children, 1979–1980; the national dental caries prevalence survey. NIH Publ. No. 82–2245. Washington, D.C., Government Printing Office, 1981. iv + 159 p.)

In addition, the survey pointed up that there are clearly regional differences in the attack rates of dental caries in children and thus it is likely that treatment patterns would vary accordingly. Figure 11–11 shows the regional distribution of dental caries by mean DMFS. Again, as with the findings from the World War II examinations of recruits on intake into the military, the Northeast Region and the Far West displayed the highest attack rates. Most likely if California had been broken out, the high attack rate would have been in the Northwest. Once again the children from the Southwest displayed the lowest dental caries attack rates, with almost half of them (44.7 percent) experiencing no dental caries whatsoever (see Fig. 11–12 and Fig. 6–4).

Their analysis also goes on to break out urban versus rural children in the various regions and points up that there are differences, as might be expected, with the children in rural areas having the higher DMFS experience. With the exception of the Northeast (the Boston area was not fluoridated until 1978), children in the urban areas had a slightly lower DMFS experience.

As might be expected, the Northeast and the Far West, with the highest total DMFS experience, had the highest number of filled surfaces per child. The proportion of DMF surfaces that had been restored was highest in the Far West and in the West Central states to the north. Those two areas also had the lowest proportion of extracted permanent tooth surfaces, whereas the Southeast had the highest number and proportion of extracted permanent

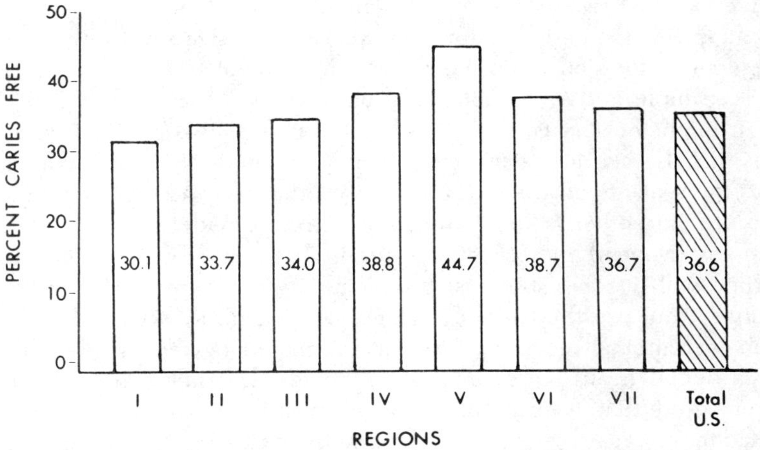

Figure 11–12. Percent of United States children who were caries free, by geographic region, 1979–1980. (From U.S. Public Health Service, National Institutes of Health, National Institute of Dental Research, National Caries Program. The prevalence of dental caries in United States children, 1979–1980; the national dental caries prevalence survey. NIH Publ. No. 82–2245. Washington, D.C., Government Printing Office, 1981. iv + 159 p.)

tooth surfaces. Thus one can observe that whereas treatment patterns tend to follow the disease patterns, they do not do so uniformly. Other influences, such as cultural factors, must be coming into play.

In addition, these findings tend to confirm those discussed in Chapter 6 about the changing patterns of dental disease not only throughout the United States but throughout the world. These changing patterns of attack rates cannot help but affect the demand for dental care and the subsequent treatment patterns—and eventually they may change the character of dental practices and public programs in those areas affected.[6, 18]

The reader is encouraged to review Chapter 6, The Epidemiology of Oral Diseases, when examining this chapter and to consider the difficulty of interpreting epidemiological findings and extrapolating from them in order to estimate treatment needs.

Initial versus Maintenance Needs

Two concepts in relation to treatment needs and the associated concept of incremental maintenance care need yet to be explored. Logically, the regularity and frequency with which one receives adequate dental care would or should decrease the amount of needs that one might accumulate over a lifetime. Quite simply, if the first carious lesion one developed were found early and restored early, the broken-down tooth with perhaps a subsequent exposure and extensive dental treatment would be avoided—or so the argument goes. Again, this argument does not always hold from a strictly cost-effective basis. There are those who argue that in a patient with a high caries attack rate the "too early" restoration of a carious fissure will only require its subsequent restoration when the associated proximal area becomes carious. A related example is the cost efficiency of applying a plastic sealant occlusally when it might be less costly to restore the one or two small pit-and-fissure lesions that the plastic sealant might have prevented. Of course, who actually applies the sealant and the cost thereof, whether the patient has a high caries attack rate, and other factors enter into the considerations.

In any event, if one accepts the thesis that routine appropriate care over a lifetime will decrease the cost of restorative care and perhaps subsequent endodontic and prosthodontic care, one might logically accept the argument that an incremental maintenance program should be the program of choice when a dental health care program is being recommended for a group of children. And that is exactly the policy position of the American Dental Association in regard to national programs of care for children. There are others who argue that a *graduated* incremental approach—starting with one age group of children and maintaining them on a regular basis annually and picking up each new group annually—is a much more logical way of proceeding, particularly when introducing a program with limited resources available. It allows the program to start on a limited scale, expand gradually, and be phased in with no large backlog of needs in eligible children at any one time. This approach has not always been accepted by some thoughtful analysts of the procedure. Some would point out that the character of the disease or attack rate and treatment needs in children is such that perhaps emphasis should be given to teenage groups. Others suggest starting with six-year-olds or the first year that children are in school as a convenient way to reach them and then reaching back to pick up four- and five-year-olds, while maintaining the six-year-olds when they become seven-year-olds and so on. Others argue that three-year-olds or preschoolers are the most crucial ones to see because of the importance of the second primary molars to the ultimate development of a healthy mouth and face (the early loss of second primary molars can often damage a dentition). A quite thorough and thought-provoking approach to this problem was carried out by Burt[5] under a contract from the Division of Dentistry of the Public Health Service.

The careful pencil-and-paper analysis with what limited data were available led to the following finding: that although not backed by a project of prospective research, the annual "front end" costs of an incremental program (that is, routine examination, radiographs, prophylaxes, reinforcement of patient education, and application of any preventive procedures that might be indicated) added up to considerably more than the costs of the accumulated restorative care. One must emphasize that the cost was in dollars and not in quality of life.

Certainly if the downward trend in caries attack continues, incremental maintenance care may not be indicated at least for extremely young children nor on as frequent a recall basis. Emphasis might be shifted to preventive visits beginning in early teenage when periodontal disease begins its subtle attack.

There are also questions being raised elsewhere about the appropriateness of the frequency of routine dental care, particularly the routine six-month recall appointment. The British scientific press recently engaged in a debate over a challenge to the appropriateness of the six-month examination as part of the British National Health Service and whether or not it should be paid for routinely without question.[45, 47] The issue has subsequently been raised in a draft of a dental program (if a dental program were to be part of a National Health Insurance Program) designed by the National Delta Dental Plans Association. Again, these points are raised not because there is an answer to them, at least not yet, but because it does raise again the question of who determines just what a dental treatment need is.

American Dental Association Surveys

In the 1950s, the American Dental Association (ADA) through its then newly formed Bureau of Economic Research and Statistics was surveying dental practices to try to gain some estimate of the treatment needs and behavior of the patients who did go to dental offices. Unfortunately, partly because of the state of the art of survey research at the time and lack of funds to do the type of survey that would have given better information, many of the data reported in early ADA surveys of dental practice were not too useful. Sometimes they were not even comparable with themselves and certainly not with data from other surveys. When collected in a similar way their own data can be compared with themselves and perhaps show a trend over time, but no external comparisons may be done legitimately. By the late 1970s, however, the ADA's reorganized Bureau of Economic and Behavioral Research, with expert consultation from professional survey research groups experienced in and capable of doing this kind of research, did the surveys with their own qualified in-house staff and on a sound sampling basis.

Data from Dental Insurance Experience

In recent years the richest potential mine of information for dental treatment needs, demands, and utilization has been the third-party carriers of prepaid dental care through commercial insurance, dental service corporations, or government sponsored or administered programs. Again, for a number of reasons, data from these sources are not easily obtained. Consumerism is a consideration, in that privacy of information and confidentiality of records prevent a number of agencies from releasing data even though proper assurances are given that (1) no individual data will be released, (2) data will only be reported in aggregates, and (3) individuals will not be able to be identified. Perhaps the carriers and agencies are simply using privacy of information and confidentiality as an excuse. In addition, some carriers frankly state that the information they have is exactly the information that their competition would be just delighted to see when making estimates of the costs and rates of a certain type of dental plan. Carriers may feel that the release of such information would take away all advantage in competitive bidding for various contracts from various purchasing groups. Suffice it to say that, for whatever reasons, actuaries keep their data close to the vest. What is known about the experience learned from this relatively new insurance type of third-party prepaid plans is reported in Chapters 12 and 13.

UTILIZATION

NORC/University of Chicago Study

Several significant publications on the utilization of dental services have appeared since the last edition of this book. The first, by Newman and Anderson,[36] recounts an unusually well-done nationwide social survey by the reliable National Opinion Research Center (NORC) of the University of Chicago. The year studied was 1964, and unfortunately, findings were not reported until 1972. In general, however, the patterns of utilization tended

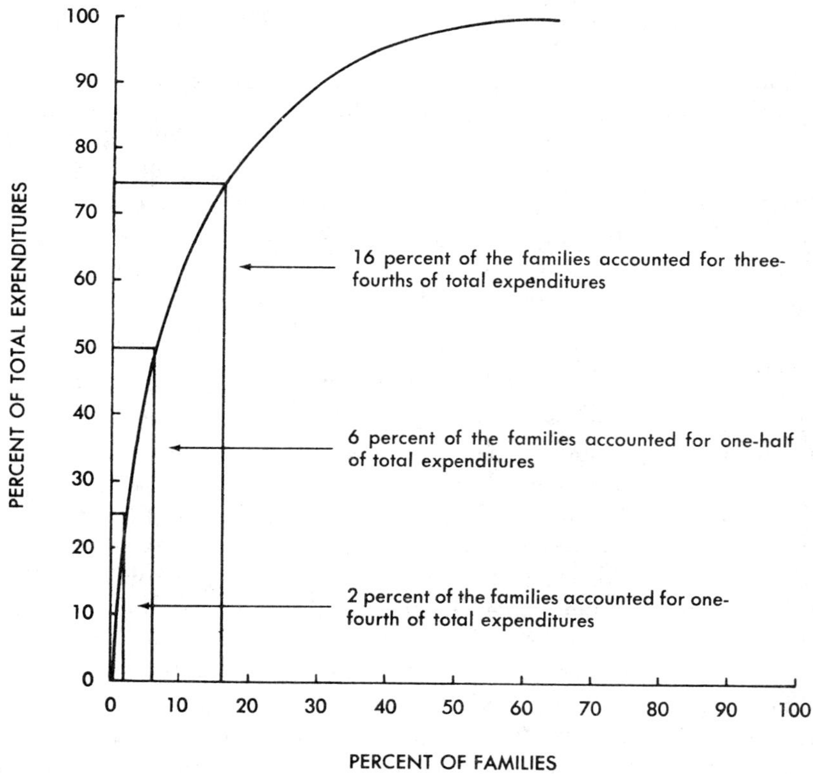

Figure 11–13. Distribution of expenditures for dental care among families, 1964. (From Newman, J. F., and Anderson, O. W. Patterns of dental service utilization in the United States; a nationwide social survey. [Chicago], University Chicago Center Health Administration Studies, 1972. xi + 127 p.)

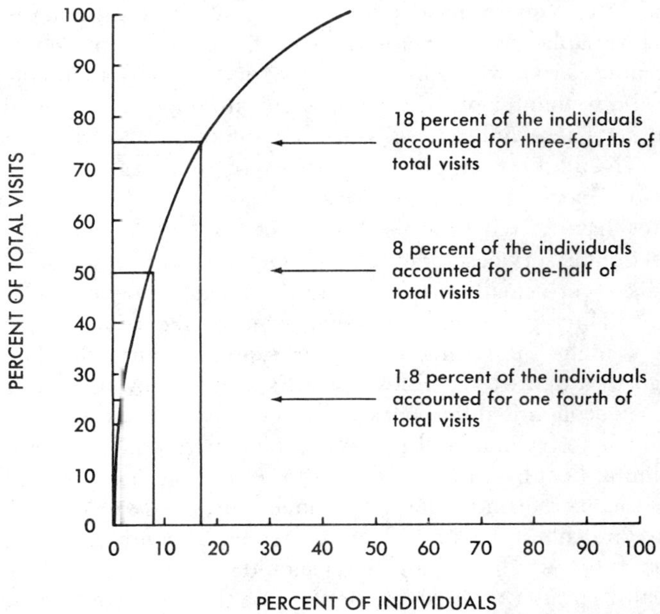

Figure 11–14. Distribution of expenditures for dental care among individuals, 1964. (From Newman, J. F., and Anderson, O. W. Patterns of dental service utilization in the United States; a nationwide social survey. [Chicago], University Chicago Center Health Administration Studies, 1972. xi + 127 p.)

to bear out previous NORC data as well as data from the National Health Survey reported in previous editions of this book. (Also Newman, 10 years later but with a different co-worker, Larsen, found essentially the same patterns. That report[49] will be detailed later in this chapter.)

The highest users of dental services were those with the highest incomes and the highest levels of education. Newman and Anderson as nondental observers were of the opinion that dental utilization had remained relatively low despite the significant increases since 1930. In the year studied, the mean number of visits per family was 4.6, the proportion of families with visits was 65 percent; the mean visits per person was 1.5, and the proportion of persons with visits was 45 percent. In terms of total number of visits and expenditures for dental care, a relatively small number of persons (or families) had accounted for a large proportion of both visits and expenditures (see Figs. 11–13 and 11–14). Utilization, when plotted against the demographic variable of age, resulted in a curve in the shape of an inverse U; that is, utilization was low for the youngest age group, highest for the teenage to young adults, and followed by a constant decline for the remaining ages. Still consistent findings were that females utilized dental services more than males, and whites more than nonwhites. Newman and Anderson speculated that the impact of dental insurance might be much less in terms of utilization than might be anticipated. But unfortunately their data, based on persons covered by dental insurance in 1964, were too few to make an extensive analysis. Race emerged as one of the crucial variables as a determinant of utilization. White-nonwhite differences remained large, with whites utilizing services more than nonwhites with respect to both amount of expenditures and number of visits and continuity of utilization. These differences were also influenced by the type of dental service received; for example, differences of more than 20 percent were observed for "cleanings, examinations and x-rays" and "fillings and inlays," with whites having a higher proportion of visits than nonwhites. For the remaining dental services (dentures, extractions, and other services) differences by race were small, and in several instances nonwhites had more visits than whites. Thus, one could infer that when the acute need for dental care is relatively high—an aching tooth, for example—an individual would be likely to go to a dentist regardless of one's attitude toward dental care. Any racial or socioeconomic differences would be small.

And finally, Newman and Anderson demonstrated the overriding importance of dental health status in relation to utilization. The presence of dental conditions means that individuals are much more likely to visit a dentist than if they have no conditions or at least no perceived conditions. These findings suggest that future studies of utilization should specify carefully the dimensions of oral health status. An index of dental health status could be constructed with different weights assigned to each condition according to the probability of making a visit (see Table 11–4).

USPHS/University of Colorado Study

An appraisal of selected literature was performed by Bauer and colleagues at the University of Colorado under contract to the U.S. Public Health

Table 11–4. Distribution of Dental Conditions and the Proportion of Persons with Conditions Who Made a Dental Visit*

Condition	Proportion with Condition	Proportion with Condition Who Made a Visit
Toothache	20% (9330)	75% (1401)
Sore or bleeding gums	8% (9302)	45% (698)
Loose permanent tooth	5% (9321)	61% (451)
Pain in tooth when drinking hot or cold liquid	14% (9302)	54% (1256)
Tartar or stains on teeth	25% (9255)	57% (2363)
Crooked teeth	7% (9311)	32% (698)

*Newman and Anderson.[36]

Service.[48] They reviewed only quantitative studies and only those after 1960. They were able to select only 44 from over 300 titles as meeting their criteria. The reviewers were extremely critical of previous studies, especially in relation to the definition of "demand" and "utilization" or the carelessness with which those terms were bandied about. They ran the studies reviewed through the gamut of the principles of research design and concluded that scarcely any study met all of the criteria for good research and that studies were often marred by one or more defects. A common defect was the widespread reliance on retrospective data, because people often inaccurately recall their utilization behavior. Patients are found consistently to embellish their recollection of frequency of visiting dentists, the amount of care received, and the amount of money paid, when their memories are checked against actual records of care.

One of the problems identified in reviews of studies on dental utilization was that the annual number of dental visits per person was the most common measure of utilization. Indeed it was the dependent variable in 70 of the 182 associations with an explanatory factor or independent variable that Bauer and his colleagues analyzed. From the point of view of economic theory and, one might add, economists, the annual number of visits is considered superior to many of the other utilization variables because it is an approximation of quantity demanded. Bauer and co-workers correctly point out, however, that its practical usefulness leaves much to be desired. For example, it gives equal weight to all visits to a dental office without regard to the type of care given or the type of provider seen. A five-minute visit for a quick checkup by an orthodontist, a two-to-three-hour appointment for a full quadrant of restorative care, and a one-hour prophylaxis by a dental hygienist are all weighted equally. Once again, dentistry is tarred with the brush that tars medicine—that is, frequently economists have studied medical utilization in terms of the number of "visits to the doctor," which can be more easily standardized and are more comparable than visits to the dental office, which frequently are not visits but actually surgical procedures of varying lengths of time.

To support this contention, a report[1] from the ADA's Bureau of Economic and Behavioral Research purports to show that while the number of dental visits per capita has remained relatively constant between 1959 and 1979, the number of dental procedures per capita has increased almost twofold (see Fig. 11–15). This report apparently was a preliminary one and no documentation was supplied.

Bauer and co-workers singled out one study to praise, that of Wan and Yates.[54] When one examines the Wan and Yates study firsthand one finds that it was conducted in a five-county area spreading across the border from New York into Pennsylvania. Whereas Wan and Yates were careful to discuss their sampling procedures, no information on the 27 percent nonrespondents from their some 3000 households was reported, all of which shows that it is easy to find fault and most difficult to plan a study without any shortcomings. The study also fell down on several of the criteria that Bauer and co-workers mentioned, namely, interviewing technics and problems of retrospective

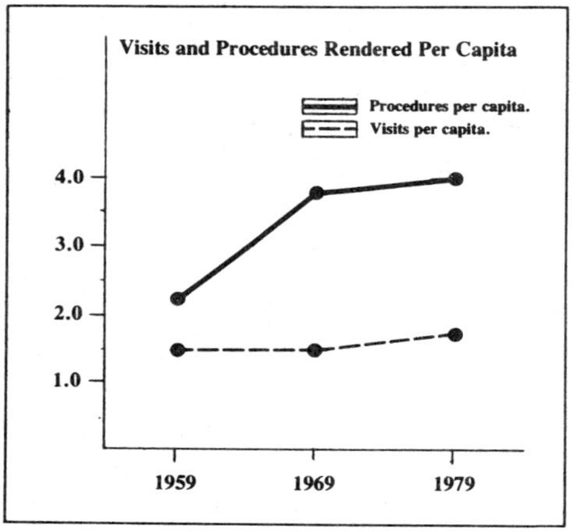

Figure 11–15. Visits and procedures rendered per capita in the United States, 1959–1979. (From [American Dental Association, Bureau of Economic and Behavioral Research.] ADA bureau report examines dental manpower issues. Am. Dent. A. News, 13:6, May 24, 1982.)

recall, among others. Economists and other social scientists who enter the dental field to conduct studies sometimes tend to use powerful statistical technics without being too careful about the quality or lack of data upon which assumptions may be based. In the parlance of today's computer world, the acronym **GIGO**—"**G**arbage **I**n **G**arbage **O**ut"—might apply. Nevertheless, the Wan and Yates study did come to some conclusions that agree with those of other studies in regard to the influence of income, social class, and dentist:population ratio—that is, the more favorable the dentist:population ratio, the more likely it is that utilization will occur. They concluded that income was the most powerful determinant of dental care utilization, with dentist:population ratio second, and social class third. None was really a powerful determinant, however. Each accounted for only 4, 2, and 1 percent of the variance, respectively.

Institute of Medicine Study

A third significant analysis of utilization conducted during the past decade is that of Douglass and Cole,[11] produced for the Institute of Medicine and funded by the Kellogg Foundation. Whereas the study presents no original data, it is a quality review of the literature and must not be overlooked. Their review shows clearly that there has been an increase between 1963–64 and 1976 in the percentage of persons visiting a dentist within a two-year period from about 55 percent to almost 62 percent. The data show further that this increase has occurred in gradual increments. Also, the number of people who have reportedly never seen a dentist has declined proportionately from about 17 percent in 1963–64 to just under 10 percent in 1976. (Data to be reported later in the chapter on the most recent National Health Interview Survey[51] show that the proportion who have never seen a dentist dropped less than a percentage point—from almost 10 percent to about 9 percent—in the two years between 1976 and 1978–79.)

In the same study, the inverse U-shaped curve with utilization by age was identified as was the fact that females consistently used dental services somewhat more than males.[11] Whites used dental services more than non-whites, even when controlling for the variables of age and sex. Just as in other analyses, as income increases, the rate of utilization increases. The education level of the head of the household is a strong predictor of utilization rates of dental services for family members, and the researchers agreed with earlier editions of this text that income and education were related independently to the frequency of dental care visits. Occupation also was a strong correlate as was socioeconomic status (SES) and social class. Place of residence and geographic region are related in that urban residents use dental services more than either farm or nonfarm rural residents, and residents in the Northeast have the highest utilization rates, and those in the South, the lowest. A number of studies have shown that there is a strong correlation between demographic and socioeconomic factors and types of dental services received. For both males and females, the teen and young adult age groups have the highest rates of utilization of prophylaxes, examinations, x-rays, "fillings" and inlays, and extractions, which corresponds with the higher overall utilization rates for these age groups. Socioeconomic factors are the strongest determinants of utilization of certain types of dental services. For example, as level of income, level of education, or status of occupation increases, utilization rates for examinations, "cleanings," and "fillings" increase while the rate of extractions decreases. They pointed out further that it is almost inevitable that an individual will visit a dentist at some time in his or her life. Several studies have indicated that less than 2 percent of persons aged 65 and older have never made a dental visit.

Health Behavior and Utilization

Health behavior in relation to utilization was analyzed by Douglass and Cole from three approaches: first, the health behavior demographic characteristics; second, the health belief model; and third, the motives for and barriers to seeking asymptomatic care. The first, the health behavior demographic characteristics, shows a relation between preventive visits and the information that the potential patients have about teeth and gums, but with no correlation with socioeconomic level. O'Shea and Gray,[40] in a related study of attitudes and behavior concerning prevention, found that attitudes about the efficacy of dental visits and of toothbrushing, which were almost universally accepted, nevertheless seemed to have little effect on actual behavior. Early childhood training and the education of parents to provide good examples seem to be the key to changing children's dental health practices. Also, preventive dental behavior is consistently associated with other preventive health behaviors.

The health belief model[19, 24, 42, 43] postulates that readiness to act, to take a voluntary asymptomatic health action, is determined by three variables: first, individuals must feel susceptible to the disease; second, individuals must feel that the disease is potentially serious in its effects in regard to them; and third, individuals must feel that a course of action that will prevent or alleviate the disease is available to them. One must add also that the course of action must not be perceived as worse than the disease: "The cure can't be worse than the disease." In the tests of the model, it was found that while most people may feel susceptible to dental disease, they do not view it as being severe.[23] Douglass and Cole concluded that the health belief model has some empirical validation and does offer a partial explanation of the socioeconomic differences seen in the utilization of preventive dental services. Further research is necessary, however, before this model can be accepted as a strong predictor of preventive health care utilization. For other views of health-going behavior, one is urged to read the study of Zola on how an individual becomes a patient.[56]

Douglass and Cole then examined the motives for and barriers to seeking asymptomatic dental care. Not all people in the higher socioeconomic levels visited dentists preventively, and minorities of the lower socioeconomic levels do make preventive dental visits. Motivation alone does not account for the incongruities in utilization of preventive dental services. The strength of motivation must be weighed against the barriers, real or perceived, to gain a clearer understanding of patterns of preventive utilization.

Based on the studies of several economists (and others),[7, 9, 13-15, 20-22, 25-27, 29, 31, 32, 37-39, 41, 53] and despite the wide range in findings, one must conclude that income and price of dental services are market forces that play a major role in the use of dental services. Other barriers to dental care include access, not only in distance and travel but also in waiting time. Anxiety and fear of pain are obvious reasons why patients may not seek dental care and account for differences of utilization of preventive care at all income levels with no differences apparent between various socioeconomic levels. Other barriers to utilization of preventive dental care may be a combination of the patient's perceived need for care, priorities in life, and acceptability generally of dental personnel and dentistry.

Finally, it seems evident that the complex relation of motives and barriers does help to explain differing patterns of preventive dental behavior. Those at a higher socioeconomic level may have more motivation to maintain healthy, attractive teeth, as well as being faced with fewer or less intense financial and access barriers. For example, they are less likely to select a dental practice on the basis of its fee schedules. Additionally, those at a lower socioeconomic level may also have fewer resources to draw from to overcome barriers; that is, the knowledge of a low-cost clinic's availability, the ability to shop around for a dentist with whom the patient feels comfortable, and an employer who will encourage or at least tolerate leave for dental visits.

Douglass and Cole speculate on what impact there might be on increased utilization through prepaid dental coverage or through insurance. Their review found substantial disagreement on what impact prepaid care will have. A variety of reports that describe particular population groups who come under dental insurance coverage generally show that (1) the effect of dental insurance coverage varied with the socioeconomic class of the insured population; (2) groups who voluntarily purchased dental insurance had the highest utilization rates, as might be expected; (3) marketing and enrollment characteristics of the plan did affect utilization substantially; and (4) after an initial marked increase, utilization rates declined as the length of time of coverage increased, with the resulting rates being 5 to 10 percentage points above the prebenefit rates; for example, a group might go from 39 percent to 49 percent utilization. Some insurance companies will refuse to write dental insurance unless the initial contract extends for at least two years to allow the company to take care of the initial surge and then benefit from the leveling off in the second and subsequent years. A different finding was reported by Glasser and Hoffman[16] (to be described subsequently).

Douglass and Cole also caution that the demand for service can increase more than the percentage of people seeking dental care increases—that is, persons already counted as seeking care can visit the dentist more often and, when they do visit, can receive a greater number of services (see Fig. 11–15), particularly if they are covered with insurance. A more detailed description of the provision and financing of dental care follows in the next two chapters.

In conclusion, Douglass and Cole are less than enchanted with the outlook for moving this country's entire population into demanding care on an effective basis. In fact, they state boldly that the outlook is bleak. Whereas they do conclude that dental insurance will shift a variable percentage of nonutilizers into that population that is demanding care and doing so effectively, they feel that an even larger percentage of nonutilizers will not take advantage of the coverage. They feel also that taking the services to the target population, as in school-based treatment programs, may guarantee that almost all persons will become users of the dental services while they are eligible for these services but that a significant number will not remain in the category of utilizers once they leave the school program. And finally and most discouraging, they point out that health education programs are not supported by any empirical evidence showing that they are effective in producing dental behavior that leads to asymptomatic dental care. The reader is referred to Chapter 15 for a more detailed description of the factors in health education.

Attractions and Blocks (or Barriers) to Dental Utilization

On occasion one gets the impression, particularly from dental personnel but also from potential patients, that if the financial barrier to dental care were lifted, the patients would rush to the dentist in droves. Disappointingly for dental professionals, the evidence does not bear out that impression.[34] Patients do not flock to the dental offices, at least from what information is available from prepaid plans in which the financial barrier has been substantially lifted.[16] True, a number of individuals will utilize prepaid plans, but the limited evidence to date suggests that where plans have gone into effect, after the initial surge the demand drops off. It is the same patients who are still coming but under a different pay system. Perhaps they are coming more often and not having to worry so much about the type of service they will receive or about having to postpone selected costly services for a while. In other words, even if payment is no longer a problem, there is still a large group of people out there who do not perceive of themselves as patients or who do not realize that they need to be patients or who do not even want to be patients. Also, they might not know that they are eligible for care at no expense to themselves.[35] There is also the contention that in order to get people to utilize a service to which they are entitled, even at no immediate cost to themselves, one has to place the service so that the potential patient will almost have to stumble over it.

A Decade of Utilization: 1964–1974

Another significant study of utilization was done by Newman and Larsen.[49] The study once again was a careful comprehensive analysis of a nationwide survey conducted ten years after Newman and Anderson's 1964 survey. The study was funded by the U.S. Public Health Service and permits analysis of the changes over the decade. The most significant finding was that there was really little change in any of the factors related to dental utilization. For example, no change had taken place in the perceived need for dental treatment on the part of the population over the 10 years. There had been changes in utilization patterns of the population in the 10-year period, however. In 1974 there were fewer families and individuals who made no visits to the dentist and there were conversely more individuals with one or two visits to the dentist. Thus, it was concluded that on an aggregate basis treatment was received by more persons in 1974 than in 1964, but that the receipt of extensive dental treatment, as indicated by the percentage of individuals with three or more visits, had not changed. The data for both 1964 and 1974 indicate that a small proportion of individuals and families account for about 75 percent of dental utilization. (See Figs. 11–13 and 11–14.)

There have also been some significant shifts in the type of dental services received between 1964 and 1974. For example, two primarily preventive services—examinations and radiographs, and prophylaxes and fluoride applications—have increased substantially since 1964. At the same time, the proportion of extractions and dentures declined slightly. Little change occurred in the proportion of people with visits for "fillings" and inlays. One aspect of the 1974 survey that was not addressed in 1964 was the scope and nature of coverage of dental insurance. By 1974 more than 10 percent of the population was estimated to be covered by insurance. Therefore, detailed data were collected. But because there were no baseline data from 1964 with which to compare them, the data collected will have to serve as a baseline for comparison with a later survey.

Once again the predisposing variables of age, sex, and race were strongly associated with dental utilization, with the young and the old having the least utilization but with utilization increasing in all age categories except ages 14–24. Females had on average more visits than males, although both females and males experienced an increase in utilization between 1964 and 1974. Nonwhites still had a substantially lower number of visits than whites, just as was found in 1964. The strong association between education and occupational levels still held, with more education and a higher occupational level correlating with greater utilization of dental services.

Anderson and Larsen also classified the variables related to utilization. In addition to the "predisposing variables," they classified another group as "enabling variables" with two major subcategories—family resources and community resources. Under family resources they include income, dental insurance coverage, and accessibility to a regular source of dental treatment, all of which go to facilitate an individual's use of dental services by reducing barriers to seeking treatment. The community resources that they feel are important are an abundant supply of dental facilities and personnel within a given area, which increases the likelihood that individuals will use those services.

Once again, family income was directly associated with utilization, and there was an increase in utilization between 1964 and 1974 in all income categories. Utilization was lowest in rural farm and rural nonfarm areas as opposed to urban areas, but individuals in rural areas increased their utilization substantially more than did city dwellers between 1964 and 1974. Dental insurance coverage had but minimal impact for the ages 2–13 and 25–44, but for the remaining age categories, insurance coverage meant that people with coverage generally had one visit more per year than those without coverage.

The third major group of variables considered as influences on the utilization of dental services includes the need for care and the self-perception of one's need for care and need for treatment. Such data were not gathered in the same fashion in 1964, so the findings from the two surveys are not contrasted here. Also, only the self-perception of the need for treatment will be considered because no professional clinical evaluation was conducted. The interviewees were asked: "If you went to the dentist today, how much work do you think would have to be done? A great deal, quite a bit, not much, or no work at all?" Perhaps surprisingly they responded inversely to their reported number of dental visits. In other words, persons whose perceived need was zero had 1.9 visits, while those reporting a great deal of perceived need had only 1.2 visits. This finding suggests that there is a relation between use of services and the person's self-perception of the need for service. It might be argued, however, that the receipt of treatment does influence the perception, so that those individuals who perceive that their current need for service is none do so because they have received more services within the last year. Those persons who responded that they had need for a great deal of treatment and who also reported that they had insurance coverage had 3.4 visits within the year; those without dental coverage but with a self-perceived need for a great deal of treatment had only 0.9 visits. This large difference of two and one-half visits is quite substantial and considerably more than the

Table 11–5. Relative Importance of Variables in Explaining Utilization*

Variable Groups	Relative Importance
Predisposing	
Demographic	Medium
Social structure	Medium
Attitudes-beliefs	†
Enabling	
Family resources	High
Community resources	Low
Need	
Perceived	Medium
Evaluated	†

*U.S. Public Health Service.[49]
†Variables not used in the analysis.

differences observed for other responses to the question of perceived need for dental treatment.

Newman and Larsen summarized the relative importance of the grouped variables, that is, the predisposing, enabling, and need variables, and assigned a relative importance to them (see Table 11–5). They concluded that the data appeared to indicate that family resource variables, particularly insurance coverage and family income, are the most important variables affecting utilization. Demographic variables (age and race in particular) and social structure (education and occupation) would be ranked lower and assigned a relative importance of medium. Self-perceptions, that is, the condition of the teeth and the actual need, were also ranked of medium importance, although they were less certain about that assessment. The relative importance of community resources as variables was judged to be low. A key community-resource variable, the dentist:population ratio, may well be a variable that would result in a change of importance from low to either medium or high.

Newman and Larsen recommended that for future research an important question to answer would be a comparison of high utilizers having coverage with high utilizers lacking coverage. It could provide some useful answers to the question: "What motivates individuals who consume a large quantity of services when financial incentives to seek treatment are present (that is, with coverage) as opposed to when they are absent (no coverage)?"

Significant in this report is that all of the variables that have been strongly associated with dental utilization still appear to be operative a decade later. Also, this report and all of the studies of utilization and all of the analyses reviewed in this chapter agree with each other for the most part.

The UAW Study of Utilization with Insurance Coverage

One of the few studies of the effects of prepayment on the utilization of dental services was reported in 1981 by Glasser and Hoffman of the United

Auto Workers.[16] The first phase, a prebenefit survey of a random sample of 506 Michigan auto workers' families, was conducted prior to the institution of the United Auto Workers' dental contract in October 1974. The prebenefit survey was carried out from June 1974 to October 1974; that is, in the four months just prior to the start of the coverage. It should be noted that the auto workers should have been aware that they had successfully negotiated a dental benefit in their last round of contract negotiations and that the benefits were not to begin until the first year of the three-year contract was up. Thus, the benefits negotiated in 1973 were not activated until a year later in October 1974.

All of the surveys were carried out in Pontiac, Michigan, or the immediate Pontiac area. A remarkably fine response rate of 97 percent of families was obtained. Of those surveyed, 46 percent reported having seen a dentist within the past year and 62 percent reported having seen a dentist within the past two years. Once again, those with higher education and higher incomes reported more visits and more preventively oriented visits, as did more females than males. Significantly, about 50 percent of the respondents said that they had delayed getting some care while waiting for the dental plan to come into effect, and 22 percent had delayed all care but emergencies.

The second phase of the study was an analysis of the actual claim forms submitted to Delta Dental Plan of Michigan for the Pontiac UAW auto workers. It should be noted that only the hourly rated UAW workers had a contract negotiated with Delta. The first three benefit years from October 1974 through September 1977 were reported. Disappointingly, Glasser and Hoffman failed to give sufficient data from which readers could make their own analyses and draw their own conclusions. Apparently they simply reported what they judged to be the findings. For example, they stated, "Several important changes were noted in the patterns of dental utilization from before to after the benefit plan went into effect." First, they contended that male and female differences were essentially eliminated. Second, more adults and families with children used the care, especially those in the child-rearing ages of 25–45. Third, the percentages of persons seeking care increased over the three-year period studied—especially for "preventive services."

Of particular interest was the absence of the "backlog of remedial work" that had been expected based on insurance industry experience. They reported that the mean number of visits was almost the same in the first two years, although the mean services used were somewhat higher in the first year than in the second year. "The so-called 'backlog phenomenon' did not occur." The percentage of the sample receiving care in the third benefit year was no different from that reported for the year prior to the plan, so they claimed. In the first three and three-quarter years of the plan, comparable percentages sought services as recalled by interviewees in the four years prior to the plan. During the plan it was reported that more children, whites, and those with higher education and income had more visits, received more services, and received more preventively oriented services.

It is unfortunate that Glasser and Hoffman do not give their data in more detail. Also, they are comparing the results of recall interviews from the prebenefit survey with the subsequent actual claim forms submitted. The problems of accurately recalling dental visits have already been mentioned earlier in this chapter.

National Health Interview Survey: 1978–79

The most recent data available on utilization of dental services come from the National Health Interview Survey,[51] conducted during 1978–79, on the volume of dental visits and the interval since the last visit. This report was based on an excellent probability sample of some 83,000 households, of which 80,000 were contacted. It estimated that 50 percent of the civilian noninstitutionalized population of the United States had made at least one dental visit

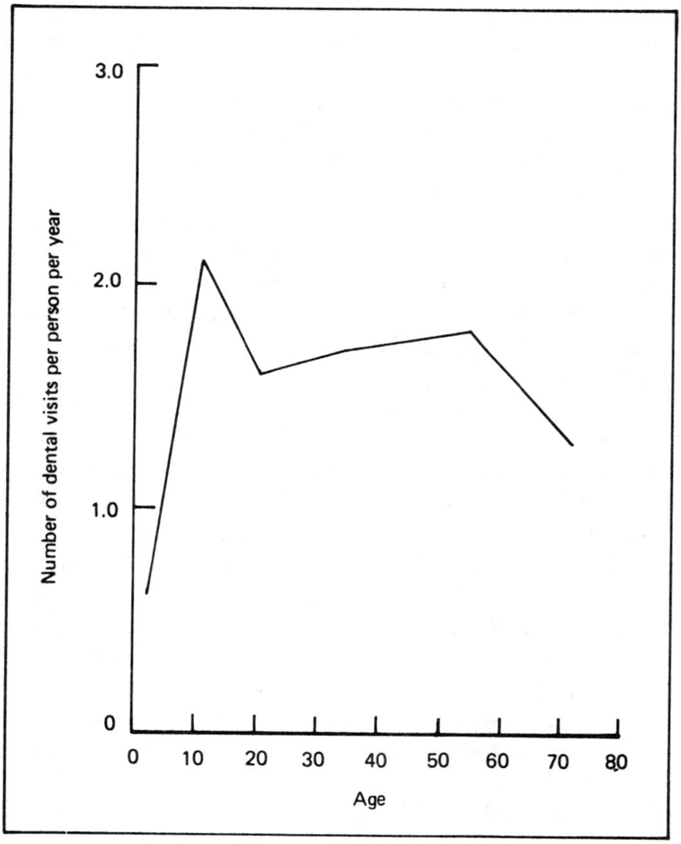

Figure 11–16. Number of dental visits per person per year, by age, United States, 1978 and 1979. (From U.S. Public Health Service, National Center for Health Statistics. Dental visits, volume and interval since last visit; United States, 1978 and 1979, by Wilder, C. S. PHS Publ. No. 82-1566–Ser. 10–No. 138. Washington, D.C., Government Printing Office, 1982. iv + 54 p.)

in the year prior to the interviews. The average person had made 1.6 dental visits in that year but about 2.9 percent of the population, aged six years and over, had never made a dental visit. Also, females once again had made more dental visits per person than males. Children aged 6–16 had the highest rate of dental visits. Whites made more dental visits than people of other races did. Persons with an average family income of $25,000 or more had the highest rate of dental visits. Persons whose head of family had 16 years of education, that is, a college education, had higher rates of utilization. Residents of metropolitan areas, once again, had made more dental visits per person than those living outside those areas. Persons living in the Northeast and Western Regions of the United States had more and higher rates of dental visits than residents of other areas of the country. The findings of these surveys are portrayed in the accompanying tables and graphs (see Table 11–6 and Figures 11–16 through 11–19).

Of interest to health planners, particularly those who are thinking about an eventual national health insurance program focusing on dental care for children (as did most of the recent national health legislation that had been introduced into Congress), are the data reported concerning school-aged children. For example, an estimated 8.8 percent of children aged 6–16 were reported as never having made a dental visit. In addition, for this same age group, over a quarter had not visited a dentist one year or more prior to the interview. Thus, about one third of the school-aged children aged 6–16 years were judged to show evidence of "neglected dental care," that is, if one accepts the conventional wisdom that going to a dentist on a regular basis makes for good dental health.

Again, the overall findings of this latest National Health Interview Survey have shown that the same patterns and associations of utilizers and nonutilizers are maintained. What is encouraging is that now at least 50 percent of the population report that they have seen a dentist within the last year—up from the 20 percent estimated to prevail in the 1930s.

COMMENTARY

In regard to *needs*, evidence is beginning to accumulate that dentistry's archenemy dental caries is on a decline: its onset is delayed and it does not appear to be attacking as many people. Those carious lesions that do occur seem to be smaller per se and confined to a smaller area of the involved tooth. If not just a temporary phenomenon or the low in a cycle of attack, there will be changing patterns of treatment needs. More teeth will be retained throughout a person's lifetime to be at risk to trauma, abrasion, erosion, staining, accretions, plaque, and loss of supporting structure. The population also is aging and still is increasing—a zero growth rate has not been attained.

As more people keep more teeth longer over their longer lifetimes, their patterns of *demand* for care and *utilization* most likely will change. The "automatic dental market" of people who "see their dentist (or dental hygienist)

Table 11–6. Percent of Population with One or More Dental Visits within a Year of Interview and Number of Dental Visits per Person per Year, by Selected Characteristics, United States, July 1963–June 1964, 1969, and 1978 and 1979*

Selected Characteristic	Percent of Population with Dental Visit within a Year			Number of Dental Visits per Person per Year		
	July 1963–June 1964	1969	1978 and 1979	July 1963–June 1964	1969	1978 and 1979
All persons†	42.0	45.0	50.0	1.6	1.5	1.6
Sex						
Male	40.1	43.8	48.3	1.4	1.4	1.5
Female	43.8	46.1	51.6	1.7	1.6	1.8
Age						
Under 5 years	11.1	11.0	14.3	0.3	0.3	0.4
5–14 years	54.9	58.8	64.2	1.9	1.8	2.0
15–24 years	55.1	55.6	56.6	2.0	1.7	1.7
25–44 years	48.5	49.5	54.3	1.9	1.6	1.7
45–64 years	38.4	42.3	48.9	1.7	1.6	1.8
65 years and over	20.8	23.2	32.5	0.8	1.0	1.3
Race						
White	44.6	47.3	52.3	1.7	1.6	1.7
All other	22.7	28.3	35.7	0.9	0.7	1.1
Family Income						
Less than $3,000	24.0	26.6	35.1	0.8	0.8	1.1
$3,000–$4,999	33.4	31.9	33.8	1.0	1.0	1.1
$5,000–$6,999	41.8	37.4	36.3	1.6	1.1	1.2
$7,000–$9,999	51.3	45.1	38.4	1.9	1.4	1.2
$10,000–$14,999	61.5	55.1	45.0	2.6	1.9	1.4
$15,000 or more	71.2	66.7	60.4	3.4	2.5	2.0

Education of Head of Family						
Less than 9 years	26.9	28.1	29.6	1.0	0.8	1.0
9–12 years	43.9	45.3	48.3	1.6	1.5	1.5
13 years or more	62.6	62.9	64.2	2.6	2.2	2.3
Usual Activity Status						
Preschool (under 6 years)	16.5	17.3	21.2	0.5	0.4	0.6
School-age (6–16 years)	56.9	60.1	64.6	2.0	1.9	2.1
Usually working (17 years and over)	43.7	46.1	52.9	1.7	1.6	1.7
Usually keeping house (female, 17 years and over)	41.1	42.0	45.3	1.6	1.5	1.6
Retired (45 years and over)	19.5	22.0	32.1	0.8	0.9	1.2
Other activity (17 years and over)	53.2	54.5	54.7	2.0	1.7	1.7
Place of Residence						
All SMSA‡	44.7	47.2	52.0	1.8	1.6	1.8
Outside SMSA:						
Nonfarm	38.1	40.9	45.3	1.2	1.2	1.3
Farm	33.7	39.9	48.6	0.9	1.1	1.2
Geographic Region						
Northeast	47.7	49.8	54.9	2.1	1.8	2.0
North Central	43.9	46.0	51.8	1.5	1.4	1.6
South	34.9	39.3	44.1	1.1	1.1	1.4
West	43.4	46.4	52.0	1.7	1.8	1.8

*U.S. Public Health Service.[51]

†Includes unknown income and education.

‡Standard Metropolitan Statistical Area.

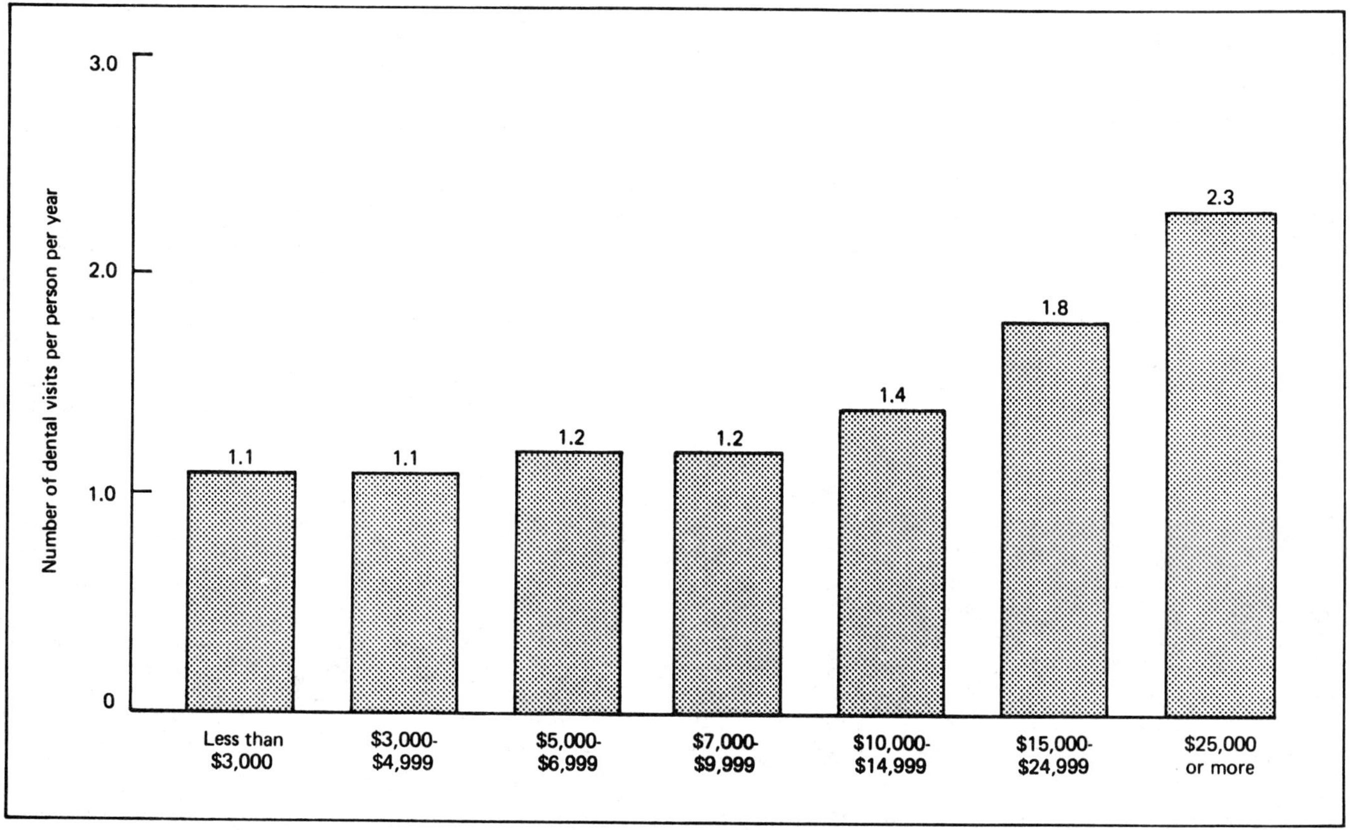

Figure 11–17. Number of dental visits per person per year, by family income, United States, 1978 and 1979. (From U.S. Public Health Service, National Center for Health Statistics. Dental visits, volume and interval since last visit; United States, 1978 and 1979, by Wilder, C. S. PHS Publ. No. 82-1566–Ser. 10–No. 138. Washington, D.C., Government Printing Office, 1982. iv + 54 p.)

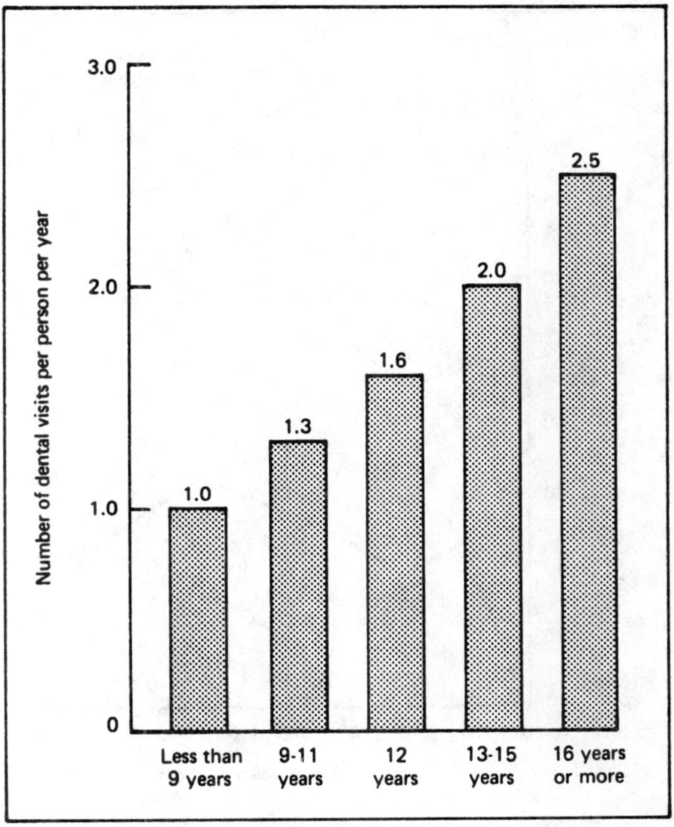

Figure 11–18. Number of dental visits per person per year, by education of head of family, United States, 1978 and 1979. (From U.S. Public Health Service, National Center for Health Statistics. Dental visits, volume and interval since last visit; United States, 1978 and 1979, by Wilder, C. S. PHS Publ. No. 82-1566–Ser. 10–No. 138. Washington, D.C., Government Printing Office, 1982. iv + 54 p.)

once a year" may now have leveled off at about 50 percent of the population. Current estimates from the National Health Interview Survey for the last few years up to and including 1980 have the percentage of the people who report having visited a dental office within the past year pegged within half a point of 50 percent. If this pattern holds and is not just a temporary plateau, the impact of increases in income, education, and dental insurance may have already been felt for the most part.

Other ways of reaching the "other half" of the population will need to be explored and tested. Dental professionals (including dental public health professionals) will need to reorient their practices, programs, and community outreach activities. Their practice focus will have to change from repairing and restoring the teeth attacked by coronal dental caries for children and young adults to preventing and controlling periodontal diseases starting with adolescents and carrying them in their practices for a half century or more.

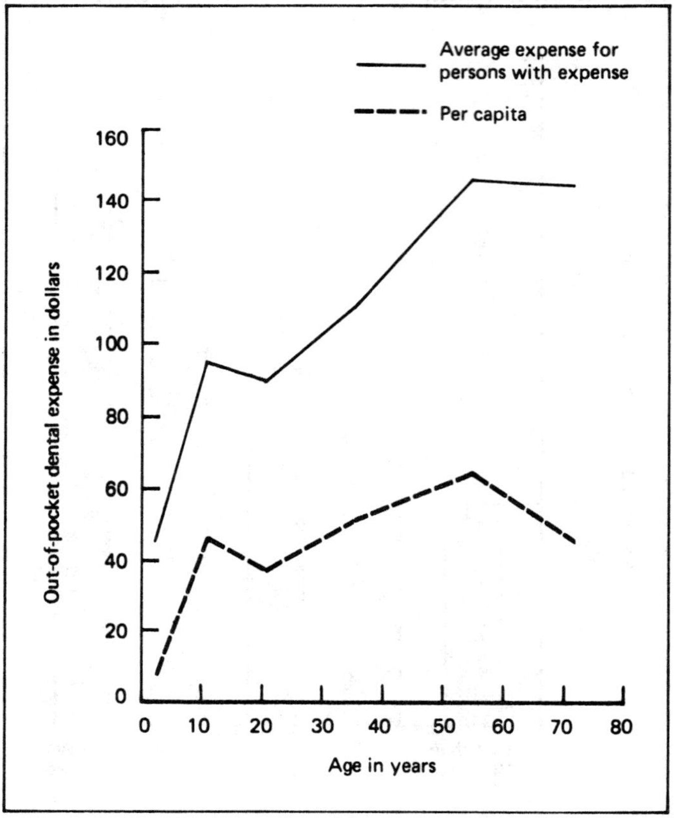

Figure 11–19. Annual out-of-pocket dental expense per person, per capita expense, and average expense for persons with expense, by age, United States, 1977. (From U.S. Public Health Service, National Center for Health Statistics. Dental visits, volume and interval since last visit; United States, 1978 and 1979, by Wilder, C. S. PHS Publ. No. 82–1566–Ser. 10–No. 138. Washington, D.C., Government Printing Office, 1982. iv + 54 p.)

The caries with which they may be concerned likely will be root caries. Their practices also will have to reach outward to the community in working with community groups, institutions, agencies, and facilities.

For dental practitioners who are wondering how to attract patients in a period of a perceived oversupply of dentists and dental hygienists, compounded by declining caries attack rates, the following is recommended:

1. Be available and accessible on days and at hours other than "usual business hours." For example, if most dental offices in your community are closed on weekends, keep yourself available on Saturdays and Sundays. Also, evening hours might well be maintained. The emergency call service of the local society (if there is one and there should be) and the local hospital emergency room service should know that you are available and accessible or at the least, "on call." Some of the most successful dental practices are open during the noon hour, in the early morning, and in the early evening to accommodate the busy executive or hourly rated blue-collar worker.

2. Offer your services to the facilities and institutions in your community where dental practitioners traditionally have not provided regular services. For example, through proper channels so as not to antagonize confreres, offer your services a half day a week or on call to local nursing homes, long-term care facilities, children's homes, senior-citizen day-care facilities and clinics, crippled children's clinics, or centers for the chronically ill, aged, and handicapped. Go to the homebound and institutionalized instead of expecting them to come to you.

Dental hygienists can be particularly useful and helpful in visiting these kinds of disadvantaged people on a regularly scheduled basis (so their visits can be expected and counted on). They can pay attention, listen to the problems, and then help screen and sort out the problems needing the immediate attention or subsequent attention of a dentist. Of course, they can be of particular value in conducting inservice dental health education for the staff of such facilities and not just for the patients or residents.

Dental professionals may not get reimbursed in dollars for these unusual out-of-office services. If they are not fully busy anyway, however, it is better to be contributing to their community than to be sitting idle. It certainly is an excellent way to build good will and enjoy good public relations. And what more legitimate way could there be to advertise?

Dental professionals are urged to work with their local dental and dental hygienists' societies on establishing:

1. Loan closets for portable dental equipment to take to bedside or to institutions without fixed dental facilities.
2. Emergency call services, especially for nights and weekends.
3. Regular referral services.
4. Dental health education and programs of prevention in the schools.

The foregoing are but some suggested approaches for the beginning dental professional in times of a perceived oversupply of dentists and dental hygienists. The need is out there. Latent demand is there. And since the dental professionals are now available in greater numbers, they must make themselves accessible.

References

1. [American Dental Association, Bureau of Economic and Behavioral Research.] ADA bureau report examines dental manpower issues. Am. Dent. A. News, 13:6, May 24, 1982.
2. Bader, J. D., Mullins, M. R., and Webster, D. B. Aspects of planning and evaluation of children's dental care in Appalachia. J. Pub. Health Dent., 39:27–34, Winter 1979.
3. Bawden, J. W., and DeFriese, G. H., eds. Planning for dental care on a statewide basis; the North Carolina dental manpower project. Chapel Hill, Dental Foundation North Carolina, 1981. xvii + 227 p.
4. Bulman, J. S., et al. Demand and need for dental care; a sociodental study. London, Oxford University Press, 1968. viii + 103 p.
5. Burt, B. A. A method of comparing the expenditures on two alternative national dental programs for persons aged 6–21. Report for PHS contract no. NO1-DH-44101. Ann Arbor, University Michigan, 1975. v + 149 p.
6. ———. New priorities in prevention of oral disease. J. Pub. Health Dent., 42:170–9, Spring 1982.

7. Conrad, D. A., and Emerson, Marie L. State dental practice acts; implications for competition. J. Health Politics, Policy, and Law, 5:610–30, Winter 1981.
8. Consumer's guide to dental health 1982. Am. Dent. A. J. (spec. issue), n.v.:1C–63C, (Mar.) 1982.
9. Doherty, Neville. Competition in the provision of dental services—impacts on providers and consumers; an introduction. J. Health Politics, Policy, and Law, 5:588–92, Winter 1981.
10. Dollar, M. L., and Kulstad, Hugo. The economic aspects of the dental health problem. p. 24–34. (In Pelton, W. J., and Wisan, J. M., eds. Dentistry in public health. Philadelphia, Saunders, 1949. xi + 363 p.)
11. Douglass, C. W., and Cole, Katherine O. Utilization of dental services in the United States. J. Dent. Educ., 43:223–38, Apr. 1979.
12. Draker, H. L. Handicapping labio-lingual deviations proposed for public health purposes. Am. J. Orthodont., 46:295–305, Apr. 1960.
13. Feldstein, P. J. Financing dental care: an economic analysis. Lexington, Mass., Heath, c1973. xvii + 261 p.
14. ———. Funding and payment of dental care; an analysis of possible alternatives. p. 193–224. (In Brown, W. E., ed. Oral health, dentistry, and the American public. Norman, Okla., University Oklahoma Press, c1974. vii + 372 p.)
15. Feldstein, P. J., and Roehrig, C. S. A national econometric forecasting model of the dental sector. Health Serv. Res., 15:415–32, Winter 1980.
16. Glasser, M. A., and Hoffman, W. S. Demand for care; the effects of prepayment on the utilization of dental services. p. 49–68. (In Bawden, J. W., and DeFriese, G. H., eds. Planning for dental care on a statewide basis; the North Carolina dental manpower project. Chapel Hill, Dental Foundation North Carolina, 1981. xvii + 227 p.)
17. Grainger, R. M. Epidemiological data. p. 311–53. (In Chilton, N. W. Design and analysis in dental and oral research. Philadelphia, Lippincott, 1967. 365 p.)
18. Graves, R. C. Aspects of the practical significance of current public health methods for the prevention of caries and periodontal disease. J. Pub. Health Dent., 42:179–87, Spring 1982.
19. Hochbaum, G. M. Public participation in medical screening programs; a sociopsychological study. Washington, D.C., Government Printing Office, 1958. 23 p.
20. Holtsman, A. G., and Olsen, E. O. The demand for dental care production; a study of consumption and household production. J. Hum. Resources, 11:546–60, Fall 1976.
21. House, D. R. Barriers to access to dental care; an economic examination. Am. Col. Dent. J., 45:160–9, 188, July 1978.
22. ———. A full-price approach to the dental market: implications for price determinations. J. Health Politics, Policy, and Law, 5:593–607, Winter 1981.
23. Kegeles, S. S. Why people seek dental care; a test of a conceptual formulation. J. Health Human Behavior, 4:166–73, Fall 1963.
24. ———. Some changes required to increase the public's utilization of preventive dentistry. J. Pub. Health Dent., 28:19–26, Winter 1968.
25. Kushman, J. E., and Scheffler, R. M. Pricing health services; verification of the monopoly pricing model for dentists. J. Hum. Resources, 13:402–15, Summer 1978.
26. Kushman, J. E. Pricing dental services; a market testing approach. J. Health Politics, Policy, and Law, 5:634–50, Winter 1981.
27. Lambert, Camille, Jr., and Freeman, H. E. The clinic habit. New Haven, College and University Press, 1967. 191 p.
28. Long, L. M., Jr., and Bawden, J. W. The estimation of treatment needs from epidemiological survey data. p. 47–8. (In Bawden, J. W., and DeFriese, G. H., eds. Planning for dental care on a statewide basis; the North Carolina dental manpower project. Chapel Hill, Dental Foundation North Carolina, 1981. xvii + 227 p.)
29. Manning, W. G., Jr., and Phelps, C. E. Dental care demand; point estimates and implications for national health insurance. R-2157-HEW. Santa Monica, Calif., Rand, 1978. xii + 57 p. (p. v, vi, 2–8, 55–7)
30. Mansfield, Edwin. Microeconomics; theory and application. 2nd ed. New York, Norton, c1975. xvi + 534 p. (p. 234–5)
31. Marquis, K. H., Marquis, M. Susan, and Newhouse, J. P. The measurement of expenditures for outpatient physician and dental services; methodological findings from the health insurance study. Santa Monica, Calif., Rand, April 1976. ix + 33 p.
32. Maurizi, A. R. Public policy and the dental care market. Washington, D.C., American Enterprise Institute Public Policy Research, 1975. 73 p. (p. 23–9)

33. McKinlay, J. B. Some approaches and problems in the study of the use of services—an overview. J. Health and Soc. Behav., 13:115–52, June 1972.
34. Metzner, C. A. Attractions and blocks; the A and B of the utilization of dental services. Am. Dent. A. J., 60:3–8, Jan. 1960.
35. Miller, Ann J. An epidemiological study of selected characteristics of utilizers and nonutilizers of dental services in a federally funded rural comprehensive care facility. Doctoral Dissertation, Ann Arbor, University Michigan, 1973. xvii + 287 p. (p. 119–20)
36. Newman, J. F., and Anderson, O. W. Patterns of dental service utilization in the United States; a nationwide social survey. [Chicago], University Chicago Center Health Administration Studies, 1972. xi + 127 p.
37. Nikias, M. K. Social class and the use of dental care under prepayment. Med. Care, 6:381–93, Sept.–Oct. 1968.
38. ———. Trends and patterns of dental care in an urban area before Medicaid. HSMHA Health Rep., 85:5–65, Jan. 1971.
39. Nikias, M. K., Fink, R., and Shapiro, S. Comparison of poverty and nonpoverty groups on dental status, needs, and practices. J. Pub. Health Dent., 35:237–59, Fall 1975.
40. O'Shea, R. M., and Gray, S. B. Dental patients' attitudes and behavior concerning prevention. Pub. Health Rep., 83:405–10, May 1968.
41. Phelps, C. E., and Newhouse, J. P. Coinsurance, the price of time, and the demand for medical services. Rev. Econ. and Stat., 56:334–42, 1974.
42. Rosenstock, I. M. What research in motivation suggests for public health. Am. J. Pub. Health, 50:295–302, Mar. 1960.
43. ———. Why people use health services. Milbank Mem. Fund. Quar., 44:94–124, (part 2) July 1966.
44. Schonfeld, W. H., and Warren-Hicks, Deborah. Estimating the need for dental care and dental health manpower in North Carolina. p. 115–65. (In Bawden, J. W., and DeFriese, G. H., eds. Planning for dental care on a statewide basis; the North Carolina dental manpower project. Chapel Hill, Dental Foundation North Carolina, 1981. xvii + 227 p.)
45. Sheiham, Aubrey. Is there a scientific basis for six-monthly examinations? Lancet, 2(8035):442–4, Aug. 27, 1977.
46. Spencer, A. J. The estimation of need for dental care. J. Pub. Health Dent., 40:311–27, Fall 1980.
47. The six-monthly dental examination. Edit. Dent. Update, 4:421, 423, 447, Nov.–Dec. 1977.
48. U.S. Public Health Service, Health Resources Administration, Bureau of Health Manpower, Division of Dentistry. Factors which affect the utilization of dental services; a review and analysis of the literature, by Bauer, J. C., Pierson, A. P., and House, D. R. DHEW Publ. No. (HRA) 78–64, Washington, D.C., Government Printing Office, 1978. v + 71 p.
49. U.S. Public Health Service, Health Resources Administration, Bureau of Health Professions, Division of Dentistry. A decade of dental service utilization 1964–1974, by Newman, J. F., and Larsen, Arne. DHHS Publ. No. (HRA) 80–56, Washington, D.C., Government Printing Office, June 1980. vii + 36 p.
50. U.S. Public Health Service, National Center for Health Statistics. Basic data on dental examination findings of persons aged 1-74 years; United States, 1971–74, by Kelly, J. E., and Harvey, C. R. DHEW Publ. No. (PHS) 79-1662-Ser. 11-No. 214. Washington, D.C., Government Printing Office, 1979. vi + 33 p.
51. ———. Dental visits; volume and interval since last visit: United States, 1978 and 1979, by Wilder, C. S. PHS Publ. No. 82-1566-Ser. 10-No. 138. Washington, D.C., Government Printing Office, 1982. iv + 54 p.
52. U.S. Public Health Service, National Institutes of Health, National Institute of Dental Research, National Caries Program. The prevalence of dental caries in United States children 1979–80; the national dental caries prevalence survey. NIH Publ. No. 82-2245, Washington, D.C., Government Printing Office, 1981. iv + 159 p.
53. Upton, Charles, and Silverman, William. The demand for dental services. J. Hum. Resources, 7:250–61, Spring 1972.
54. Wan, T. T. H., and Yates, Ann S. Prediction of dental services utilization: a multivariate approach. Inquiry, 12:143–56, June 1975.
55. Young, W. O., and Striffler, D. F. The dentist, his practice, and his community. 2nd ed. Philadelphia, Saunders, 1969. xvi + 346 p. (p. 193)
56. Zola, I. K. Pathways to the doctor—from person to patient. Soc. Sci. Med., 7:677–89, Sept. 1973.

CHAPTER 12

THE PROVISION OF DENTAL CARE

Brian A. Burt

INTRODUCTION

Dental professionals know that the need for dental care services ranges from minor in some individuals to extreme in others. The demands that people make to have their needs treated, however, are dependent on a number of factors in addition to their specific dental needs. Age, sex, race, income, education, and place of residence are all important, as are the attitudes of individuals regarding dental health and how they perceive their own susceptibility to dental disease.[57] These factors are described in detail in Chapter 11. Yet other factors influencing demand are the type of "delivery system" available and whether the individual finds it an accessible and acceptable form of care.[47, 57]

What is meant by the expression "delivery system"? One definition states that a *system* is an organized group of related and interdependent activities that can be bound together because they are designed to accomplish a purposeful objective.[93] The objective of what has come to be called a *dental delivery system* is the resolution of explicit dental needs through the delivery or provision of dental services[93] by means of these organized and interdependent activities.*

A delivery system in health care is a complex entity involving numerous interdependent elements, the most important of which are:

1. The structure of the system—that is, the organizational arrangements by which patients and providers get together for the provision of health care services.
2. The financing arrangements by which the care services are paid.
3. The supply of provider personnel of various types.

While other elements of a delivery system such as physical facilities and

*The word "delivery" is widely used in the United States to mean the provision of services; the terms "delivery" and "provision" are synonymous in this context.

record keeping can be identified,[93] the three areas listed are the fundamentals. They are interdependent, meaning that changes in any one of them can affect the others as well. The division of the subject into three chapters that separately examine the provision of care, financing, and personnel is therefore an artificial but convenient way to give these issues the consideration they deserve.

Dental personnel owe it to themselves to understand, as well as they can, both the delivery system in which they work and the society in which they live. Many in the profession do not and become bewildered and even angry about social changes and the effects of these changes on their practices. The consumer movement, inflation, and increasing governmental activity in the health care field all have an impact. So do other social developments, such as changing rates of population growth, migration patterns, the women's movement, and changes in the general affluence and expectations of society. These social forces are likely to remain the major influences on the structure of health care for quite some time.

Organized dentistry has two primary goals. One is to seek to improve the dental health of the public; the other is to preserve the autonomy and economic well-being of the profession. There is nothing necessarily wrong with that second aim—every politically organized group in society has a similar one. Dentistry can get caught in the conflict of change, however, when its efforts to secure its own well-being are perceived as not being in harmony with the public interest, or when public efforts to improve the dental health of society are seen by dentistry as being antagonistic to its self-interest. This type of conflict will continue to occur; just and acceptable outcomes are more likely if the dental profession understands the social forces that lead to these conflicts. The theme that dentistry's means of achieving its goals can lead to clashes with governmental and consumer groups will be touched on a number of times throughout the next three chapters.

The Historical Context of Health Care Provision

Health care services throughout the world have traditionally been provided by the "two-party" arrangement, a private contract in which the only persons involved are the provider and the recipient of services. This financing arrangement remains the essence of private practice, which is still a major mechanism of health care provision in most countries.

With the advent of industrialization in Europe and North America in the eighteenth and nineteenth centuries, societies became more urbanized and complex. The Industrial Revolution brought major disruptions to previously stable patterns of life. The traditional pattern of health services (such as they were at the time) grew strained; new disease problems appeared with the new urban-industrial life and affected large numbers of people. New methods of providing services evolved or had to be devised. One such model was National Health Insurance (NHI), introduced in Germany by Bismarck in the 1880s, in Britain by Lloyd George in 1910, and in other industrialized countries in subsequent years. All of these plans were part of broad systems of social security, and many have become considerably expanded since their introduction. While humanitarianism was a factor in their development, a more powerful stimulus was probably the awareness that a healthy and secure society led both to political stability and to greater economic and industrial strength. For example, Britain's introduction of NHI in 1910 was at least partly spurred by anxiety about the rapidly growing industrial capacity of Germany, for it had become accepted in Britain that the national investment made by Germany in the health and security of its citizens was paying off handsomely.[52] With NHI widely perceived today in the United States as a "liberal" issue, it is worth remembering that it was first introduced in a highly conservative monarchy—Germany of the 1880s—for the main purpose of preserving the status quo.

NHI is primarily a financing mechanism by which health care services are paid for from a publicly organized fund or funds. It does not necessarily imply a change in the existing system. A National Health Service (NHS), on the other hand, is a system in which both the financing and the structure of the care system are publicly organized and administered. Some countries have developed systems somewhere between the two; the British National Health Service, for example, is publicly financed, but many aspects of the previous care system have been left virtually unchanged.

Limited forms of NHI such as Medicare have been introduced in the United States, with specific services available to specific groups (see Chapter 13). The introduction of generalized NHI in the United States has been attempted many times;[56] it is strongly opposed in many quarters and just as strongly supported in others.[31] The fundamental issue is probably whether access to health care is considered a right or a privilege, and therefore whether responsibility for providing health care rests with the individual or with society. Dental personnel should seriously consider this issue before reaching a decision on it. The emotional rhetoric surrounding "socialized medicine" (a subject discussed later in this chapter) is best avoided and the issue judged on its merits.

Individual versus Social Responsibility

Health care has always been rationed in one way or another.[68] The traditional rationing method has been fee-for-service, meaning that those who can afford care can get it, while those who cannot afford it do not. With any shift from individual responsibility to social responsibility for health care, more equitable though inevitably more complicated means of rationing will be sought.

While it may be a cliché to say that America is an individualistic society, it is nonetheless true that individualism has probably been a more powerful cultural force in the United States than it has been in other countries.[27] Many of the settlers who first emigrated to America (white settlers, at least) were voluntarily leaving rigid social or political systems, and they naturally brought with them a desire to live free of the constraints they had left behind. An abundance of natural resources and a seemingly limitless frontier gave rise to the attitude that people could "be themselves" in America, presumably meaning that they could mold their own destinies largely by their own efforts.[27] That belief is probably only partly true, but one need only look around at advertisements today ("No one tells me what to smoke," "Express your own unique lifestyle by driving a ______," "We do it all for you") to see that the culture of individualism is still very much alive.

The high point of unfettered *laissez-faire* capitalism in Western Europe occurred around the middle of the nineteenth century and in the United States about a generation later. By the early years of the twentieth century, however, attitudes in European countries were turning away from individualistic philosophies toward those based more in community or society-wide programs. By the 1970s, national state-operated social programs were the norm in Europe, especially in the fields of health, education, social security, and housing. Similar programs existed in the United States, though to a lesser extent, and it is interesting to speculate on why this was so. One reason suggested is that the relative isolation of the United States from external political turbulence during its formative years allowed the development of a more introspective national character than was the case in European societies.[99] In addition, catastrophic events have a way of hastening social change. The effects of two wars in the first half of the twentieth century probably hastened the development of social welfare programs in Europe; the United States largely escaped the social devastation of those wars. It should be remembered, however, that the United States' first Social Security Act was passed in 1935, in the midst of a social catastrophe—the Great Depression.

Another major contribution to individualism in American society comes from what is referred to as the "puritan ethic," which historians consider to have arrived with the earliest English colonists.[32] Essentially, this is a set of beliefs and attitudes that holds that God rewards man for his honest toil in this life as well as in the next and that individual wealth or poverty is justified and largely controllable by one's own efforts. It follows that the accumulation of great personal wealth can be seen as a reward for virtue and hard work, just as poverty can be seen as a punishment for immorality or laziness. That the "puritan ethic" is still alive and well is evident in the higher priority given by some to the punishment of "welfare cheats" rather than to the alleviation of genuine human distress.

The first serious questioning of the culture of individualism in the United States only came during the widespread social distress caused by the depression of the 1930s. Additional revelations of the extent and consequences of poverty in the United States during the early 1960s led to a series of acts passed by the 89th Congress in 1964 and 1965. The legislative measures, principally the Medicare and Medicaid health programs (discussed in Chapter 13), the Civil Rights Act, the Economic Opportunity Act, the Model Cities

Act, and the Elementary and Secondary Education Act, represented efforts to achieve greater equity for all citizens of the United States. The more conservative mood of the 1980s, which developed out of an economic recession, a growing awareness of limited resources, and a loss of faith in the government's ability to solve complex problems, brought this trend to a halt. Only history will show whether the renewed emphasis on individualism in the early 1980s was a permanent or temporary phenomenon.

American attitudes, shaped by individualism and the puritan ethic, are evolving more slowly to the belief, long held by other countries, that access to health care is a right rather than a privilege.[24, 31] The "right to health care" is an emotional and often misunderstood concept, one frequently interpreted as "the right to health." Of course, no one has a right to health. Health, an elusive entity to define, is a dynamic state influenced by such factors as genetic endowment, nutrition, housing and environment, life habits, personal attitudes and beliefs, and medical care received, probably in that order of importance. While medical care has been overvalued by Western society as a determinant of health,[24, 43, 54] most individuals at some time in their lives have a need for it and that need is sometimes urgent. Should access to at least a basic level of health care be the right of all Americans, regardless of means, education, or place of residence, or should individuals be expected to make whatever arrangements they want or are able to?

DELIVERY SYSTEMS FOR DENTAL CARE

The essential feature of dental care delivery in the United States is the diversity of practice modes and their constant evolution within the overall rubric of a private practice philosophy. Most people in the United States still receive their dental care through a traditional fee-for-service arrangement, but private practice has moved a long way from purely fee-for-service care since the mid-1960s. This adaptability in a rapidly changing world is a major strength of American private practice and ensures its continuing development. Whether the changes resulting from the process of adaptation to social demands are for better or worse can be argued.

This chapter will describe and discuss the various modes of dental practice, both the private and public, within the United States. There will also be discussion of different systems of dental care used in some other countries, which have aroused American interest. The chapter will conclude with a commentary on potential future trends in dental care.

The Private Practice of Dentistry

Traditionally, health care in the United States has been delivered by independent private practitioners. It was estimated by the American Dental

Association (ADA) in 1976 that almost 90 percent of all active dentists were in private practice.[10]

Private practice has endured and will continue to endure because it has a number of inherently desirable features. One advantage to both provider and patient is flexibility. A dental practitioner can provide care for as many hours per day as he or she chooses and for as many days per year. When demand for care in a locality increases, private practitioners can respond if they wish by working longer hours, by increasing their productivity to meet it, by increasing their fees, by some combination thereof, or by doing nothing different. There is a built-in economic incentive to be as efficient as possible in private practice, since it represents a big investment of private capital in facilities and equipment; the return on that investment is the practitioner's profit. Choice of equipment, materials, and employees therefore is made carefully, and all can be chosen to suit the tastes of the individual dentist.

Private practice is overwhelmingly the method of dental care delivery preferred by dentists. That is an important factor to consider, presuming that dentists work more satisfactorily in the system they prefer. This article of faith is perhaps best expressed in the policies of the ADA relating to dentistry's position in a national health program, in which it is stated:

> It is the dental profession's firm belief that the dental component of any national health program should be founded upon the traditional efficient private system of delivery of dental care.[14]

There are probably several reasons why private practice is the practice mode preferred by dentists. It could be that dental students are sensitized to the belief that it is practically the only suitable way to provide care. Or perhaps the cultural perceptions of private practice are such that the majority of applicants to dental school can already see themselves as private practitioners after graduation, so that the process of selecting dental students from these applicants ensures self-perpetuation.

It is accepted practically without question by most dentists that private practice allows the provision of the highest quality of dental care, as well as providing the most personal and pleasing environment for the patient. Beliefs of this nature are difficult either to substantiate or to refute in any objective manner; whether or not they are universally true is probably less important than the fact that many dental professionals firmly believe them to be true.

Private practice allows free choice of dentist by the prospective patient, and conversely, the dentist is free to treat or not to treat anyone seeking care. "Free choice" can become an emotion-laden subject, carrying as it does the overtones of free enterprise, healthy competition, and the absence of regulatory constraints. There is little doubt that the ability to choose one's own dentist is valued among patients in higher socioeconomic groups. These patients are more accustomed to regular dental visits[57] and for the most part come from the same socioeconomic strata as do their dentists. Patients in higher socioeconomic groups also live and work in localities where dentists tend to be more available,[10] so that changing one's dentist when desired usually is not difficult.

It is by no means certain, however, that "free choice" is as prized among patients in lower socioeconomic groups. All too often, in the inner-city and rural communities where such groups live, there is little choice of a dentist because few practitioners usually choose to practice in such areas. Because dentists are self-employed business people, they tend to establish their practices in localities where they can be reasonably sure of demand for their services; these localities are typically higher-income suburban areas. There is a clear relation between the availability of dentists and the per capita income of an area.[10] Rural areas and poorer areas of cities are less attractive sites for a private dental practice, because private practitioners are attracted to areas of high demand in order to show a return on their investment of capital. As a consequence, maldistribution of dentists is a standard feature of the private practice system. It is unlikely that there will ever be private practitioners available to serve the needs of many communities that are either geographically remote, economically depressed, or both.

Even within communities that are well-served by dentists, there are groups who are not readily treated by private practitioners. Treatment of the behaviorally difficult preschool child, for example, requires time and patience to an extent that is often uneconomical for a general practitioner, and pedodontists are either unavailable or too expensive for many families. At the other end of the age scale, many elderly persons, especially those on modest fixed incomes, cannot afford the periodontal and prosthetic care that they need, and many have difficulty in traveling around because of physical infirmities. In addition to the old and young, there are persons who are chronically ill, mentally retarded, or physically handicapped, or who have systemic illnesses that require them to be treated in a hospital. Private practice is poorly geared to care for such groups, and as a result their dental treatment in the United States has tended to be neglected.

Poorer groups thus often have a double problem: care is relatively less available to them, and when it can be found it is relatively expensive. It is hardly surprising that persons in low socioeconomic areas are often thought "not to value dental care." That belief is unlikely to be true; rather, the circumstances of their lives do not always permit the disadvantaged the luxury of "valuing dental care" the way that dentists like their patients to value it.[36] Given this situation, "free choice" can be most accurately described as a middle-class value.

"Free choice" also cuts the other way; dentists are free to reject patients if they wish. Some practitioners may feel that they are treating a sufficient number of patients and therefore may accept no new patients of any kind. Others may reject patients whose care is financed by public programs such as Medicaid. This rejection may be based on the dentist's belief that such programs offer inadequate compensation or have too much "red tape," or it may be based on the dentist's inability to accept the attitudes, values, and needs of low-income persons. The dentist may feel that such persons may not be "good patients."

Regarding the dentist's right of choice of patient, the ADA's Principles of Ethics state that

> While dentists, in serving the public, may exercise reasonable discretion in selecting patients for their practices, dentists shall not refuse to accept patients into their practice or deny dental service to patients because of the patient's race, creed, color, sex, or national origin.[22]

Several ethical questions about the "free choice" issue, however, still remain. One is whether a dentist is ethically justified in turning away any patient in pain. A second question is what happens to the patient's "free choice" when rejected by the dentist he or she has chosen.

From the community viewpoint, the principal advantages and disadvantages of private practice as a delivery system relate to economics. Private funds are used to build the facilities, buy equipment, hire auxiliary staff, and pay for some (though by no means all—see Chapter 14) of the expensive education of personnel. Dentists set their own fees. Many dentists also traditionally practice "price discrimination," meaning that they charge well-to-do patients higher fees than they charge poorer ones. Wealthier patients in these practices therefore subsidize the poorer ones.

The complaint of some consumer groups that dentists' fees are too high is often unfair, for such complaints often fail to take into account the facts of life in private practice. The solo dental practitioner is a self-employed businessperson and thus has certain fixed overhead costs to meet: utilities, rent, equipment, supplies, staff payroll, insurance for premises and equipment, as well as personal insurance for income protection in the event of illness or accident. It is interesting to compare the dental practitioner's position with that of the medical surgeon, whose community provides the operatory and the hospital bed. Malpractice insurance, though not yet the massive expense it has become in many medical specialties, is rising steadily for dentists. These expenses must be met regardless of whether patients come or not, or whether bills are collected or not. In addition, the dentist is a highly trained and qualified professional and thus is deemed by American culture to be entitled to a reasonably high level of personal income. Dentists are increasingly being graduated from dental school heavily in debt[40] because of the high costs of their education and have a strong incentive to begin showing profits immediately after they begin practice.

While business aspects of dental practice can be too readily forgotten by some critics of the dental profession, the fact remains that they are frequently incompatible with the need to provide for the dental treatment requirements of *all* people. Regardless of whether "price discrimination" is still practiced, dental fees remain too high for many persons. This cost barrier is not necessarily a sign of the insensitivity of dentists to public needs; rather, it is an inherent feature of private practice.

To summarize, private dental practice is a delivery mechanism of major importance, since much of the demand for dental care is only met by private practice. Both its advantages and its disadvantages relate to economics; it is flexible but necessarily expensive for many potential patients.

Group Practice

The term "group practice" simply means a number of dentists practicing together under certain organizational arrangements. There are a number of definitions proposed, stemming from the variety of types of groups. The definition adopted by the ADA is as follows:

> Group practice is that type of dental practice in which dentists, sometimes in association with the members of other health professions, agree formally between themselves on certain central arrangements designed to provide efficient dental health service.[4]

The number of dentists involved in this definition is not specified. Frequently, two dentists working together are considered to be in a partnership rather than a group. A partnership is a number of dentists working together under a contractual agreement, each of them being an equal principal in the practice. There are numerous forms of looser business association in which the dentists are more correctly called "associates." A 1971 survey by the U.S. Public Health Service used this definition of group practice:

> A group dental practice is defined as a practice formally organized to provide dental care through the services of three or more dentists, using office space, equipment, and/or personnel jointly.[95]

General practice groups are those composed entirely of general practitioners, single-specialty groups are those in which all members of the group are of the same specialty, and multispecialty groups contain practitioners in two or more specialty fields of practice.[95]

The 1971 survey identified 715 group practices (defined as having three or more dentists) in the United States, involving 3,148 dentists and 7,358 auxiliaries.[95] These figures mean that only a little more than 3 percent of active dentists in the United States were in group practice at that time, and growth since 1971 has probably not been rapid. More than half of the practices identified in the 1971 survey were three-person groups. Eight practices were found that had more than 20 members each; most of them were multispecialty practices. Although the greatest number of group practices, and dentists working in group practices, was found in California, the greatest concentration of group practices was found in the northeastern section of the United States. The most common form of organization found was partnership, followed by corporation, and then sole ownership.[95]

Dentists in group practices seem to enjoy higher income levels than their solo colleagues,[8, 17, 21, 46] either because group practice is more efficient than solo practice[55] or because the more managerially efficient type of dentist tends to go into group practice.

Several advantages for the dentist who practices in a group, as opposed to solo practice, have been cited. These benefits relate to better ways of organizing one's life—vacations and continuing education leaves can be planned more readily, because colleagues in the practice can temporarily care for a dentist's patients during that time.[58] There is less disruption in the practice caused by illness to a dentist or an auxiliary, and consultation with colleagues is readily available. Quality of care is said to be improved because of the built-in peer review. Finally, financial fringe benefits, such as sick leave and pension plans, can be built into a group organization more readily than into a solo practice, thus easing some of the day-to-day economic concerns of dental practice.[58] Obviously, of course, economies of scale through the sharing of personnel, equipment, and other resources are the major advantages in group practices.

The greatest problems for the dentist considering group practice appear to be related to personality.[58] It is essential that dentists in a group be temperamentally compatible. Because individual decision-making becomes subjugated to decisions made by the group, similar philosophies of patient care are clearly necessary. When a dentist chooses to join an existing group practice, or when several dentists decide to form one, it is conventional wisdom to have a trial period of three to six months before binding organizational arrangements are made. This approach is used to allow any incompatibilities to surface, so that if necessary a dentist can leave the practice without the complications of breaking a legal agreement.

In contrast to physicians, dentists are taught to work independently. Indeed, dentistry probably attracts many who enjoy working by themselves. This desire for independence is one reason suggested for the slow growth of dental group practice in the United States. Another is the historical but groundless suspicion that group practices are somehow unethical; the ADA has made it clear that there is nothing in its Principles of Ethics that should inhibit the growth of group practices.[22, 59]

Open and Closed Panels

Most group practices treat patients on the traditional fee-for-service basis and only a few administer prepaid programs.[95] Some of these group practices operate as *closed panels* and are a continuing source of concern to organized dentistry. Closed-panel practice under a prepayment plan is defined by the ADA as existing if patients eligible for dental services in a public or private program can receive these services only at specified facilities from a limited number of dentists.[12] If the services are provided in a group practice facility and are prepaid by an organization, the practice is more precisely termed "prepaid group practice."[12]

The definition given by the U.S. Public Health Service is less satisfactory. It states that closed-panel practice exists when a group of dentists who share office facilities provide stipulated services to an eligible group for a set premium.[97] For beneficiaries of plans using closed panels, choice of dentists is limited to panel members, and dentists must accept any beneficiary as a patient.[97] This definition seems too narrow, because the dentists concerned do not necessarily have to share office facilities and there is some choice of dentists (if the patient desires) from those within the panel.

Much of the profession's concern about closed panels is that patients are denied free choice of dentists,[16] though as noted earlier in the chapter, this "free choice" argument can become a bit rhetorical. The closed panels that seem to cause most concern are those set up by union groups for the treatment of the union's members and staffed by salaried dentists who treat only the union group and their dependents.[86] When a union is considering providing a dental health program for its members, organized dentistry frequently tries to present an alternative prepaid plan in which dental care would be provided by private practitioners.

Closed-panel clinics have aroused a lot of emotion at various times; it has been charged that they are unethical and that they deliver care of inadequate quality. The "quality" question cannot be substantiated, but the ethics of closed panels have been argued. Some contend that dentistry's opposition to closed panels is based on economic grounds and that dentists are really more concerned about the possible loss of their patients to the closed panel. Feldstein argues that interest groups invariably try to restrict competition and try to provide "good" reasons for doing so.[39] If dentistry's opposition to closed panels is perceived in that light, the profession is in the position of having its policies seen only as protection of self-interest.

Lindahl's argument that there is a place for closed panels and that the ADA should cease its rigid opposition to them is well-reasoned.[62] Lindahl, a respected figure in dentistry, thinks that dentists' opposition to closed panels is economic and that charges of poor quality are baseless. On the issue of free choice, he states: "It is becoming increasingly obvious that some consumers prefer a limited choice of practitioner if they feel that qualified practitioners have been selected for them."[62] Lindahl's argument, presented in 1971, shows little sign of being accepted by the ADA's House of Delegates.

A legitimate concern among dentists is who controls a closed-panel practice. It is thought that a dental care facility set up by a union, for example, may be administered by lay persons to the extent that some areas of clinical management, properly the concern of the dentists, are dictated by the lay administrators. Dentists in such a facility, for example, could be instructed to extract teeth and provide dentures to adult patients, rather than to exercise their clinical judgment. If such instances do occur, clearly the quality of the care provided may not be adequate and the dentists involved are practicing unethically. On the other hand, there are many examples of so-called closed panels in which the dentist exercises the same degree of clinical freedom as a solo practitioner.

Open-panel practice, considered acceptable by the dental profession, is characterized by three features, according to the definition of the U.S. Public Health Service: any licensed dentist may participate, the beneficiary has choice from among all licensed dentists, and the dentist may accept or refuse any beneficiary.[97] *Prepaid group practice* is the term given to a group practice that provides dental services on a prepaid basis.[12] Such groups are now generally regarded as open panels, though this has not always been so.

The line of distinction between closed and open panels can become blurred at times. For example, a prepaid dental care program provided by a private practitioner may have signed up relatively few participating dentists in the community; a closed panel may have a large number of dentists from which a patient can choose. It is not clear just how many dentists must be available before "free choice" exists. It can be argued, for example, that dentists participating in Delta Dental Plans, which were originally developed by organized dentistry (see Chapter 13), constitute a closed panel. Because much ADA policy is based on preservation of "free choice," dental personnel should give this subject much thought.

A new dental or auxiliary graduate, when considering whether to enter a group practice, should be properly concerned with the administrative and clinical quality of the practice rather than with the often emotional rhetoric about "closed" or "open" panels. Once the graduate is satisfied about the quality of the practice, the decision rests on personal preference.

Health Maintenance Organizations (HMOs)

The concept of the Health Maintenance Organization (HMO) is as much based on financial arrangements as it is on structure, so the material in this section overlaps with that in Chapter 13 to some extent.

The idea of HMOs is not new, but the implementation of the idea was given formal encouragement with the passage of the Health Maintenance Organization Act of 1973 (PL 93-222). This act made federal funds for the development of HMOs available under certain conditions, with the intention that they would provide an acceptable alternative to the private practice system and help restrain the costs of care, both through the inherent features of the HMO delivery system and by competing with the private delivery sector.

An HMO is defined in the 1973 Act as " . . . a legal entity which provides a prescribed range of health services . . . to each individual who has enrolled in the organization in return for a prepaid, fixed, and uniform payment."[90] Usually, but not always, the HMO looks like a large group practice with a number of services available under one roof. Myers[70] described an HMO as having five essential elements: a managing organization, a delivery system, an enrolled population, a benefit package, and a system of financing and prepayment. HMOs use a *prepaid capitation* system of financing medical services. Only a small proportion of HMOs offer dental services. If dental services are offered, they are (1) included in the capitation premium, (2) subject to a separate premium, or (3) paid for by fee-for-service. Some HMOs begin their dental plans with fee-for-service until they can develop an "experience rating" from which to establish a capitation premium. (Prepaid dental group practices sometimes use prepaid capitation with their group contracts, whereas dental insurance plans usually use prepayment for fee-for-service reimbursement.) In 1977, the median family monthly medical premium for membership in an HMO was $89.[48]

The 1973 Act defined certain basic services that an HMO was required to provide in order to qualify for federal support funds. Originally, required dental care in these basic services was limited to preventive services for children up to age 11, services that came to be interpreted as prophylaxis, topical applications of fluoride, and prescription of systemic fluoride. The Act also defined supplemental services, which could be provided at a contracted premium in addition to the basic services. Some dental care was included among the items listed in the supplemental services, although this requirement could be waived if dental personnel were unavailable to deliver it.[90] Regulations to the Act allowed a phase-in period of three years for the basic services, but even before the end of that period, the limited required dental care in the basic services was removed and made a supplemental service.

In 1977 there were 165 HMOs—42 of which were eligible for federal support funds—with 6.3 million members.[48] Only a small number of the HMOs offered dental services. A survey by the ADA reported that by September 1978 there were 203 HMOs—69 of which were qualified to receive federal support funds—serving 7.5 million members. Only 21 of these 69 federally qualified HMOs were identified as providing "comprehensive" dental services.*

There is not much difference between prepaid group practice and an HMO, because an HMO that qualifies for federal funds is really a group practice that meets certain statutory conditions. Since the 1973 Act, a number of existing prepaid medical group practices have been able to become certified as HMOs without much change in their structure and thereby to qualify for federal funds. There have been HMO-type organizations in existence for years, the best-known of which are probably the Kaiser-Permanente Plans on the West Coast, the Health Insurance Plan of New York, and the Group Health Association (GHA) of Washington D.C. Of these three, only the last-named offered dental care to its enrollees. A study of the GHA's prepaid dental care program showed that the cost of operating it greatly exceeded expectations, but this could have been due at least in part to the high socioeconomic status of the voluntary enrollees.[87] In other words, the demands of this group were higher than would be found in a representative sample of the public, thus driving up costs.

The possibility that such "adverse selection" would affect a prepaid plan was studied in New York, where voluntary enrollees were compared with a nonvoluntary group who received dental care as a fringe benefit.[73] The voluntary group utilized dental services to a greater degree, but did not necessarily have greater dental needs. They did however have a higher "dental consciousness."

Some opposition to HMOs by dentists has received wide publicity. For example, in Massachusetts, an HMO called the Harvard Community Health

---

*American Dental Association, Council on Dental Care Programs. Dental care in federally qualified HMOs. Am. Dent. A. J., 99:672–96, Oct. 1979.

Plan (HCHP) announced plans to expand in the Newton-Wellesley area west of Boston.[34] The HCHP, which began in 1969 with 88 members, had 78,000 enrollees by 1978. Its expansion plans included a dental treatment center to house from three to ten dentists, who would initially provide care on a fee-for-service basis until a prepaid plan could be established. Opposition from local dentists was reported by a Boston newspaper to be heavy and based exclusively on economic arguments.[34] But the competition the dentists obviously opposed is exactly what the HMO promoters were seeking.

One of the principal advantages of HMOs, as a method of providing health care, is that they claim to reduce the cost of care for those enrolled.[30] These savings are purportedly due to the greater emphasis on ambulatory care and consequently on reduced hospital utilization. "Unnecessary" hospitalization, principally for routine diagnostic tests and minor surgery, is thereby curtailed. Dental care, however, already is classified as ambulatory care and few dental procedures require inpatient hospitalization. The major advantage of the HMO concept therefore seems to have little applicability to dentistry.

Also of note is that in 1977 there were 25 commercial insurance companies involved in 50 operational HMOs, 26 of which were federally qualified.[51] The insurance industry is said to be exploring further investment in HMOs. If the insurance industry has the political strength ascribed to it[72] and if it retains its interest in HMOs despite the likely reduction of federal funds available for them during the 1980s, HMOs should continue to develop.

The ADA has partly accepted HMOs, though without any enthusiasm. The Association's policy states that while it does not oppose the HMO concept, it does oppose their preferential treatment by the federal government.[16] It regards dental care under HMOs as an experimental delivery system and states that the HMO approach " . . . has not been demonstrated to be more economical, efficient, or otherwise better in the delivery of dental services."[16] The "dual choice" provision of the 1973 law has upset many dentists. The provision states that employers with 25 or more employees must offer the option of membership in a qualified HMO if one is available when they offer health care contracts as fringe benefits to their employees. Because qualified HMOs can receive federal funds for their support, dental practitioners may be justified in claiming the competition is unfair. However, federal funds are available precisely because it is thought to be in the public interest to support HMOs and thus provide a competitive alternative to private practice.

With the extensive cuts in selected areas of federal spending enacted by the Reagan administration, continued federal support for qualified HMOs is in jeopardy. If it is withdrawn, some HMOs will probably close their doors. But because only about one in three HMOs was receiving federal funds, many will presumably continue as before. Much will depend on their degree of public acceptance and the extent to which interests like the insurance industry choose to continue their support. The future of dentistry in HMOs is difficult to predict. Removal of federal support for HMOs, and with it presumably the "dual choice" provision, should effectively alleviate the ADA's concerns.

Dental Personnel in HMOs

There are four basic organizational modes under which dental care is provided in an HMO: the staff model, the group model, the independent practice association (IPA), and the primary care capitated network or direct contract model. These basic organizational modes are evolving rapidly and need careful study by dental professionals who come in contact with them. The proliferation of models is another example of how traditional private practice can successfully adapt to changes in society while still preserving its identity.

Staff Model. Dentists, dental hygienists, and dental assistants are salaried employees of the HMO and work the same way as other salaried dentists, dental hygienists, and dental assistants do in a closed panel. There may or not be a dental director. The staff model is the only one of these four modes that affects auxiliary personnel directly, because in the other three the terms of their employment in dental practices are not directly affected.

Group Model. In this instance, the HMO contracts directly with a group practice, partnership, or corporation for the provision of dental services. The group concerned receives a regular capitation premium from the HMO. Dentists in the group receive their income according to the usual way a group practice is run, so the method of payment to the individual dentists is usually not affected by the HMO contract, though the amount may be.

Independent Practice Association (IPA). The IPA is an association of independent dentists (or physicians in the medical analogue) that develops its own management and fiscal structure for the treatment of patients enrolled in an HMO. The IPA can also contract with other prepaid agencies, such as health service corporations or Delta plans, to provide dental services to specific groups on a capitation basis. The American Dental Association considers the IPA to be an open panel,[12] since all dentists in a community are supposedly free to join. In practice, however, the IPA may be selective, thus blurring yet again the distinction between "open panel" and "closed panel" practice. Dentists remain in their own offices and continue to treat their fee-for-service and other patients. The IPA receives its capitation premium from the HMO (or other prepayment agency) and in turn reimburses the individual dentists on either a modified fee-for-service basis or a capitation basis. In many instances the dentist is "at risk" to provide the specified services. IPAs seem to be growing rapidly.

Primary Care Capitated Network or Direct Contract Model. The network is similar to the IPA, except that the HMO contracts directly with the individual provider for provision of services. The provider again is "at risk."

Assumption of Risk

The essence of the capitation system of payment is that the provider receives an established or previously agreed upon sum per patient enrolled, regardless of whether or not the patient seeks care. In return, the provider agrees to provide specified services as necessary for a predetermined period of time.

Clearly, the concern of the provider is that the amount of money received (which is known before a contract is signed) be sufficient to cover the services needed (which are unknown, though they often can be reasonably estimated). If the cost of the services required exceeds the income received through the contract, the provider loses—"cost overruns" are not permitted. Conversely, if the services required are less than the income provided by the contract, the provider gains. It follows that in some contracts there is the potential for undertreatment and discouragement of service utilization, raising a concern related to both ethics and the quality of care received.

It is therefore understandable that both the ADA and individual dentists are cautious about the "assumption of risk." Of course, risk is assumed by an HMO when it establishes its monthly premium for its enrollees, just as it is assumed by a third-party carrier in a prepaid care plan (see Chapter 13). The IPA and capitated network models, however, bring the concept of assuming risk directly to the dentists, either collectively or individually.

As experience grows and more empirical data become available, the extent of the risk involved in HMO and other capitation contracts should become better defined. In the meantime, dental providers are wise to be cautious when they enter into contracts requiring them to assume risk directly.

The Future of Group Practice

Dentistry, for the most part, tends to be suspicious of any departure from traditional fee-for-service private practice. Schoen, however, has had much experience with prepaid group practice and is a strong proponent of the concept.[81-85] He argues that prepaid group dental practice could move the dental profession closer to the moral and ethical ideals of dentistry than typical fee-for-service solo practice can, and that the quality of care improves when the dentist does not have to worry about the patient's ability to pay. He also judges that the HMO concept is well-suited to the provision of dental care, because the maintenance of dental health in their patients is an ideal of most practitioners. Schoen, however, does visualize some problems with integrating dental care into HMOs: (1) public attitudes are not conducive to health maintenance and (2) those who need the HMOs are those who can least afford the premium payments. Schoen also suggests that dental health maintenance over a lifetime is probably more costly (in direct dollar expenditures) then total neglect.[85] Dental care providers naturally do not like to accept this latter argument, but it does refer only to direct expenditures; the costs in the lower quality of life that results from dental neglect are undoubtedly real, though difficult to quantify.

It is likely that group practice in dentistry will continue to grow slowly, unless legislative changes or trends in the economy make it more attractive to dentists. As stated earlier, HMOs are not likely to disappear completely with the withdrawal of federal support.

Hospital Dentistry

Dental departments in hospitals have been increasing in number. The ADA's 1977 survey of hospital dental departments found that some 53 percent of all hospitals provided some form of dental services, at least as indicated by the presence of one or more dentists on the dental staff.[19] Some 40 percent of all hospitals reported having some physical dental facility in 1976.[20] An estimated 38,604 dentists, 35 percent of all active dentists in 1977, were members of hospital dental staffs, though only about one quarter of the nominal dental staff were actually working in a formal full-time or even part-time capacity.[19] Many of the remaining dentists with hospital privileges use them only occasionally.

General practice residencies in hospitals are growing rapidly, and by 1977 there were 753 positions in 266 residency programs.[18] With the greater emphasis placed by the 1976 Health Professions Educational Assistance Act (discussed in Chapter 14) on the training of general practitioners rather than specialists, these programs can be expected to continue growing.

Dental care provided in hospitals is often for those special situations in which general anesthesia and the other resources of a hospital are required, such as oral surgery to remove carcinomas, cleft palate repair, and maxillofacial prosthetic treatment for victims of burns or trauma in the head and neck region. In addition, some routine dental care is provided in hospitals for patients who are suffering from serious systemic disease, patients for whom the risk of being treated in the private dental office would be unacceptably high. The success of the ADA in gaining corporate membership and a seat on the board of the Joint Commission for the Accreditation of Hospitals in January 1980 should help improve the status of departments of hospital dentistry.

Department Store Clinics and Franchised Practices

In the late 1970s, several major department store chains, such as Sears and Montgomery Ward, opened dental clinics in some of their stores and announced their intention to open more. These clinics operated during usual store hours and were perceived by the stores' management as a further step in "one-stop" shopping. The stores' management viewed the dental clinics as an extra service for their customers, no different from the pharmacies and optical departments that have been in chain stores for some years.

The dental clinic space in department stores is usually leased by a dentist because most state laws do not allow dental practices to be owned by a nondentist. To date, the stores' management seems to have kept out of clinic management, other than to stipulate that they remain open during shopping hours. While organized dentistry has greeted "department store dentistry" with suspicion, the indications are that it is a form of practice that will continue to develop. Dental care administered in these clinics seems little different from that provided in other practice modes, and dentists practicing in them seem to enjoy full clinical freedom. Many such clinics operate on more of a "walk-in" basis than do traditional practices, so they may attract more patients who might otherwise not approach a dental office. As long as the quality of care provided remains as high as that available in the traditional office, department store clinics seem to offer a number of advantages. If they attract new nontraditional patients without taking regular patients from established practices, their development is to be welcomed.

Considerable change in practice development may occur if state dental laws change to allow more ownership of dental practices by nondentists. For example, department stores could own their clinics and hire dentists as salaried employees. Other business entrepreneurs, with an eye toward maximizing profit, might operate chain dental practices ("franchised" practices) with more ruthless efficiency and less concern for patient welfare than do most dentists. The legitimate concern about such developments is that business managers may want to eliminate less profitable services and perhaps less profitable types of patients, meaning that the dentists may lose their clinical freedom. In such circumstances, quality of care in its broadest sense may be threatened. Some of these developments await the outcome of the Federal Trade Commission's inquiry into dentistry (to be discussed).

Organized dentistry views all of these developments with understandable concern. Rather than automatically opposing or accepting them, dental professionals should consider each development on its merits. Some of them may be inevitable social trends, so that again dentistry should do its best to ensure that the best interests of the public and the providers are protected as these practice models evolve.

Public Programs

Private practice is usually not able to meet the dental demands of all people. There are a number of public programs, therefore, aimed at meeting the needs of specific groups of recipients in this diverse society.

A distinction must be made between a *delivery system* and a *financing mechanism*. There are a number of programs sponsored by the federal government, especially those in which the government provides all or most of the funds, in which care is delivered by private practitioners. The practitioners treat the patient in the usual way, except that they bill the government, rather than the patient, for their services. These financing mechanisms are discussed in detail in Chapter 13.

There are some dental care programs sponsored by the government, however, in which specific delivery systems are employed in addition to a funding mechanism. Many of these programs are now sponsored by the federal government, but many remain under the control of state and local health departments. All are under considerable strain from the federal budget cuts in social services enacted in the early 1980s.

The oldest health care programs of the federal government are directed either at certain groups of its own employees or at other specific groups for whom it has an obligation or who would find it difficult to get care anywhere else. Each branch of the armed forces, for example, provides dental care for its own personnel and sometimes for the dependents of personnel. Care is provided for the most part by dentists who themselves are members of the armed services, and is dispensed from clinical facilities wholly owned and maintained by the service concerned. Some care is contracted out to private dentists, especially care for eligible dependents who can be treated under CHAMPUS (Civilian Health and Medical Program of the Uniformed Services).

The U.S. Public Health Service is responsible for the dental care provided to American Indians, federal prisoners, Coast Guard personnel, Coast and Geodetic Survey personnel, Merchant Marine personnel, merchant seamen, and those persons suffering from Hansen's disease. Some of these groups are treated in specific clinical facilities staffed by salaried dentists, and some are treated by private practitioners under a financing mechanism. The Indian Health Service, for example, maintains its own clinical facilities on most Indian reservations in the western part of the United States. Many of these facilities are in remote areas far from any other source of dental care. In less remote areas, private practitioners treat American Indians on a contractual basis.

Community health centers often are federally funded group practices, chiefly medical but with a dental component, established to meet the needs of groups in particular geographical areas. Included under this title are Neighborhood Health Centers, Family Health Centers, and Rural Initiative Systems. These centers are established in areas where access to private care is limited, and they employ salaried dental personnel. Another program aimed at making care available in areas unattractive to private practice is the National Health Service Corps. This program, discussed more fully in Chapter 14, provides salaries for dentists in remote areas who treat patients in much the same way as private practitioners. Dental care for veterans, under the aegis of the Veterans Administration, is now limited to inpatient care provided in the agency's hospitals.

Many states, counties, and cities have had dental care programs operating for years. Such programs, often administered by an agency of the state or local government, have been principally aimed at providing care for indigent and medically indigent persons (see Chapter 13) eligible to receive some form of public welfare. The services and quality of these programs vary widely. Many state and local dental treatment programs, which for years have had their own facilities and salaried personnel, continue to treat the same group as they always have; the only change is that they can now bill their state's Medicaid program for services provided.

The budget-cutting at federal, state, and local levels in the 1980s has put many of these programs in jeopardy. There are some long-standing public programs that have been terminated; others have been drastically reduced. With similar budget reductions in Medicaid (see Chapter 13), many people are now unable to receive the dental care they need. While the future of these public programs is uncertain, the effect on the dental health of many people must be detrimental.

Auxiliary Based Dental Care Programs

Certain systems of dental care in which auxiliary personnel provide most services have developed in other countries and have aroused some interest in the United States.

While the ADA remains strongly opposed to such plans,[7, 15] all dentists and auxiliaries should be knowledgeable about these delivery systems so that they can make their own analyses.

The New Zealand School Dental Nurse

The New Zealand school dental nurse plan was introduced in 1921 and has acted as a model for the development of similar or slightly modified programs in many other countries.

New Zealand is a nation of some three million people in the South Pacific Ocean, some 1,500 miles off the eastern coast of Australia. Its economy is predominantly rural, with little industrialization, and living standards are high. New Zealand was a world leader in a number of social programs: old-age pensions, visiting maternal and child health nurses, and interestingly enough, the secret ballot at political elections. A number of these programs began in the late nineteenth century, about the time that social security programs were initiated in Bismarck's Germany. Given these traditions, the introduction of the school dental nurse plan was probably not as radical an innovation as it seems, though there was some concern among dentists at the time.[89] The stimuli for the program were the extensive dental diseases found in army recruits in World War I (1914–18) and the concomitant resolve at government level that action was required to alleviate this problem. Dentists were in short supply, and treatment of young children was not as accepted an area of dental practice at that time as it is now. Dental caries was and still is highly prevalent in New Zealand.[25, 26]

When the service began, care was offered only to younger school-age children, but eligibility now extends to all preschool children and all children in primary and intermediate school (2½ to 13½ years of age). Children up to age 16 are eligible for treatment by private practitioners at public expense, but beyond that age dental care is provided through traditional private practice, with some exceptions for special groups who receive public assistance. School dental clinics are attached to primary and intermediate schools throughout the country, and an extensive reequipping program of installing modern equipment began in the mid-1970s. (See Fig. 12–1.)

There is only one dental school, but until recently there were three training schools for dental nurses in New Zealand. The nurses' training course is two years long. Nurses learn a certain amount of basic science as well as

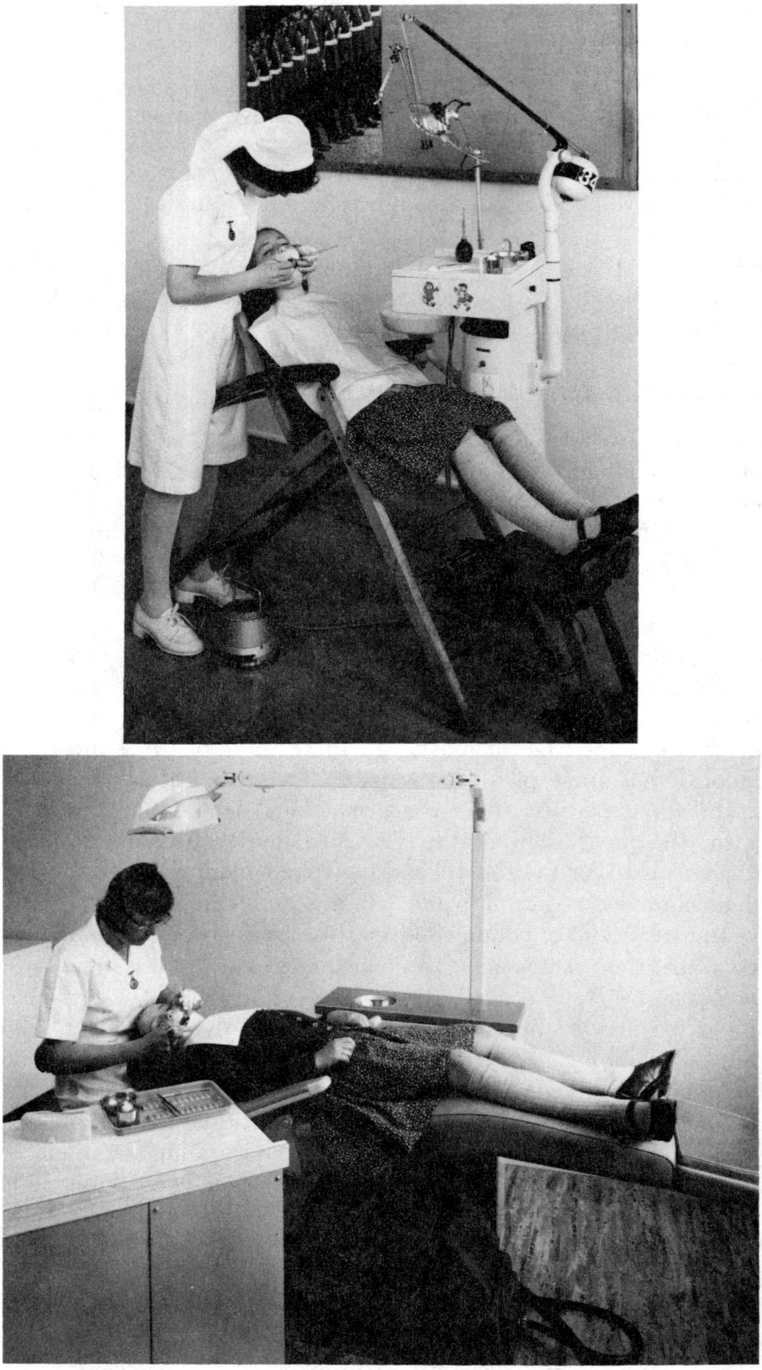

Figure 12–1. The old and the new. New Zealand school dental nurses treating patients in an older clinic (upper) and in a more modern clinic (lower). (Photograph courtesy of New Zealand Department of Health.)

technical procedures, and considerable emphasis is placed on learning to recognize conditions that are beyond their competence to treat, which are referred to a private practitioner.

Nurses' clinical duties are listed by the New Zealand Department of Health, Division of Dental Health, as follows:[64]

1. Oral examination.
2. Prophylaxis.
3. Topical fluoride application.
4. Advice on dietary fluoride supplements.
5. Administration of local anesthetic.
6. Cavity preparation, and placement of amalgam and silicate fillings in primary and permanent teeth.
7. Pulp capping.
8. Extraction of primary teeth (not permanent teeth).
9. Individual patient instruction in toothbrushing and oral hygiene.
10. Classroom and parent-teacher dental health education.
11. Referral of patient to private practitioners for more complex services, such as extraction of permanent teeth, restoration of fractured permanent incisors, and orthodontic treatment.

These duties have changed only slightly from those originally set in 1921, with only topical fluoride applications, advice on dietary fluoride, treatment of permanent anterior teeth, and classroom dental health education added since then. Extraction of permanent teeth has been removed as a duty, because as the dental health of the child population improved, there were too few permanent teeth requiring extraction for trainee nurses to learn the procedure.

There is one supervising public health dentist for approximately 50 nurses, so nurses function with a high degree of independence.[64] Many young children in New Zealand are examined and treated totally by dental nurses and never see a dentist until their teenage years. While this fact has disturbed some American observers,[49, 76] there is no evidence that the dental or general health of the children suffers as a result. One measure of the acceptance of the service is the high degree of utilization among the target population; some 98.5 percent of the primary and intermediate school population are treated by the service, as are 64 percent of preschool children.[64] Comparable figures for the utilization of dentists in the United States are 58.8 percent and 11 percent.[94]

For several reasons the school dental nurse program in New Zealand is now in the process of organizational adjustment. One is that after many years of steady growth, staffing is saturated. Married nurses are remaining in employment longer, as are married women in other countries. In addition, widespread fluoridation is now reducing the need for restorative treatment on a national scale,[64] and the rate of population growth is declining, again as it is elsewhere. As a result of these influences, the intake of new trainees at the three training schools dropped from 280 in 1960 to 122 in 1976[64] and then down to 30 by 1981, when two of the schools had closed. In time, program administrators intend to shift the nurses' duties further in the direction of prevention and health education.

School Dental Nurse Programs in Other Countries

The New Zealand school dental nurse plan has attracted tremendous attention in dental circles all over the world. By 1970 there were at least 15 other countries and jurisdictions that had adopted similar plans,[71] most of which were based on the New Zealand concept, with modifications to suit the local environment.

In Canada, all 10 provinces have publicly funded dental care plans for children,[33] most based on provision of care by dentists. The province of Saskatchewan introduced its plan, whereby children aged 3 to 12 were to be treated by dental nurses, in September 1974. By 1976–77, there were approved positions for 134 dental nurses and 18 dentists.[61] Each nurse was expected to provide complete treatment annually for 446 children; this was anticipated to increase to 550 children in time. Children are being phased into the program from the younger age groups; older ages will be included as the number of trained nurses increases.

Saskatchewan dental nurses receive two years' training in the one training school in Regina. Care is delivered on a team basis, with one dentist supervising several teams of nurses in a particular location.[74] The nurses, however, are trained as independent operators. They receive direct supervision from the dentist during the first two months and then work with a more experienced dental nurse for the third month. If their performance is satisfactory, they then work without direct supervision. The supervising dentist carries out all initial examinations of newly enrolled children, meets with each nurse at least once per week, and monitors each nurse's productivity. The supervising dentist also provides the care when procedures outside the scope of the nurse's duties are required. Services are provided free of direct charge. The plan is popular with the public and by 1976 nearly 80 percent of eligible children were enrolled.[61]

In Britain, the first operating auxiliaries based on the New Zealand school dental nurse model were graduated in 1962.* They are generally known as "New Cross" auxiliaries, because the one training school is located in the New Cross area of south London. New Cross auxiliaries are deployed more conservatively than either New Zealand or Saskatchewan nurses; they are not trained to work as independent operators. They may work only in community dental clinics operated by local government or in hospital settings. Supervision is more direct, and completed care must be checked by the supervising dentist before the patient is dismissed. There are still only a few hundred New Cross auxiliaries in Britain, compared with over 20,000 dentists.

It should be recognized that Britain had a long-established school dental

*In this context "operating" means legally allowed to carry out direct intraoral treatment procedures.[38]

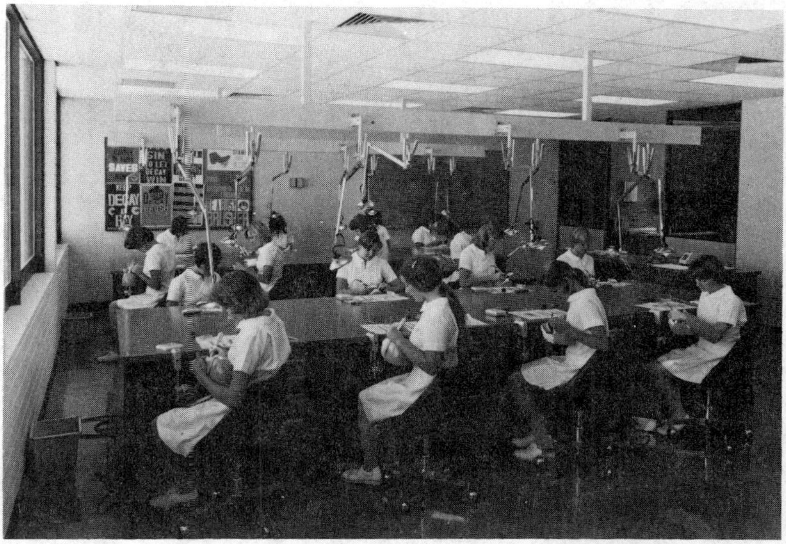

Figure 12–2. Trainee dental therapists learn restorative procedures at the Somerton Park School of Dental Therapy, Adelaide, South Australia. (Photograph courtesy of South Australian Department of Public Health.)

service, with salaried dentists and its own facilities, well before the introduction of New Cross auxiliaries. Although their introduction was met with noticeable opposition from some dentists, this resistance has largely dissipated as the quality of care provided by the auxiliaries has become accepted as excellent.[2] However, the residual resistance to New Cross auxiliaries, probably based chiefly on economic grounds, is a likely reason for their relatively conservative deployment.

Several Australian states now have statewide dental plans in which direct patient care for children up to 15 years of age is provided by auxiliaries, called "dental therapists."[41] South Australia began its plan in 1969 and by 1976 had 110 therapists supervised by 20 dentists.[79] (See Fig. 12–2.) Each therapist is expected to treat annually some 800 children in fluoridated areas and 500 in urban nonfluoridated areas. They are trained to work as independent operators after the supervising dentist has carried out the initial examination of new patients. Public acceptance again is high, with some 90 percent of eligible children enrolled. There is supporting evidence from research studies to show that trained therapists are as capable as dentists of recognizing treatment needs in recall patients.[78] In the state of Western Australia, dental therapists are employed in a generally similar fashion to that of South Australia, though they may also be employed by private dental practitioners. In the mid-1970s, Western Australia appeared to be the only jurisdiction in the world where operating auxiliaries, permitted to cut and restore dental hard tissues, could be employed in private practice as well as in public service. (See Fig. 12–3.)

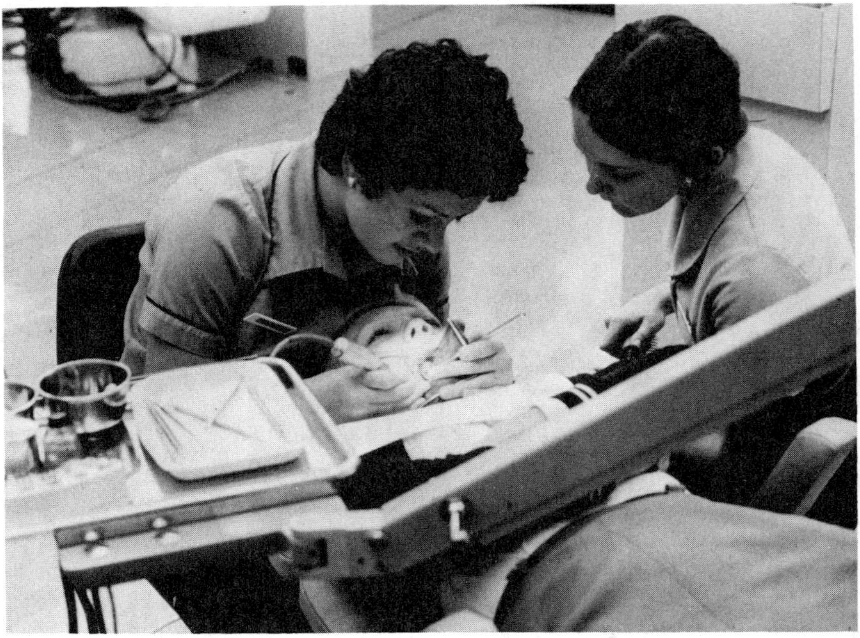

Figure 12–3. A school dental therapist in Western Australia treats a patient in a school-based clinic. The dental assistant is at the right of the picture. (Photograph courtesy of Dr. John Prichard, Principal Dental Officer, Western Australia Department of Public Health.)

Analysis of Auxiliary Based Dental Care Delivery Programs

The well-accepted dental nurse/therapist (terminology is by no means standard) programs in New Zealand, Saskatchewan, and South Australia are all in localities with some features in common. All three are jurisdictions with a history of government-sponsored social welfare plans, so the introduction of dental nurses was probably not a radical departure from social and cultural traditions. All have, or had, a perceived shortage of dentists, and all three have democratically elected governments that were responding to a perceived need when the plans were introduced.

The principal advantage of centrally administered school dental nurse plans is that care can be provided to children in areas where no care would otherwise be available. Rural towns and remote areas that would never be able to support a private practitioner can receive a dental nurse team, thus alleviating the problem of availability of care for children. In New Zealand, dental care is available to all children, regardless of how remote their homes may be. More so than New Zealand, both Saskatchewan and South Australia are characterized by vast distances and sparse populations outside the major urban area, and in both places dental care is steadily becoming available to all children. In these three localities, the dental nurses work as independent operators and, except for the visits of their supervisor, they are not dependent on the presence of dentists in order to be effective. In Britain, however, the New Cross auxiliaries have had less impact, because the legal necessity for them to work under a dentist's supervision means that they can only be employed where salaried dentists are also employed. Since Britain suffers from a marked maldistribution of dentists,[47] the New Cross auxiliaries are unable to fulfill one of the purposes for which they were introduced—namely, to make dental care available to children in areas where there are insufficient dentists. If dental nurses are to be effective, therefore, it seems that they need to be legally permitted to act as independent operators, at least to the extent that they do not have to have a dentist physically present for their day-to-day operations.

Dental nurses are presumed to provide care more cheaply than dentists. Obviously they are less expensive to train than dentists, because they receive only a two-year education in a limited range of dental procedures. In employment, their salaries are similar to those of physical therapists and schoolteachers without advanced degrees. On the other hand, there is a high attrition rate for dental nurses; it has been suggested that this rate is high due to marriage. In South Australia, loss of therapists from the field has averaged 12.5 percent per year, consistent with the average eight-year working life span of dental nurses noted in New Zealand.[79] Changes in marriage and childbearing practices, together with the trend for wives to work outside the home, are beginning to increase the working life of the South Australian therapist. Additionally, an increasing number of males are likely to be trained as dental therapists in South Australia.

Many Americans are skeptical about the value of programs such as New Zealand's on the grounds that recipients do not develop self-responsibility for seeking health care. This belief has been strengthened by studies such as one carried out in 1964 in Brookline, Massachusetts, that used the phrase "the clinic habit" to sum up the perceived problem.[60] It concluded that the use of public dental services in childhood does not lead to the same children's seeking care from private practitioners when they are no longer eligible (because of age) for the public clinic's services. The phrase "the clinic habit" means that while public facilities are used when they are readily available, this usage fails to inculcate habits of personal responsibility for subsequent health care. However, this study could be interpreted as having a cultural bias. If children use a dental clinic, then seek little dental care after they leave the clinic program, are they better or worse off than if they had never used the clinic at all? Is it assumed that children of lower socioeconomic parents would visit private practitioners if the clinic program did not exist? And what is self-responsibility anyway? Is a person who depends on a practitioner's recall card to make an appointment that different from a clinic patient who has a program available at school? The answers to these questions are often based upon cultural assumptions.

Another debatable issue is whether increased availability of less expensive care leads to decreased quality of care. Many dentists are convinced that dental nurses cannot provide the same quality of care as dentists can. Some derisively refer to dental nurses as "half-trained dentists," to which the usual reply is that they are not half-trained dentists but fully trained auxiliaries, competent to carry out the duties for which they have been trained. The New Zealand dental nurse program has been visited by a large number of dental delegations from other countries, and at least five of these visits have been made by dentists from the United States.[37, 41, 44, 49, 76] The conclusions of these visitors about the quality of care provided varies and seems to correlate with the preexisting attitudes of the visitors or the political purpose of the visits. All, however, made subjective assessments of quality, without set criteria or standards, and thus allowed considerable room for personal biases to enter into their conclusions. The report of one such group of visitors, a delegation from the California Dental Association, is a case in point.[76] This visit was made at a time (1972) when the position of dental auxiliaries in California was under examination by a committee appointed by the Governor. The leader of the California delegation to New Zealand had only recently written: "I am unequivocally opposed to paradental personnel performing irreversible procedures or working without the direct supervision of a dentist."[75] This attitude, reflecting the position of organized dentistry in the United States,[7, 15] makes it difficult to see how the visitors could examine a system like New Zealand's in an unbiased fashion.

It is true that most New Zealand children reach the age of 15 without having seen a dentist.[64] What degree of significant oral pathological conditions is thereby missed is unknown. Yet 29.5 percent of American children under 17 years old have never visited a dentist at all.[98] Because dental nurses are trained to refer conditions beyond their own treatment competency, it becomes difficult to argue that more oral pathological conditions go unrecognized in New Zealand than they do in the United States.

The quality argument can go on and on. Studies in the United States and Canada have shown that dental auxiliaries can be trained to carry out a limited number of technical functions,[1, 3, 23, 50, 63, 65, 66, 80, 88] and there is little reason to doubt that auxiliaries trained to work independently operate at an adequate level of technical skill. Until more satisfactory methods of evaluating the overall quality of care, not just the technical standards, are developed, the debate will continue to be subjective and emotional, with positions adopted on political grounds.

There are other administrative concerns about dental care plans in which care is delivered by auxiliaries. Development of a career structure is one; a competent auxiliary may not want to remain in a job that holds little room for career advancement. (One interesting effort at developing a career structure for auxiliaries in the Canadian province of Ontario is described in Chapter 14.) Geographical isolation is another problem; few auxiliaries (or dentists, for that matter) want to remain in a remote area for long periods. Questions of remuneration and conditions of service are certain to arise, and job dissatisfaction can lead to poor morale and hence to low productivity. The increasing unionization of dental auxiliaries in many countries can lead to special problems in program administration. A possible oversupply of school dental therapists has been seen in several well-established programs. While these problems also arise in other groups such as schoolteachers, they do require skillful and sensitive administration for satisfactory resolution and continued successful delivery of dental care.

PROVISION OF DENTAL CARE IN THE 1980s

It is generally realized that the "old days" of dental practice—a time perceived as a more stable and orderly existence, when patients came to their dentists, were treated, and paid for the service received—are gone. It is acknowledged that third-party payment is here to stay. But what about the other issues in the provision of dental care, especially that array lumped under the heading of "government intervention"? Moore summed up the situation as follows:

> . . . there is the growing lack of public confidence and respect for health professionals of all kinds. They are increasingly perceived as selfish exploiters of disease and disability when in fact most are merely frightened small businessmen who do not understand why everyone wants to get involved in their business.[69]

The ADA has long held that all citizens should have access to dental care, regardless of age, income, or any other factor. This principle was restated in Resolution 165 H-1976, passed by the 1976 House of Delegates,[14] which included the statement: "The dental profession is actively engaged in efforts to ensure that available dental care services are sufficient to serve the effective demand of the people of the nation, *providing access to dental care for all.*" (Italics added.) The ADA developed this theme further with the issuance of its Access Program in 1978.

Few dentists would argue philosophically that dental care should not be accessible to all, yet some policies of the ADA seem inconsistent with this principle. For example, the ADA insists that private practice be the foundation for practically all dental care programs,[5, 14] whether publicly or privately funded. Clearly, this policy stems from the Association's perception of the superiority of private practice, though more skeptical observers might view it as a selfish defense of vested interest.[39, 69]

The development of care systems to treat special groups, such as the poor, the old and young, the mentally disabled, the handicapped, and the chronically ill and homebound, usually requires public financing. As discussed earlier, private practice is not structured for treatment of such groups. A number of states have mobile dental units staffed by salaried dentists for the purpose of treating some geographically remote populations. Provision of dental treatment in depressed inner-city areas is a different kind of problem. Apart from action by some dental schools[28] and progressive city health departments, dental care often joins the other services that inner-city residents have to do without. Community health centers and the National Health

Services Corps, mentioned earlier, have had only a small effect in inner-city areas.

For treatment of the chronically ill and homebound, the U.S. Public Health Service showed in a demonstration project in Kansas City in 1960 that such programs were entirely feasible.[92] Despite the evident success of this project, few public agencies have instituted similar programs. Drastic cutbacks in public funds virtually preclude the establishment of such programs in the 1980s, but some agencies might be faulted for not having set them up in earlier years, when funds were more plentiful.

ADA Response to Perceived Threats

The private practice of dentistry received more public scrutiny during the 1970s than ever before. Dentistry did not enjoy being in the spotlight and perceived the attentions of governmental agencies and consumer groups as a threat to private practice. In 1976, the president of the ADA[35] listed five major concerns facing the dental profession:

1. Containing the cost of dental care
2. Federal involvement in professional education
3. Federal involvement in manpower policies
4. Federal intrusion into professional ethics
5. Denturism

All five concerns were perceived as direct or indirect threats to the private practice of dentistry. The president of the ADA in 1977 stated that:

> The very fiber of our American dental practice—our principles of ethics, our dental laws, our private practice delivery system—is being challenged. It is imperative that the dental professional act positively, aggressively, and with haste to meet these challenges.[29]

One method of meeting the perceived challenges began in January 1975, when the ADA launched an expensive public relations effort known as PEP, an acronym for Public Education Program.[11] PEP included such activities as advertising in national newsmagazines to promote private practice, increasing the appearances of dental speakers on radio and television talk shows, special training for many dentists in public speaking and radio and television speaking, and the issuance of numerous booklets on dental service delivery intended for both dentists and patients. The aim of this ambitious program was to convince the public and its legislative representatives that private practice was the dental care system of choice and should be preserved. The underlying assumption was that private practice was in danger of extinction.

Some observers may not view PEP-type efforts the same way that the profession does. In a provocative assessment of the record of health professions in the political arena, Feldstein states that all health professions act in their own interest,[39] as do most groups in society. Feldstein, a health economist, contends that the health professions in the United States, including dentistry, work to preserve their monopolistic positions, which ensure the preservation of autonomy and continuance of high income.[39] In the absence of obvious public evidence that dentists' incomes are dropping,[8, 17, 21] (although real income for dentists was purported to drop between 1967 and 1974,[77] a period that included price controls and a recession), some may have viewed PEP as a selfish attempt to preserve an unjustified monopoly. Some evidence that this may be so came in the elections of 1978, when Oregon voted overwhelmingly to license denturists* to practice in that state. Some persons believe that the vigorous campaign by the dentists in Oregon to oppose this development may have had the opposite effect from that intended.

In July 1976 and January 1977, a direct challenge to the traditional private practice of dentistry came from an agency of the federal government, when the Federal Trade Commission (FTC) initiated three separate actions against the ADA and several of its constituent and component societies. These actions followed a complaint filed by the FTC against the American Medical Association (AMA) in 1975, in which the FTC alleged that the AMA was practicing illegal restraint of trade. During this period the FTC aggressively sought to discover restraint of trade, unfair trade practices, and restriction of competition in what it called the "dental care industry." The first action, in July 1976, was an investigation into state laws and regulations restricting denturism. The FTC's objective was to establish trade rules regarding the provision of dentures. In 1978, the FTC proposed a trade regulation rule that would abrogate state laws prohibiting nondentists from designing and furnishing complete dentures to edentulous persons. FTC staff members were reported to have concluded tentatively that denturism is a desirable alternative to current methods of providing dentures.[29] By 1981, there were threats of Congressional action to curb the FTC's jurisdiction over state-regulated professions and the investigation seemed to have slowed down, though it remained unresolved.

The second action, in January 1977, was a complaint alleging that the ADA's ethical provisions that prohibited advertising were in fact a restraint of trade, which unfairly restricted competition among dentists. This inquiry followed the 1975 decision of the U.S. Supreme Court (*Goldfarb* v. *Virginia State Bar*), which stated that the learned professions were not exempt from antitrust legislation. The reaction of organized dentistry was naturally one of deepest concern, but with the decision of the Supreme Court in June 1977 (*Bates and O'Steen* v. *State Bar of Arizona*), dentistry was obliged to accept that advertising by practitioners was legal. Prior to that decision, a number of states had specifically prohibited advertising in their dental practice acts. These prohibitions could no longer be enforced after *Bates*, as a test case in

---

*A "denturist" is a term applied to a person, usually a dental laboratory technician, who wishes to provide denture care directly to patients rather than remain as a valuable dental auxiliary. This treatment is usually complete dentures, which technicians normally fabricate in the dental laboratory under the prescription of the dentist. The ADA defines a "denturist" as a person who is educationally unqualified and not licensed, for the necessary protection of the public, to practice dentistry in any form on the public.[9] Denturism is discussed more fully in Chapter 14.

Louisiana soon made clear.[67] Even in those states that did not legally prohibit it, advertising by dentists had long been subject to ethical restraint. However, after the 1977 Supreme Court decision, the ADA somewhat reluctantly had to revise its code of ethics to permit some forms of advertising.[22, 53] (The effects of advertising are discussed in more detail in Chapter 13.)

The FTC order against the AMA's "restraint of trade" was sustained in court, and on appeal went to the U.S. Supreme Court. In March 1982, the Supreme Court split 4–4 on its decision in the AMA case, but denied an AMA petition for a rehearing. The effect of this denial for a rehearing was to let stand the lower court's decision. Prior to this decision by the Supreme Court, the FTC and the ADA had reached an interim agreement in 1979, pending the outcome of the Supreme Court's decision in the AMA case. The 1979 agreement prohibited the ADA from declaring any truthful advertising by dentists as unethical, though disciplinary action could be taken against "false and misleading" advertisers. A final order issued by the FTC against the ADA in August 1982 confirmed the 1979 interim agreement on advertising. The ADA and AMA remained deeply unhappy with the role of the FTC in regulation of the professions, and in the early 1980s were actively promoting legislation that would remove state-regulated professions from the jurisdiction of the FTC.

The third action, launched by the FTC's San Francisco office in January 1977, was perhaps the most far-reaching of all, though it seemed to receive less publicity at the time than the advertising affair. The FTC probe into the "dental care industry," an expression that dentists find repugnant, signifies the FTC's belief that provision of health care is a service industry like any other. Practices being investigated by the FTC were listed by the ADA[42] as:

1. Those affecting the disclosure of information, including price information, relating to dental services.
2. Those affecting ownership of dental practices, including restrictions on who can own practices.
3. Those affecting the mobility of dentists and hygienists among states, including recognition or the refusal to recognize other states' licenses.
4. Those affecting the duties that can be performed by dental hygienists.
5. Those affecting entry into the practice of dentistry and dental hygiene, such as citizenship and language requirements, accreditation and ownership of schools training dentists and dental hygienists, and examination and licensing of dentists and hygienists trained outside the state of examination.

Although the existence of an investigation does not necessarily imply that violations of law have occurred, the potential outcome of this inquiry could be profound. After some years of hearing testimony and gathering other material, the FTC retreated a little when it announced in 1980 that it was dropping its investigation into how state laws restrict independent practice by hygienists. A final resolution of all the issues may be affected by Supreme

Court decisions, the outcome of proposed legislation to curb the FTC's activities, and the passage of time.

The FTC, established in 1914, has the task of protecting the public from anticompetitive practices. Its investigations into dentistry and other health professions are spurred by its perception that true competition in the provision of health care is inhibited by state laws governing the practice of health care and by ethical codes of the professional associations. In pursuit of its charge, can the FTC override state laws on professional practice? This is a delicate question, one that will probably require specific legislation and perhaps judicial inquiry to resolve. Reaction by the professions accompanied by increased political lobbying against the FTC in 1980 resulted in a narrow loss for Congressional legislation that would have kept the FTC out of state-regulated professions. Additional threats of Congressional cuts in the FTC's appropriations probably accounted for the apparent moderation of the FTC investigations in 1980. Further legislation defining the limits of the FTC is pending in Congress. Another variable is the ambivalent position of the Reagan administration regarding the FTC—that is, support for private practice, but with encouragement of competition in the marketplace. The future is far from clear.

Regardless of the outcome of the FTC investigation, private practice has already changed as a result of it. Advertising has been a major reason behind the growth of department store clinics and franchised dental practices. Further changes regarding independent practice for hygienists and perhaps for denturists cannot be ruled out.

"Socialized Dentistry"

The aggressive (to dental eyes) posture of the FTC in the late 1970s did nothing to allay American dentistry's time-honored fear of "socialized" health care. What is perceived as "socialized" dental care is common in Europe and in other countries, but is violently opposed by dentists (and other health professions) in the United States for cultural and political reasons. Indeed, the fear of "socialized dentistry" is so strong that many practitioners perceive any move to promote alternative care systems as sinister machinations of the federal government to "drive the private practitioner out of business."

Actually, the use of the terms like "socialized dentistry" or "nationalized health care systems" in public debate over delivery systems is often not very helpful; the expressions are open to a wide range of individual interpretations and thus lead to more confusion than clarification. For example, in a 1976 publication the ADA made the following statement:

> American dentistry is recognized as the world leader, and American dental health is the best in the world. In Great Britain, which is considered to have one of the better nationalized health care systems, the percentage of adults who have lost all their teeth is twice that in the United States.[13]

This statement is presumably put forward to support the contention that the quality of care under private practice in the United States is higher than that delivered by general practitioners and salaried dentists in the National Health Service in Britain, but in that context the statement is misleading. The first sentence is certainly open to debate; its acceptance depends on what is meant by "dental health." Whether Great Britain has one of the "better nationalized health care systems" is also debatable. Whereas the statement about tooth loss is true,[47, 96] the implication that the difference in proportions of edentulous persons in each country is attributable to current systems of care is false, because more than half of the edentulous population in Britain lost all their teeth *before* the introduction of the National Health Service there in 1948.[47] The type of delivery system is but one of many factors contributing to the extent of total tooth loss in a population; cultural factors and traditional attitudes and values are at least of equal importance. In its efforts to defend private practice, the ADA does its cause little good by propagating such slanted information.

Probably few health providers are opposed to all "socialized medicine," defined as: "Medical and hospital services for the members of a class or population administered by an organized group (such as a state agency) and paid for from funds obtained usually by assessments, philanthropy, or taxation."[100] Yet, compulsory enrollment in a system of National Health Insurance, a service included in this definition, is opposed by organized dentistry.[6] Other forms of "socialized medicine," such as care provided to less affluent countries through the U.S. Agency for International Development, or health care provided to military personnel on active duty, are clearly desirable and noncontroversial. The type of governmental intervention most feared by the dental profession in the United States is *state medicine*, defined as: "Administration and control by the national government of medical and hospital services provided to the whole population and paid for out of funds raised by taxation."[100]

While the professions may not actively set out to oppose the public interest, their own goals plainly come first. Opposition to "denturism," for example, can be seen as clearly based on protecting the profession's economic well-being,[39] though many dentists have no doubt that licensing "denturists" is truly not in the public interest. Dentistry can adopt the posture of wanting "to protect people from themselves," such as in the case of denturism. It could be, however, that the public sees the dental profession as "trying to overregulate people's lives." It would be ironic if people began to view the dental profession, which perceives itself as a staunch opponent of government "overregulation," in the same light as governmental regulatory agencies.

The Future of Dental Care in the United States

Nations adopt care systems that are socially and culturally acceptable. The traditional culture of individualism in the United States had led to the development of private practice, an entrepreneurial approach to the provision of care. But the diversity of the United States means that private practice is unable to meet the needs of all people who demand dental services; therefore, other systems of care are evolving and will continue to evolve, to serve the public.

There seems little doubt that the private practice of dentistry will continue to be the principal method of providing dental care. Private practice is acceptable to a large part of the American public and will continue to be demanded. But while much private practice will remain in its traditional role, other practitioners will be more involved in IPAs, capitation plans, department store and franchised practices, and no doubt other modifications of private practice. Even though not all these developments are welcomed by dentists, the profession has shown by its almost universal adoption of third-party prepayment plans that it can adapt to changing social circumstances. There is no doubt it can continue doing so, and indeed must do so if it wishes to preserve private practice. Changes in the system of providing health care will come from social forces such as population changes, economic developments, and public attitudes and values. The dental profession by itself cannot dictate what the system should be. All dental professionals must view their professions as a part of a large and complex social order that is in a constant state of evolution. If that viewpoint were accepted, dentistry would be in a better position to offer leadership in the development of health care systems and to assist in their administration.

References

1. Abramowitz, Joseph, and Berg, L. E. A four-year study of the utilization of dental assistants with expanded functions. Am. Dent. A. J., 87:623–35, Sept. 1973.
2. Allred, Harry, ed. A series of monographs on the assessment of the quality of dental care. London, The London Hospital Medical College, c1977. xi + 242 p.
3. Ambrose, E. R., Hord, A. B., and Simpson, W. J. A quality evaluation of specific dental services provided by the Saskatchewan Dental Plan: final report. Regina, Saskatchewan Department Health, 1976. 19 p.
4. American Dental Association, House of Delegates. Am. Dent. A. Tr., 110:305–6, 1969.
5. ———. Guidelines for dentistry's position in a national health program. Am. Dent. A. Tr., 112:492–517, 1971.
6. American Dental Association, Task Force on National Health Programs. Dentistry in national health programs: a report with recommendations. Am. Dent. A. J., 83:569–600, Sept. 1971.
7. American Dental Association, House of Delegates. (Res. 78-1972-H.) Am. Dent. A. Tr., 114:707–9, 1973.
8. American Dental Association, Bureau of Economic Research and Statistics. The 1973 survey of dental practice. Chicago, The Association, n.d. 39 p.
9. American Dental Association, House of Delegates. (Res. 97-1973-H.) Am. Dent. A. Tr., 114:743–4, 1973.
10. American Dental Association, Bureau of Economic Research and Statistics. Distribution of dentists in the United States by state, region, district and county. Chicago, The Association, c1977 iii + 63 p.
11. American Dental Association, Public Education Program. Reviewing 1975 and anticipating 1976. Am. Dent. A. J., 91: 750–5, Oct. 1975.

12. American Dental Association, Council on Dental Care Programs. Glossary of dental prepayment terms. Am. Dent. A. J., 98:601–4, Apr. 1979.
13. American Dental Association, Public Education Program. Do you believe in private practice? Chicago, The Association, 1976. 12 p. (p. 4)
14. American Dental Association, House of Delegates. (Res.165-H-1976.) Am. Dent. A. Tr., 117:908, 1976.
15. ———. (Res. 40-H-1976). Am. Dent. A. Tr., 117:839, 1977.
16. American Dental Association, Council on Dental Care Programs. Policies on dental care programs. Chicago, The Association, 1977. 45 p.
17. American Dental Association, Bureau of Economic Research and Statistics. Survey of dental practice 1975. Chicago, The Association, 1977. 43 p.
18. American Dental Association. Advanced dental education: annual report 1977/78. Chicago, The Association, 1978. 48 p.
19. American Dental Association, Bureau of Economic Research and Statistics. The 1977 survey of hospital dental departments. Chicago, The Association, c1978. 26 p.
20. American Dental Association, Council on Hospital and Institutional Dental Services. Accredited hospital dental services. Chicago, The Association, 1978. 18 p.
21. American Dental Association, Bureau of Economic Research and Statistics. The 1977 survey of dental practice. Chicago, The Association, 1978. 50 p.
22. American Dental Association, Council on Bylaws and Judicial Affairs. Principles of ethics and code of professional conduct. Am. Dent. A. J., 105:493–5, Sept. 1982.
23. Baird, K. M., Purdy, E. C., and Protheroe, D. H. Pilot study on advanced training and employment of auxiliary dental personnel in the Royal Canadian Dental Corps: final report. Canad. Dent. A. J., 29:778–87, Dec. 1963.
24. Banta, D. What is health care? p. 12–39. (In Jonas, Steven, ed. Health care delivery in the United States. New York, Springer, 1977. xvii + 492 p.)
25. Barmes, D. E. Features of oral health care across cultures. Internat. Dent. J., 26:253–66, Sept. 1976.
26. Beck, D. J. Dental health status of the New Zealand population in late adolescence and young adulthood. Wellington, New Zealand, National Health Statistics Centre Special Report no. 29, 1968. 106 p.
27. Billington, R. A. Frontiers. p. 75–90 (In Woodward, C. V., ed. The comparative approach to American history. New York, Basic Books, c1968. xi + 370 p.)
28. Bissell, G. D., O'Shea, Robert, and Perez-Bode, Rene. Dental students in a neighborhood clinic: a review after six years. J. Pub. Health Dent., 37:47–56, Winter 1977.
29. Board asks $75 dues increase to meet critical challenges facing private practitioner. ADA Information Bul., June 1977.
30. Califano, J. A., Jr. Remarks made at the National HMO Conference. J. Dent. Educ., 42:556–9, Oct. 1978.
31. Chapman, C. B., and Talmadge, J. M. The evolution of the right to health concept in the United States. Pharos of Alpha Omega Alpha Honor Society, 34:30–51, Jan. 71.
32. Cooke, Alistair. America. New York, Knopf, 1974. 400 p.
33. Curry, T. M. Dental care plans for children in Canada, by province. Ottawa, 1976, 21 p. typescript.
34. Dietz, Jean. Harvard plan growth vexes the competition. Boston Globe, n.v.: Oct. 9, 1978.
35. Dr. Shira calls for unity of national dental groups. ADA Leadership Bul., 6: n.p., Aug. 16, 1976.
36. Dummett, C. O. Understanding the underprivileged patient. Am. Dent. A. J., 79:1363–7, Dec. 1969.
37. Dunning, J. M. Deployment and control of dental auxiliaries in New Zealand and Australia. Am. Dent. A. J., 85:618–26, Sept. 1972.
38. Elderton, R. J. Dental ancillaries. p. 202–20 (In Slack, G. L., and Burt, B. A., eds. Dental public health: an introduction to community dentistry. Bristol, Wright, 1974. ix + 338 p.)
39. Feldstein, P. J. Health associations and the demand for legislation: the political economy of health. Cambridge, Mass., Ballinger, c1977. xii + 255 p.
40. Financial situation of dental students: an interview with Harry W. Bruce. Am. Dent. A. J., 92:862–6, May 1976.
41. Friedman, J. W. The New Zealand School Dental Service: lesson in radical conservatism. Am. Dent. A. J., 85:609–17, Sept. 1972.
42. FTC issues complaint against ADA. ADA News, Jan. 24, 1977.

43. Fuchs, Victor. Who shall live? Health, economics, and social choice. New York, Basic Books, c1974. vii + 168 p.
44. Fulton, J. T. Experiment in dental care: results of New Zealand's use of school dental nurses. World Health Organization Monograph series no. 4. Geneva, the Organization, 1951. 87 p.
45. Gibson, R. M., and Fisher, C. R. National health expenditures, fiscal year 1977. Soc. Sec. Bul., 41:3–20, July 1978.
46. Gift, Helen C., and Schaid, Karen. A. Patterns of dental practice in the United States: solo vs. group practice. Am. Dent. A. J., 91:148–52, July 1975.
47. Gray, P. G., et al. Adult dental health in England and Wales in 1968. London, Her Majesty's Stationery Office, 1970. vi + 294 p.
48. Group Health Association of America. National HMO census survey, 1977. Summary. Washington D.C., The Association,. 1977. 38 p.
49. Gruebbel, A. O. A study of dental public health services in New Zealand. Chicago, American Dental Association, 1950. 59 p.
50. Hammons, P. E., Jamison, H. C., and Wilson, L. L. Quality of service provided by dental therapists in an experimental program at the University of Alabama. Am. Dent. A. J., 82:1060–6, May 1971.
51. Health Insurance Institute. Source book of health insurance data, 1977–78. Washington D.C., The Institute, 1978. 80 p.
52. Hannock, E. P. Social security: a system emerges. p. 19–21. (In Origins of the Social Services: a series from New Society. London, New Society Publications, 1968. 34 p.)
53. House approves revisions of "Principles of Ethics." ADA Leadership Bul., 8:2, Nov. 6, 1978.
54. Illich, Ivan. Medical nemesis: the expropriation of health. New York, Bantam, c1976. xviii + 300 p.
55. Jerge, C. R., et al. Group practice and the future of dental care. Philadelphia, Lea & Febiger, 1974. xv + 420 p. (p. 103–22)
56. Jonas, Steven. National health insurance. p. 434–66 (In Jonas, Steven, ed. Health care delivery in the United States. New York, Springer, c1977. xviii + 492 p.)
57. Kegeles, S. S. Adequate oral health: blocks and means by which they can be overcome. p. 73–122. (In Brown, W. E., ed. Oral health, dentistry, and the American public. Norman, Okla., University Oklahoma Press, c1974. vii + 372 p.)
58. Kerr, I. L. The potential of group practice. Paper presented at the 20th National Dental Health Conference, American Dental Association, Chicago, Illinois, April 14–16, 1969.
59. ———. Legislation and professional regulations affecting group practice and the adoption of new methods of care delivery. p. 206–28. (In Jerge, C. R., et al. Group practice and the future of dental care. Philadelphia, Lea & Febiger, 1974. xv + 420 p.)
60. Lambert, Camille., Jr., and Freeman, H. E. The clinic habit. New Haven, College University Press, c1967. 191 p.
61. Lewis, M. H. Personal communication. Aug. 23, 1976.
62. Lindahl, R. L. A place for the closed panel. Mass. Dent. Soc. J., 20:178–83, Summer 1971.
63. Lobene, R.R., et al. The Forsyth experiment in training of advanced skills hygienists. Dent. Hyg., 48:204–13, July–Aug. 1974.
64. Logan, R. K. Personal communication. July 12, 1976.
65. Lotzkar, S. J., Johnson D. W., and Thompson, Mary. B. Experimental program in expanded functions for dental assistants. Phase I: baseline, and phase 2: training. Am. Dent. A. J., 82:101–22, Jan. 1971.
66. ———. Experimental program in expanded functions for dental assistants. Phase 3: experiment with dental teams. Am. Dent. A. J., 82:1067–81, May 1971.
67. Louisiana Dental Act ban on advertising ruled unconstitutional. ADA Leadership Bul., 9:1–2, Jan. 15, 1979.
68. Mechanic, David. Rationing medical care. The Center Magazine, 11:22–31, Sept.–Oct. 1978.
69. Moore, T. G., Jr. The present system as viewed by the consumer. p. 61–9. (In Jerge, C. R., et al. Group practice and the future of dental care. Philadelphia, Lea & Febiger, 1974. xv + 420 p.)
70. Myers, Beverlee A. Health maintenance organizations: objectives and issues. HSMHA Health Rep., 86:585–91, July 1971.
71. Myers, S. E. WHO and dental auxiliaries around the world. Am. Dent. Hyg. A. J., 45:32–9, 4th Quar., 1970.
72. Navarro, Vicente. Medicine under capitalism. New York, Prodist, c1976. xvi + 230 p.

73. Nikias, Mata K. Prepaid dental care: patterns of use and source of premium payment. Am. J. Pub. Health, 59:1088–1103, July 1969.
74. Province of Saskatchewan, Department of Health. Saskatchewan Dental Plan: report of first year of operation, September 1, 1974, to August 31, 1975. Regina, Department Health, 1976. 27 p.
75. Redig, D. F. Can expanded duties work in private practice? Calif. Dent. A. J., 48:2–7, Fall 1972.
76. Redig, D. F., et al. Delivery of dental services in New Zealand and California. Southern Calif. Dent. A. J., 41:318–50, Apr. 1973.
77. Rest-Mincberg, Carol. The relation between organized dentistry's positions on manpower policy issues and present and future states of the market for dental services. Paper given at the 106th annual meeting of the American Public Health Association, Los Angeles, Calif., Oct. 1978.
78. Roder, D. M. Diagnosis, treatment planning and referral by school dental therapists. Austral. Dent. J., 19:242–9, Aug. 1974.
79. ———. Personal communication. June 11, 1976.
80. Romcke, R. G., and Lewis, D. W. Use of expanded function hygienists in the Prince Edward Island manpower study. Canad. Dent. A. J., 39:247–62, Apr. 1973.
81. Schoen, M. H. Group practice in dentistry. Med. Care, 5:176–83, May–June 1967.
82. ———. Group practice and poor communities: dental care. Am. J. Pub. Health, 60:1125–32, June 1970.
83. ———. External forces encouraging group practice. Dent. Clin. N. Am., 16:265–74, Apr. 1972.
84. ———. Methodology of capitation payment to group dental practice and effects of such payment of care. Health Serv. Rep., 89:16–24, Jan.–Feb. 1974.
85. ———. Dental care and the health maintenance organization concept. Milbank Mem. Fund Quar., 53:173–93, Spring 1975.
86. Smith, Q. M., et al. Dental care in a group purchase plan: a survey of attitudes and utilization at the St. Louis Labor Health Institute. PHS Publication no. 684. Washington, D. C., Government Printing Office, 1959. vi + 68 p.
87. Smith, Q. M., and Pennell, E. H. Service requirements in dental payment: predictability and adverse selection. Pub. Health Rep., 76:11–18, Jan. 1961.
88. Soricelli, D. A. Implementation of the delivery of dental services by auxiliaries: the Philadelphia experience. Am. J. Pub. Health, 62:1077–87, Aug. 1972.
89. The state dental scheme and the New Zealand Dental Association. Edit. N. Z. Dent. J., 16:145–8, Jan. 1921.
90. U.S. Congress, Senate. Health Maintenance Organization Act of 1973. Pub. Law 93-222, 93rd Cong., 2nd sess., 1973. Washington, D. C., Government Printing Office, 1974. vii + 72 p.
91. U.S. Department of Health, Education and Welfare, National Center for Social Statistics. Medical recipients characteristics and units of selected medical servies, 1972. DHEW Publication no. (SRS) 75-03153, NCSS Report B-4 (Fy 1972) Supplement. Washington, D. C., Government Printing Office, 1974. n.p.
92. U.S. Public Health Service, Division of Dental Public Health and Resources. Dental care for the chronically ill and aged: a community experiment. Washington, D. C., Government Printing Office, 1961. vi + 54 p.
93. U.S. Public Health Service, Division of Dentistry. Dental delivery systems terminology. DHEW Publ. No. (HRA) 77-6. Washington, D. C., Government Printing Office, n.d. 9 p.
94. U.S. Public Health Service, National Center for Health Statistics. Dental visits: volume and interval since last visit, United States, 1969, by Wilder, C. S., DHEW publication no. (HSM) 72-1066, Ser. 10, no. 76. Washington, D. C., Government Printing Office, 1972. iii + 37 p.
95. U.S. Public Health Service, National Institutes of Health. Group dental practice in the United States, 1971, by Brusseau, Louise. S., Hoggard, F. M., Jr., and Gribble, J. L. DHEW Publication no. (NIH) 73-189. Washington, D. C, Government Printing Office, 1973. vi + 55 p.
96. U.S. Public Health Service, National Center for Health Statistics. Edentulous persons, United States, 1971, by Burnham, C. E. DHEW Publication no. (HRA) 74-1516. Washington, D. C., Government Printing Office, 1974. iv + 31 p.

97. U.S. Public Health Service, Division of Dentistry. Prepaid dental care: a glossary, by Paquin, Nancy. A., Albertini, T. F. and Brusseau, Louise. DHEW Publication no. (HRA) 75-20. Washington, D. C., Government Printing Office, 1975. 31 p.
98. U.S. Public Health Service, National Center for Health Statistics. Current estimates from the Health Interview Survey, United States, 1977, by Howie, L. J. and Drury, T. F. DHEW Publication no. (PHS) 78-1554, Ser. 10, No. 126. Washington, D. C., Government Printing Office, 1978. ix + 98 p.
99. Woodward, C. V. The comparability of American history. p. 3–17. (In Woodward, C. V., ed. The comparative approach to American history. New York, Basic Books, c1968. xi + 370 p.)
100. Woolf, H. B., ed. Webster's new collegiate dictionary. Springfield, Mass., Merriam, c1973. 32a + 1536 p.

CHAPTER 13

FINANCING FOR DENTAL CARE SERVICES

Brian A. Burt

INTRODUCTION

Health care services traditionally have been provided on a fee-for-service basis, whereby the patient receives specific services and pays the provider for them directly. This "two-party" system is a private contract in which the only parties involved are the provider and the recipient of services.

Methods of financing health care in the United States, however, have progressed far beyond the traditional private payment system since the mid-1930s, and especially so since 1965. The fundamental change has been the emergence of "third parties," so that the financing of health services is no longer a matter of a purely private contract between provider and recipient. In 1977, for example, 70 percent of the total outlay for health care was administered through a third party and 42 percent of all health care services were paid for by government agencies.[31]

Dentistry's entry into the third-party system has been relatively recent, but third-party dental care is now a major and still expanding part of dental practice. Dental graduates need an understanding of the variety of mechanisms for financing dental care, because these mechanisms will be an integral day-to-day part of their practices. As the costs of health care continue to rise, methods will be sought to ease costs either by legislation or by the development of a variety of funding approaches. Dental personnel owe it to themselves and to their patients to develop the clearest possible understanding of the social forces at work in this complex situation. This chapter examines and discusses the various methods of financing health care services in the United States.

The Costs of Health Care

The costs of health care services have risen sharply in all industrialized countries in recent years,[39] but nowhere does this seem to have become such

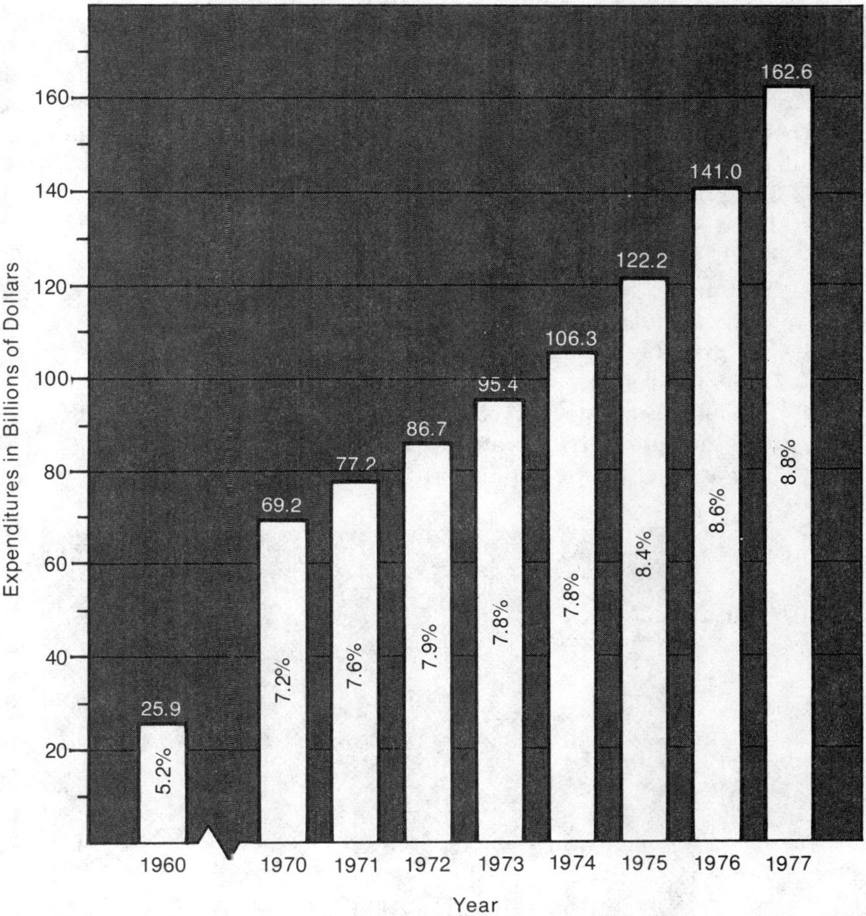

Figure 13–1. National health expenditures in billions of dollars and as a percentage of the gross national product, United States, 1960, 1970–1977. (From the Social Security Administration.[31])

a matter of deep public concern as in the United States. As an illustration of how rapidly health care costs have risen, the average American in 1977 spent $737 on personal health care services,[31] compared with only $290 in 1970.[30] Figure 13–1 shows how the rate of expenditure for health care services is increasing and also how health care costs are absorbing a greater proportion of the gross national product. The total amount spent on health care in 1977, $162.6 billion,[31] is more than double the amount spent in 1971.[30] By 1979, total health care expenditures had risen to $212.2 billion—9.0 percent of gross national product and an average of $943 per person.[32]

This trend of spiraling health care costs is expected to continue. Projections show that barring any fundamental change in the health care system, total health expenditures are expected to reach $462 billion in 1985 and $821 billion in 1990.[26] The 1990 figure represents 10.8 percent of gross national product, compared with the 9.0 percent recorded for 1979. This doubling of health care expenditures at five- or six-year intervals considerably exceeds the general inflation rate, which is why the subject of controlling rising health care costs has become a political issue.

The acceleration in the rate of increase of health care costs has been attributed to a number of factors,[24] principally:

1. The public's increasing demand for health services.
2. The ever-growing technology of health care.
3. The lack of incentives in medical care to keep costs down—for example, treatment carried out in the hospital that could be reasonably provided to the ambulatory patient.
4. The probably higher quality of care now being delivered.
5. General inflation.
6. The increasing practice of "defensive medicine," in which diagnostic tests and prescribed treatment are aimed at avoiding lawsuits rather than at meeting the patients' real needs.

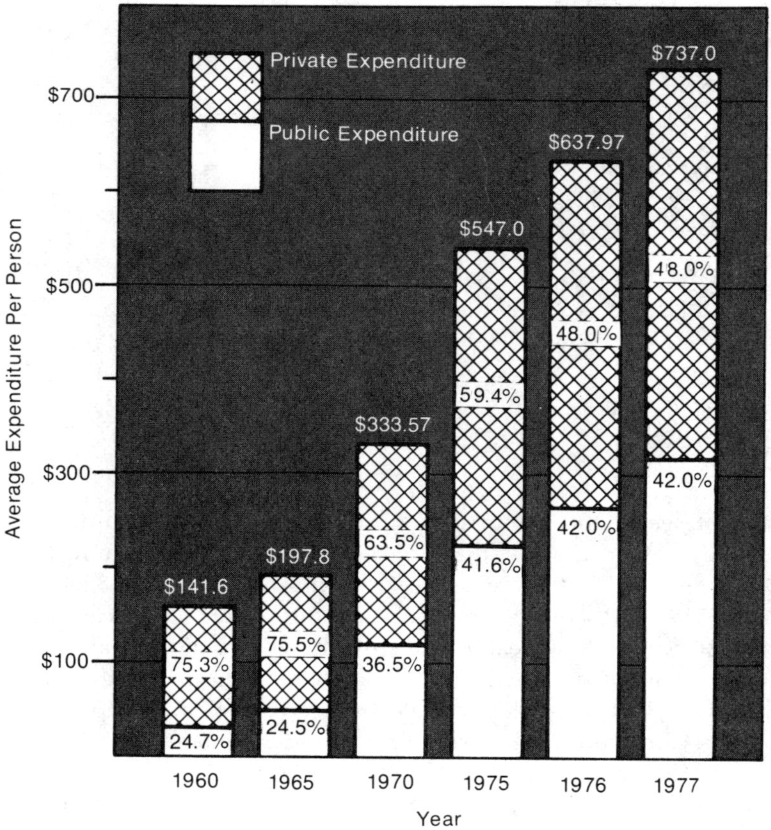

Figure 13–2. Average expenditure for all health care per capita (including personal services, education, construction of facilities, and research), United States, 1960–1976, showing the proportionate expenditure of private and public funds. (From the Social Security Administration.[31])

7. A marked increase in expenditures of public funds for health care.
8. An excessive number of hospital beds and subsequent underutilization of them.
9. An unnecessary duplication of resources resulting from unplanned growth of facilities and proliferation of the more expensive forms of personnel.

To illustrate just one of these factors, the increase in public expenditures for health care is shown in Figure 13–2. In 1976 and 1977 over 42 percent of all monies expended for health care were government expenditures.[30, 31] Only 12 years before that, government spending accounted for less than a quarter of all monies expended for health care.[31] This proportion of public expenditure is projected to hold through 1990,[26] although reductions in federal expenditures on social services could alter that projection.

The Costs of Dental Care

The total expenditure on dental care by Americans was $10 billion in 1977[31] and $13.6 billion by 1979.[32] These figures represent about 6.4 percent of all health expenditures, a proportion that has remained fairly steady since 1965, though it has declined in the long term (see Fig. 13–3). Figure 13–3 also shows the increase in average per capita spending on dental care from $21.56 in 1970 to $45.41 in 1977. Average per capita expenditure on dental care is projected to reach $126 in 1985 and $210 by 1990.[26]

Fees for dental care have not been rising as rapidly as those in other areas of health care. In fact, the American Dental Association (ADA) claims that dental fees in recent years have risen no more than the overall cost of living.[4] The ADA states that although demands for dental care have been rising considerably in recent years, increases in the productivity of dentists and good preventive practices have helped to "hold the line" on dental fees. This argument is based on statistics issued by the U. S. Department of Labor, Bureau of Labor Statistics, which uses the Consumer Price Index (CPI) to measure changes in the purchasing power of the urban consumer's dollar. Estimates by the federal government's Health Care Financing Agency support the ADA's statement. From 1969 to 1979 dental fees increased at an annual rate of 6.7 percent, which is roughly equal to the general inflation rate.[26] Increases in dental fees in that period accounted for more than half of the total expenditure increase for dental care, while a greater intensity of services used per visit accounted for 26.5 percent. Presumably additional patient visits (which does not necessarily mean more patients—it could be more visits for existing patients) accounted for the rest of the expenditure increase.

In view of these figures, dentists are often puzzled when patients and the public complain about "the high cost of dental care." One possible explanation for these complaints, in light of the facts just given, is that 39 percent of all *out-of-pocket* expenses for health care go for dental care.[19] Insurance covers the bulk of medical payment, and patients are more aware of out-of-pocket payments than they are of insurance premiums.

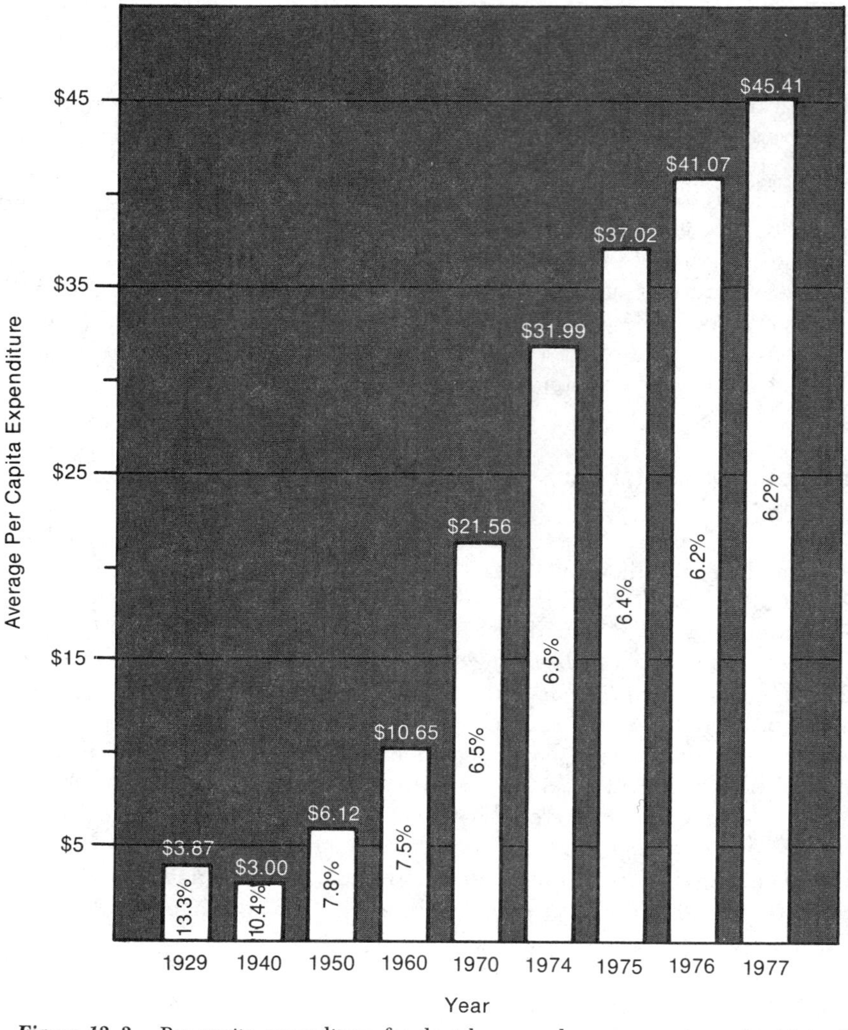

Figure 13–3. Per capita expenditure for dental care and as a percentage of total health expenditure, United States, selected years 1929–1977. (From the Social Security Administration.[31])

Table 13–1 shows how the increases in dentists' fees from 1967 to 1979, as measured by the CPI, compare with increases in medical care and with all goods and services. Figure 13–4 depicts how dental fees have risen at a slower rate than have physicians' fees and the cost of a semiprivate room in a hospital.

It seems likely that the rate of increase in the cost of health care will continue to spiral, at least in the foreseeable future. The subject is extremely complex, but as a matter of concern to everybody, it is certain to attract increasing political attention—especially in view of reductions in federal

Table 13–1. Relative Changes in Prices for Dental Care, Medical Care, and All Goods and Services, 1967 and 1972–80, as Measured by the Consumer Price Index (CPI)*

Year	Dentists' Fees	Medical Care	All Goods and Services
1967	100	100	100
1972	132.2	132.5	125.3
1973	136.4	137.7	133.1
1974	146.8	150.5	147.7
1975	161.9	168.6	161.2
1976	172.2	184.7	170.5
1977	185.1	202.4	181.5
1978	198.1	219.4	195.4
1979	214.8	239.7	217.4
1980	240.2	265.9	246.8

*U.S. Department of Labor, Bureau of Labor Statistics. *Monthly Labor Review*, various issues. *Health Care Financing Trends*, various issues.

spending on health programs during the 1980s. While the rising costs of dental care are not in themselves a great matter of political concern, dentistry could be affected by actions to control the overall costs of health care.

MECHANISMS OF PAYMENT FOR DENTAL CARE

The mechanisms by which dental practitioners receive payment for their services can be grouped into the following general categories:

1. Private fee-for-service.
2. Postpayment plans.
3. Private third-party prepayment plans.
   a. Commercial insurance companies.
   b. Nonprofit health service corporations, such as Delta Dental Plans and Blue Cross/Blue Shield.
   c. Prepaid group practice, including health maintenance organizations and independent practice associations.
   d. Capitation plans.
4. Salary.
5. Public programs.

Private Fee-for-Service

Private fee-for-service, the two-party arrangement, is the traditional form of reimbursement for dental services, not only in the United States but in most other countries as well. Although alternative forms of payment for dental

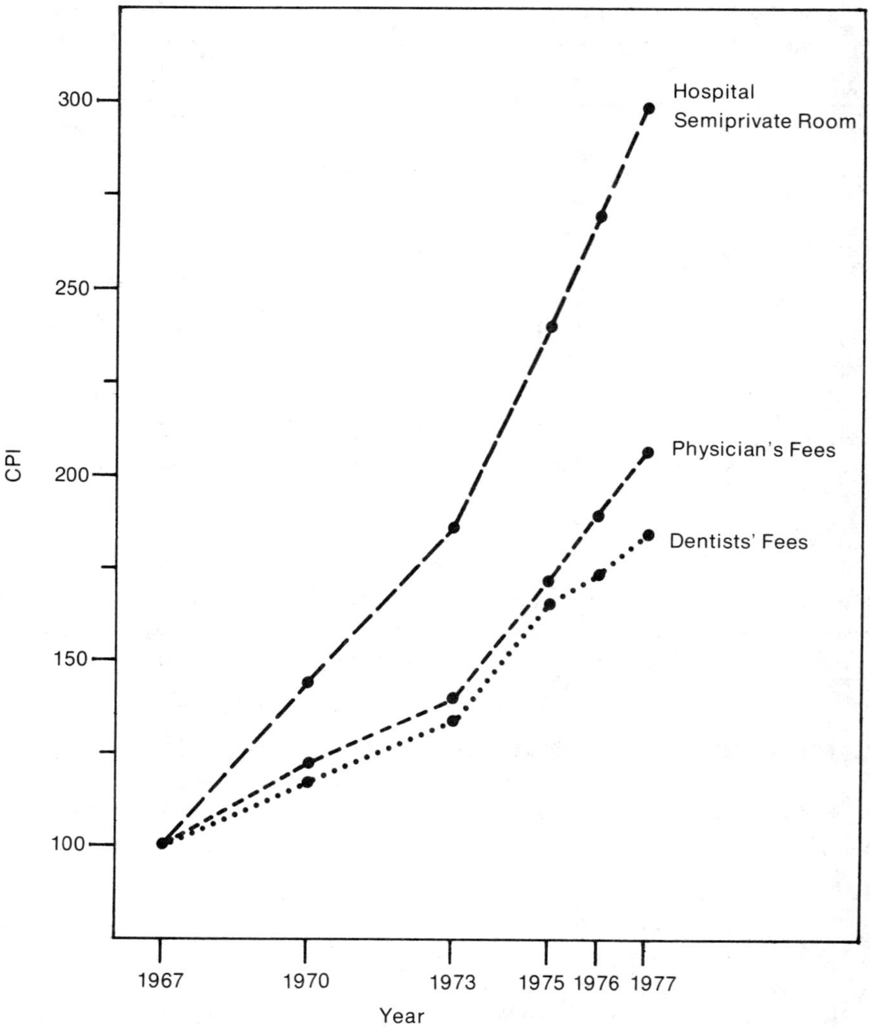

Figure 13–4. Changes in three factors of the medical care component of the Consumer Price Index, United States, 1967–1977. (From the U.S. Department of Labor, Bureau of Labor Statistics. Monthly Labor Review, various issues.)

services are growing rapidly, at present the private fee-for-service arrangement is still the method by which most American dental patients pay for their care.[31] Nearly 80 percent of all payment for dental services in 1977 was by direct private payment.[31] Dentists overwhelmingly prefer to practice under the fee-for-service arrangement, and the ADA defends fee-for-service as the most efficient way of financing and providing dental care.[6] Fee-for-service care is an integral part of private practice as a delivery method (see Chapter 12).

There are a number of advantages to the private fee-for-service system. The first advantage is that it is culturally acceptable; the concept of the individual establishing a fee for the service rendered is inherent in the American way of doing business. The second advantage of the fee-for-service system is its flexibility. Fees can be changed in accord with market conditions; and the dentist is also able to practice what is called "price discrimination," meaning that some patients pay more than others for the same service. (This practice is a time-honored one among dentists, who have viewed it as a kind of "Robin Hood" approach in which fees charged to wealthier patients can subsidize treatment provided to poorer ones.) The use of fee-for-service is also administratively simple, since in the traditional practice of the system, dentists rarely keep a written list of fees for procedures. Yet another advantage of private fee-for-service is that this is the only system under which some forms of dental care likely will ever be provided. Unusual or extremely expensive types of treatment for the most part will only be provided under a private fee-for-service contract.

There seems little doubt that fee-for-service practice will continue to flourish. There will always be patients who do not fit into any of the groups around which alternative payment methods are being developed, and there are and will continue to be both the means and the preference to demand dental services on a fee-for-service basis in the United States. Despite flexibility and price discrimination, however, there are still some potential patients who simply cannot afford the dental care offered. These persons would thus be unable to receive dental care if private fee-for-service were the *only* financing mechanism for dental care.

Fee-for-service private practice is sometimes referred to in dental circles as "the free-enterprise system of dental care." Use of the term "free enterprise" in this context is quite erroneous and should therefore be avoided. Fee-for-service private practice as currently constituted, in fact, is the antithesis of free enterprise. This subject will be discussed more fully later in this chapter.

Postpayment Plans

Postpayment, or budget-payment plans, are not true third-party financing plans but rather mechanisms for the individual purchase of service. While dentists have frequently arranged to allow payment for dental care to be made at intervals over a period of time, the first steps to offer this service through an organized dental society plan were taken in the late 1930s by local dental societies in Pennsylvania and Michigan.[1] A number of local dental societies followed in succeeding years in establishing similar plans.

Under a budget-payment plan, the patient borrows money from a bank or finance company to pay the dentist's fee at the time that the agreement to receive care is made. After the application is approved by the lending institution, the dentist is paid the entire fee less a discount charge, which is placed in a special loss-reserve fund to reimburse the bank for any uncollectible notes. The patient then repays the loan (with interest, of course) to the bank in budgeted amounts. The balance of the loss-reserve fund not used to reimburse the bank for delinquencies is the property of the dental society or the participating dentists.

At the time that they were developed it was hoped that budget-payment plans would bring the benefits of routine dental care to a large segment of the population, but it is hardly surprising that they have not done so. Studies of two of these plans showed that the budget plan was used primarily by people of middle income rather than low income and it was used primarily to finance prosthetic treatment.[67, 68] Although some in dentistry clearly saw postpayment plans as a successful financial mechanism,[51] there were still problems associated with defaulted loans.[67] Low-income patients would also have more difficulty being accepted as credit worthy by the lending institutions.

More recent methods of credit payment for services have tended to bypass postpayment plans. By the late 1970s, many dentists were accepting credit cards, and many patients now use this mechanism for purchasing their dental care in much the same way as they use them for purchasing other goods and services. Given the current trend of the widespread use of credit cards, it is unlikely that postpayment plans will develop any further.

Private Third-Party Prepayment Plans

Third-party payment for dental services is defined as payment for services by some agency rather than directly by the beneficiary of those services.[72] The dentist and the patient are the first and second parties and the administrator of the finances is the third party, defined as the party to a dental prepayment contract that may collect premiums, assume financial risk, pay claims, and provide administrative services.[10] The third party is also known as the carrier, insurer, underwriter, or administrative agent.* The purchaser of the plan can be an organized private group such as a union, or it can be an employer, a union-employer welfare fund, or a public agency, such as an agency of the federal government. Usually, however, the term "third party," without further qualification, refers to a private carrier such as an insurance company; when the government acts as the third party it is more commonly referred to as public financing.

Private third-party plans are now almost totally *prepayment* plans. This form of prepayment is frequently referred to as dental insurance, though strictly speaking, the use of the term "insurance" in this context is incorrect. Traditionally, insurance involves a group of people making small payments in order to cover the risk of any one of them suffering catastrophic loss, such as the loss of a home through fire. Prepayment, on the other hand, is a mechanism

*It can be debated just who actually pays for third-party care. A union that negotiates a dental plan as a fringe benefit is choosing to accept the plan rather than cash, so the union members pay for it in wages foregone. Ultimately, if the companies employing the union members increase the price of their products to finance the plan, the purchasers of those products pay for it. Reference to the third-party agency as the "payer for services," though common, is incorrect; nor are the union members getting "free" care, even if they do not pay directly out of pocket.

to spread the financial load of dental care over a group, because prepayment plans apply to *groups* of people—most commonly, employed groups such as a particular union or the teachers in a school system. There has been little growth of so-called true dental insurance, in which a person can purchase an individual policy.[37] What individual policies are available are characterized by high premiums and limited benefits; this is the carriers' method of countering the risk of high utilization and "adverse selection" (to be discussed).

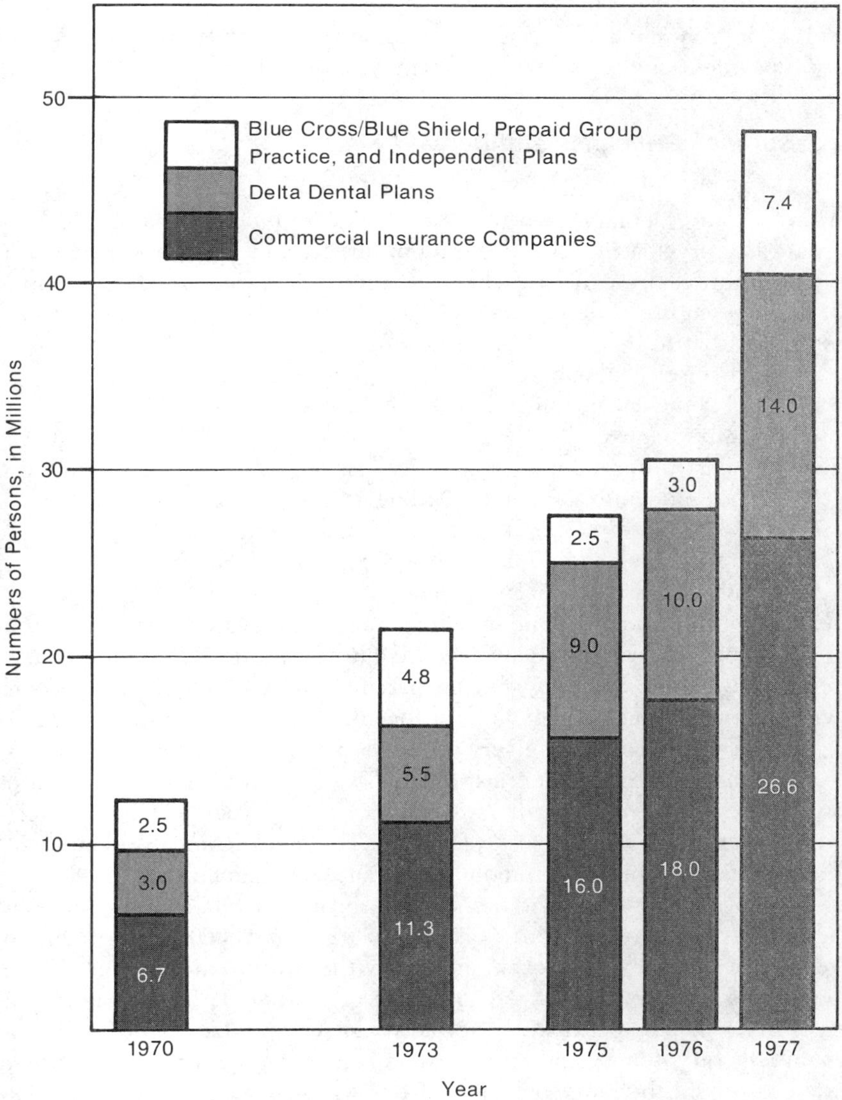

Figure 13–5. Growth in numbers of persons covered by dental prepayment plans, United States, 1970–1977. (From the American Dental Association, Council on Dental Care Programs.[9])

The rapid growth of prepayment plans during the 1970s has changed the nature of dental practice. The growth is illustrated in Figure 13–5, which shows that the number of persons covered by prepayment plans practically quadrupled from 12.2 million in 1970 to 48 million in 1977, and reached 68 million by 1979.[9] The potential market may be double that figure, so that all dental graduates are likely to be affected by prepayment in their practices. While it has been suggested that third parties constitute an intrusion into the dentist-patient relation,[49] the majority of dentists have clearly adapted to them readily. "Insurance patients" are now a standard feature of many dental practices.

It is appropriate at this stage to examine the principles behind insurance and prepayment and to see how they apply to dental care.

Insurance Principles and Dental Care

During the years after World War II, when medical insurance was growing rapidly, dental care was one of the "fearful four" areas of health care (dental care, psychiatric care, prescription drugs, and long-term care) considered uninsurable by carriers. This reasoning was based on the assumption that the very nature of dental need violated the basic principles of insurance.[22] These state that to be insurable, a risk must:

1. Be precisely definable.
2. Be of sufficient magnitude that if it occurs, it constitues a major loss.
3. Be infrequent.
4. Be of an unwanted nature, such as destruction of a home through fire.
5. Be beyond control of the individual.
6. Not constitute a "moral hazard," which means that the presence of insurance itself should not lead to additional claims.[22]

All health insurance violates some of these principles. For example, illness is not predictable for the individual, and health care is usually a wanted service. Insurance carriers found they could get around these problems in several ways. One way is by having patients pay part of the cost of some services, hence using an economic disincentive to overutilization of service. The portion of the cost of the service that a patient pays is either *deductible* or *coinsurance*. A deductible is a stipulated flat sum that the patient must pay toward the cost of treatment before benefits of the program go into effect,[10] sometimes called a "front-end" payment. The most familiar example of a deductible is probably in automobile insurance. A deductible of $200 means that if damage is sustained, the first $200 of repairs must be paid by the owner whether the total cost of repairs comes to $250 or $1000. Copayment (the term is synonymous with coinsurance), on the other hand, means that the patient pays a percentage of the total cost of treatment.[10] For example, if a patient is to pay 20 percent of the daily cost of hospital care, the absolute amount will vary depending on the hospital and type room chosen. Insurance carriers also limit the range of health care services covered: some are available and some not, according to the plan. This is termed "limitation of benefits."

A third way that insurance carriers fitted health care into the insurance model was by offering health insurance at first only to groups. This was done because illness experience is reasonably predictable in a group, though not for an individual. The risk of "adverse selection," which means that the plan selected only high-risk beneficiaries, was thereby reduced because group insurance "averaged out" the risks. The probability of adverse selection was also reduced by the use of waiting periods after enrollment before any benefits became available. The waiting period ensured that persons with existing disease were not simply going to use the plan to have that disease treated and then drop out. As experience with the administration of health insurance grew, carriers were able to offer individual policies. Today, many commercial and nonprofit insurance carriers make individual policies available for hospital and major medical coverage, although premiums are considerably higher and benefits are invariably more limited than for group policies. As mentioned earlier, individual dental insurance policies are available but uncommon.[37]

After looking at the list of insurance principles, it can be seen why dental care was for a long time considered uninsurable. Nearly everyone has some dental treatment needs, and they tend to be frequent rather than infrequent. In addition, the cost of necessary treatment is rarely catastrophic, as it can be for hospital care.

By the late 1960s, however, with some 85 percent of the American population covered by hospital and surgical expense insurance,[37] coverage for dental expenses emerged as an area for future negotiation by labor groups seeking additional fringe benefits.* Growth of dental prepayment plans through the 1960s and especially the 1970s can therefore be seen as a natural social development. In addition, evaluations of some of the earliest group prepayment plans indicated that dental care indeed was insurable because cost was shown not to be the only barrier to dental care.[57-59] Even with the cost barrier removed, potential patients did not pour in as many had previously expected; while utilization of dental service was increased, it stayed well short of 100 percent. In other words, although all members of the group needed dental care and all were paying a premium toward it, only some members were seeking treatment. Subsequent experience has confirmed that the degree of utilization in any given group is reasonably predictable.

Reimbursement of Dentists in Prepayment Plans

The ADA has consistently supported the concept of *usual, customary, and reasonable (UCR) fee* as the preferred method for reimbursement† for dentists in prepayment plans.[2, 3, 6] The Association is opposed to *capitation*

*Passage of the Taft-Hartley Act in 1947 allowed labor unions to seek fringe benefits through collective bargaining.

†ADA resolutions that UCR fees should be the preferred method of reimbursement were rescinded on legal grounds in 1975, following the U. S. Supreme Court decision in June 1975 in *Goldfarb* v. *Virginia State Bar et al.* This decision ruled that learned professions were not exempt from antitrust laws.

and *fee schedules* as the sole forms of reimbursement in prepayment plans, arguing that where such mechanisms exist they should be on an equal footing with UCR fees, so that prospective patients have a choice. Probably this choice is of more interest to the purchaser of the group contract than it is to the individual patient. Apart from UCR fees the only other form of payment that the ADA considers acceptable in prepayment plans is a *table of allowances.*[6]

These terms require definition. First, the usual, customary, and reasonable fees:

Usual Fee. The fee usually charged for a given service by an individual dentist to private patients—that is, his or her own usual fee.

Customary Fee. A fee is customary when it is in the range of the usual fee charged by dentists of similar training and experience for the same service within the specific and limited geographic area (socioeconomic area of a metropolitan area or a county).

Reasonable Fee. A fee is reasonable if it meets these two criteria or if in the opinion of the responsible association's review committee, it is justifiable considering the special circumstances or the particular patient in question.[10]

The definition for "usual fee" is clearly less than satisfactory and was under review by the ADA in 1981.* When third-party dental programs first began, many dentists were opposed to them on the grounds that they would be "regimented" or forced to adopt lower fees than those that they usually charged. The evolution of the UCR fee concept as a mechanism acceptable to dentists and to carriers has allowed third-party dental care to be provided while still permitting the individual dentist to charge what he or she believes the services are worth. It is fair to suggest that dental prepayment plans would never have developed to the extent they have without the UCR fee concept.

A *table of allowances* is defined as a list of covered services that assigns to each service a sum that represents the total obligation of the plan with respect to payment for such service, but that does not necessarily represent a dentist's full fee for that service.[10] For example, if a third-party plan permits a fee of $8 for a particular service for which the dentist's usual fee is $10, the dentist will then carry out the service, pick up the $8 from the carrier, and may charge the patient $2 to make up the usual fee. Under UCR fees, on the other hand, the plan pays the dentist's usual fee in full (less, of course, any required patient copayment), in this case, the $10. (Other possible deductions, such as withholdings for reserves and research and development plus over-90th percentile fees, are described later in this chapter.)

The table of allowances, as a method of reimbursement, has not proved to be entirely satisfactory, because patients are often unaware that the plan to which they subscribe may not cover them in full for dental care. The term "table of allowances" is sometimes used as a synonym for a *fee schedule,* a confusing practice that should be avoided. A fee schedule is defined as

*The new definition of "usual fee", adopted by the ADA at its annual meeting in 1981, reads as follows: The usual fee is the fee that the dentist most frequently charges and accepts as payment in full for dental services.

maximum dollar allowances for dental procedures that apply under a specific contract.[10, 72] The difference is that a fee schedule is usually taken to mean payment in full, whereas a table of allowances, as just explained, may not. Fee schedules for dental care in the United States are established by some public programs such as the Veterans Administration program and the Medicaid programs in some states. Dentistry's opposition to fee schedules is based on: (1) their potential inflexibility, meaning that the fees listed can soon be below customary fees, particularly in times of rapid inflation; (2) the implicit assumption that all dentists' treatment is of the same quality and therefore worth the same fee; and (3) the fear that autonomy is threatened, especially if the fee schedule is not controlled by the dentists. Sometimes a group of dentists in a community will agree to treat specific patients for fees set in a schedule; for example, in some Head Start programs. This action is usually confined, however, to a limited group of patients, and is considered a semiphilanthropic gesture by the dentists concerned.

The ADA is opposed to the use of a *capitation fee* as the only method of payment in third-party programs.[6] A capitation fee is defined as a fixed monthly or yearly payment paid by a carrier to a dentist in a closed panel, based on the number of patients assigned to the dentist for treatment.[72] The dentist receives so many dollars per head per year, regardless of whether the participants in the plan receive no care, a little care, or a great deal of care. The distrust of capitation by dentists is based on the fear that high utilization and demands for expensive forms of care could rapidly outrun the capitation fee that the plan will pay and that therefore dentists will be at an economic disadvantage. Schoen has argued that capitation works every bit as well as fee-for-service and that with proper planning data it is a highly efficient method of financing group dental care, especially for less affluent groups.[54-56] Despite Schoen's claims of success with capitation in his own group practice, dentists and the ADA remain cautious (see Chapter 12).

Delta Dental Plans

In June 1954, the Seattle District Dental Society in Washington state was approached by the International Longshoreman's and Warehouseman's Union-Pacific Maritime Association (ILWU/PMA) with a request that the Society submit a proposal for a comprehensive dental care program for children up to 14 years of age. The union was requesting their employers to add a program of dental care for children to the union members' fringe benefits; the idea was for the program to begin in Seattle and then spread to the smaller port areas throughout Washington. It was clear that a statewide program was really being requested, so the Washington State Dental Association soon became involved. The proposal requested by the union would have required information on administration, fees, methods of operation, dental care provided, and control of quality, and at that time there was almost no previous experience or data upon which to draw. If, however, the Dental Association wished to discourage the union from setting up its own closed-panel clinics with salaried dentists providing care for the children, its only alternative was to devise a plan whereby the children could be treated in the offices of private dentists. Shortly thereafter, the first dental service corporation was born.* Within a few years there were also dental service corporations formed in Oregon and California, and in subsequent years the idea of the dental service corporation spread from the West Coast. By the mid-1970s there were 42 dental service corporations active throughout the United States.[9]

A dental service corporation is a legally constituted nonprofit organization incorporated on a state-by-state basis and sponsored by a constituent dental society to negotiate and administer contracts for dental care.[10] Dental service corporations are usually subject to the insurance laws of the state in which they are constituted.[74] As the number of corporations grew through the early 1960s and the size of the groups for which dental care benefits were negotiated grew in size, the need for a national organization of dental service organizations became apparent. Accordingly, the National Association of Dental Service Plans (NADSP) was formed in June 1966, with staff and financial help from the ADA. The NADSP changed its name to Delta Dental Plans Association in April 1969,[33] and the member corporations became known as the Delta Plan for the particular state. The terms "Delta Plan" and "dental service corporation" are therefore synonymous for all practical purposes.

The underlying philosophy of the Delta Dental Plans is that the dental practitioners can adapt their traditional patterns of practice to meet the demand for group purchase of dental care. In this sense, Delta plans have followed the lead of the professionally sponsored Blue Cross and Blue Shield hospital and medical plans. The majority of the board of directors of most Delta plans are dentists, who are elected from a slate approved by the state dental society. Other board members represent the worlds of finance, insurance, and labor and consumer groups. Delta plans employ experienced actuaries and administrators to guide them in what is now a highly competitive field.

Delta plans also have specific approaches to ensure the quality of care provided and to keep a program's costs within its limits. Quality of care is monitored by a series of posttreatment examinations, whereby a sample of individual patients who have received care through a Delta plan is examined by a panel of disinterested dentists to ensure that (1) the care claimed and paid for has in fact been provided and (2) that it is of "acceptable" quality.† Mechanisms for cost control include coinsurance, preauthorization procedures for certain treatment, and annual limits on specific items of care that can be expensive, such as orthodontic care.

Reimbursement of Dentists in Delta Plans

Because of Delta's traditionally close association with organized dentistry, Delta plans use the UCR concept almost exclusively.[5] The way in which a

---

*Full details of the early development of dental service corporations are given in: U. S. Public Health Service. The dental service corporation; a new approach to dental care. PHS Publ. No. 570, Washington, D.C., Government Printing Office, 1961. v + 70 p. Although this publication is no longer in print, copies can still be found in many dental libraries.

†For a further discussion of quality control mechanisms, see Chapter 2.

dentist is reimbursed depends on whether the dentist is participating or nonparticipating (often called a "nonpar" dentist) in the plan. A participating dentist is defined as any duly licensed dentist with whom a Delta plan has a contractual agreement to render care to covered subscribers.

Delta plans encourage all dentists to participate. Those who do generally agree to conditions similar to the following:

1. Prefiling of their usual and customary fees.
2. Acceptance of payment for their services at the 90th percentile of fees as payment in full, which means they will not assess the patient for any further charges.
3. Fee audits by auditors from Delta, who may check their office records from time to time. The purpose of these audits is to ensure that the dentists are indeed charging their Delta Plan patients the same fees as they charge their other patients.
4. Posttreatment inspection of randomly chosen patients, whom they have treated, by other dentists. The participating dentists agree to abide by decisions regarding quality of care rendered.
5. The withholding of a small amount of each fee, usually less than five percent, to go into the Delta capital reserve fund. Adequate reserves are required by state insurance commissioners in most states. This withholding is expected to be gradually reduced as reserves reach the required level. Some small percentage is retained for research and development.

Nonparticipating dentists can also treat patients covered under Delta plans and be reimbursed by Delta. They do not need to prefile their fees and are not subject to fee audits. However, nonparticipating dentists are usually paid at a considerably lower percentile than the 90th, often at the median, or 50th percentile.

The 90th Percentile

The percentiles of a set of data divide the total frequency into hundredths, so that the 90th percentile is that value below which 90 percent of the observations lie. To illustrate how percentiles are applied, suppose in a given area there are 100 participating dentists who have filed their fee for a particular service. Naturally, the fee filed for this service will vary from one dentist to another. In this particular instance, the range of fees charged for the service runs from \$9 to \$20. If each of these filed fees is spread out in a frequency distribution from the lowest to the highest, the result will be a redistribution like that shown in Figure 13–6. Only 10 of the dentists charge \$9 for their service, 20 of them charge \$10 or less, 30 of them charge \$11 or less, and so on. According to the graph, 90 percent of the dentists charge \$14 or less for this particular service. In this set of data, therefore, \$14 is the 90th percentile fee. There are a few dentists who charge considerably more for this service. In this example, the 95th percentile is at \$18 and the 100th percentile is at \$20. If it can be assumed in Figure 13–6 that the dentists are neatly distributed in groups of 10—that is, if 10 dentists charged \$9, another 10 charged \$10, and so on (which would be unlikely to happen in real life)—the mean fee for the service would be \$12.78. The median fee, which is equivalent to the 50th

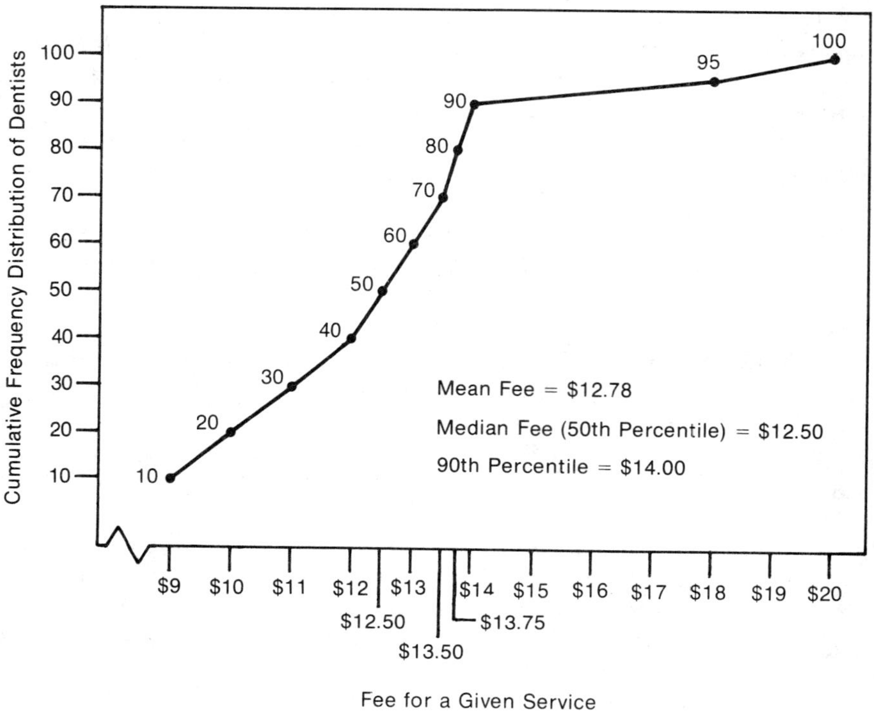

Figure 13–6. Cumulative frequency distribution of hypothetical fees for a given dental service, to illustrate the 90th percentile.

percentile by definition, in this case would be $12.50. The key point to note is that if payment is made at the 90th percentile, 90 per cent of the participating dentists receive their full fee for the service (less withholding) and only 10 percent of the participating dentists would be paid at somewhat less than their usual fee. "Nonpar" dentists frequently are paid at the 50th percentile.

The rationale behind paying at the 90th percentile is to exclude from payment those few dentists at the top end of the scale who charge fees considerably higher than the norm for an area; it fits the definition of "customary." Thus, it is a cost-control mechanism usually written into the Delta plan contract.

Commentary on Delta Dental Plans

In comparison to the giants of the commercial insurance world, the Delta plans are small. And yet they have managed to grow to a healthy state and to compete quite successfully in what is now a highly competitive marketplace. (See Fig. 13–5.)

A group or organization wishing to purchase a prepaid dental care plan seeks bids from interested carriers. Delta's attractiveness as a carrier rests on a number of aspects that commercial insurance companies either do not possess or do not choose to employ. These are:

1. Control of costs, achieved through preauthorization, fee audits, and payment for participating dentists at the 90th percentile and for nonparticipating dentists at a lower percentile. Delta is also a nonprofit organization.
2. Quality assurance procedures, principally posttreatment clinical examinations of treated patients.
3. That individual patients know they will not have to pay extra for their treatment, since participating dentists agree to receive payment in full from Delta. Copayment or deductibles are clearly stated in the benefit policy.

In addition, Delta's attractiveness to potential purchasers depends on its wide support from dental practitioners. A high proportion of practicing dentists—around 80 percent—are participating dentists in the states with the most active Delta plans, such as California and Michigan. As a result, potential purchasers know that care is readily available for the members of their group and under set terms and conditions.

The close ties between dentists and Delta plans allow *benefit packages*, that is, the services available to the members of the purchasing group, to be established according to dental health principles. Benefit packages in Delta plans tend to include accepted preventive services and services that are appropriate for different age groups as well as to encourage regular attendance and maintenance of good dental health by varying copayments with the type of service. For example, in many Delta plans now there is no copayment for annual examination and fluoride applications, a 20 percent copayment for restorations, and a 50 percent copayment for prosthetic care. The financial incentive in these plans is to seek regular care and maintain dental health. As well as fulfilling one of dentistry's aims, that of using improved access to dental care to improve the dental health of the public, this type of practice is more satisfying to the dentist.

Dentists also avoid difficult collections with Delta, though the dentist still has to recover copayments from the patient. Some dentists find the withholding irksome, but most are prepared to accept it. (It should be remembered that a dentist who accepts credit cards also is subject to a withholding.)

By the late 1970s, dissatisfied rumblings about Delta were being heard both in dental circles and in the public arena as well. It was claimed by some dentists that the participating/nonparticipating arrangements were unfair and possibly even unconstitutional and should therefore be removed.[50] The ADA's House of Delegates in 1977 went so far as to recommend ". . . the elimination of patient benefits on the basis of the providing dentists' 'participating' or 'nonparticipating' status in any prepayment program."[7] In addition, the growing consumer movement was threatening the traditional dominance of Delta's governing boards by dentists, because government was suggesting that those who have a financial interest in the policy decisions of health care carriers should not be in a position to make those decisions.

One possible outcome of these movements is that Delta could follow the lead of Blue Cross/Blue Shield and become just another carrier, formally separated from the profession that gave it birth. That would be a pity, since the Delta experience has shown that the profession has been able to accept a degree of self-regulation in the public interest. A divorce of Delta from organized dentistry would tend to reinforce the view of those who believe that health professions are unable to act in the public interest, and it would not be in the best interests of preserving dentistry's own autonomy. Dentists would be well-advised to accept the minor irritations that participating status with Delta can bring,[21] because these inconveniences must be matched against the long-term interests of the profession and society.

Health Service Corporations

The health service corporations, of which Blue Cross/Blue Shield is the most important, have for years offered limited dental coverage as a part of hospital/surgical/medical policies. Dental coverage was usually limited to services provided in a hospital, which constitute a minor proportion of all dental care provided. Health service corporations showed no enthusiasm for going any further into dental prepayment, on the grounds that it was a poor insurance risk, but their attitude changed once dental prepayment was shown to be feasible. This development was to be expected, for Blue Cross/Blue Shield was heavily involved in the rapid growth of hospital/medical/surgical group coverage in the years following the enactment of the Taft-Hartley labor law in 1947.

Blue Cross/Blue Shield dental plans have adopted many of the cost-control features pioneered by Delta plans. Many now use prefiled UCR fees from dentists, either to reimburse the dentists in the same way Delta does or to establish "fee profiles" or "fee screens" for different geographic areas as a basis for reimbursement. In some states, it is difficult to distinguish Blue Cross/Blue Shield dental plans from Delta plans, in terms of benefits and administration.

In some states, Blue Cross/Blue Shield plans are also showing interest in organizing independent practice associations (IPAs) for marketing capitation plans. IPAs, described in Chapter 12, can be connected with health maintenance organizations (HMOs), private entrepreneurial capitation plans, and now Blue Cross/Blue Shield. If IPAs prove to be successful and accepted by dentists, Delta plans also will virtually have to become involved with them.

Commercial Insurance Plans

More persons have dental insurance from commercial insurance carriers than they do from any other type of carrier (see Fig. 13–5). Once it was clear that prepaid dental plans were viable and that they were likely to be a rapidly growing section of the prepaid health care market, commercial insurance companies developed an interest in prepaid dental care plans as a profitable area of business. The fundamental difference between commercial insurance companies and Delta plans is that commercial insurance companies operate for profit; Delta does not. It could be expected, therefore, that commercial insurance carriers would need to charge higher premiums than would Delta plans, in order to allow for the profit margin. In practice, however, they have become competitive through a variety of other mechanisms. One way is that a commercial insurance carrier can be more selective about the group to which it chooses to offer dental insurance. Commercial insurance companies claim no obligation toward the dental health of the community, whereas Delta does, since Delta primarily reflects the views of the dental profession. As a result, Delta plans may get saddled with more adverse risks than commercial insurance carriers would. Commercial carriers sometimes arrange an *indemnity* program, which provides specific cash payment reimbursement for specified covered services.[10] These payments can be made directly to the patient (which gives no guarantee to the dentist that his fees are going to be paid), or they can be *assigned* by the patient to be paid directly to the dentist. In practice, most dentists naturally insist on assignation before commencing treatment. Fee payments in these programs are usually based on a table of allowances.

Commercial insurance companies also organize their levels of reimbursement differently. Dentists in most cases do not file their UCR fees with a commercial insurance company, but rather the carrier operates *fee profiles*; that is, they work out the "going rate" for particular services from their unverified reported experience of fees in the area, and dentists are paid at that rate. This arrangement is somewhat more haphazard than the reimbursement methods used by Delta or usually by Blue Cross/Blue Shield and consequently can create frustrations among some dentists.

However, many dentists also see advantages in dealing with commercial companies. Many do pay the dentist directly for provision of covered services (a service plan[10]), and some dentists report that this payment is quicker and more "hassle-free" than dealing with Delta.[21] Commercial companies also do not conduct fee audits and posttreatment dental examinations to assess the quality of care delivered, though many use preauthorization and annual expenditure limits. Preauthorization procedures by commercial companies, especially where radiographs are requested, have irritated enough dentists to lead to the passage of a resolution by the ADA's House of Delegates in 1976 that provides guidelines for submission of radiographs to third-party carriers.[6]

Commercial insurance companies can compete successfully with Delta Dental Plans because their expertise in promotion and marketing allows them to present attractive total health package plans to potential purchasers. In addition, their large financial reserves allow them, if necessary, to offer a reduced dental premium to a particular group as a "loss-leader," in order to get a toehold on the market.

Commercial companies have no organizational ties with the dentists who provide the services, and the profession has no voice in the determination of their policy. Furthermore, commercial coverage ordinarily does not encourage utilization of professional services (indeed, their profit motive acts to discourage utilization), whereas many Delta plans try to encourage utilization through the absence of copayments for regular recall services. But dental prepayment is a business, highly competitive and increasingly lucrative. The fact that commercial insurance companies can offer attractive total health insurance packages to potential groups of purchasers means that their share of the market is almost certain to continue growing.

Prepaid Group Practice

Group practice, as a method of delivering dental care services, was defined and described in Chapter 12. Some specific points about the financing of care in group practices, however, should be reiterated here. There is no inherent relation between group practice and prepaid care or between group practice and any other form of financing arrangements, for that matter. Net income in a group practice can be divided equally or prorated according to patient load, years of service, and specialty status, while some group practices make all their dentists salaried.[54] Whereas the majority of patients who receive care through group practices do so on the usual private patient fee-for-service basis, larger group practices have resources and personnel that make it feasible for them to offer contracts to consumer groups on a prepaid, capitation basis, and a few do so.[71] In fact, in the early 1960s, the largest number of persons enrolled in prepaid dental care plans received their dental care services from group practices.[68] Since then the rapid growth of Delta plans and commercial insurance coverage has caused the proportion of the population that receives its prepaid care through group practices to drop considerably.

Health Maintenance Organizations

Health Maintenance Organizations (HMOs) were described as a delivery method in Chapter 12. Essentially they are prepaid, capitation-based group practices, which may differ from other prepaid group practices only in that they must meet certain statutory requirements if they wish to be eligible to receive federal subsidies. The principal difference between HMOs and fee-for-service group practices is that the prospective reimbursement feature on a fixed capitation premium in an HMO sets up different financial incentives. Although it has not yet been tested with respect to dentistry, it is possible that the mix of services received by patients in an HMO differs from that seen in fee-for-service practice. It is likely that the future growth of dental care in HMOs will be principally associated with the development of IPAs (Chapter 12).

Capitation Plans

By 1980, dental providers in many states became aware of the increasing proportion of their patients who were enrolled in various capitation plans. The basis of capitation, as previously described, is that the contracting provider, whether an HMO, group practice, IPA, or individual dentist, receives an established, negotiated sum on a monthly or yearly basis for each eligible patient. The money is paid regardless of whether the patients utilize care or not. In return, the patient is entitled to receive a prescribed set of services over a specified period. The ADA distinguishes between a capitation "fee," paid to a dentist in a closed panel by a third party, and a capitation "premium," paid to an organization such as an HMO.[10] The principle is the same in either case.

Apart from the development of HMOs, other third-party carriers and even private entrepreneurs (including dentists) are becoming involved in the marketing of capitation plans. Some have "open enrollment," meaning that plans are not purchased by specified groups but that an individual can "buy in." Many of these plans offer only limited services (such as examination, prophylaxis, radiographs, and treatment plan) and may be more saleable to participating dentists because the risk assumed is low. Dentists might even find these limited capitation plans attractive because they provide the chance to recruit new fee-for-service patients. In areas of the country where there is a real or perceived oversupply of dentists, these capitation plans could be attractive to both purchaser and provider.

Capitation plans have sprouted, in all their permutations and combinations, at such a rapid rate that reliable information on them is difficult to find. Their continued growth and evolution, however, seem certain. They may be necessary, in some form, to preserve third-party payment during times when the national economy is under stress.

Controlling the Costs of Third-Party Dental Care

If third-party dental plans are to continue to grow, mechanisms for restraining cost increases within them must be employed. A number of such mechanisms have been described and are in common use; others may need to be developed. If cost controls are not routinely and successfully incorporated, dental plans may become a target for legislative action aimed at cost control. An even less desirable outcome would be that dental plans could become priced out of the market or so restricted in services offered that they would have little appeal to purchasers. Hospital, major medical, and surgical coverages, after all, are essential; dental coverage, in many people's view, is not. For their own sake as much as for the public's, dental professionals should support the development of acceptable cost-control mechanisms.

The expression "cost control" to many dentists is synonymous with poor quality of care. That association should not be made, for appropriate methods of cost control do not demand the use of inferior materials or technics. Instead, cost control should be based on a concept of cost effectiveness—that is, how can a purchasing group best spend its money in order to gain maximum dental health benefits for its members?

Bailit and colleagues developed a thoughtful approach to this question, based on the results of their research in prepaid dental care.[12] They base their suggestions on the premise that the dentist has substantial control over the services provided among third-party patients presenting for treatment. This situation is analogous to that of medicine, in which there is little financial incentive to minimize costs[20, 23] once an insurance patient presents for treatment. If the prepaid plan substantially covers the cost of care, the patient will tend to accept most treatment plans suggested.

Prereview is the assessment of all estimates for treatment above a set dollar amount (during the 1970s, usually $100 to $150) conducted before the treatment is carried out, in order to determine (in part) if the same quality of treatment can be provided at less cost.[10] While prereview occurred in 20 percent of the claims reviewed by Bailit and colleagues, prereviewed cases constituted 80 percent of all expenditures. Bailit considers prereview mechanisms important, but of limited value in controlling the costs of a program. The main value may be in dentists' knowing there is a prereview process.

Bailit and associates also considered the development of prepaid group practice to be a useful cost-control mechanism; but as described in Chapter 12, group practices are developing slowly in the United States. The most promise for cost control, Bailit contends, lies in the structure of the benefit plan. For example, research showed that whereas only 10 percent of patients received crowns and bridges, that 10 percent absorbed 30.4 percent of program costs. (A related finding by Douglass and Day was that 34.5 percent of all dental care expenditures in 1977 were for fixed prosthetics and that crowns and bridges have now become the largest single item of expenditure in dental care.[19]) The question is whether these services are cost-effective, because if they continue to be provided at this rate they can rapidly drain a group purchaser's funds, which may have been better spent elsewhere. Bailit does not go so far as to suggest that crown-and-bridge services be restricted, but such controls may become more common until the appropriate cost-effectiveness studies are carried out. Other limitations on services—notably orthodontic services—are a feature of many plans.

Determination of cost-control mechanisms requires making decisions that many dentists find distasteful. *Third-party plans do not remove the cost barrier to dental care; they merely change its nature.* The amount of care a plan can finance is still finite; the object of controls is to try to use that financing to best advantage. The more that dentists are able to accept that philosophy, the better they will be able to work with purchasers and administrators to devise cost-control mechanisms. It is better that such mechanisms come from dentists in the first place, rather than be imposed by well-intentioned but less clinically knowledgeable persons.

Less satisfactory methods of cost-control involve selling contracts that are cheap in every sense. For example, table-of-allowance plans are usually less expensive than UCR plans, so they can appear more alluring to a purchaser. However, the "table" plan may be cheaper because it offers unrealistically low allowances, excludes many needed services, or has other restrictive clauses. Participants in this plan may then be chagrined to find that they do not get what they expected and still personally have to finance a lot of their care. As in many other areas of life, purchasers of dental plans get what they pay for. Depending on what the purchaser is looking for, the initially higher price of a UCR plan may turn out to be better value over time.

With a degree of economic stringency expected to linger through much of the 1980s, some merging of the UCR and capitation concepts is likely to occur. For example, a plan could offer a package of diagnostic and preventive procedures at a capitated rate (without patient copayment), while other treatment services could be reimbursed under the UCR mechanism. It is likely that pressures to control costs will lead to growth and evolution of the capitation concept in the 1980s.

Salary

Dentists in some group practices (especially closed-panel clinics), those in the armed forces, and those employed by public agencies are salaried. A new graduate beginning a career as an associate in an established practice may draw a salary for a temporary period until a decision is reached about whether or not to enter into more binding arrangements.

Salaried service has the advantage of allowing a dentist to be largely free of the business concerns of running a practice, and thereby allows the dentist to concentrate on clinical matters. Fringe benefits are also often attractive. The main disadvantage of salaried practice could be the lack of financial incentive that some dentists need to be highly productive. It is often advisable for new dental graduates to take their first job in a salaried position, at least for a time, because they can obtain good clinical experience free from the concern that their inexperience may be financially costly. On the other hand, salaried positions rarely permit the accumulation of the kind of wealth that a gifted dentist with a flair for management can achieve in private practice. Probably the choice for a dental graduate is a matter of temperament; many chafe in a salaried post while others prefer it.

Public Financing of Dental Care

Only 5.0 percent of all expenditures for dentists' services in 1977 were from public funds,[31] whereas 42 percent of *all* health expenditures come from public funds.[31] Figure 13–7 shows the proportionate expenditures between public and various types of private payments for different areas of health care in 1977; it can be seen from this figure that direct private payments still constitute nearly 80 percent of all expenditures for dental care. While this latter percentage has been diminishing in recent years, it is because of the growth of private prepaid care rather than public programs. The proportion of expenditures for dental care made from public funds has remained fairly constant for some years.[30, 31, 46, 75] (See Fig. 13–8.)

The proportion of total public expenditures on health care services in

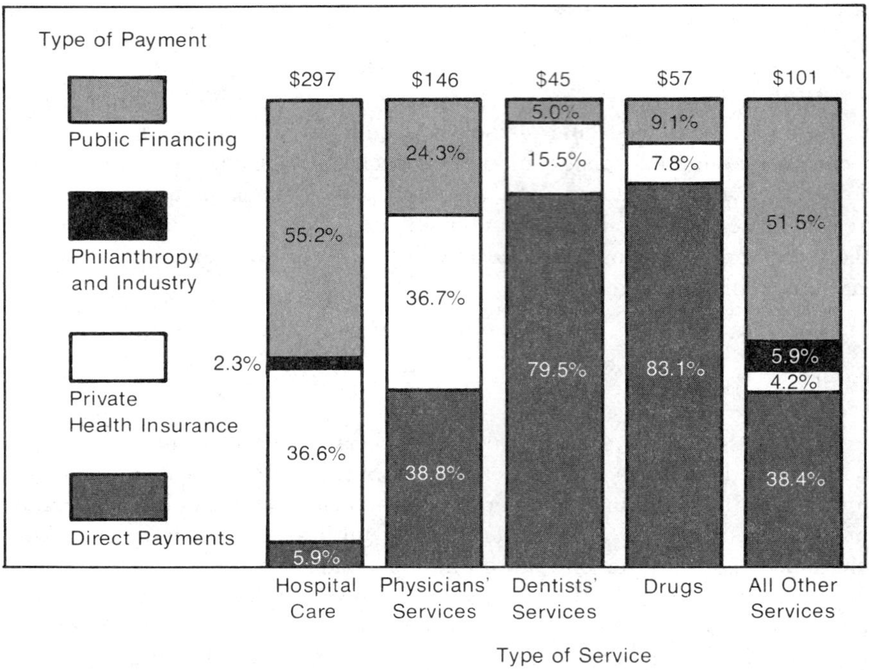

Figure 13–7. Proportionate expenditures on various categories of health services, by type of payment mechanism, and average per capita expenditure by type of service, United States, 1977. (From the Social Security Administration.[31])

1977 that went to dental care was very small, well under 1 percent. Over half of all public expenditures for health care went toward hospital care; the other major areas of public expenditures were physician's services, nursing home care, research, and the construction of health care facilities.[31]

Public financing of health care services can arouse an emotional response among health care providers, many of whom perceive it as "socialized medicine" as opposed to the traditional "free enterprise" health care delivery in the United States (see Chapter 12). While it should be understood that the private practice of medicine or dentistry is not true free enterprise, some who see private practice as being threatened often persist in using the term "free enterprise health care system" synonymously with private practice; for example, as in ". . .our voluntary health system, under a banner of free enterprise, has withstood the test of time and is alive and well."[25] Such a view encourages a polarized perspective; health care provision in the United States is usually depicted in terms of a confrontation between "free enterprise" (which stands for individualism, hard work, efficiency, high quality, a caring relation, and a fundamental aspect of the American way of life) and "socialism" (which signifies laziness, inefficiency, dreary standardization, impersonal care, poor quality, and foreign and somehow sinister ideals). So long as these attitudes prevail, health care providers cannot objectively analyze social trends and how they

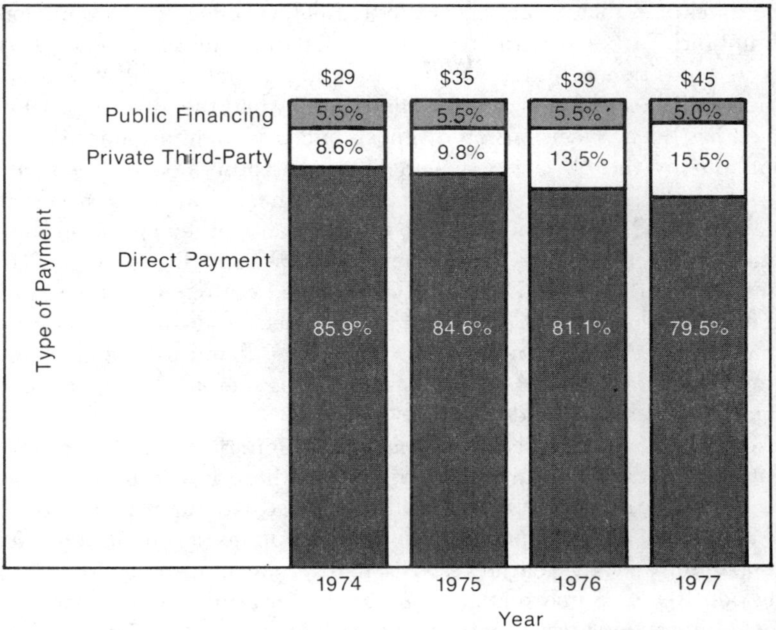

Figure 13–8. Proportionate expenditures on dental care by type of payment mechanism, and average annual per capita expenditures for dental services, United States, 1974–1977. (From the Social Security Administration.[31])

are affected by them. For that reason, a brief discussion of "free enterprise" is in order.

"Free Enterprise" Health Care

Free enterprise implies the purchase and sale of goods and services in a perfect, competitive marketplace. A perfect market is one in which:

1. Buyers and sellers have full knowledge of the products being purchased and sold.
2. Price is a regulator of supply and demand.
3. There are many participants, with no single one so powerful that he or she can significantly influence the market or other competitors.
4. There is ready entry into and exit from the market.
5. There must be no difference in the quality of the product; that is, it must be standard or homogeneous.[43]

All of these conditions rarely exist in real life, though with many products and services a certain departure from them—that is, "imperfect competition"—will still result in a market in which price is the major determinant of supply and demand.[36]

It has been pointed out, however, by a number of economists in health care,[11, 27, 41, 48, 60] that the health care marketplace departs so far from a perfectly competitive one that price has little regulatory effect on production and consumption. To begin with, patients are far from fully informed. They are rarely in a position to judge whether their treatment has been appropriate, whether the fees charged are justified, and what the quality of the care received has been. Decisions on diagnosis and treatment are not made by the patient, but by the physician, whom Fuchs has described in this context as "the captain of the team."[28] While the growth of health insurance has improved access to medical care, it provides no incentives to either physician, hospital, or patient to keep the cost of treatment down.[20] Patients are hospitalized for diagnostic tests that could quite easily be carried out on an ambulatory basis, often because the costs of the tests are covered by insurance only for the hospitalized patient. In dentistry, fees have been found to be higher in areas with a relatively *greater* supply of dentists,[42] thus seeming to oppose the usual economic law of supply and demand.

Not only is the medical care market so imperfect that price is a poor regulator of production and consumption, but there is also little competition in the medical care market.[23, 43] An ill or injured patient is in no position to make a rational choice among the available options for treatment. Even a dental patient seeking routine care is hardly encouraged to "shop around" among dentists. Fee information is generally not available, and dentists tend to be contemptuous toward prospective patients who ask, "How much does a filling cost?" Not only can the prospective patient find price information difficult to obtain until a treatment plan has been prepared, but the patient also has no way of distinguishing between the quality of treatment offered by different dentists. Indeed, organized dentistry goes to some length to point out that receiving dental care is not the same as purchasing a new car or washing machine. While there is good reason for this stance, it gives credence to the view that dental care is not a "free-enterprise" system, because "shopping around" *is* encouraged before buying the car or washing machine. It has been argued that health care's professional groups try to restrict competition rather than encourage it.[23] If the health provider groups do strive to maintain their monopolistic positions (and it can be argued that they should indeed do so in the public interest), that is another reason why the health care delivery system is not governed by "free enterprise."

There is also no free entry into the health care marketplace. Strict laws define who may provide medical and dental care, and such privileges are only attained after a long and arduous period of education in institutions that cannot accommodate all who wish to be trained in them.[34] Again, this monopolistic position is strongly upheld by dentistry and is probably in the public interest, but again it is not "free enterprise."

In June 1977, the U.S. Supreme Court ruled that lawyers cannot be prohibited from advertising in newspapers the fees they charge clients for routine legal services. This case, *Bates and O'Steen* v. *State Bar of Arizona*, has had a profound impact on all the professions.[14] In dentistry, it led to passage of two resolutions by the 1977 House of Delegates of the ADA, which in effect removed disciplinary constraints against dentists who advertise ". . .in the public press the availability of their services and the fees which they would charge for routine dental procedures."[8] Such dentists would also not be barred from joining the ADA solely because of their advertising.[8] While the long-term effects of advertising by dentists cannot be predicted,[14] the greater availability of fee information may introduce some competition into the provision of dental services. It is interesting to note that in a Minnesota survey, 63 percent of a random sample of the public thought that advertising would reduce dental costs, while only 25 percent of dentists thought so.[45]

It is difficult to argue that the health professions are doing themselves or the public a favor by describing their services as "free-enterprise" health care; the professions might be better advised to make the case that a monopoly in the provision of health care services is in the public interest. True "free enterprise" health care would mean that any number of people (such as denturists, independently practicing hygienists, and even totally unqualified persons) could set up as health care providers and charge fees for their services. While such a situation might be acceptable in a fully informed and educated society, the public generally is not in a position to make intelligent choices among the various options that might result. The dental profession certainly opposes any such development. The professions should therefore be able to argue that their monopoly is in the public interest and abandon their misplaced stance on "free enterprise."

Monopolies in the United States, such as utility companies, are usually subject to public regulation. Some segments of society by the late 1970s were apparently viewing health care as a type of public utility, distasteful though the health professions may find such a view. The health professions should seriously consider, however, whether a regulated monopoly position is not preferable to true "free enterprise" in health care, both in their own interests and in the interests of the public they serve.

The Development of Public Care Programs

It was stated earlier in this chapter, and in the previous one, that American society is not unanimous on what constitutes the appropriate role for government in the financing and provision of health care. Dental professionals should develop their own attitudes on a basis of available knowledge, and a good starting point is to examine the historical role of government in health care in the United States.

The English Model

The early development of public care programs in the United States naturally reflected the English experience. The earliest structured form of social services in England was conducted by the monastic orders during the eleventh to fifteenth centuries.[62] These orders maintained systems of social relief, conducted hospitals for the sick and mentally ill, and provided food and shelter for the poor. During his power struggle with the papacy in the 1530s King Henry VIII dissolved these monasteries in an attempt to weaken the power of the Pope in England. As can happen with some legislation, however, action intended to have one result led to a quite different outcome. In this case the result of the dissolution of the monasteries was widespread destitution. In an attempt to deal with this problem, the "Poor Laws" were first established in 1601 under Queen Elizabeth I. These laws made it the duty of the local community to provide for the poor, the lame, the blind, and others whose families were unable to support them. England at this time was an agricultural community in which movement from one area to another was extremely difficult. People on the whole were born, lived, and died in the same village or community. Hence, the responsible role of the local community in these laws made sense, since it reflected the way of life at the time.

The Poor Laws came under great strain with the advent of the Industrial Revolution in the middle of the eighteenth century, for industrialization in England was a true social revolution on a massive scale.[62] Mass migration to the cities encouraged overcrowding, disease, and epidemics, while the *laissez-faire* economic attitudes of the time led to unemployment, starvation, and squalid living and working conditions for the masses, as well as enormous wealth for a few. Men, women, and children underwent appalling hardships in the mines and factories, which frequently led to disease, disability, and premature death. The Poor Laws, which dealt only with the relief of destitution, were inadequate to handle this new kind of problem.

The ideology of *laissez-faire* economics, combined with an acceptance of Malthusian theories of population growth, favored no action to improve the lot of the poor. Malthus, an English country clergyman living in the nineteenth century, wrote that unrestricted growth of population would eventually exceed the expansion of food supply.[44] The growth of population therefore needed to be checked, either by "moral restraint" or by the inroads of starvation, disease, or other disasters, which he grouped under the heading of "misery and vice." Malthus also wrote that the existence of terrible living conditions was not the result of unjust socioeconomic development but rather the consequence of necessary natural laws. Given this view, new public welfare programs that were as degrading as possible were perceived as being in the public interest as well as being sanctioned by a Higher Power.

At a time when there was little mass communication, it took the works of writers like Dickens to arouse the conscience of the growing middle class. Early epidemiological research demonstrated the link between poor living conditions and disease (see Chapter 5), and the pragmatic Victorians became aware that toleration of widespread destitution was not in the national interest. The first public health legislation in England came in the 1850s and evolved steadily, though not without considerable political conflict, to National Health Insurance in 1910 and to a National Health Service in 1948.

The forces that led to the introduction of the National Health Service in 1948 were far more complex than this brief outline has space to analyze. The results of the two world wars, economic trends, and political forces that reflected the emergence of a more egalitarian society were all powerful factors. Interested readers are referred to texts by Willcocks, Titmuss, and Lindsey listed at the end of this chapter under Additional Readings.

American Public Welfare Programs

The earliest welfare efforts in English colonial America were based firmly on the English poor law tradition. Industrialization in the United States followed the same pattern of social disruption as had occurred earlier in England.[17] Even now, dislocations following automation of industry illustrate how individuals who are willing and able to work may become unemployable because the skills they possess are no longer needed. Industries move abruptly from one state to another or to another country for economic or political reasons, leaving workers in communities in which they were located with no obvious source of employment. These disruptions take place now in a highly mobile society, where the old poor law mentality that local communities should provide for themselves is quite obsolete. In modern-day industrial society such problems are national in scope and should be treated that way.

There are several reasons why the American approach to public welfare differs from the English approach. One is that the "puritan ethic" appears to have had a more sustained influence on public policy in the United States than it did in England and Europe. Another is the tradition of individualism in the United States (see Chapter 12). In addition, many of the early pioneers in America were nonconformist religious groups from England and Europe, who brought with them Calvinistic and other rigid beliefs about the nature of man. These attributes of the early pioneers led to the development of some fundamental American traditions and also allowed ready acceptance of the nineteenth-century philosophy of *laissez-faire* economics.[17]

Often overlooked is the original and continuing influence of Spanish colonial America, especially in the Southwest, which antedated the 13 original colonies on the eastern seaboard. An older but still valuable reference on this subject is the thoughtful appraisal by Lyle Saunders in the book *Cultural Difference and Medical Care; the Case of the Spanish-Speaking People of the Southwest*, published by the Russell Sage Foundation. This book points up the cultural tradition of reliance upon the "patron," the owner of the hacienda, for most economic wants—including health care. With the increasing number of Spanish-speaking peoples in the United States, the effect of the puritan ethic may be countered to some degree; government now may be perceived as the "patron" and looked to for assistance in some instances. In other instances the tradition of the Spanish-speaking peoples of the Southwest is to turn to the family (and the extended family) for assistance. It has been estimated that over half of the people in the Southwest will be members of Spanish-speaking families by the year 2000.

Another difference in the development of the American and European social welfare models is that in the United States general welfare relief and payment for health care services for the indigent remained linked together longer than they did in European countries.[61]

Dentistry did not play a significant part in the early development of public medical care programs. Oral health was of relatively little concern in a period when the population was decimated periodically by typhoid, diphtheria, cholera, smallpox, and gastroenteric diseases. Although a few public clinics were established on a voluntary basis by dentists as early as the mid-nineteenth century, public dental care facilities remained almost nonexistent for many years.[52] The U.S. Public Health Service, for example, did not employ dentists on a regular basis until 1919,[53] and the well-known philanthropic dental clinics such as Eastman, Forsyth, Guggenheim, and Strong-Carter all opened in the period from 1910 to 1930.

The Federal Government and the Direct Financing of Health Care

The federal government has been involved in the direct financing of health care almost from the time of its inception. In 1798 the U.S. Congress established the Marine Hospital Fund, the forerunner of the U.S. Public Health Service, to provide medical care for merchant seamen. The rationale was that merchant seamen were an important group who had special health and safety hazards attached to their work, and few had a permanent residence on land. More pragmatically, it was accepted that the seamen posed a threat to the public health because they could transmit communicable disease from one port city to another. The federal government gradually accepted responsibility for the provision of health care services to certain other groups. (For example, military and Coast Guard personnel, American Indians, Alaskan natives, and inmates of federal penitentiaries all receive their health care services through federal facilities.) *This limited and carefully defined role of the federal government in providing direct care only to such special groups was seen for a long time as the right and proper function of the federal government in the provision of health care.*

The relation between the various levels of government in the United States was permanently changed in 1935 with the passage of the first Social Security Act. This act was passed in the midst of the Great Depression, with its unprecedented problems caused by mass unemployment and widespread destitution. The act created a system financed from compulsory employee-employer contributions to provide income maintenance for the elderly. The Old Age Insurance Provisions (OAI) of the original Act of 1935 became extended to the Old Age and Survivors Insurance (OASI) in 1939, and then to the Old Age, Survivors, and the Disabled Insurance (OASDI) in 1960.[61] All the provisions of the Social Security System until then were related to income security, rather than to the financing of health care services per se. In addition, public welfare payments at that time were made directly to the recipients only. The size of the monthly check was determined by a formula that attempted to determine "minimum costs" for living, though the total dollar amount was ordinarily so low that most individuals could have afforded only limited emergency care. Furthermore, the choice was left to the recipient about whether to buy health care or some other item judged to be a necessity. It is perhaps not surprising that under this system, recipients of public welfare tended to seek health care only when they perceived themselves or a member of their family to be seriously ill.

A significant change in methods of federal financing for health care came with the passage of the so-called Kerr-Mills bill in 1960. This legislation, supported by both the ADA and the American Medical Association, linked the health care needs to the general welfare of the aged indigent by a program know as Medical Assistance to the Aged (MAA). Although the effects of this program were relatively disappointing,[61] the Kerr-Mills bill introduced to the public welfare system the use of "vendor payments"—that is, payments directly to those who provided service—while still maintaining the means test. This procedure removed payment of health care from the area of elected choice by the recipient. The plan also served as the predecessor to the major changes brought about in the 1965 amendments to the sections of the Social Security Act relating to public health programs.

The 1965 amendments to the Social Security Act were in their own way as landmark a piece of legislation as the original act 30 years before. Title XVIII, known as Medicare, provided for the receipt of health care services by all persons aged 65 and over, irrespective of the economic means of the recipient. Although it could be seen as a natural extension of Kerr-Mills legislation, Medicare cut across traditional cultural boundaries by removing any form of means tests for the recipients. The resultant uproar tended at first to obscure the provisions of Title XIX of the 1965 amendments, known as Medicaid. Medicaid intended to bring access to health care to those indigent and medically indigent* sections of the population. Both Medicare and Medicaid will be discussed in detail in a later section of this chapter.

In order to understand how the federal government became involved in the vendor payments financing of health care through the 1965 amendments to the Social Security Act, it is first necessary to review the established federal-state-local pattern of some 30 years duration that preceded them.

Public Financing of Dental Care, 1935–1965

The Social Security Act of 1935 provided no funds expressly for the provision of health care. At the time of the Great Depression, however, the inability of the vast majority of the public to purchase health care in the traditional way was recognized as one of the major social problems of the time. The system of *grants-in-aid* was developed around this time as a method of using federal finances for needed health care services without disturbing the traditional federal-state relation.

Grants-in-aid were monies allocated among the states according to specified formulas. In order to receive these grants, the states had to expend their own funds for the same objectives as those supported by the grant-in-aid, often in the ratio of one dollar from state or local sources to two dollars from

*Medically indigent refers to that portion of the population that, although not dependent on public welfare to meet the basic necessities of life, does not have available income to purchase health care through the usual private practice channels. It has been suggested that this concept was and is meaningless, as costly new developments in the diagnosis and treatment of previously untreatable diseases can make anyone medically indigent.[61]

federal sources.[29] Grants-in-aid during this period were available only for general support of specific categories of needy individuals, such as the blind, dependent children, permanently and totally disabled, and the aged.

Those who did not qualify for aid under one of these four categories, even though they might be equally needy, were included in a catch-all program known as general assistance, which was financed entirely by state and local funds and therefore usually funded at a lower level of support. Although payment for health services was frequently supposed to be covered under general assistance programs, often only the most basic medical services actually were. The primary aim of welfare administrators was often to save as much as possible of the limited state and local funds earmarked for health services rather than to ensure that health care needs were met. As funds were usually inadequate to cover much beyond basic services for the indigent anyway, the medically indigent could expect little help. This system also ensured that the provision of health care services for the needy remained firmly locked to their general support, thus helping to ensure that "the poor got sicker and the sick got poorer."

The dental care pattern during this 30 years can be seen then as one in which limited direct care was provided by the federal government and a great variety of dental care programs were financed and administered by state and local communities, frequently with the help of federal monies through the grant-in-aid system.* These programs varied from good to nonexistent, the overall pattern being one of inconsistency and usually inadequate financing. It was the growing public awareness in the early 1960s of the problems of poverty and of the ill-health resulting from poverty that set the stage for the 1965 amendments to the Social Security Act.

Public Financing of Dental Care since 1965

Medicare

Title XVIII of the Social Security amendments of 1965 is the program known as Medicare. As originally conceived, this program removed all financial barriers for hospital and physician services for all persons over age 65, regardless of their financial means. As is often the case, however, expenditures on the Medicare program in the first few years of operation were considerably higher than estimated, and it was not long before some financial constraints were introduced in the program. By the mid-1970s, Medicare had two parts: Part A, hospital insurance, and Part B, supplemental medical insurance. Both parts contain a highly complex series of service benefits available, and both parts also require some payment by the patient. These payments are a deductible for each hospital episode in Part A and a flat premium in order to qualify for benefits under Part B.

Medicare was brought into being because the voluntary health insurance

---

*Many state health department dental public health programs got their start via such grants-in-aid through the then Children's Bureau and focused on maternal and child health (MCH).

system was unable to provide adequately for persons over age 65. The health insurance industry primarily operates for profit, and those over 65 are a high-risk group in terms of general health care needs. The risk of adverse selection by the insurance carrier was therefore very high. Additionally, because the income of persons aged 65 and older is usually considerably less than for those in the employed population, they have limited funds to spend on health care. Hence, there were twin problems of high health care needs and low income. The MAA program of 1960 attempted to meet these problems, but was too cautious to be successful.[61]

The uproar that surrounded Medicare's birth in 1965 has subsided as the public has come to realize that it has filled a necessary gap in the financing of health care. In 1977, some 26 million Americans were enrolled in the Medicare program, and expenditures for the program were $20.7 billion, of which public financing paid $17.6 billion.[31] In 1979, Medicare expenditures totaled $29.3 billion.[32]

The dental segment of Medicare is limited to those services requiring hospitalization for their treatment, usually surgical treatment for fractures and cancer, and hence constitutes a negligible proportion of the program. Dentists generally would like to see at least the provision of dentures allowed under Medicare, both to allow them to provide a better service for their older patients and to help head off the threat of "denturism" (see Chapter 14).

Medicaid

Medicaid, the name given to Title XIX of the Social Security Amendments of 1965, differs from Medicare in several important aspects. The original intent of the program was to provide funds to meet the health care needs of all indigent and medically indigent persons. Medicaid is a joint federal-state program, with the federal government providing between 55 and 83 percent of the finances for the program in any one state. By the mid-1970s, all states had authorization for the Medicaid program and only Arizona had not implemented it.[64] In all states with the Medicaid program, welfare recipients are automatically covered. Twenty-one states, however, had not covered the medically indigent by 1975. Eligibility standards vary widely from state to state, as do the expenditures on authorized services. In 1974, for example, the average national Medicaid expenditure for a child who was receiving aid to dependent children (ADC) welfare payments was $190 nationally. This varied, however, from $50 per child in Mississippi to $460 per child in New York.[64]

Expenditures for the Medicaid program grew at a more rapid rate from 1970 to 1977 than did the total expenditures for all health care, though its proportion of total expenditures has tended to level out since 1972. Figure 13–9 shows the expenditures for Medicaid from 1970 to 1977 in dollars and as a proportion of total expenditures for personal health services. Medicaid expenditures by type of service are shown in Figure 13–10, which shows that 3 percent of total expenditures were for dental services. (Yet Medicaid in 1977 accounted for nearly 80 percent of all public expenditures for dental services.[31]) The number of recipients in Medicaid is hard to determine because of the

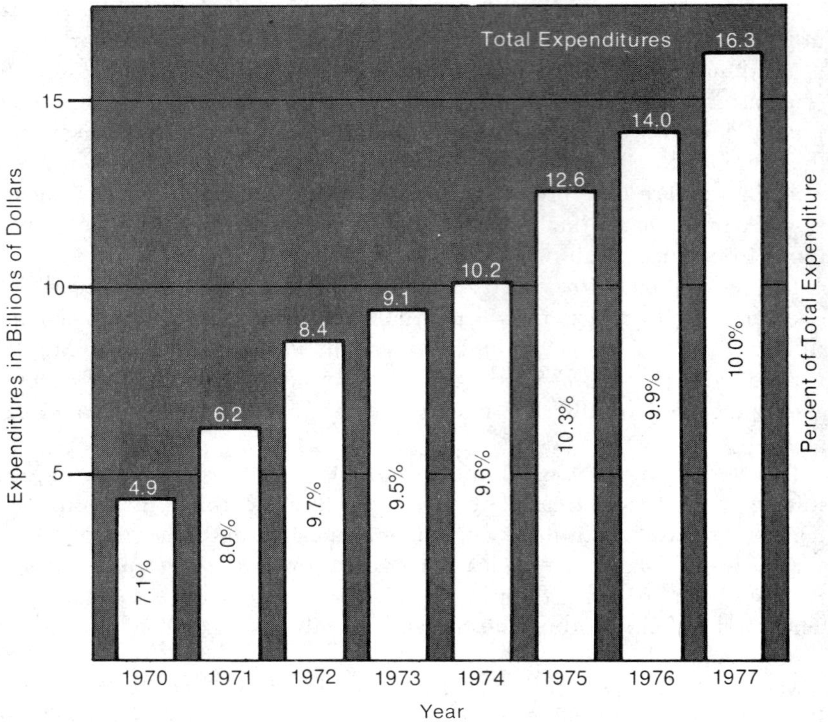

Figure 13–9. Expenditures on the Medicaid program from federal, state, and local sources, in billions of dollars and as a percentage of total expenditures on personal health services from all sources, United States, 1970–1977. (From the Social and Rehabilitation Service,[64] Social Security Administration.[31])

relative speed at which people can move in and out of eligibility, but the best available data indicate that in 1972 there were over 18 million persons who utilized Medicaid services.[63] By 1976, the estimated number of recipients had increased to 24.6 million, of whom 4.4 million had received dental services.[65]

In order to qualify for the federal government's share of Medicaid financing, every state Medicaid program must cover at least these basic services for everyone receiving federally supported financial assistance: inpatient hospital care, outpatient hospital care, laboratory and x-ray services, skilled nursing facility services, and home health services for individuals aged 21 or older.[64] In addition, amendments to the Medicaid program instituted in 1968 required that states offer early and periodic screening, diagnosis, and treatment (the so-called EPSDT program) for individuals under 21, family planning services, and physician services. Federal financial participation is also available to states electing to expand their Medicaid programs by covering additional services or by including people eligible for medical care but not for financial assistance. For this latter group, states may offer the services required for financial assistance recipients, or they may substitute a combination of

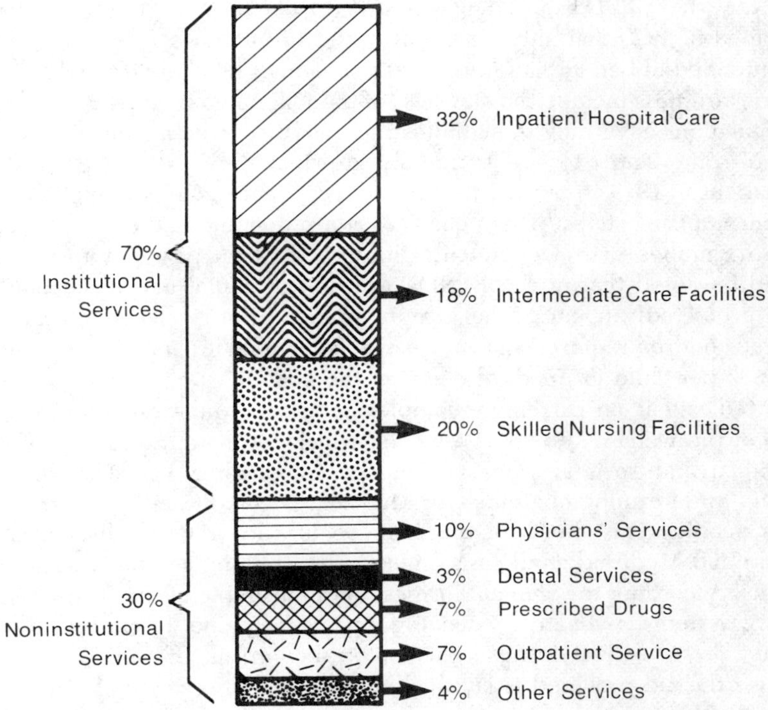

Figure 13–10. Proportion of Medicaid expenditures going to various services, United States, 1974. (From U.S. Department of Health, Education and Welfare.[63])

seven services. Dental care is not a mandatory service except for persons under 21 (part of the EPSDT program). By 1975, a total of 34 states plus Guam and Puerto Rico had a dental service of some kind, but again the type and quality of these dental services varied widely from one state to another.[64]

To what degree Medicaid has been successful is a subject open to debate. Certainly it has made some beneficial impact.[18] For example, the infant mortality rate, widely regarded as a good general measure of the adequacy of health services, dropped sharply in the United States between 1965 and 1975.[73] More rigorous evaluation of the Medicaid program is made difficult by the structure of the program, which complicates the keeping of accurate records. Individual recipients can float in and out of eligibility for the program quite regularly. For example, an unemployed person could register for Medicaid, get a job a few weeks later and thus be ineligible, and then be laid off a few months later and therefore become eligible again. This individual could then be registered several times and in different places.

The EPSDT program, enacted into law in 1968, was supported by the ADA because for the first time a federal program mandated dental care for indigent children. EPSDT therefore had the potential of bringing into the dental care system millions of indigent children and youth. Unfortunately, however, the EPSDT program was slow to get off the ground, and it was estimated in 1975 that only 4 percent of the 13 million needy children that it was intended to benefit had in fact been screened, let alone treated.[47] Reasons for this tardiness include the slowness of the federal government in publishing its regulations governing the administration of the program and the unwillingness of some states to add to rapidly growing Medicaid costs.[47] Additional regulations in 1979 attempted to increase compliance by increasing the penalty to noncompliant states. This penalty was a reduction in the federal share of Aid to Families with Dependent Children (AFDC) payment to states.[66] It should be noted that in the EPSDT age group, dental needs (as could have been predicted) appear to be a more urgent priority than medical needs. Treated children required an average of $90 per child for dental care, compared with $35 per child for medical needs in the mid-1970s.[16]

Medicaid is an extremely complex program. Many of its problems are those of the welfare system as a whole, which result from the clash between individual and societal values (discussed in Chapter 12). The application process to determine eligibility for Medicaid is complicated and confusing to many people. The effects of this may be to encourage families to stay on welfare and Medicaid at all costs, since redetermining eligibility again can be tedious. According to some authorities, an undesirable effect of the American welfare system has been to encourage many recipients to cling to the small amount of security it brings. This unforeseen result of welfare occurs not because the aid provided is lavish, but because the security of some regular income and access to health care under Medicaid ceases as soon as the affected individual "breaks out" and finds employment.

Although the program has reached a large number of people, inevitably there are loopholes. Certain groups, such as widows under 65 and families without children, have been identified as not being eligible for the benefits of Medicaid; indeed, some 28 percent of the poor are without Medicaid coverage.[18] The economic recessions of the early 1970s and the 1980s sharply increased the number of persons on the Medicaid caseload, and because this happened during a period of rapidly increasing medical care costs, the higher costs of the Medicaid program were seen as excessive by some states. As a result, some states have been cutting back on eligibility, reducing the availability of services and the levels of payment to providers. Unfortunately, dental services are often included among the first of these cutbacks. Many dentists, frustrated by rapidly changing eligibility standards for prospective patients, reductions in available services, changes in percentile fees paid, and delays in payment for services rendered, have refused to treat new patients under Medicaid. Hence the classic vicious circle is complete, and the outcome is that many needy persons are still unable to receive the dental care they require.

From its inception, Medicaid has been plagued by political scandal and allegations of corruption and abuse. Public officials in New York City, for example, estimated in 1970 that between 5 and 10 percent of Medicaid claims in New York City showed evidence of either fraud or poor quality care.[13] A fair proportion of this criticism was directed at the dental profession.

The future of Medicaid in the 1980s remains clouded. The Reagan administration is cutting federal spending in the social services, and Medicaid is a prime target for substantial reductions. While the administration seeks to move responsibility for Medicaid to the states, the states already feel overburdened by Medicaid costs and are resisting. Whatever the outcome, the most likely losers are the Medicaid recipients, who are threatened with loss of access to health services provided by private practitioners.

Low-income persons also appear likely to suffer the loss of traditional publicly funded public health services, because these programs are also being severely curtailed by budgetary restrictions. The Reagan administration's philosophy of turning social welfare programs over to the states is likely to cause loss of needed services if finances for these services are not also made available to already stretched state budgets. The substitution of "block grants," in which previously categorical federal funds (evolved from the grant-in-aid days) are lumped together to be used at a state's discretion, is unlikely to help dentistry. The total sum of federal funds received by the state is reduced, and there are heavy political pressures to use the funds for other health-related purposes. The immediate future for traditional public health programs does not look optimistic, though philosophies may change yet again when large numbers of people are unable to get needed health care.

Other Programs of Public Financing for Dental Care

The Veterans Administration (VA) program provides some dental care to eligible patients through its system of hospitals. The VA programs absorbed 12 percent of all public expenditures for dental care in 1977.[31] The federal government also provides financing for dental treatment of children in Head Start, the preschool child development program, and of enrollees in the Job Corps, the training program for young adults from disadvantaged backgrounds. Both of these programs were initiated under President Lyndon Johnson's "war on poverty" in the mid-1960s. In both programs, private dental practitioners provide care to enrollees and are paid by local administrators of the programs. Because arrangements for care and for payment are made locally, practitioners are wise to ensure that all arrangements for payment for care to providers are mutually understood.

Rehabilitative care for children born with cleft lips and palates has long been financed cooperatively by state funds and grants-in-aid from the federal government, because it was recognized that just about everybody is "medically indigent" when it comes to treatment of cleft lip and palate. As cleft palate only occurs in approximately one in 700 live births in the United States,[35] however, the total public funds required for this rehabilitation are not excessive. All states have some resources available for team treatment of cleft lip and palate (Chapter 9); dental personnel should be aware of resources available in or near their community.

Unfortunately, public financing for the dental care of persons with other handicapping conditions, for example, those who are cerebral palsied, mentally retarded, or paraplegic or quadriplegic, has never been as forthcoming. While some states do have reasonable programs for the treatment of children with these conditions, few have any kind of financing available for the dental treatment of these persons when they become adults. The dental treatment of chronically ill and homebound adults has also been neglected almost completely. The U.S. Public Health Service financed and organized a demonstration project in Kansas City in 1960 designed to provide dental care to more than 3,300 chronically ill patients.[69] This demonstration showed that such projects are feasible and that patients with limited mobility can be successfully treated. Despite this successful demonstration project, however, organized community programs to provide care for chronically ill and homebound individuals are by far the exception rather than the rule.

Financing under National Health Insurance (NHI)

Although the idea of NHI in the United States is not new,[15] the mounting pressure for some such program during the 1970s was largely a reaction to the high costs of health care services. However, if NHI is perceived as simply a financing mechanism without any restructuring of the care system, the rate of cost increases is not going to diminish.[40] Indeed, it is highly likely that the rate of increase in direct expenditures would far exceed present levels. It was precisely this realization that largely accounted for the hesitancy in enacting NHI during the mid-1970s. In the 94th Congress (1974–1976), some 20 proposals for NHI were introduced—this in itself is evidence of widespread public interest. The scope of these proposals ranged from modest increases in catastrophic health insurance to virtually comprehensive care for everybody, and most of the proposals included dental care—usually for school-age children—in some form or another. Suggested methods of financing NHI mostly centered around joint employer-employee contributions, increases in Social Security payments (for those plans that would be administered through the Social Security Administration), and financing through general revenues. It is highly likely that the private health insurance industry would also have a role.

Opponents of NHI said that the program would be inflationary because utilization of services would increase sharply and the increase in demand would raise prices for care. Supporters of NHI say that while the global costs of health care services would be likely to increase, the load would be more equitably distributed and the end result would more likely be a healthier, more secure, and more productive society.

While the economic cost of introducing NHI must be balanced against the social costs of not introducing it, there seems little likelihood of NHI in the early 1980s. Discussion in government circles centers around a "competitive" type of health insurance, for which purchasers could theoretically "shop around" for the "best buy." From the earlier discussion on free enterprise, it can be questioned just how qualified most purchasers are to select the "best buy."

FUTURE DEVELOPMENTS

Private fee-for-service dentistry is likely to remain the predominant method of financing dental care in the foreseeable future. Other methods of financing care received through the private practitioner, however, are likely to become more common. More and more practitioners are likely to have a mix of patients financed by prepaid fee-for-service and capitation plans in addition to their privately financed patients. More of these same practitioners may be members of IPAs. More and more prospective patients may have the choice of financing their care through existing prepayment plans, HMOs, or other capitation plans, in addition to paying private fee-for-service.

Prepayment plans mushroomed in the 1970s to the extent that "dental insurance" is now an accepted part of dental practice—almost a traditional part, so rapidly have changes come. Prepayment plans are likely to continue growing, though at a slower rate because the biggest groups are already included. The cloud on the horizon for prepayment plans is the general state of the economy—just as dental care was among the last fringe benefits to be added, so it can be the first dropped when the economy gets rough. In addition, the "competition" approach to NHI may price out dental plans if some of the proposals under discussion become enacted.

Capitation plans seem to be growing, despite dentistry's reluctance to support them. But the profession was also suspicious of prepayment in the early 1960s and has adapted well. There is no reason why the profession cannot also adapt to capitation. Finally, practitioners should expect that variations of the prepayment-capitation-IPA approach will continue to be developed and presented. All should be examined on their merits.

Because it depends on public funding, traditional public health practice is less adaptable than private practice. The budget-cutting climate of the early 1980s has been hostile to public health, and there is no question that many programs will suffer as their funds disappear into "block grants" and are used for other purposes. With the apparent continued attrition of Medicaid, however, there will be many Americans denied access to needed dental care. The traditional public health approach may need to be modified to use a mixture of public and private funds if the dental needs of all people are to be met. Dental personnel can be certain that the financing of dental care is a dynamic area with further rapid evolution still in store.

References

1. American Dental Association, Council on Dental Health. Budget payment plans for the individual purchase of dental care. I. Am. Dent. A. J., 55:446–51, Sept. 1957.
2. American Dental Association, House of Delegates. (Resolution 9–1966–H.) Am. Dent. A. Tr., 107:311, 1966.

3. ———. (Resolution 30–1968–H.) Am. Dent. A. Tr., 109:305–6, 1968.
4. American Dental Association, Bureau of Economic Research and Statistics and Bureau of Public Information. Dentists' fees and inflation. Am. Dent. A. J., 93:129–33, July 1976.
5. American Dental Association, Council on Dental Care Programs. Supplemental report 2; Delta Dental Plans. Am. Dent. A. Tr., 117:32–57, 1976.
6. ———. Policies on dental care programs. Chicago, The Association, 1977. 45 p.
7. American Dental Association, House of Delegates. (Resolution 34H–1977.) Am. Dent. A. Tr., 118:911–2, 1977.
8. ———. (Resolutions 71H–1977; 72H–1977.) Am. Dent. A. Tr., 118:947–8, 1977.
9. American Dental Association, Council on Dental Care Programs. Personal communication, Aug. 4, 1980.
10. ———. Glossary of dental prepayment terms. Am. Dent. A. J., 98:601–4, Apr. 1979.
11. Arrow, K. J. The welfare economics of medical care. p. 13–48. (In Cooper, M. H., and Culyer, A. J., eds. Health economics. Harmondsworth, England, Penguin, 1973. 396 p.)
12. Bailit, H. L., et al. Controlling the cost of dental care. Am. J. Pub. Health, 69:699–703, July 1979.
13. Bellin, L. E., and Kavaler, Florence. Policing publicly-funded health care for poor quality, overutilization, and fraud—the New York City Medicaid experience. Am. J. Pub. Health, 60:811–20, May 1970.
14. Block, L. E. The advertising of dental services. Dent. Surv., 54:12–8, Mar. 1978.
15. Chapman, C. B., and Talmadge, J. M. The evolution of the right to health concept in the United States. Pharos of Alpha Omega Alpha Honor Society, 34:30–51, Jan. 1971.
16. Children's Defense Fund. EPSDT; does it spell health care for poor children. Washington, D.C., Washington Research Project, Inc., c1977. xv + 304 p.
17. Cooke, Alistair. America. New York, Knopf, 1974. 400 p.
18. Davis, Karen. National health insurance: benefits, costs, and consequences. Washington, Brookings Institution, c1975. xiii + 182 p.
19. Douglass, C. W., and Day, J. M. Cost and payment of dental services in the United States. J. Dent. Educ., 43:330–48, June 1979.
20. Eisenberg, J. M., and Rosoff, A. J. Physician responsibility for the cost of unnecessary medical services. New Eng. J. Med., 299:76–80, July 13, 1978.
21. Eklund, S. A., Malvitz, Dolores M., and Striffler, D. F. Report on a study of the automobile employees' dental benefits. Part 2: Attitudes of dentists in three Michigan counties after one and two years. Mich. Dent. A. J., 59:636–47, Dec. 1977.
22. Faulkner, E. J. The role of health insurance. p. 523–32. (In Gregg, D. W., ed. Life and health insurance handbook. Homewood, Ill., Irwin, 1959. xxxiii + 1060 p.)
23. Feldstein, P. J. Health associations and the demand for legislation: the political economy of health. Cambridge, Mass. Ballinger, c1977. xii + 255 p.
24. Foley, H. A. Cost containment begins at home. Edit. Pub. Health Rep., 93:n.p., July–Aug. 1978.
25. Franklin, D. R. External factors leading to the loss of professional control of the delivery of oral health care. Am. Col. Dent. J., 45:36–51, Jan. 1978.
26. Freeland, M. S., and Schendler, Carol E. National health expenditures: short-term outlook and long-term projections. Health Care Financing Rev., 2:97–138, Winter 1981.
27. Fuchs, V. R., ed. Essays in the economics of health and medical care. New York, Columbia University Press, 1972. 239 p.
28. Fuchs, Victor. Who shall live? Health, economics, and social choice. New York, Basic Books, c1974. vii + 168 p.
29. Gerrie, N. F. Grants-in-aid in federal-state dental public health program relationships. Am. Dent. A. J., 54:182–8, Feb. 1957.
30. Gibson, R. M., and Mueller, Marjorie S. National health expenditures; fiscal year 1976. Soc. Sec. Bul., 40:3–22, Apr. 1977.
31. Gibson, R. M., and Fisher, C. R. National health expenditures, fiscal year 1977. Soc. Sec. Bul., 41:3–20, July 1978.
32. Gibson, R. M. National health expenditures, 1979. Health Care Financing Rev., 2:1–36, Summer 1980.
33. Goetz, James. The plan name and symbol. Am. Dent. A. J., 78:706–9, Apr. 1969.
34. Graham, J. W. Dental education; summary of the 1977–1978 Annual Report of the Council on Dental Education. Am. Dent. A. J., 96:767–71, May 1978.

35. Greene, J. C. Epidemiology of congenital clefts of the lip and palate. Pub. Health Rep., 78:589–602, July 1963.
36. Haveman, R. H., and Knopf, K. A. The market system. 2nd ed. New York, Wiley, 1970. 227 p. (p. 140–3)
37. Health Insurance Institute. Source book of health insurance data, 1977–78. Washington, The Institute, 1978. 80 p.
38. Hogeboom, F. E. Practical pedodontia or juvenile operative dentistry and public health dentistry. 6th ed. St. Louis, Mosby, 1953. 642 p.
39. Hu, Teh-Wei, ed. International health costs and expenditures. DHEW Publ. No. (NIH) 76–1067. Washington, D.C., National Institutes Health, 1976. 383 p.
40. Jonas, Steven. National health insurance. p. 434–66. (In Jonas, Steven, ed. Health care delivery in the United States. New York, Springer, c1977. xviii + 492 p.)
41. Klarman, H. E. The economics of health. New York, Columbia University Press, 1965. 200 p.
42. Kushman, J. E., and Scheffler, R. M. Pricing health services: verification of a monopoly pricing model for dentistry. J. Hum. Resources, 13:402–15, Summer 1978.
43. McCarthy, Carol. Financing for health care. p. 247–88. (In Jonas, Steven, ed. Health care delivery in the United States. New York, Springer, c1977. xviii + 492 p.)
44. Malthus, T. R. An essay on the principle of population. 7th ed. (1872, reprinted) New York, Kelley, 1971. xv + 551 p.
45. Meskin, L. H. Advertising of dental services: a consumer and dentist attitude survey. Am. Col. Dent. J., 45:247–53, Oct. 1978.
46. Mueller, Marjorie S., and Gibson, R. M. National health expenditures, fiscal year 1975. Soc. Security Bul., 39:3–20, 48, Feb. 1976.
47. Murray, Jamie B. Whatever happened to EPSDT? Am. Dent. A. J., 90:545–8, Mar. 1975.
48. Mushkin, Selma J. Toward a definition of health economics. Pub. Health Rep., 73:785–93, Sept. 1958.
49. Nelsen, R. J. Interface of the dental profession and the public. Am. Col. Dent. J., 43:176–85, July 1976.
50. Niemann, W. W. Time for reassessment. Mich. Dent. A. J., 60:518–9, Oct. 1978.
51. Ryan, K. J. Complete dental coverage through postpayment and prepayment. Am. Dent. A. J., 68:60–4, Jan. 1964.
52. Salzmann, J. A. Principles and practice of public health dentistry. Boston, Stratford, c1937. xvi + 584 p.
53. Schmekebier, L. F. The Public Health Service. Baltimore, Johns Hopkins, 1923. 298 p. (p. 66–7)
54. Schoen, Max. Group practice owned by a partnership using some salaried dentists and contracting directly with purchasers of group dental care. Am. Dent. A. J., 62:392–8, Apr. 1961.
55. Schoen, M. H. Group practice and poor communities: dental care. Am. J. Pub. Health, 60:1125–32, June 1970.
56. ———. Methodology of capitation payment to group dental practice and effects of such payment on care. Health Serv. Rep., 89:16–24, Jan.–Feb. 1974.
57. Smith, Q. E., et al. Dental care in a group purchase plan: a survey of attitudes and utilization at the St. Louis Labor Health Institute. PHS Publ. No. 684. Washington, D.C., Government Printing Office, 1959. vi + 68 p.
58. Smith, Q. E., and Pennell, E. H. Service requirements in dental prepayment: predictability and adverse reaction. Pub. Health Rep., 76:11–8, Jan. 1961.
59. Smith, Q. E., Mitchell, G. E., and Lucas, Gertrude A. An experiment in dental prepayment: the Naismith Dental Plan. PHS Publ. No. 970. Washington, D.C., Government Printing Office, 1962. iv + 31 p.
60. Sorkin, A. L. Health economics. Lexington, Mass., Heath, c1975. xvi + 205 p.
61. Stevens, Rosemary, and Stevens, Robert. Medicaid: anatomy of a dilemma. Law and Contemporary Problems, 35:348–425, Spring 1970.
62. Trevelyan, G. M. English social history. London, Pelican Books, 1967. 649 p. (First published by Longman Green in 1942.)
63. U.S. Department of Health, Education, and Welfare, National Center for Social Statistics. Medicaid recipients' characteristics and units of selected medical services, 1972. DHEW Publ. No. (SRS) 75–03153, NCSS Report B–4 (FY 1962) Supplement. Washington, D.C., Government Printing Office, 1974.

64. U.S. Department of Health, Education, and Welfare, Social and Rehabilitation Service. Personal communication. Nov. 18, 1976.
65. U.S. Department of Health, Education, and Welfare, Health Care Financing Administration. Medicaid state tables: fiscal year 1976; recipients, payments, and services. Washington, D.C., Government Printing Office, 1978. vi + 160 p.
66. ———. Medicaid requirements for state programs of early and periodic screening, diagnosis, and treatment of individuals under 21. Fed. Register, 44:29420–7, May 18, 1974.
67. U.S. Public Health Service, Division of Dental Resources. Budget payment plan of the Nevada State Dental Society. Washington, D.C., Government Printing Office, 1959. iii + 18 p.
68. ———. A dental society reports on budget payment. Washington, D.C., Government Printing Office, 1960. 28 p.
69. U.S. Public Health Service, Division of Dental Public Health and Resources. Dental care for the chronically ill and aged; a community experiment. Washington, D.C., Government Printing Office, 1961. vi + 54 p.
70. U.S. Public Health Service, Division of Dental Health. Fact sheet on privately sponsored prepaid dental care. 1966, 1 p. duplicated.
71. U.S. Public Health Service, National Institutes of Health. Group dental practice in the United States, 1971, by Brusseau, Louise S., Hoggard, F. M., Jr., and Gribble, J. L. DHEW Publ. No. (NIH) 73–189. Washington, D.C., Government Printing Office, 1973. vi + 55 p.
72. U.S. Public Health Service, Division of Dentistry. Prepaid dental care: a glossary, by Paquin, Nancy A., Albertini, T. F., and Brusseau, Louise S. DHEW Publ. No. (HRA) 75–20. Washington, D.C., Government Printing Office, 1975. 31 p.
73. U.S. Public Health Service, National Center for Health Statistics. Health in the United States, 1975. DHEW Publ. No. (HRA) 76–1233. Washington, D.C., Government Printing Office, 1976. 60 p.
74. U.S. Public Health Service. Insurance regulations affecting prepaid dental care plans; a state-by-state analysis. DHEW Publ. No. (HRA) 78–8. Washington, D.C., Government Printing Office, 1978. viii + 217 p.
75. Worthington, Nancy. National health expenditures, 1929–74. Soc. Security Bul., 38:3–20, Feb. 1975.

Additional Readings

Lindsey, Almont. Socialized medicine in England and Wales: The National Health Service 1948–61. Chapel Hill, University North Carolina Press, 1962. 561 p.

Titmuss, R. M. Essays on the welfare state. New Haven, Yale University Press, 1959. 232 p.

———. Commitment to welfare. New York, Pantheon, 1968. 272 p.

Willcocks, A. J. The creation of the National Health Service; a study of pressure groups and a major social policy decision. London, Routledge and Kegan Paul, 1967. vii + 118 p.

CHAPTER **14**

DENTAL PERSONNEL IN THE UNITED STATES

Brian A. Burt

INTRODUCTION

Social forces are the principal determinants of the structure and process of health services. The types of dental personnel in a society are part of the structure; their numbers and distribution are part of the process. Accordingly, dental personnel need an understanding of these social forces—their history, current development, and likely future direction—if concerns about supply and distribution of personnel are to be alleviated or even understood. This chapter examines the factors influencing the supply and distribution of the various types of dental personnel in the United States, and attempts to provide an understanding of how these patterns are influenced by various social forces.

Dentistry is ultimately accountable to the public it serves, and the most basic facts about that public are its numbers, growth rates, age, and geographic distribution. For that reason, this chapter begins with a brief consideration of population growth and distribution in the United States. Assessment of the types, numbers, and distribution of dental personnel should then be made against this background.

Population Trends in the United States

The population of the United States was estimated by the 1980 Census as 226.5 million,[94] which constitutes between 5 and 6 percent of the world's population. The rate of increase each year during the 1970s was generally less than 1.0 percent. By contrast, the annual average growth rate around the turn of the century was 2.0 percent; in the 1950s, 1.7 percent; and in the 1960s, 1.24 percent.[100] For a global perspective, the contrast between population growth rates in some economically developed Western countries and those in some developing nations of Latin America and Africa is shown in Figure 14–1.

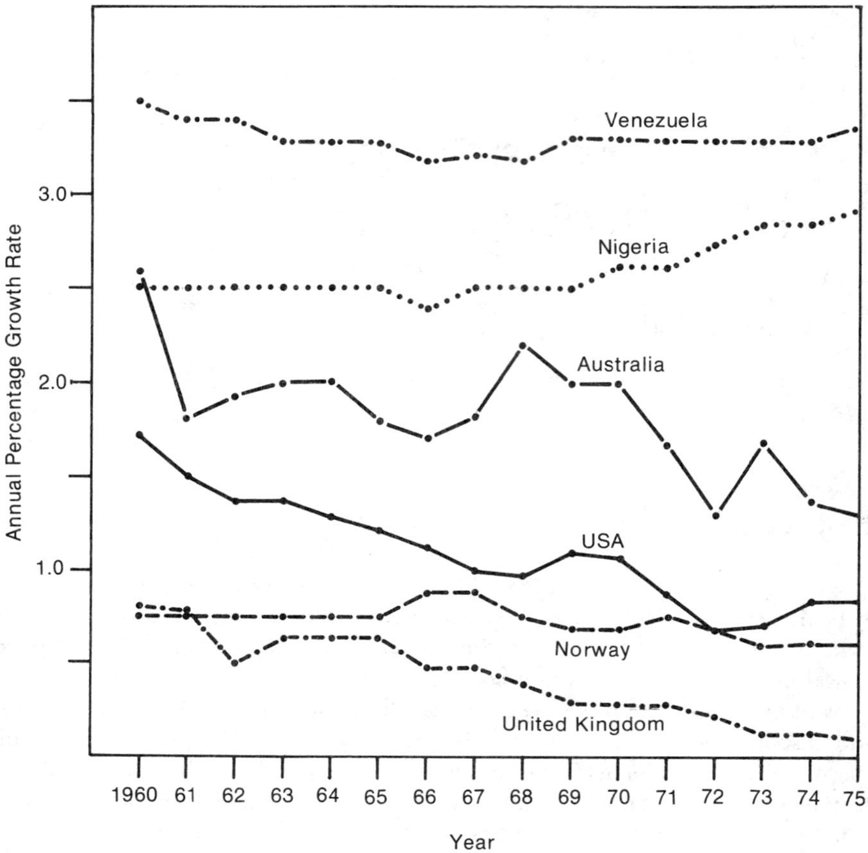

Figure 14–1. Growth in population in six countries, expressed as the annual percentage rate of growth, 1960–1975. (From the U.S. Department of Commerce, Bureau of the Census. World Population, 1975.)

In the United States, the life expectancy of 72.8 years in 1977 was the highest ever, and the crude death rate of 8.8 per 1,000 persons was the lowest ever.[102] The infant mortality rate of 15.2 per 1,000 live births in 1977 was also the lowest ever (though still considerably higher than in a number of other countries[98]), as was the crude birth rate of 14.8 births per 1,000 persons, though this low birth rate has been relatively constant for some years.[102]

Because the number of women in the childbearing years is increasing, the recent relative constancy of the *birth* rate indicates that the *fertility* rate (number of live births per 1,000 females aged 15–44) is still declining. It is this latter phenomenon, probably associated with the availability of birth-control technology, the women's movement, and changing social attitudes, that has received widespread publicity. Whether this decline in the fertility rate is a permanent change in society or whether it is merely one extreme of the swing of the pendulum is unknown. Even a moderate increase in the fertility rate, however, would produce a sharp population increase because of the ever-growing number of women in their childbearing years.

Despite the low fertility rate, what is sometimes called "zero population growth" (in which population stabilizes because increases through births and immigration equal decreases through death and emigration) has not been achieved in the United States. Total population therefore continues to grow, although at a slower rate than in earlier years.

One effect of the demographic trends just described has been to produce an older population; in 1979 the age group 65 and over constituted 11.2 percent of the population, the highest ever, and it is likely to increase further.[101] This aging trend will have an important bearing on the types and distribution of dental services and therefore the types of personnel required in future years. For example, there could be a greater need for periodontic and prosthetic care at the expense of pedodontic care.

Distribution of Population

The major population centers of the northeastern and north central regions grew at a slower rate than the western, mountain, and southern states during the 1970s; New York, Rhode Island, and the District of Columbia actually declined in population from 1970 to 1980.[94] Figure 14–2 shows the proportional increases in population in different regions from 1970 to 1980. It can be seen that the biggest proportional increases came in the mountain and western states, the Southwest, and the South. To give these changes more

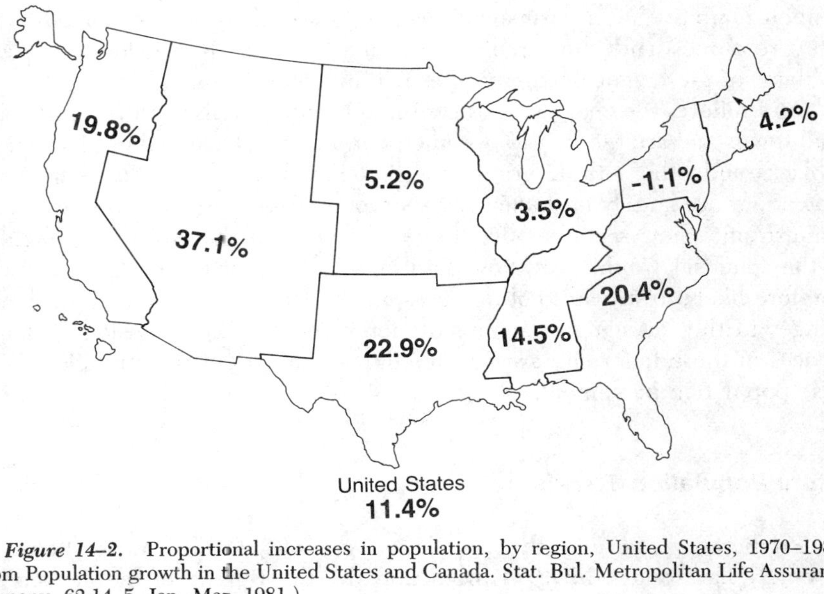

Figure 14–2. Proportional increases in population, by region, United States, 1970–1980. (From Population growth in the United States and Canada. Stat. Bul. Metropolitan Life Assurance Company, 62:14–5, Jan.-Mar. 1981.)

Table 14–1. The Five States with the Greatest Proportional Increase in Population, and the Five with the Least Proportional Increase, 1970–80*

State	Population in Thousands (Rounded) *1970*	*1980*	*Change*	*Percent Change*
Nevada	489	799	+ 310	63.5
Arizona	1,775	2,718	+ 943	53.1
Florida	6,791	9,740	+2,949	43.4
Wyoming	332	471	+ 139	41.6
Utah	1,059	1,461	+ 402	37.9
New York	37,213	36,788	− 425	− 1.1
Rhode Island	949	947	− 2	− 0.3
Pennsylvania	11,801	11,867	+ 66	0.6
Massachusetts	5,689	5,737	+ 48	0.8
Ohio	10,657	10,797	+ 140	1.3

*Statistical Bulletin of the Metropolitan Life Assurance Company.[94] Does not include the District of Columbia, which lost 15.7 percent in the years 1970–80.

perspective, Table 14–1 lists the five states with the greatest proportional increases and the five with the least proportional increases in the period 1970 to 1980. This table, which shows absolute as well as proportional changes, illustrates how percentage changes by themselves can be misleading. For example, Wyoming showed a 41.6 percent increase in population and Ohio only 1.3 percent. The *absolute* increase in Wyoming, however, was 138,000, whereas Ohio's absolute increase of 140,000 was actually greater.

Reasons for this "sunbelt migration," which reverses the trends of more than a century, are primarily economic. Inflation is driving many industries to the less unionized southern states, and many of the "sunbelt" states are richer in energy resources. It cannot be certain, however, whether the "sunbelt migration" is a permanent change. Some of these states have limited water resources and their rapidly growing cities may develop the social problems of the bigger northern cities within a generation.

At a different level, big cities continue to lose population to suburbs and small towns and are tending to become poorer and to have higher proportions of blacks and other ethnic groups in their populations.[100] Because minority populations are largely in the lower socioeconomic groups, the cities' tax bases diminish and their revenues dwindle. The "crisis of the cities," highlighted by the financial troubles of New York and Cleveland in the late 1970s, is therefore likely to spread to other cities unless American society makes major changes in the financing arrangements for its cities. The provision of dental services in these inner-city areas is one of many functions that are affected by these population movements.

Future Population Trends

Prediction regarding the population growth of the United States is extremely hazardous; the 1974 projections by the Bureau of the Census for the year 2000 range from 250 million to 300 million,[100] depending on the assumptions used as a base for the projections. Prediction of population *distribution* within the country is even more uncertain. Some predictions, however, must be made when decisions about dental personnel are required: Are there too many dentists and should some dental schools be closed? Are more auxiliary schools needed? Should long-term priority be given to young patients or old patients, and how will the services required, and hence perhaps the types of personnel, be affected? These are difficult questions certainly, but they are questions that demand responses, for in the long run they affect everyone in dentistry.

TYPES OF DENTAL PERSONNEL

Only about one dentist in six still apparently practices alone or with only one auxiliary,[28] because the profession now recognizes that several different categories of personnel are fundamental to the efficient provision of care. In fact, the concept of the "dental team" is used to describe the providers of dental care, all of whom have different roles, functions, and periods of training and combine to provide care to dental patients. The "dental team" can mean different things under different circumstances, for example, whether all its members operate under the direct control of a dentist or not. Although it has been promoted for years by agencies such as the World Health Organization,[118] the "dental team" remains a concept rather than a precisely defined term.

Dentist. A *dentist* is a person licensed to practice dentistry under the laws of the appropriate state, province, territory, or nation. These laws ensure that to become licensed a prospective dentist must satisfy certain qualifications such as (1) completion of an approved period of professional education in an approved institution, (2) demonstration of competence, and (3) evidence of satisfactory personal qualities. Dentists are concerned with the prevention and control of the diseases of the oral cavity and the treatment of unfavorable conditions resulting from these diseases, from trauma, or from inherent malformations. They are legally entitled to treat patients independently, to prescribe certain drugs, and to employ and supervise auxiliary personnel. Dentists (and dental hygienists) must be both *licensed* and *registered.*

Licensure is the process by which an agency of government grants permission to persons meeting predetermined qualifications to engage in a given occupation and use a particular title or by which it grants permission to institutions to perform specified functions.[91] *Registration* is the process by which qualified individuals are listed on an official roster maintained by a governmental or nongovernmental agency.[91]

After successfully completing examinations set by a state's licensing body and meeting other specified requirements, dentists in the United States become licensed to practice dentistry under the laws of that state. They must also be registered by their state board of dentistry. In many other countries, registration and licensure can be secured after receiving a degree from a recognized dental school and without further examination by the licensing body. Recognition by one licensing authority (state, province, or nation) of qualifications received in another can be a complicated and politically sensitive process.

Dental Auxiliary. *Dental auxiliary* is a generic term for all persons who assist the dentist in treating patients. It includes the categories of dental assistant, dental hygienist, assistant or hygienist with expanded functions, dental laboratory technician, receptionist, and secretary. Auxiliaries can be usefully classified as *operating* and *nonoperating*,[119] depending upon whether they carry out any intraoral procedures in the direct treatment of patients. The corresponding generic term in Britain is "dental ancillary."

Auxiliaries of all types operate under varying degrees of supervision by dentists. Even those auxiliaries who appear to operate more or less independently, such as the school dental nurse of New Zealand described in Chapter 12, work under some form of supervision. The definition of the degree of supervision required for various types of dental auxiliary remained confusing until the American Dental Association (ADA) defined four degrees of supervision of auxiliaries in 1975.[14] Always with the assumption that ultimate responsibility was assumed by the licensed dentist, these degrees of supervision were defined as follows:

1. *General supervision:* The dentist has authorized the procedures, and they are being carried out in accordance with the diagnosis and treatment plan completed by the dentist.
2. *Indirect supervision:* The dentist is in the dental office, authorizes the procedure and remains in the dental office while the procedures are being performed by the auxiliary.
3. *Direct supervision:* The dentist is in the dental office, personally diagnoses the condition to be treated, personally authorizes the procedure, and before dismissal of the patient, evaluates the performance of the dental auxiliary.
4. *Personal supervision:* The dentist is personally operating on a patient and authorizes the auxiliary to aid treatment by concurrently performing supportive procedures.[14]

Dental Assistant. A *dental assistant* is a nonoperating auxiliary who assists the dentist or dental hygienist in treating patients but who is not legally permitted to treat patients independently. A dental assistant may only work under the supervision of a licensed dentist, carrying out duties prescribed by the dentist or by a dental hygienist employed by the dentist. Traditionally, these duties include immediate chairside assistance in the handling of dental equipment and materials used by the dentist or dental hygienist in treating patients.

Voluntary certification programs for dental assistants exist in many countries. *Certification* is the process by which a nongovernmental agency or association grants recognition to an individual who has met certain predetermined qualifications specified by that agency or association.[91] A dental assistant is not required, however, to be legally certified, registered, or licensed or to have completed any particular duration or amount of education. The vast majority of the world's dental assistants are trained "on the job."

Dental Hygienist. A *dental hygienist* is an operating auxiliary licensed and registered to practice dental hygiene under the laws of the appropriate state, province, territory, or nation. To be licensed, hygienists, like dentists, must satisfy certain qualifications, such as (1) completion of an approved period of education in an approved institution, (2) demonstration of competence, and (3) demonstration of satisfactory personal qualities. Hygienists are recognized auxiliaries in a number of countries in which their duties and deployment are essentially similar.

Dental hygienists are concerned with prophylaxis (or "cleaning" teeth), the health of the supporting structures of the teeth, and prevention of further diseases by direct clinical procedures and by the education of individual patients and groups. Hygienists work under the supervision of dentists, either in private dental practice or in institutional settings such as health departments or school dental programs.

Expanded-Function Dental Auxiliary. The *expanded-function dental auxiliary* (EFDA or EDDA*—the terms are synonymous) is a more recent development in operating auxiliaries in the United States and Canada. An EFDA is a dental assistant, or a dental hygienist in some cases, who has received further training in duties related to the direct treatment of patients, though still working under the direct supervision of a dentist. Not all states in the United States recognize EFDAs, and the duties permitted by those that do vary considerably.

Dental Laboratory Technician. A *dental laboratory technician* is a nonoperating auxiliary who fulfills the prescriptions provided by dentists regarding the extraoral construction and repair of oral appliances and bridgework.

Denturist. Denturist is a term applied to those dental laboratory technicians who are permitted in some states in the United States and elsewhere to fabricate dentures directly for patients without a dentist's prescription. These denturists must be licensed and registered. Illegal denturists are also known to operate in other jurisdictions; the term has strong political overtones in jurisdictions where denturists have not achieved legal recognition. Denturists are legally recognized in most Canadian provinces and some Australian states, and by 1980 denturists were legally recognized in four states in the United States (Maine, Arizona, Colorado, and Oregon). There is a possibility that other states may sooner or later recognize denturists.

Dental Nurse and *Dental Therapist.* The *dental nurse* and *dental therapist* are more or less synonymous terms that describe an operating auxiliary who in some countries is legally permitted to treat special population groups, usually children, with little direct supervision from a dentist. The extent of their duties varies from one system to another, as does the degree of supervision required, but all dental nurses and therapists require specific

*EDDA (Expanded-Duty Dental Auxiliary) is an older term.

training, licensure, and registration. *Preventive dental nurses/therapists* are trained in some countries to provide preventive services only, usually in a school dental service. Because their period of training is short and their duties limited, these auxiliaries can provide preventive services to specified groups at lower cost than can dentists or hygienists.

These varieties of dental personnel will be discussed in more detail throughout this chapter.

SUPPLY OF DENTISTS IN THE UNITED STATES

Table 14–2 shows the numbers of persons per dentist in 16 countries in order to provide some perspective for the discussion of dentist availability in the United States. The major point illustrated is the difference between economically developed countries and economically developing countries.

Counting dentists anywhere is not as easy as it might seem. Sources of head counts in the United States are usually state licensing boards and the ADA's *American Dental Directory*, but invariably these lists are not completely accurate; some dentists retain their licenses after retirement and some dentists are licensed in more than one state. Whatever the source, enumeration is usually made in terms of *active* dentists, *practicing* dentists (which customarily excludes those dentists in full-time teaching, research, or government service), or *all* dentists.

Table 14–2. Population-to-Dentist Ratios for 16 Countries in Various Geographic Locations, at Varying Stages of Economic Development, and with Varying Political Systems*

Country	Population†	Dentists	Population-to-Dentist Ratio‡
Norway	4.0	3,605	1,100
Argentina	24.3	13,300	1,800
United States	214.5	106,740	2,000
Switzerland	6.4	2,544	2,500
U.S.S.R.	249.8	97,200	2,600
Japan	108.3	39,229	2,800
Canada	22.1	7,611	2,900
United Kingdom	55.9	15,479§	3,600
Australia	13.1	3,477	3,800
Turkey	37.9	3,789	10,000
Mexico	54.3	5,101	10,600
Ecuador	6.7	253	26,600
India	574.2	9,000	63,800
Thailand	39.8	389	102,300
Kenya	12.5	65	192,000
Nigeria	59.6	84	709,600

*American Dental Association, taken from the Statistical Yearbook of the United Nations, editions 1972, 1973, and 1974.

†In millions.

‡Rounded to the nearest hundred.

§Dentists contracting with the National Health Service, probably 80 to 90 percent of total active dentists.

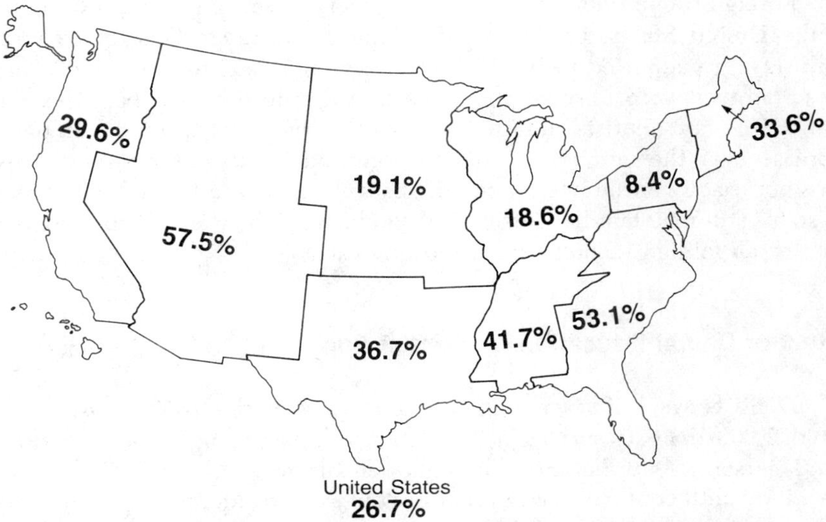

Figure 14–3. Proportional increases in numbers of dentists, by region, United States, 1970–1980. (From U.S. Public Health Service, Division of Health Professions Analysis. Unpublished data on dental personnel, June 1979–Feb. 1981.)

Dentists are the fourth largest group of health professionals in the United States.[112] (The first three are nurses, physicians, and pharmacists.) In 1980, it was estimated that there were 121,240 active civilian dentists in the United States,[107] an increase of 26.7 percent since 1970. Figure 14–3 shows the proportionate increase in the numbers of dentists in each region from 1970 to 1980.

Only some 3.5 percent of dentists in the United States are female, a proportion that is remarkably similar to that of 1920, when women constituted 3.0 percent of all dentists.[97] The reasons why there are so few women dentists in the United States appear to be social and cultural, because in other countries women comprise a higher proportion of dentists—for example, women account for 75 to 80 percent of dentists in Poland, Russia, and Finland; 40 percent in Denmark and Sweden; 25 percent in France; and 15 percent in Britain. With the changing role of women in American society and spurred by affirmative action programs, however, an increasing number of dental students are women. In 1969–70, women constituted only 1.3 percent of first-year enrollment in dental schools,[61] but in 1980–81, the first-year class was 19.8 percent female.[62] Women constituted 1.9 percent of all American dental students in the 1971–72 academic year and 17.0 percent in 1980–81.[62] Clearly, the percentage of dentists who are women should slowly rise over time.

In 1970, only 2.3 percent of dentists were black and another 1.3 percent were of Spanish heritage.[109] More minority students are slowly finding their way into dentistry, again assisted by affirmative action requirements; 4.2 percent of dental graduates in 1977 were black and another 4.8 percent were members of other minority groups.[115] Minorities constituted 11.5 percent of all dental students in 1980–81.[62]

Foreign-trained dentists have never been present in significant numbers in the United States, unlike foreign medical graduates. Only 5,759 foreign dentists were admitted to the United States from 1955 to 1976, and many of these dentists were unsuccessful at passing a state licensing board examination.[113] The 552 dentists admitted in 1976, however, constituted a 12 percent increase over the number of dentists admitted in 1975. American dentistry does not exactly encourage foreign dentists to immigrate to the United States; 35 states still maintain barriers against graduates of nonaccredited schools[31, 113] (that is, all foreign schools except those in Canada).

Effect of Dental Education on Dentist Supply

Dentists were first enumerated separately in the 1850 Census, which listed 2,900 dentists serving a population of 23 million, or one dentist per 7,931 persons. As the number of dental schools grew during the latter part of the nineteenth century, the number of dentists expanded until by about 1900 there was one dentist per 2,565 persons in the United States. By 1930, this ratio was down to one dentist per 1,732 persons.[106]

This steady increase in the relative supply of dentists was caused principally by changes in dental education. Although many dentists in the second half of the nineteenth century were still being trained under an apprenticeship system, proprietary dental schools grew rapidly as a free-market response to demand. Apparently they were profitable ventures, for there were 14 such schools by 1880 and 57 by 1900.[81] Operating as they did, without restrictions on either admission policies or length and type of curriculum, the quality of these proprietary schools was highly variable. Enough poorly trained practitioners emerged from them, however, to stimulate the establishment of the Dental Education Council in 1909 for the purpose of upgrading and standardizing the quality of dental education. The Council recognized the proprietary schools and periodically rated them, as well as those schools that were attached to universities, according to merit. These procedures led to continuing unrest and dissatisfaction, especially among the faculties of those dental schools in the universities that were strongly opposed to recognition of proprietary schools.

The publication of the Flexner report[51] on medical education in 1910 acted as a precedent for the report by William Gies[56] on dental education in 1926. The Gies report is rightly seen as a landmark in American dental education. It led to the establishment of a minimum requirement of one year of college prior to admission to a four-year dental school. As well as promoting educational standardization, the report also hastened the demise of the proprietary dental schools. Some of the proprietary schools survived by becoming part of a university, many simply closed, and the last one became a public trust in 1929.[81]

The continuing dissatisfaction with the work of the Dental Education Council led to the restructuring of that body as the Council on Dental

Education of the ADA in 1937. The Council on Dental Education remains a standing committee of the ADA, and it continued as the accrediting agency for dental schools until January 1, 1975, when the Commission on Dental Accreditation took over the function of accrediting dental and auxiliary training schools and graduate programs in dentistry. The Commission is a more broadly based agency of the ADA; it includes auxiliaries, public members, and a student representative, as well as representatives of the Council on Dental Education.

Accreditation is the process by which an agency or organization evaluates and recognizes a program of study or an institution as meeting certain predetermined qualifications or standards.[91] It applies only to institutions and their services or their programs of study.

Accreditation is said to be unique to the United States,[88] though the system used in Canada is very similar. The federal government has no jurisdiction over education, and there are considerable differences among states in the priority given to education. For these and related reasons, accreditation evolved as a voluntary, self-regulatory means of establishing and maintaining nationally acceptable standards of educational quality. In other countries, schools for dentists and auxiliaries are periodically checked by the relevant government or licensing bodies to ensure maintenance of standards.

These activities over nearly a century can be viewed either as an example of the profession's regulation of itself to produce a superior practitioner in the

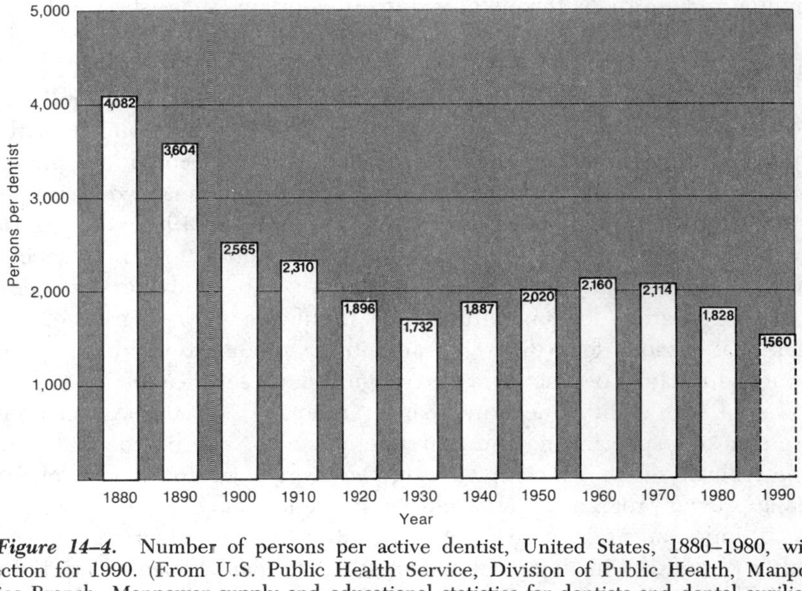

Figure 14–4. Number of persons per active dentist, United States, 1880–1980, with a projection for 1990. (From U.S. Public Health Service, Division of Public Health, Manpower Studies Branch. Manpower supply and educational statistics for dentists and dental auxiliaries. Division of Dental Health, Bethesda, 1972; U.S. Public Health Service, Division of Dentistry. Unpublished data; U.S. Public Health Service, Division of Health Professions Analysis. Unpublished data on dental personnel, June 1979–Feb. 1981.)

public interest or more cynically as an example of the profession's efforts to protect itself.[49] In any event, a by-product was a reduction in the number of dentists relative to population following the demise of the proprietary schools. As Figure 14–4 shows, the number of dentists relative to population increased fairly steadily to 1930, but following the extinction of the proprietary schools and influenced by the Great Depression and World War II, the trend was reversed until the 1970s.

Dental Specialists

The early development of dental specialists was quite informal. Some dentists took graduate training, or a residency, before limiting their practices. Others undertook a formal "preceptorship" by working in the offices and under the direction of recognized specialists. Still others developed additional skills through practice, short continuing education courses, and study of the literature. When these individuals were confident of their own skills (and perhaps of their ability to secure referrals from other practitioners), they announced to former patients and colleagues in the profession that they were limiting their practices to a certain area of dentistry. Varying patterns developed as each specialty grew and matured relatively independently. Examining boards that certified specialty competence came into being, as well as specialty societies, such as the American Academy of Pedodontics and the American Association of Orthodontists, that maintained educational and experiential qualifications for membership. In addition, some states established specialty licensure following a special examination by the state board of dental examiners. By 1979, 14 states offered specialty licensure.[31]

During the early 1960s, the ADA attempted to develop an overall pattern which would be both logical and equitable. The Judicial Council, with the approval of the House of Delegates, ruled that one could not announce limitation of practice in a special area unless the educational requirements set by the Council on Dental Education were met. In 1961, the House of Delegates[3] established that the basic educational preparation for all specialties would require a minimum of two academic years of graduate study beyond the dental degree, leading either to a certificate or a degree. During a transitional period, four different methods of qualification for the right to announce limitation of practice were recognized: (1) certification as a diplomate by one of the eight American boards authorized by the Association; (2) possession of a specialty license from one of the 14 state boards that examine in the specialty fields; (3) completion of two years of advanced academic study in an approved program; or (4) exclusive limitation and ethical announcement of such limitation prior to 1965.[7] As a result of this "grandparent clause," the number of dentists in limited practice is higher than available data indicate, though the number of these "informally limited" practitioners is diminishing over time as their ranks are thinned by death and retirement. In all instances, the individual must limit his or her practice exclusively to the specialty. As of 1980, minimum criteria for those entering a specialty are full-time limitation in addition to either the completion of two years of approved advanced study or specialty licensure by a state board, if relevant.

Under guidelines originally set by the ADA House of Delegates and the Council on Dental Education and now maintained by the Commission on Dental Accreditation, examining boards have been established in each of the eight areas of specialty practice recognized by the profession: dental public health, endodontics, oral pathology, oral and maxillofacial surgery, orthodontics, pedodontics, periodontics, and prosthetics. Certification as a diplomate by one of the boards is not a prerequisite for limitation of practice. The stated purpose of a board is to provide leadership in the elevation of standards for the practice of the specialty and, through examination and certification, to recognize those individuals who have demonstrated unusual competence.

Unlike the situation in medicine, in which 79 percent of practitioners in the late 1960s practiced as specialists,[95] most dentists—about 87 percent—still practice as general practitioners. However, there was a sharp increase in the proportion of specialists and a proliferation of specialty training programs during the late 1960s and the early 1970s. The growth of training programs presumably reflected an increasing desire among dental graduates to become specialists and was a "market response" rather than a planned occurrence. In 1960, 4.7 percent of dentists were specialists, but by 1970 this proportion had grown to 10.0 percent[106] and in 1977 it was 13.7 percent.[115]* The proportion of dentists who are specialists then leveled off—it was 13.6 percent in 1980.[107] Two thirds of all specialists are orthodontists or oral surgeons, which are the two most long-established specialties.

As a result of the sharp growth in specialty training programs from 1960 to 1976, the attitude of many dental leaders now is that a further increase in the number of specialists would not benefit either the profession or the public.[67] This view is based on the general acceptance of the contention that one of the chronic problems in the American health care system is "fragmentation," the dispersal of many medical specialists and the frequent absence of coordination between them.[54, 69] "Fragmentation" is not seen as a problem in dental care provision, but it could become a quite unnecessary one if specialist growth continues at the rate seen between 1960 and 1976.

The Health Professions Educational Assistance Act of 1976 (PL 94–484) was specifically designed to limit the growth of specialists in dentistry as well as medicine. The 1976 Act mandated that dental schools, as a condition of receiving federal capitation awards, must have at least 70 percent of new residency positions (over those in the 1977–78 school year) in general dentistry or pedodontics.[116] It is interesting to note that the growth rate of specialists may have been slowing anyway, since the number of students enrolled in specialty programs prior to the 1976 Act was reduced slightly from previous years.[21] In fact, the number of first-year specialty students was stable from

*For 1977, the ADA's Survey of Dental Practice reported that 89.5 percent of the dentists responding identified themselves as general practitioners.[28]

1971–1980, so that the proportion of specialists in dentistry not only should not rise much in the foreseeable future, but also may even diminish as the total number of dentists continues to grow. Enrollment in general practice residencies continued to increase during 1971 to 1980.[62]

Distribution of Dentists

In 1980 there were 1,828 persons per active civilian dentist in the United States.[107] However, the geographical distribution of these dentists was uneven.[24] This problem is unique neither to dentistry as a health profession nor to the United States, for it is found wherever a relatively free choice of practice location can be exercised. Figure 14–5 shows the number of persons per dentist for each region of the United States in 1980. It can be seen that the regions of the West Coast and the Northeast are quantitatively the best served in terms of dental personnel. Table 14–3 provides data for the five most favorable and five least favorable states in terms of availability of dentists in 1980. The population-to-dentist ratio ranges from 1,348 persons per dentist in Washington state to 3,067 persons per dentist in Mississippi. Nevertheless, every state had a more favorable ratio in 1980 than it had in 1970.[107] Figure 14–6 illustrates the apparent maldistribution of dentists at a more local level. The seven-county Health Services Area of Southeastern Michigan includes urban, suburban, small city, and rural areas and is therefore typical of many such localities in the United States. Even in this small area there is a more

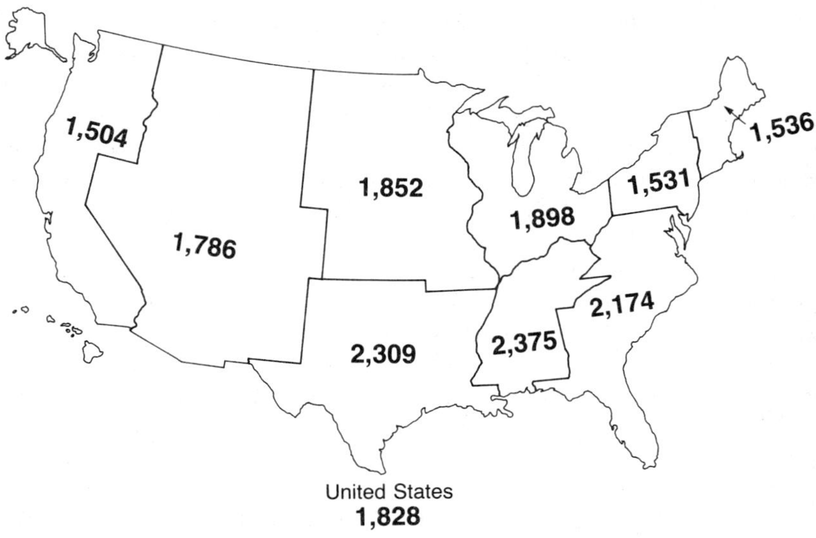

Figure 14–5. Number of persons per active dentist, by region, United States, 1980. (From U.S. Public Health Service, Division of Health Professions Analysis. Unpublished data on dental personnel, June 1979–Feb. 1981.)

Table 14–3. The Five States with Most Favorable Population-to-Dentist Ratios, and the Five States with the Least Favorable Ratios, United States, 1980*

State	Number of Dentists	Population-to-Dentist Ratio†
Washington	2,683	1,348
Connecticut	2,290	1,368
Oregon	1,779	1,372
New York	12,841	1,397
Utah	917	1,439
North Carolina	2,203	2,591
Alabama	1,380	2,725
South Carolina	1,086	2,732
Arkansas	793	2,801
Mississippi	786	3,067

*U.S. Public Health Service, Division of Health Manpower Analysis.[107] Does not include the District of Columbia, where the population-to-dentist ratio was 1208 to 1.

†Ratios were based on population estimates made by the Census Bureau prior to the 1980 Census. These estimates for national population were low by some 2 percent. Depending on how accurate the count of dentists is (see text), the ratios may be underestimates.

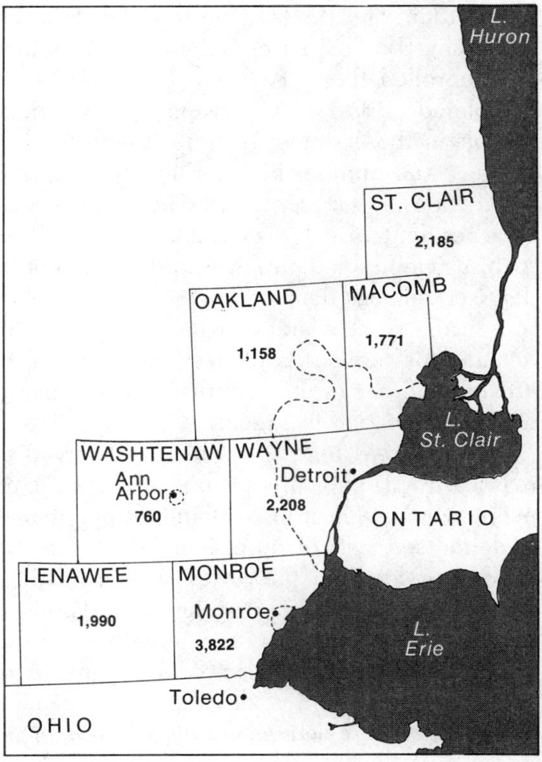

Figure 14–6. Number of persons per dentist in seven counties of southeastern Michigan, 1975. (From Michigan Health Council, 1976 Report.)

than threefold difference in numbers of persons per dentist from the most favored to the least favored county.

Data showing maldistribution of manpower, such as those in Table 14–3 and Figure 14–6, must be interpreted with some caution, because they do not automatically mean reduced accessibility to care in the lesser-favored areas. Many other factors such as traditional traffic patterns and market areas must also be considered, as should the demographic composition of the population. For example, Florida's ratio of 2,083 persons per dentist in 1980 is less favorable than the national ratio, but it is likely that much of the increase in Florida's population between 1970 and 1980 (2.9 million, see Table 14–1) was made up of elderly people, whose dental needs are relatively few. Florida has 18.1 percent of its population aged over 65, easily the highest proportion for any state.[101] (The next generation of elderly people, however, may have considerably greater dental needs because of greater and longer tooth retention—see Chapters 6, 9, and 11. With an aging population and greater life expectancy, there will be more such people to treat.)

There are a number of reasons for this uneven distribution of dentists. The most fundamental is the relative freedom a dentist has in choosing a practice location. It is therefore perfectly natural that dentists make this choice much as other people do, that is, for reasons of personal preference—attachment to a home town, good schools, or convenience to social, cultural, or recreational facilities.[11] Second, the location of dental schools also influences distribution, and the 60 American dental schools are located in only 34 states (including the District of Columbia and Puerto Rico). Seven of those schools have enrolled their first class since 1972, and four of them (the Universities of Colorado, Florida, Mississippi, and Oklahoma) are the first modern dental schools in those states. In time, the presence of these newer schools should improve the number and perhaps the distribution of dentists in their states and regions. Most dental schools are in state universities, where tuition for state residents usually is considerably less than that for out-of-state residents. A third reason for the uneven distribution of dentists is that the availability of dentists reflects demand for services to a considerable extent, a "market response," so that areas of high income and educational attainment where demand for services is highest, such as well-to-do suburbs, have a relatively greater number of dentists than do poorer areas, such as inner cities. Some of the information in Figure 14–6 can be interpreted in this light.

Rural areas tend to be less well-served than suburban areas for several reasons. First, population counts of areas classified as rural often include many people who live near or work in metropolitan areas and thus have ready access to dental services; second, demand for care is often lower in rural areas (this is partly related to the lower socioeconomic status of rural residents); and third, as mentioned, dentists and their families have an understandable desire to be near the attractions and amenities of urban-suburban areas. The uneven distribution of dentists has produced some legislative and regulatory responses from government, not all of them received enthusiastically by the dental profession. These actions are discussed later in the chapter.

State Practice Acts and Maldistribution

The necessity to pass a licensing examination in each state inhibits the movement of dentists (and also licensed auxiliaries) from one state to another.[82] In addition, it has been suggested that certain states have adopted deliberately restrictive policies in their licensing examinations, in an effort to prevent what they see as too many dentists, or dentists "of the wrong kind," from practicing in the state.[49, 82] A perusal of results of state board examinations shows a wide disparity in proportions of applicants failing—from zero to 55 percent in the 1977 exams, for example.[31]

The answer to these perceived restrictions, many argue, is *reciprocity*, that is, licenses awarded by one state are universally recognized by all states. Some go as far as to say that the very existence of individual state practice acts (and what is seen as parochial jealousies in their administration) is a major cause of maldistribution and that the problem would be greatly alleviated by reciprocity. Regional multistate boards help facilitate interstate movement. Others argue that reciprocity could well make maldistribution worse, as great numbers of dentists would then swarm to desirable locations.

There is little doubt that the presence of individual state practice acts is an inhibiting factor in the free movement of licensed dental personnel, but whether relaxing this policy would improve distribution is a moot point. Australia, for example, is a federation of states like the United States. It has long had reciprocity among states, but still has a severe maldistribution problem both among states and between city and rural areas.[33] In Britain, where there is one central licensing body for dentists, there are nearly twice as many persons per dentist in Wales and the southwestern region of England as there are in the more affluent London and southeastern region.[64] Personal residential preference and socioeconomic determinants of public demand for care appear to be the major forces influencing dentists' locations in Britain and Australia, just as they are in the United States.

Some states have moved to provide a degree of reciprocity. For example, Illinois recognizes licenses from eight other states; New Jersey, from two; and South Dakota, from states participating in the Central Regional Dental Testing Service. More developments may be expected from *licensure by credentials*, which is the licensing of dentists previously licensed in another state, without examination but on the basis that their credentials meet specific criteria of the state board of dental examiners. Sixteen states had this provision in 1979.[31]

Shortage or Surplus?

The magnitude and meaning of the 26.7 percent increase in the number of dentists between 1970 and 1980 are interpreted in different ways by different people; dentists with unfilled appointment books say "too many dentists," while public agencies frequently hear of people unable to receive care and of towns with an insufficient number of dentists.[41]

For many years after World War II, both the dental profession and the public accepted that a shortage of dental personnel was imminent if not actual. It was expected that significant increases in demand, stemming from rising affluence and rapid increases in population, would outstrip the ability of the dental profession to provide all the care expected. The influential final report of *The Survey of Dentistry,*[120] published in 1961, based some of its recommendations calling for marked increases in the number of dental graduates and auxiliaries on gloomy assumptions of personnel shortages in the future. In 1960, the House of Delegates of the ADA passed this resolution:

> *Resolved,* that the dental schools be requested to give consideration to programs under which an increased number of dentists and dental auxiliary personnel could be trained to meet reasonable estimates of future needs based on an increased population and a greater public appreciation of dental health services, and be it further
>
> *Resolved,* that the Council on Dental Education be requested to advise institutions of higher learning and other agencies of the need to give consideration to the development of additional facilities for educating dental students and dental auxiliaries in order to assist in meeting the needs of the nation for an adequate supply of dental personnel.[4]

In 1963, the ADA referred to ". . . the impending shortage of health personnel . . ." as ". . . probably the most critical problem in the health field today,"[32] and again foresaw shortages in 1965.[8] These views were still in evidence in 1971, when the ADA's Task Force on National Health Programs stated as a basic assumption: "The United States faces a shortage of dental personnel in the next 20 years and the shortage will occur whether or not there is a national dental health program."[9]

By the mid-1970s, however, many in dentistry did not accept the existence of a personnel shortage.[37, 58] The double-barreled effect of a 51 percent increase in the numbers of graduates between 1961 and 1975 (see Table 14–4), chiefly as a result of increased federal support of dental schools, and the abrupt drop in the rate of population growth led to an increase in the relative supply of dentists (see Fig. 14–4). The ADA's Bureau of Economic Research and

Table 14–4. Number of Dental Schools and Dental Graduates, United States, Selected Years 1931–1980, with Projection for 1985*

Year	Dental Schools	Dental Graduates
1931	38	1,842
1941	39	1,568
1951	42	2,830
1961	47	3,290
1965	49	3,198
1970	53	3,749
1975	59	4,969
1980	60	5,256
1985	60	5,400

*U.S. Public Health Service Division of Dentistry,[106, 110] American Dental Association,[21, 62] U.S. Public Health Service, Bureau of Health Manpower.[115]

Statistics in 1973 agreed that the relative supply of dentists was going to increase considerably by 1985,[10] a notable reversal from its position only eight years before.[8] Some dentists became concerned that an oversupply of dentists was imminent,[58, 74] which they believed could lead both to a diminution in the quality of care and to economic losses within the profession. They also believed that an oversupply of dentists could make it easier for the profession to be "regimented and controlled" by the federal government, and any suggestion of "outside control" cuts to the heart of that autonomy that dentistry holds most dear. In 1976 the House of Delegates of the ADA rescinded the 1960 resolution that recognized the existence of a manpower shortage.[18] Those who fear an oversupply of dentists look with apprehension at developments in medicine, where the impending "physician glut" is more pronounced and even less questioned.[79] Joseph Califano, the Secretary of Health, Education, and Welfare in the late 1970s, alluded to the oversupply of physicians and medical specialists on several occasions[38, 39] and promised that federal policy would counteract it.*

In the climate of deep mistrust of government that characterized the health professions during the late 1970s, some voices in dentistry saw the potential "oversupply" of dentists as a result of a long-standing deliberate policy on the part of the federal government.[52] Such an attitude seems unnecessarily extreme, including as it does an assumption of a monolithic governmental policy traversing six presidential administrations during a turbulent period of American history. It also ignores the ADA's strong support of the federal Health Professions Education Act of 1963[5, 32, 45] and the fact that this legislation not only rescued many dental schools from financial crises[55] but also allowed the quality of dental education to be elevated.

With the benefit of hindsight, it may be true to state that the massive support given by the federal government to dental education from 1963 to about 1980 was at least partly misdirected.[47] The principal reason, however, for the current concerns is simple—no one in the early 1960s foresaw the dramatic drop in fertility rates and the consequent lowering of the rate of population increase. It seems unreasonable to expect that anyone should have, any more than one can predict with assurance in 1980 what the rate of population increase will be in the United States by the year 1995.

Additional reasons for a relative oversupply of dentists, if there is one, are related to the sluggish economy of the late 1970s and early 1980s, which probably inhibited patients from seeking care. In addition, there was a sharp decline in dental caries incidence (see Chapter 6). Dentists are also more productive, a factor that has helped to slow down the rate of increase in dental fees (see Chapter 13).

A 1977 projection by the Division of Dentistry of the U.S. Public Health Service indicated that the supply of dentists would slightly exceed demand by 1990.[111] Assumptions made in this projection were that population growth

*The number of physicians in the United States increased from 143 per 100,000 population in 1960 to 177 per 100,000 in 1975, and was expected to reach 242 per 100,000 in 1990.[39]

would continue at the 1977 rate, that between 43 and 50 percent of the population would be covered by dental prepayment, and that the number of dental graduates would peak at 5,460 in 1982 and then remain stable through 1990. (This figure of 5,460 dental graduates is a reduction from the earlier estimates made in 1972[106] and 1975,[110] but a little higher than that made in 1979[115] and shown in Table 14–4.) Of course, if any assumptions prove to be faulty, so will the projection. There was evidence by 1981 that dental school enrollments were being reduced,[59] so the number of graduates from 1985 on likely would be less than was previously estimated. Predictions are a hazardous business.

It is likely that the number of persons per dentist will continue to decline for the foreseeable future (barring sudden increases in the rate of population growth), but it is also quite possible that increasing demands for care will keep the demand-supply balance stable. There is no absolutely correct number of persons per dentist in the population; what may have been the "right" number of dentists in one decade is not necessarily right in the next. Policy, such as the Health Professions Education Act of 1963 and its successors, must be established even though it takes at least 10 years before the fruits of that policy are seen—schools built, faculty established, the first new classes graduated. Table 14–4 suggests that the 1963 Act began to have real impact on the number of practicing dentists in the years 1970 to 1975.

If one assumes some continuance of the economic growth characteristic of post–World War II America (even if at a slower rate than in the first 25 postwar years), demands for dental care should continue to increase. Third-party payment (see Chapter 13) is introducing a whole new segment of the population to dental care. Other developments in modes of dental practice, such as "department store dentistry," may also help introduce new patients to regular dental care. It should be remembered that only half of the American population visited a dentist for any reason in 1979;[114] new modes of practice may help bring many of the "other half" to dental care.

In summary, while the population-to-dentist ratio is likely to continue to decrease before leveling out, one hesitates to assert that the resulting number of dentists will be enough, too few, or too many—and judged by whose standards?

Measuring Dental Personnel Requirements

Supply of dentists traditionally has been measured by the population-to-dentist ratio. Apart from the definition of whether active, practicing, or all dentists are being counted, this measure is simple, is usually easy to determine with a fair degree of accuracy, and makes a fair basis for comparative study. Similar ratios have been used for years in measuring the supply of personnel in other areas, both health-related and outside of health. Population-to-dentist ratios have been used as a basis for national policy; for example, they were used in the framing of the Health Professions Education Act of 1963.

In time, however, it became clear that the population-to-dentist ratio was inadequate for use in policy determinations.[48] One disadvantage is that it does not make allowance for the varying *productivity* of dentists; some dentists work part-time only, some increase their output by more efficient use of auxiliaries, and older dentists approaching retirement often prefer to see fewer patients than do younger dentists who are building their practices. Second, the ratio makes no allowance for specialists, whose patterns of practice may be quite different from those of general dentists. Third, where operating auxiliaries treat patients, as in those states where EFDAs are permitted, the population-to-dentist ratio by itself can give a misleading picture of personnel available to provide care. Fourth, it does not address the distribution of dentists, which must be considered along with numbers. Fifth, the population-to-dentist ratio gives no indication at all what the "ideal" number of dentists in a particular community should be; there is no "standard" ratio. To illustrate this last point, the testimony of the ADA before Congress in 1962 was aimed at persuading the government to maintain the population-to-dentist ratio of that year into the future.[32] The implied assumption was that the ratio of 1962 was somehow "correct," presumably meaning that most demands for care were being met, that most people seeking care did not have an undue waiting period, and that most dentists neither were harried by high demands nor burdened by excess spare time. In retrospect, it can be seen that there was no justification for many of these assumptions.

Much of the anxiety in some dental circles about an oversupply of dentists is based on the belief that a ratio of about 2,000 to one is somehow "correct," while a ratio of 1,600 to one would be an "oversupply," and 2,400 to one a "shortage." It should be evident by now that this kind of numbers game is not fruitful, though its influence still lingers. Consider again Figure 14–6, the population-to-dentist ratios in southeastern Michigan. Washtenaw County has 760 persons per dentist; Monroe County has 3,822. Does this difference mean a surplus of dentists in Washtenaw and a shortage in Monroe? One simply cannot judge from these figures alone. The Washtenaw figure is heavily influenced by the presence of a large dental school at Ann Arbor, the faculty and graduate students of which affect the ratio without necessarily increasing the availability of care. Perhaps many residents of Monroe County work in the Detroit or the Toledo, Ohio, areas, and are able to receive dental care there. The Wayne County ratio of 2,208 persons per dentist looks reasonable enough, but there are whole tracts of inner-city Detroit where there is literally no dental service available and whose residents have to travel some distance, at considerable inconvenience, to receive care.

Even a brief consideration of these factors indicates that the population-to-dentist ratio, as applied to specific political units such as a nation, state, or county, has limited application when used alone. Instead, it should be an introduction to a wider consideration of the factors that affect the demand for dental services and dental productivity: the distribution of dental personnel and of population, transportation, and traffic patterns; and the extent and the effectiveness of the various health care systems in the community under study.

In practice, however, the population-to-dentist ratio will probably continue to be used as a measure of personnel requirements for some time, because methods of determining the other factors mentioned, while being explored,[86] are still in their infancy. One such method examined by the ADA in the mid-1970s is the Dental Planning Information System (DPIS), which attempts to match productivity and demographic data supplied by dentists with factors influencing the demand for care—all in a complex series of equations that interrelate as part of a larger computer-based analysis. The DPIS was intended to be employed at national, state, and local levels, but difficulties with collecting the required data have hindered its application, illustrating the practical problems in applying a good theoretical system. Valid measurement of personnel requirements still has a long way to go; subjective judgments based on population-to-dentist ratios seem likely to remain the principal method for some time yet.

SUPPLY OF DENTAL AUXILIARIES IN THE UNITED STATES

Dental Hygienists

Dental hygiene is a relatively young profession; the first training course was established in 1914. Since that time, dental hygiene has become accepted as an integral part of dentistry in the United States, where the profession originated, and in a number of other countries as well.

In 1980 there were estimated to be 38,400 active dental hygienists in the United States, a 250 percent increase since 1970.[107] Table 14–5 shows the growth in the number of active hygienists from 1950 to 1980 and in particular the extremely rapid growth of the early 1970s. Most of the new schools in this period were established in two-year colleges and reflect both the demand for

Table 14–5. Number of Active Hygienists, Hygienists per 100 Dentists, Dental Hygiene Training Schools, and Students, for Selected Years, United States, 1950–1980*

Year	Number of Active Hygienists	Active Hygienists per 100 Active Dentists	Schools of Dental Hygiene	Students
1950	3,190	4.0	18	1,091
1955	4,160	4.9	31	1,938
1960	8,800	9.8	34	2,237
1965	11,600	12.1	53	3,502
1970	15,100	14.8	100	5,931
1975	26,900	24.0	173	10,084
1978	32,200	28.0	196	11,055
1980	38,400	30.4	204	10,932

*U.S. Public Health Service Division of Dentistry,[110] Bureau of Health Manpower,[115] Division of Health Professions Analysis.[107]

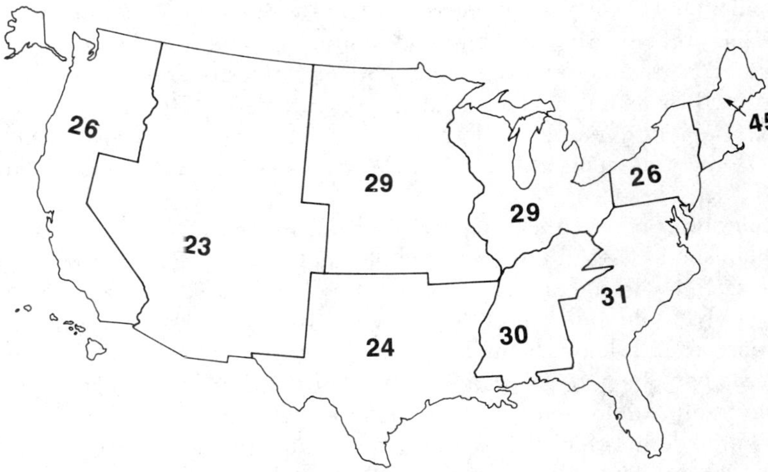

Figure 14–7. Number of active hygienists per 100 active dentists, by region, United States, 1977. (From U.S. Public Health Service, Bureau of Health Manpower. Dental manpower fact book. Government Printing Office, Washington, D.C., 1979.)

training schools and the availability of federal funds for their establishment. The earlier schools of dental hygiene were usually found in university dental schools, but these programs are now greatly outnumbered by the two-year community college programs.

This sudden large increase in the number of hygienists raises questions of how many and of what kind are needed, and whether the growth of training programs will continue at the rate set in the early 1970s. The potential market for hygienists should still be reasonable,[20] because the 1975 Survey of Dental Practice[22]* showed that only 21.9 percent of responding dentists employed at least one full-time hygienist and 19.5 percent employed one part-time, thus leaving over 58 percent who did not employ a hygienist at all. While there are signs that the market for hygienists is approaching saturation,[73, 80] recent dental graduates moving into practice are more likely to have been trained to work with auxiliaries in dental school than were many of their older colleagues. On the other hand, decreasing dentist "busyness" in times of economic recession is an inhibiting factor for hygienist employment. Table 14–5 might indicate a reduction in the number of dental hygiene students, though data for subsequent years would be needed to see if there really is a trend in that direction.

Dental hygienists in the United States are distributed unevenly, as shown in Figure 14–7. Their distribution is measured relative to dentists rather than

*The ADA's 1977 Survey of Dental Practice did not distinguish between full-time and part-time hygienists. It did continue to show that 57.9 percent of responding dentists did *not* employ a hygienist.[28]

to population. Hygienists are relatively most numerous in New England, where the profession had its beginings, and in the South. They are least well-distributed in the middle of the United States. Minority groups are as sparsely represented in dental hygiene as they are in dentistry; in the 1970 Census, only 3.3 percent of employed hygienists were black or of Spanish heritage.[109] In 1977 only 4 percent of dental hygiene students were members of minority groups.[19]

The duties of a dental hygienist are similar in most countries where they are established. These duties, carried out under the supervision of a dentist, are associated with the preventive aspects of dental care: scaling and polishing teeth, applying fluorides and other preventive agents, and educating patients to practice sound dental habits. In more recent years, "expanded duties" for hygienists have been developed in some states in the United States, meaning that the training of hygienists is extended to teach them to carry out additional duties in the dental office. These duties are frequently categorized as *reversible* or *irreversible*. Reversible procedures are those that can be reversed without permanent changes in the oral status of the patient, such as the application of a rubber dam. Irreversible procedures are those that can or do leave a permanent change, such as preparing cavities and giving local anesthetic injections. Many dentists appear willing to allow some extension of reversible duties for hygienists, if legally permitted, but not irreversible procedures.[57] Much debate centers around in-between procedures, such as the packing and carving of amalgam into cavities prepared by the dentist. In a resolution passed by the 1975 House of Delegates,[15] the ADA strongly opposed the performance of these duties by hygienists, despite research evidence from a study at Forsyth Dental Clinic that hygienists were quite capable of doing them adequately.[76] (There is a fuller discussion of expanded-function auxiliaries later in this chapter.)

Outside of the armed services, dental hygiene is almost a completely female profession, for reasons that appear to be cultural and traditional. Like many traditionally accepted conditions, however, this situation is now being seriously questioned[40] and is beginning to change. Even if the dental hygiene profession continues to be essentially a female preserve, the traditional passiveness of hygienists may not remain. Hygienists, licensed and regulated by state boards of dentistry, are showing increasing dissatisfaction at not having a voice in their own licensing. For example, in Michigan, efforts by the Michigan Dental Hygienists' Association to have voting representation on the State Board of Dentistry resulted in a court case that was based on the premise that dental hygiene was a separate profession. The case was successful in the Circuit Court, but on appeal was returned by the Michigan Court of Appeals to the lower court and subsequently dropped.[68] The appellate court judge's ruling was that dental hygiene was not a separate profession, since hygienists could not practice independently but only under supervision of a dentist. The judge also ruled, however, that hygienists are "professional persons within the practice of dentistry."[68] Subsequent negotiation resulted in the hygienists' gaining representation on the reconstituted Michigan State Board of Dentistry, along with dental assistants and the lay public.

It is likely that similar outcomes will be seen in other states. The assertiveness of hygienists[40] has surprised and alarmed some dentists but should be seen as an outgrowth of the hygienists' perceived frustration about the lack of career opportunities[75] and perhaps also the lack of recognition, appreciation, and respect for their abilities. It perhaps also is related to the women's movement. Dental hygienists have expressed concern about their lack of career structure and perceived job insecurity in some cases.[73, 75] Rates of pay (usually salary, sometimes commission) vary greatly, even within a limited geographical area.[73] The apparent absence of a reasonably standard pay-scale means that a hygienist, regardless of competency and seniority, could feel threatened if there were other hygienists available who were willing to work for less. Instances of arbitrary dismissal have been reported[73] and may increase if the rapidly increasing supply of hygienists causes intense competition for jobs.

A majority of hygienists receive some form of fringe benefits,[73] but perhaps dentistry as a profession and dentists as individual employers might be advised to devote more attention to job satisfaction among hygienists.

Independent Contractual Practice of Dental Hygiene

Concerns about job security and professional status are threatening to lead to some fundamental changes in the practice of dental hygiene. Dental practice acts in every state require hygienists to work under the supervision of a dentist, with direct supervision implied if not actually stated. But in December 1976, a California hygienist, Linda Krol, opened her own office next door to that of two dentists whose patients she was treating on a contractual basis. Her action was based on their interpretation of the state dental practice law. Following the lodging of a complaint, the California Board of Dental Examiners ruled in 1978 that hygienists may not practice independently in their own offices. In agreeing to the Board's ruling, Krol accepted that her office would be considered an extension of the setting in which the dentists practiced, and the case appeared settled. Krol continues to practice adjacent to her supervising dentists and has stated that ". . . appropriate supervision, whether general or direct, is well provided for with this arrangement."[71]

What Krol pioneered is *independent contracting*, in which the hygienist has a formal agreement regarding supervision with a specific dentist or dentists and often a financial arrangement too. Hygienists may practice in an office in or (as in Krol's case) adjacent to the dentist's office, paying their own fixed and variable costs and collecting their own fees from patients. Because the dentist is a "supervisor," at least the letter of most state laws is preserved.[117] Proponents of independent contractual practice for hygienists state that it is both financially and professionally more rewarding than traditional practice. The number of independent contractors seems to be growing, though just how many there are is unknown.

Independent Practice

An even more radical departure from tradition is *independent practice,* in which the hygienist selects a site, rents or purchases space, and secures equipment and supplies. There is no agreement with a dentist regarding supervision; the hygienist hangs out a shingle and goes it alone.[117] Independent practice clearly flirts around the periphery of existing law, though the partners in an independent hygiene practice in Colorado Springs were satisfied after two years that all legal requirements had been met.[90] There are a handful of other hygienists in independent practice around the United States. These hygienists naturally have aroused the attention of their state boards, and court actions to end independent practice have been launched in several states.

The future of independent practice is uncertain. Resolutions passed by the American Dental Hygienists' Association in October 1980 were worded in such a way that they appeared to support the concept. These resolutions, which aroused the concern of the ADA[2] and were perceived as provocative by dentists, may have been encouraged by the inquiry of the Federal Trade Commission (FTC) into the subject of independent practice for hygienists (see Chapter 12). However, the FTC dropped this inquiry in late 1980.[53] A bill to legalize independent practice for hygienists in the state of Washington died in committee in early 1981;[70] the Washington State Dental Association testified against the bill. Other states have similar legislation pending.

Future Developments

From all this ferment, it is obvious that the practice of dental hygiene is changing, though it is difficult to know what will be the final outcome in the United States. The move toward professional autonomy and independent practice, the attitude and reactions of organized dentistry, the role of other auxiliary groups, the issue of expanded function, and the rapid increase in the supply of hygienists (along with the realization that their working life appears longer than previously estimated)[73] are all factors that will affect the result. The long-term developments could range from a continuation of the present system of practice to an acceptance of independent practice. The issues that graduating dentists and hygienists must deal with are what effects these future developments—or lack of them—will have on accessibility to dental care, the quality of services delivered, the well-being of the professions themselves, and the ultimate effect on the dental health of the public.

Dental Assistants

Dental assistants are the most numerous of all dental personnel groups in the United States and along with dental laboratory technicians are the most long-established auxiliaries. They began to be employed with regularity in dental practices toward the latter part of the nineteenth century. The first assistants were trained on the job by their dentist-employers to aid in receiving patients and performing "housekeeping" chores and the clerical procedures of the office. Many assistants today still follow this same pattern, for formal training for dental assistants is not required in any licensing jurisdiction in the United States or elsewhere.

It was estimated that in 1977 there were 155,500 active dental assistants in the United States, or 123 per 100 active dentists;[107] the 1975 Survey of Dental Practice stated that 87.8 percent of the respondents reportedly employed full-time assistants.[22] The number of assistants has increased sharply in recent years, for in 1965 there were an estimated 87,350 assistants, or 91 per 100 active dentists.[103] The increase can be largely attributed to the establishment within dental schools of specific training programs, originally encouraged by federal funds, in which dental students were taught how to use assistants effectively. As more and more of these students are graduated, they naturally seek to employ more auxiliaries. Another measure of increased utilization of assistants can be seen in the same 1975 survey,[22] in which over one third of all respondents reported employing at least two full-time assistants. This figure probably gives some measure of the extent to which "four-handed" dentistry is practiced. The effective use of assistants this way greatly improves the productivity of a well-managed practice and probably is a more satisfying way of working for both dentist and assistant. There are apparently more tangible rewards as well; dentists' reported incomes, both net and gross, are associated with the reported numbers of auxiliaries employed.[22]

Although dental assistants are not legally required to be licensed, the ADA and the American Dental Assistants' Association have jointly approved minimum educational standards recommended for assistants. It is estimated that 26 percent of active assistants in 1980 have been graduated from formal programs, and the number is expected to increase steadily because of the growth in the number of training programs to certify assistants. In 1978, for example, there were 273 institutions offering training programs, more than double the number in 1968.[115] The number of enrolled students in 1978 was 9,429, also a doubling of the 1968 enrollment.[115] The 1970 Census showed that assistants were 98 percent female, and 6.9 percent were members of minority groups.[109] In 1977, the proportion of minority students in training programs for assistants was 14.3 percent.[19]

The winds of change seem to be blowing through the dental assistants' organization, even if not quite as strongly as among hygienists. In 1976, the American Dental Assistants' Association issued a press release in which it urged state legislatures to move toward licensure or registration of dental assistants, formulated on ADA educational standards. This suggestion is in opposition to ADA policy, which, although it encourages the concept of educationally qualified dental assistants, does not favor the idea of licensure. While this difference of opinion did not appear to grow into a bigger issue, it presumably represented a move by the assistants to improve their status. Perhaps, too, these efforts by the assistants are symptomatic of deeper frustrations with their job conditions,[35] frustrations that perhaps have been present for a long time though unrecognized by dentists, and that the social climate of the 1970s has allowed to bubble to the surface. While some assistants do not look upon their jobs as careers, and many dentists will always prefer to teach their own assistants, all dentists would be prudent to consider the job satisfaction as well as the tangible rewards offered to the assistants they employ.

In most states, dental assistants are now legally allowed to carry out more than their traditional duties; state laws and regulations have been changed to allow "expanded functions" of assistants. There is a bewildering and constantly changing variety of tasks, however, that are permitted from one state to another.[23, 72] While the acronym of EFDA (Expanded-Function Dental Auxiliary) has become widely used in North American dentistry, it can mean different things to different people. There have been a number of research studies that clearly demonstrate that a dental assistant can be trained to carry out a number of duties that have traditionally been the preserve of the dentist and to carry them out competently and well.[1, 65, 77, 78, 93]

Expanded-Function Dental Auxiliaries

Although dental assistants were used in the nineteenth century, it was not until the shortage of civilian dentists during World War II, due to the enlistment of many dentists in the armed services, that serious consideration was given to their more efficient use. The introduction of the high-speed air-turbine dental hand-piece in the 1950s removed much of the drudgery from cavity and crown preparation and made greater productivity much more achievable. Development of "four-handed" dentistry, with the dentist and assistant both seated, was a natural consequence, and with it came sweeping changes in design of dental chairs, operating equipment, access to instruments, and layout of the dental office.

This continued development in equipment, materials, and procedures is constantly making the role of the dental assistant more complex; the "four-handed" assistant in a busy office must know instruments and understand procedures well if this type of practice is to work. As a result, the assistant is becoming an increasingly more vital part of dental practice; a skilled "four-handed" assistant's role can reasonably be compared with that of the chief nurse in a hospital operating room. In the interest of greater operating efficiency, it was therefore inevitable that these assistants began to do more and more intraoral procedures. As stated, research into the subject has shown that both hygienists and assistants are capable of carrying out a wide range of extra duties at a good level of quality[1, 65, 76–78, 93] and that the productivity and income of dentists can be greatly improved as a result.[34, 84, 87]

The studies with EFDAs were done in a variety of special institutional settings, though considerable pains were taken to simulate the characteristics of the private office. Limited special studies in a few private offices have been conducted in California and North Carolina,[42, 85] and despite some difficulties in adjusting office routine, they confirm that EFDAs can be successfully

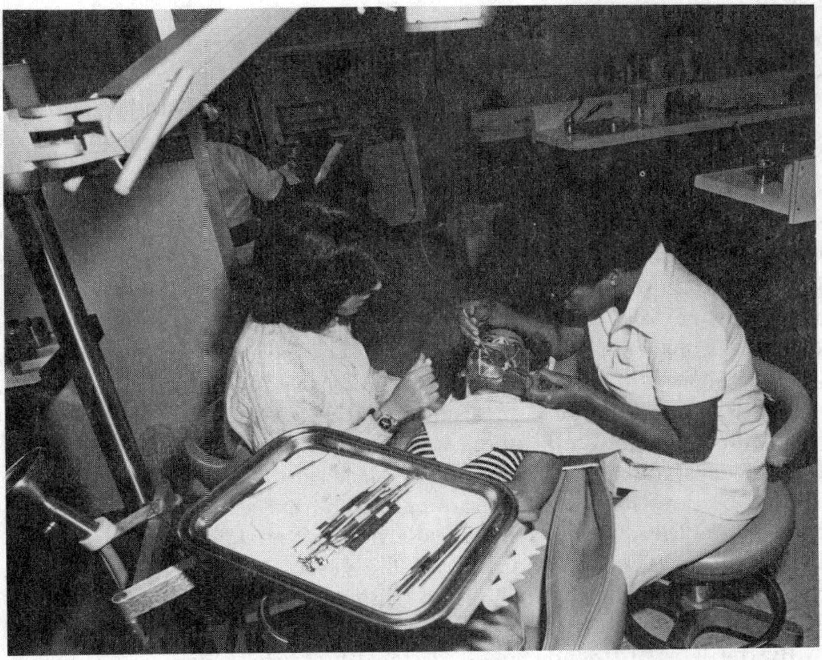

Figure 14–8. Philadelphia technotherapist (left) completing a restoration, aided by a dental assistant. The supervising dentist can be seen (background, right) in the adjoining operatory. (Photograph courtesy of Philadelphia Department of Public Health.)

utilized there. EFDAs are routinely utilized in the Indian Health Service and the Philadelphia City Department of Health (see Fig. 14–8) and by some private practitioners in states where they are permitted.[23] There are no data available to show just how many dentists are employing EFDAs, but indications are that in 1980 it was a small number.

Moves toward utilization of EFDAs were given impetus during the 1960s, at the time when a critical shortage of dental personnel was seen as imminent. If the country is to be short of dentists, the reasoning went, at least let those in practice be as productive as possible. Federal money became available for dental schools to operate Dental Auxiliary Utilization (DAU) programs, which essentially trained dental students in four-handed dentistry, and later for Training in Expanded Auxiliary Management (TEAM) programs, which taught dental students to work with auxiliaries who carried out an even wider range of functions, including packing and carving amalgams in cavities prepared by the students.

The federal government's interest in promoting EFDAs has always been ahead of that of the rank and file of the dental profession. The government's interest is in increased productivity and in the subsequent supposedly lower cost of care to the public. Many practicing dentists, on the other hand, are suspicious of changes in the status quo, and in the "oversupply" climate of

1980 they are not much interested in hiring more auxiliaries. Why should they increase productivity and overhead costs, they reason, if they already are not busy enough?

The translation of favorable results from experimental studies in the 1960s into practice was inhibited by state dental practice acts, many of which expressly prohibited auxiliaries from carrying out certain duties. These laws, for the most part, were written during an earlier period before EFDAs were even thought of. A period of legislative activity then followed. By the end of 1973, there were only seven states that had no legal provisions on expanded functions and 39 states that had provisions both authorized and implemented.[72] Further change has taken place since 1973,[23] and there is much variation in these provisions from state to state. Most states allow expanded functions for both hygienists and assistants; a few specify one or the other. Some states prescribe "open" functions, meaning that the dentist can delegate any duty not specifically prohibited; others have a list of itemized functions for auxiliaries. Seven states allow hygienists to place and carve amalgams in cavities prepared by dentists; six of this same group permit assistants to do so as well. However, another 15 states specifically prohibit auxiliaries from carrying out this procedure. The debate on reversible versus irreversible procedures for auxiliaries still goes on in much of the United States. Readers should be aware that the legal situation is constantly changing.

By the late 1970s, however, six states had established special categories of EFDAs who can (or will, when plans are fully developed) receive special training and testing before they are permitted to perform certain expanded functions.[23] In one of these states, California, a Registered Dental Assistant in *Extended* Functions (a step beyond *expanded* functions) will be an auxiliary who upon completing postlicensure training and passing an examination set by the state dental board will be permitted to perform the following duties:

1. Retraction of gingivae for impression procedures.
2. Take impressions for cast restorations.
3. Take impressions for space maintainers, orthodontic appliances, and occlusal guards.
4. Preparation of teeth for bonding by etching.
5. Determining root length and endodontic file length.
6. Fitting of trial endodontic filling points.
7. Application of pit-and-fissure sealants.[23]

Similarly, a Registered Dental Hygienist in Extended Functions in California, after training and examination, will be permitted to perform the following functions:

1. Retraction of gingivae for impression procedures.
2. Take impressions for cast restorations.
3. Take impressions for space maintainers, orthodontic appliances, and occlusal guards.
4. Temporary stabilization procedures.
5. Debridement of the periodontal surgical site.
6. Placement of intraoral sutures.[23]

It is expected that arrangements will be ready for these auxiliaries in California by 1985.

Developments in the training and duties of EFDAs in the Canadian province of Ontario during the 1970s provide an example of an attempt to build a logical career structure for assistants and hygienists. Four levels of training and qualification were recognized in 1974.[44]

Certified Dental Assistant: A training course of eight months' duration was available in all community colleges and a few secondary schools. The assistant was taught traditional chairside duties; the only intraoral duty was exposing radiographs

Preventive Dental Assistant: The trainee had to be a certified dental assistant. Full-time courses were of three to six weeks' length in some community colleges. Preventive dental assistants were permitted to (1) polish the coronal portions of teeth without instrumentation, (2) take impressions for study models, (3) topically apply caries-preventive agents, (4) place and remove rubber dams, and (5) maintain a patient's oral hygiene.

Dental Hygienist: A student had to be a certified or a preventive dental assistant. The eight-month training program in most community colleges allowed hygienists to: (1) carry out scaling; (2) conduct a preliminary examination of the oral cavity, including taking a case history, a periodontal examination, and recording clinical findings; (3) provide a complete prophylaxis, including scaling, root planing, and polishing of fillings; (4) apply and remove a periodontal pack; and (5) apply fissure sealants.

Dental Hygienist with Expanded Duties: Training at two or three community colleges was open to dental hygienists who had at least one year's practical experience. The training course was of four months' duration and permitted these auxiliaries to carry out the additional duties of: (1) removing sutures; (2) placing, finishing, and polishing restorations of amalgam, silicate, and resin; (3) placing and removing matrix bands; (4) placing cavity liners; (5) retracting gingiva for impression taking; (6) fitting and removing orthodontic bands; (7) separating of teeth prior to banding by a dentist; (8) cementing temporary crowns previously fitted by a dentist; and (9) placing temporary fillings.[44]

All of these auxiliaries were permitted to work only under the direct supervision of a dentist; the pattern of development in Ontario follows the philosophy of the use of EFDAs in the United States rather than that of the independently operating school dental nurse in Saskatchewan (see Chapter 12). This logical career pattern was intended to allow greater job satisfaction and career flexibility for the auxiliaries concerned, because they could follow their training through the four levels or stop at any desired level.

By 1979, however, it was anticipated that no more preventive dental assistants would be trained, since those already trained were having difficulties finding employment. An oversupply of hygienists was also apparent, so there was a reduction in the number being trained and a proposed realignment of duties between hygienists and hygienists with expanded duties. It appears that dentists in Ontario did not accept the new auxiliaries to the extent that had been hoped. Similar moves in the United States, therefore, should be carefully planned, because regardless of how logical and well-intended a career-ladder plan may be, its outcome will be largely determined by employment opportunities.

The ADA and EFDAs

A complicating factor in the legal status of EFDAs in the United States has been the position of the ADA, which although it does not directly or legally control state boards must obviously have some influence. During the mid-1960s, ADA policy encouraged experimental projects. By the early 1970s, however, when many became concerned about the possible oversupply of dentists, ADA policy reversed itself to oppose such experimentation. This policy reversal was defined by one health economist in these terms: If the increase in EFDAs comes at the same time as an increase in dentists, clearly it will have a negative impact on the dentists' willingness to employ such personnel.[46]

Because most of the research studies on the use of EFDAs were based in dental schools, some dental educators became irritated at what they perceived as the ADA's efforts to interfere with academic freedom. However, ADA policy continued to become more opposed to experiments with EFDAs, and the 1975 ADA House of Delegates passed the following resolution:

> *Resolved,* that in the training, education and utilization of dental auxiliaries for the purpose of assisting the dentist in providing high quality dental care through expanded functions, it shall be the policy of the American Dental Association that expanded functions shall be performed under the direct supervision of the dentist and that auxiliaries shall perform only those functions as defined in state dental practice acts for which they have had appropriate education and training, and be it further
>
> *Resolved,* that final decisions related to dental practice and utilization of dental auxiliaries rest with the state society and the state board of dentistry, and be it further
>
> *Resolved,* that the American Dental Association oppose the preparation of teeth, the placement, carving and contouring of dental restorations and the injection of local anesthetics by dental auxiliaries, and be it further
>
> *Resolved,* that the American Dental Association opposes any program, or the funding of such program, of training, education or utilization of dental auxiliaries that is not in accord with these policies, and be it further
>
> *Resolved,* that the Board of Trustees take action to effect intent and purpose of this resolution through appropriate legislative efforts.[15]

The unequivocal language and intent of this resolution meant that ADA policy was in opposition to the laws of some states, to the policies of many of its own constituent (state) dental societies, and to the exercise of what many educators saw as academic freedom. This uncomfortable situation is indicative of the contrasting and at times confused views held on the subject, as well as the high emotions it engenders. At a 1976 workshop on dental auxiliary utilization, the views of government and educators on one hand and private practitioners on the other remained far apart.[17]

On one aspect of expanded functions, however, there has been little division of opinion. Dentistry in the United States has remained uniformly hostile to any suggestion that independent or quasi-independent operating auxiliaries should be utilized; the whole discussion of auxiliary duties in the United States is firmly in the context of auxiliaries working under the direct supervision of a dentist. ADA policy recognizes three categories of auxiliary—hygienist, assistant, and laboratory technician—and is opposed to the development of new auxiliaries. There was an attempt to introduce New Zealand–type school dental nurses (see Chapter 12) in Massachusetts in the late 1940s, but swift and effective political action by organized dentistry ended the plan.[43]

Similar controversy about auxiliaries and their roles has occurred in American medicine, but at present even the quasi-independent nurse-practitioner is becoming common in some areas of the United States. Law tends to follow custom. Some dentists are said to be allowing their auxiliaries to carry out duties that at present are illegal.[36] If so, such duties may become legal in due course. It appears certain that expanded-function auxiliaries are here to stay, though their path of development is not easy to plot in view of the preoccupation of dentistry with a perceived oversupply of dentists in a time of economic stress.

Dental Laboratory Technicians

The dental laboratory technician, like the dental assistant, has been a part of dentistry for a long time. The technician's task is to fabricate crowns, bridges, dentures, and orthodontic and other appliances on the prescription of the dentist. Many of these tasks require high precision, and the technician's skill weighs heavily on the ultimate success of the treatment. The technician is entitled to receive from the dentist a clear written prescription or work order of what is required, together with adequate quality casts, models, plans, and measurements necessary to carry out the prescribed mechanical procedures. Most dentists do relate to their technicians this way, but unfortunately there appear to be some who are happy to "leave it to the lab," when "it" is an element of treatment planning that is properly a responsibility of the dentist.

Traditionally, technicians were directly employed by dentists and worked in a laboratory in the same suite of offices as the dentist. Over time, however, this arrangement became uneconomical for most dentists. In addition, some technicians have become "specialists" whose skills are properly at the disposal of many dentists. Most technicians now are employed by independent commercial laboratories,[20] which provide their services to dentists. In the 1977 Survey of Dental Practice, only 7.5 percent of dentists responding directly employed a laboratory technician either full- or part-time.[28]

It was estimated that in 1977 there were 45,100 active technicians in the United States, or 38.3 per 100 active dentists.[115] The number of technicians continues to grow, though not at the same explosive rate as that of hygienists and assistants. In 1980 there were 56 institutions offering accredited dental laboratory technology training programs, with a total of 2,665 students enrolled,[107] but it has been said that this number may not be enough to meet the growing demand for technicians' services.[66]

Denturists

There is a restiveness and a desire for autonomy among dental laboratory technicians, just as there is among hygienists and assistants. The form these desires take, however, fills organized dentistry with alarm and even fury, because many dental technicians are working to have state dental practice acts changed to allow them to treat the public directly. These technicians call themselves "denturists" and their craft "denturism." The ADA defines denturism as ". . . the fitting and dispensing of dentures illegally to the public,"[13] a definition both clear and brief. As previously noted, attempts to legalize denturism were made in a number of states by the end of the 1970s and with success in Maine, Arizona, Colorado, and Oregon. Denturists are confident that it is only a matter of time before more states legalize their activities.

Why has the denturists' movement surfaced in the United States at this time? Partly it is stimulated by events in Canada, where by the mid-1970s seven of the ten provinces had legalized denturism. Another reason is the rising cost of dentures; with less of an investment in education and lower overhead, denturists claim to supply dentures at lower fees than dentists can. It is likely that there is a large number of older people who need dentures but are unable to afford them, so a "market" for denturists' services could be said to exist. (Medicare, the national health insurance program for persons aged 65 and over, makes no provision for dentures at all. Medicaid varies from state to state, but many states do not include any dental care for adults; public aid for dentures is therefore limited.) Many dentists, too, may have unwittingly given the impression that dentures are "made" by the technician, so some patients may see the dentist as little more than an unnecessary middleman in the provision of dentures. Some researchers have commented on a prevalent public feeling of hostility toward health professionals, mainly directed at physicians but extending to dentists by implication, which is associated with growing public impatience with the problems of cost and access in health care. Whether this feeling is rational or not is hardly relevant, but if it exists to any degree, legislation opposed by dentistry can be more easily passed. Finally, the social climate of the times is again a factor. All kinds of groups want recognition, status, autonomy, and no doubt, higher income. The dental profession is no more or less immune than any other group to being affected by these social forces.

The ADA has vigorously opposed the denturist movement at the political level. The Association's principal argument is that denturists are unqualified to treat patients and that poor-quality care and even actual harm could result to patients. While the soundness of this argument may be evident in dental circles, it may not be so clear to the public and the legislators they elect. This fact was made painfully clear in the Oregon election of November 1978. Supporters of denturism had put the subject on the election ballot through the statewide initiative process, which meant that if it succeeded, the measure automatically became law. Not only was it successful, but also the 3–1 margin of victory stunned organized dentistry. The ADA's postmortem analysis[29] came to some sobering conclusions, which should be thoughtfully considered by all dental personnel. The principal conclusions reached were:

1. The public viewed denturism as a consumer issue, not a health issue.
2. The public believed that dentistry's campaign was spurred by economic self-interest.
3. There were some votes based on sympathy for the elderly.
4. Denturism provided consumers with freedom of choice.
5. The media campaign organized by dentistry through a public relations firm was widely perceived as tasteless and unprofessional.

Some local dental societies have now established low-cost denture clinics for the elderly in an effort to hold back denturism, and the ADA has established criteria for the fabrication of good quality dentures at reduced cost.[26] These services are referred to as "professional quality denture treatment."[27] If Medicare were to be amended to include provision for dentures, that would also be a major step toward easing the cost of professionally made dentures, but there is little sign of that happening.

It is not unlikely that the denturist will become a recognized operating dental auxiliary in the future; the FTC, in its inquiry into dentistry (see Chapter 12), apparently considers this development desirable.[83] The ADA postmortem analysis in Oregon hinted at this likelihood when it noted that dentistry needs to recognize that political compromise is not always unsavory and that "part of the art of politics is knowing how long to hold off the inevitable."[29] On the other hand, with declining rates of total tooth loss, the issue may fade away.

LEGISLATIVE INFLUENCE ON SUPPLY AND DISTRIBUTION

Legislators presumably respond to what they see as society's needs in the health care field. One area that has received considerable attention at the federal and state levels in the United States is improvement of the supply of health personnel through economic incentives and controls. It is not surprising that political actions in these areas are frequently not well received by organized dentistry and private practitioners, who see these actions as potential threats to their autonomy or economic well-being.

Most programs enacted have been designed principally to provide financial aid to training institutions and to students; the object has been simply to increase the *supply* of certain types of graduates. Only in the 1970s did legislation attempt to regulate the *distribution* of health manpower, because it had become generally accepted by then that there was an uneven distribution of dentists in the United States. What should be done about maldistribution, however, is still a subject of debate. Some say that free-market forces will allow the problem to sort itself out; with the relative increase in the supply of dentists (see Fig. 14–4), some popular areas will become oversupplied, and some dentists will be forced to move into currently undersupplied areas. Some of this movement will probably occur, but it will take time and may still be only partially effective; dentists will move to slightly undesirable areas rather than highly undesirable ones. Others believe that only significant changes in the dental care system will solve the problem and that if dentists are left as free as they now are to choose a practice location, maldistribution will continue.

The National Health Service Corps

One federally sponsored program aimed directly at easing maldistribution of health manpower is the National Health Service Corps (NHSC), the result of legislation enacted in 1971.* The NHSC is designed mainly for physicians, but dentists are also included. In brief, the program provides for dental student scholarships and for recent graduates to become commissioned officers in the U.S. Public Health Service, after which they can be assigned to designated shortage areas for a period of time, usually two years. Local communities, whether urban or rural, ask the federal government to designate them as shortage areas, and certain criteria are then applied to see if the communities qualify. Most requests for designation come from the Health Systems Agency for the area (to be discussed) or from community health centers. If the area does qualify as a shortage area, the physician or dentist is assigned and facilities are provided. Fees, those usual for the community, are charged for services provided and go to the government, from whom the professional receives a salary. The professional is expected to become licensed in the state concerned, in the hope that the professional will remain in the community when the service term is completed. About 10 to 15 percent of NHSC sites had evolved into independent private practices by 1979.[30]

By mid-1976, there were 83 dentists placed in designated shortage areas; this number had increased to 250 dentists placed and 689 dental shortage areas designated by 1979.[30] By 1980 there were 2,944 dentists serving 881 designated dental shortage areas.[107] Shortage areas were no longer only rural outposts; urban areas and institutions were also included by 1980.

When the NHSC began, the federal government designated shortage areas in consultation with the local dental societies concerned. Naturally, there were frequently disagreements over the designation of a shortage area,

*An engrossing and highly readable account of how the National Health Service Corps bill became law is given in: Redman, Eric. The dance of legislation. New York, Simon and Schuster, 1973. 319 p.

disagreements that pointed up the shortcomings of the population-to-dentist ratio as a measure of availability of dental care. A statement on the NHSC, issued by the ADA in November 1976,[16] accepted the NHSC as a "temporary method" for relieving personnel shortages. The statement went on to specify that NHSC dental offices should be as similar to private offices as possible and that the government agencies involved should call on the local dental societies for consultation and cooperation. When criteria for designation of shortage areas were published in 1978,[103] however, there was only a statement that when an area was designated as a shortage area, written notice should be given to ". . . appropriate public or nonprofit private entities which are located in or which have a demonstrated interest in the area so designated."[103] Subsequent rules proposed that comments from health professional societies in the area be one of four factors taken into account by the Secretary of the Department of Health, Education, and Welfare before assigning an NHSC professional, but that it should receive least weight of the four.[104] Organized dentistry was naturally not pleased about receiving only this token recognition.

The criteria for designation of a shortage area were defined in 1980 as follows:

1. The area is a rational area for the delivery of dental services.
2. One of the following conditions prevails in the area:
   a. The area has a population-to-dentist ratio of at least 5,000 to 1, or
   b. The area has a population-to-dentist ratio of less than 5,000 to 1 but greater than 4,000 to 1 and has either unusually high needs for dental services or insufficient capacity of existing dental providers.
3. Dental manpower in contiguous areas is overutilized, excessively distant, or inaccessible to the population of the area under consideration.[105]

Specific methods are provided for applying these criteria, including some fairly complex formulae. Although these criteria have dropped the use of set jurisdictions, such as counties, for "rational areas," a modified population-to-dentist ratio is still being used as a method of determining a shortage. Presumably it will continue to be used until a better method can be demonstrated.

Many graduates from dental schools and auxiliary schools are likely to be affected by the NHSC in one way or another. Threats to its existence were heard during the administration's search for social service areas to be financially cut in fiscal year 1980–81, but the NHSC seems popular enough to survive, even though it may be scaled down. Organized medicine and dentistry would be happy to see the scope of the NHSC reduced. Some 40 dental graduates with NHSC scholarships were being placed annually by the end of the 1970s, and at that time scholarship graduates were expected to outnumber volunteers as the program expanded.[30] But with a two-thirds reduction in the number of NHSC scholarships in the early 1980s (part of the reduction in federal spending in the social services) probably few of the remaining scholarships will be allocated to dentistry.

The operation of the NHSC is a good example of how the government's perception of a problem differs from that of organized dentistry. With its concerns about a relative oversupply of dentists, dentistry believes that some shortage areas have been inappropriately designated by a distant bureaucracy and that NHSC dentists have been needlessly placed. The government sees itself as responding to a public need for dental care. With the reduction in scholarships and the likelihood of a greater role for professional societies in designation of shortage areas, dental activity may not develop much more in the NHSC.

Health Systems Agencies

The National Health Planning and Resources Development Act of 1974 (PL 93–641) was enacted ". . . to ensure the development of a national health policy and of effective State and area health planning and resources development programs. . . ."[99] The Act divides the country into 204 Health Service Areas (HSAs), each with its own health planning agency called a Health Systems Agency (also HSA).[108] The governing body of this HSA must have a majority of consumers, and it must also represent all health provider professionals, health care institutions, health insurers, and professional schools.

Each HSA, in conjunction with its State Health Planning and Development Agency, has a broad range of functions aimed at:

1. Improving the health of the residents of its area.
2. Increasing the accessibility, acceptability, continuity, and quality of the health services provided.
3. Restraining increases in the cost of care resources.
4. Preventing unnecessary duplication of resources.

This latter function is the "certificate of need" requirement by which HSAs have become best known. New hospitals, for example, require a "certificate of need" before they can be constructed. This certificate has sometimes been refused if the HSA considers that the area has sufficient hospital beds, because unnecessary duplication is considered a major factor in excessive health care costs.

Dentists' offices have been exempt from certificate-of-need requirements. Since the future of health planning legislation has remained uncertain in the Reagan administration, dentists do not seem likely to be affected much by HSAs in the near future. New graduates, however, are well advised to become involved in the activities of the HSA in the area of their practice location.

Subsidies to Dental Schools and Dental Students

Before and since the NHSC, governmental programs to increase the supply of dental manpower existed in the form of financial incentives to dental schools and subsidies to dental students. Most dental schools are constructed and largely supported by state governments. Their object is to supply dentists for the state concerned, as indicated by the standard practice of charging higher rates of tuition for out-of-state residents.

While some federal money has gone into dental schools for decades, the proportion of federal money supporting dental schools rose dramatically in the years up to the early 1970s. The Health Professions Education Act of 1963 was designed to alleviate the perceived shortage of health personnel, including dentists. This legislation subsidized existing schools, provided funds for new construction and renovation, and provided direct aid to students, all with few strings attached. One effect of this legislation was an increase in dental graduates (see Table 14–4), though Feldstein's thoughtful economic analysis indicates that the act was only partly effective.[47] Feldstein argues that the increase in the number of dentists was greater than would have been achieved without the act, but that an increase in the supply of dental personnel could have been greater for the same public expenditure if there had been enrollment increases and curriculum changes.

The comprehensive Health Manpower Act of 1971 continued financial aid to schools, but with some stricter provisions for the use of the money attached. This act was followed by a period of financial recession, inflation, slower population growth, and growing belief in some dental circles that the perceived shortage of manpower was tending toward an oversupply. Hence, the Health Professions Educational Assistance Act of 1976 (PL 94–484) was enacted in a different atmosphere from that of 1963 and concentrated on improving the supply and distribution of *primary-care personnel* rather than on simply increasing numbers of personnel. Part of the Act's requirements are that dental schools could only qualify for federal support funds if they either (a) increased enrollment of first-year students by a specified proportion or (b) provided "off-site" training for dental students. Both options were intended to increase manpower supply in currently undersupplied areas, though the rationale for enrollment increases was not clear.

The 1976 Health Professions Educational Assistance Act was due to be renewed in 1980. Congress did not get to it, however; it was renewed by a *continuing resolution,* that is, extended for another year in its present form. Indications are that the policy in the Reagan Administration will be to end federal financial support to medical and dental schools altogether, the culmination of several years of reduced support. Some limited loan support to students may still be available.

The Health Professions Educational Assistance Act of 1976 led to some bitterness among the dental profession. Many saw it as a major step toward federal "control" of dentistry, others as unprecedented interference in academic freedom. Six dental schools in fiscal 1979 (Alabama, Case Western Reserve, Emory, Michigan, Oregon, and Pittsburgh) declined federal aid rather than accept the conditions under which it was offered.[92] The opposing argument is that better access to dental care, a continuing goal of government, will never be achieved under the supposed free-market approach to practice location and that some directed approach is required. Federal funds for student loan support were already diminishing at the time of the 1976 Health Professions Educational Assistance Act, and tuition was rising sharply throughout the mid-1970s.[50, 61] The end result of these trends could only be that of restricting dental education mostly to the affluent,[50] a development that few see as socially desirable.

A major factor in this problem is economic inflation, with the financial burdens it places on both schools and students. The cost of maintaining dental schools is becoming staggering, and states are finding it increasingly difficult to provide the necessary financial support. Most dental schools are part of state universities. The few remaining totally private schools receive some limited government support. Tuition at these schools, naturally, is considerably higher than at state schools.[62]

It is worth remembering that student tuition, high as it is and with a median indebtedness of $12,000 to $14,000 per graduate in 1980,[63] pays only a small fraction of the cost of a dental student's education at a state-supported dental school. Even that fraction is shrinking: in 1967 tuition paid for 14.1 percent of the cost of a student's education and in 1974 it was down to 11.6 percent.[60] The taxpayer pays the rest.

Associated with the increases in tuition costs was a decline in the number of applicants to dental schools in the late 1970s. Applications fell from 15,500 in 1974–75 to 10,000 in 1978–79, and candidates taking the Dental Aptitude Test (DAT) dropped from 21,367 to 14,467 over the same period.[96] The long-term result of this trend, if it continues, is seen by many to be in the interests of neither the profession nor the public.[89] If soaring costs of dental education are barring suitable applicants and if taxpayers are financing nearly 90 percent of a dental student's education anyway, it would seem more equitable for society to assist dental students with tuition and living costs when necessary and to require some public service commitment from *all* newly graduated dentists in return. A period of service, not only in designated NHSC areas but also in institutions and public health programs, seems preferable to requiring financial repayment of loans; forcing financial repayment of loans can simply drive more graduates into high-demand affluent areas in order to make as much money as possible in a short time, thus aggravating the present problems. Greater development of the "service-payback" approach seems the best legislative solution to the financial stress of dental students, and it could also help alleviate the access problems of many people. NHSC scholarships follow this philosophy, but they currently only reach a fraction of dental students.

As far as the financial burdens of the schools are concerned, some schools will find continued survival difficult with the end of a generation of federal support and continuing inflation. It is possible that some schools may have to close. Enrollment cuts have been seen in four schools in 1981;[59] others may follow. Perhaps the resulting drop in numbers of graduates will in time ease the projections of "oversupply" (the 1985 projection in Table 4–4 already looks too high). Who knows, in time there might even be a perceived shortage of dentists and then the whole cycle can start again.

FUTURE DEVELOPMENTS

Predicting the future is a thankless task at best, and the task of attempting to predict future developments in health care in the United States for the years 1980 to 1990 is more thankless than most. Rate of population growth, types of health care systems that evolve, economic developments, consumers' demands, and legislative action will all be major factors in shaping the future of the dental care system. Within dentistry, the growth of specialists, the ability to increase productivity in the dental office, and the apparent growing restlessness of auxiliary groups will all exert their influences. The demands of society may mean that the cherished autonomy of the dental profession may be curtailed to some extent.

It was stated at the beginning of Chapter 12 that division of the subject of provision of dental care into methods, financing, and personnel was artificial because the three are interdependent. It is hoped that these three chapters have served to make that point as well as to illustrate the complexities of the numerous social forces affecting the provision of dental care.

References

1. Abramowitz, J., and Berg, L. E. A four-year study of the utilization of dental assistants with expanded functions. Am. Dent. A. J., 87:623–35, Sept. 1973.
2. ADA officers respond to dental hygiene issue. ADA News, May 4, 1981.
3. American Dental Association, Council on Dental Education. Specialists and specialties. Am. Dent. A. Tr., 102:219, 1961.
4. American Dental Association, House of Delegates. (Resolution 9–1960-H.) Am. Dent. A. Tr., 102:206–7, 1961.
5. American Dental Association, Council on Dental Education and Council on Legislation. Federal support for dental education. I. Am. Dent. A. J., 64:272–6, Feb. 1962.
6. American Dental Association, Council on Legislation. American Dental Association witnesses support federal grants-in-aids on dental education before Congressional Committee. Am. Dent. A. J., 64:555–61, Apr. 1962.
7. American Dental Association, Council on Dental Education. Qualifications for examination by specialty boards. Am. Dent. A. Tr., 106:390–3, 1965.
8. American Dental Association, Bureau of Economic Research and Statistics. Number of dental graduates required annually to 1985. Am. Dent. A. J., 71:697–8, Sept. 1965.
9. American Dental Association, Task Force on National Health Programs. Dentistry in National Health Programs: a report with recommendations. Am. Dent. A. J., 83:569–600, Sept. 1971.
10. American Dental Association, Bureau of Economic Research and Statistics. Growth in population and numbers of dentists to 1985. Am. Dent. A. J., 87:901–3, Oct. 1973.
11. ———. Survey of recent graduates. II. Factors related to selection of a practice location. Am. Dent. A. J., 87:904–6, Oct. 1973.
12. American Dental Association, House of Delegates. (Resolution 78–1972-H.) Am. Dent. A. Tr., 114:707–9, 1973.
13. ———. (Resolution 97–1973-H.) Am. Dent. A. Tr., 114:743–4, 1973.
14. ———. (Resolution 48–1975-H.) Am. Dent. A. Tr., 116:695, 1975.
15. ———. (Resolution 50–1975-H.) Am. Dent. A. Tr., 116:701–2, 1975.
16. American Dental Association. Statement on National Health Service Corps. Chicago, The Association, 1976 2 p. duplicated.
17. American Dental Association, Council on Dental Education. Special report on dental auxiliary utilization and education. Am. Dent. A. Tr., 117:208–38, 1976.
18. American Dental Association, House of Delegates. (Resolution 162H-1976.) Am. Dent. A. Tr., 117:903–4, 1976.

19. American Dental Association, Division of Educational Measurements. Annual report on dental auxiliary education, 1977/1978. Supplement 1: minority report in dental auxiliary education. Chicago, The Association, n.d. 5 p. duplicated.
20. ———. Annual report on dental auxiliary education, 1977/78. Supplement 2: employment of recent graduates of dental auxiliary education. Chicago, The Association, n.d. 16 p. duplicated.
21. American Dental Association. Advanced dental education: annual report 1976/77. Chicago, The Association, 1977. 49 p.
22. American Dental Association, Bureau of Economic Research and Statistics. Survey of dental practice 1975. Chicago, The Association, 1977. 43 p.
23. American Dental Association, Council on Dental Education. Legal provisions for delegating expanded functions to dental hygienists and dental assistants. Chicago, The Association, 1977. 55 p.
24. American Dental Association, Bureau of Economic and Behavioral Research. Distribution of dentists in the United States by state, region, district and county. Chicago, The Association, 1979. 66 p.
25. American Dental Association, House of Delegates. (Resolution 40H-1976.) Am. Dent. A. Tr., 117:839, 1977.
26. American Dental Association. Final report from the Ad Hoc Committee for the Delivery of Quality Prosthetic Care for the Financially Disadvantaged. Am. Dent. A. J., 95:1024–38, Nov. 1977.
27. ———. Recommendations concerning professional quality denture services. Am. Dent. A. J., 96:393–5, Mar. 1978.
28. American Dental Association, Bureau of Economic Research and Statistics. The 1977 survey of dental practice. Chicago, The Association, 1978. 50 p.
29. American Dental Association, Bureau of Economic and Behavioral Research. The Oregon lesson: results of postelection research. Am. Dent. A. J., 98:749–54, May 1979.
30. American Dental Association, Council on Dental Health. National Health Service Corps (NHSC) dental summary. Dent. Planning Newsletter, 3:3, May 1979.
31. American Dental Association, Bureau of Economic and Behavioral Research. Facts about states for the dentist seeking a location. Chicago, The Association, 1979. 33 p.
32. Association testifies in support of Educational Assistance Act. Am. Dent. A. J., 66:389–91, Mar. 1963.
33. Australian Department of Labour and National Service. Professional and technical manpower study no. 1: dentists. Melbourne, Advocate Press, 1970. 69 p.
34. Baird, K. M., Purdy, E. C., and Protheroe, D. H. Pilot study on advanced training and employment of auxiliary dental personnel in the Royal Canadian Dental Corps: final report. Canad. Dent. A. J., 29:778–87, Dec. 1963.
35. Blair, K. P. Dental assistants: why do so many leave dentistry? Edit. Calif. Dent. A. J., 6:8, Nov. 1978.
36. Butts, H. C. Stretching the law by a few hurts us all. Edit. Am. Dent. A. J., 92:841, May 1976.
37. ———. Dental manpower shortage? Edit. Am. Dent. A. J., 93:507, Sept. 1976.
38. Califano, J. A., Jr. Remarks made before the Association of American Medical Colleges, New Orleans, Louisiana, Oct. 24, 1978.
39. ———. The government-medical education partnership. J. Med. Educ., 54:19–24, Jan. 1979.
40. Darby, Michele L., and Schwartz, Susan. Status of dental auxiliaries: an issue of gender? Am. Dent. Hyg. A. J., 51:271–5, June 1977.
41. Douglas, B. L., and Babeaux, W. L. The dental manpower demands-versus-needs dilemma. Ill. Dent. J., 46:77–82, Feb. 1977.
42. Douglass, C. W., et al. Expanded duty dental assistants in solo private practice. Am. Col. Dent. J., 43:144–63, July 1976.
43. Dunning, J. M. Extending the field for dental auxiliary personnel in the United States. Am. J. Pub. Health, 48:1059–64, Aug. 1958.
44. Ellis, R. L. Personal communication. Feb. 17, 1977 and June 19, 1979.
45. Federal funds for dental education. Edit. Am. Dent. A. J., 64:241–2, Feb. 1962.
46. Fein, Rashi. Health manpower: some economic considerations. J. Dent. Educ., 40:650–4, Oct. 1976.
47. Feldstein, P. J. Financing dental care: an economic analysis. Lexington, Mass., Heath, c1973. xvii + 259 p. (p. 116–33)

48. ______. A preliminary evaluation of federal dental manpower subsidy programs. Inquiry, 11:196–206, Sept. 1974.
49. ______. Health associations and the demand for legislation: the political economy of health. Cambridge, Mass., Ballinger, c1977. xii + 255 p.
50. Financial situation of dental students: an interview with Harry W. Bruce. Am. Dent. A. J., 92:862–6, May 1976.
51. Flexner, Abraham. Medical education in the United States and Canada: a report to the Carnegie Foundation for the Advancement of Teaching. New York, Carnegie Foundation, 1910. xvii + 346 p.
52. Franklin, D. R. External factors leading to the loss of professional control of the delivery of oral health care. Am. Col. Dent. J., 45:36–51, Jan. 1978.
53. FTC closes investigation of independent hygienists. ADA News, Dec. 15–29, 1980.
54. Fuchs, Victor. Who shall live? Health, economics, and social choice. New York, Basic Books, c1974. vii − 168 p.
55. Galagan, D. J. Back from the brink—how and why U.S. dental schools rebuilt. Dent. Survey, n.v.:14–5, 18, May 1978.
56. Gies, W. J. Dental education in the United States and Canada. New York, Carnegie Foundation, 1926. xxi + 692 p.
57. Gilmore, N. D., et al Consumer and provider attitudes toward dentist and expanded auxiliary functions. Am. Dent. A. J., 93:614–21, Sept. 1976.
58. Goodman, S. E. The dentist shortage that never was. Dent. Management, n.v.:33–8, July 16, 1976.
59. Government panel approves school enrollment cut. ADA News, May 11, 1981.
60. Graham, James. Dental education, 1975–1976: summary of the ADA annual report. Am. Dent. A. J., 92:880–3, May 1976.
61. ______. Dental education: summary of the 1977–1978 Annual Report of the Council on Dental Education. Am. Dent. A. J., 96:767–71, May 1978.
62. ______. Dental education 1980–1981. Am. Dent. A. J., 102:823–5, June 1981.
63. ______. Indebtedness of dental school graduates and the effects on the type and location of their dental practice. Am. Dent. A. J., 102:836–9, June 1981.
64. Gray, P. G., et al. Adult dental health in England and Wales in 1968. London, Her Majesty's Stationery Office, 1970. vi + 294 p.
65. Hammons, P. E., Jamison, H. C., and Wilson, L. L. Quality of service provided by dental therapists in an experimental program at the University of Alabama. Am. Dent. A. J., 82:1060–6, May 1971.
66. Harrison, Alan, and Stephens, A. P. A survey of accredited dental technology education programs in the United States. Am. Dent. A. J., 92:952–5, May 1976.
67. Hillenbrand, Harold. The necessity for trained advanced dental professionals. J. Dent. Educ., 45:76–87, Feb. 1981.
68. Hygienists' ruling overturned in appellate court. Mich. Dent. A. J., 59:573–4, Nov. 1977.
69. Illich, Ivan. Medical nemesis: the expropriation of health. New York, Bantam, c1976. xviii + 300 p.
70. Independent hygiene practice bills fail in Washington state legislature. ADA News, May 11, 1981.
71. Interview with Linda Krol. RDH, n.v.:30–4, May–June 1981.
72. Johnson, D. W., and Holz, F. M. Legal provisions on expanded functions for dental hygienists and assistants, summarized by state, 1973. DHEW Publ.No. (HRA) 75–21, 2nd ed. Washington, D.C., Government Printing Office, 1974. v + 97 p.
73. Judge, Susan P., and Malvitz, Dolores M. The survey of dental hygiene in Michigan: availability of jobs, salaries and benefits, job security. Mich. Dent. Hyg. A. Bul., 6:9–13, June 1976.
74. Kaplan, R. I. Are we producing too many dentists? Edit. Am. Col. Dent. J., 44:15–6, Jan. 1977.
75. Lebowitz, Ann, ed. A study of the participation of women in the health care industry labor force: executive summary report. DHEW Publ. No. (HRA) 77–644. Washington, D.C., Government Printing Office, 1977. iii + 15 p.
76. Lobene, R. R., et al. The Forsyth experiment in training of advanced skills hygienists. Dent. Hyg., 48:204–13, July–Aug. 1974.
77. Lotzkar, S. J., Johnson, D. W., and Thompson, Mary B. Experimental program in expanded functions for dental assistants: Phase 1, baseline, and phase 2, training. Am. Dent. A. J., 82:101–22, Jan. 1971.

78. ______. Experimental program in expanded functions for dental assistants. Phase 3: experiment with dental teams. Am. Dent. A. J., 82:1067–81, May 1971.
79. Louria, D. B. Coping with the approaching doctor glut. New Eng. J. Med., 300:1047–9, May 3, 1979.
80. Malvitz, Dolores M., and Judge, Susan P. The survey of dental hygiene in Michigan: distribution of employed hygienists. Mich. Dent. Hyg. A. Bul., 6:6–8, Mar. 1976.
81. Mann, W. R. Dental education. p. 239–422. (In Hollinshead, B. S., dir. The survey of dentistry: the final report. Washington, D. C., American Council Education, c1961. xxxiv + 603 p.)
82. Milgrom, Peter. Regulation and the quality of dental care. Germantown, Maryland, Aspen, 1978. xv + 251 p.
83. Oppose any FTC rules adversely affecting public. ADA Leadership Bul., 8:3, Nov. 6, 1978.
84. Pelton, W. J., et al. Economic implications of adding one therapist to a practice. Am. Dent. A. J., 86:1301–9, June 1973.
85. Redig, Dale, et al. Expanded duty dental auxiliaries in four private dental offices: the first year's experience. Am. Dent. A. J., 88:969–84, May 1974.
86. Renton, David, and McClendon, B. J. Summary proceedings: projecting dental manpower requirements: productivity and demand indices workshop, Dec. 12–13, 1973. Bethesda, Division Dentistry, 1973. Various pagings, duplicated.
87. Romcke, R. G., and Lewis, D. W. Use of expanded function hygienists in the Prince Edward Island manpower study. Canad. Dent. A. J., 39:247–62, Apr. 1973.
88. Santangelo, M. V. The dental accrediting process. J. Dent. Educ., 45:513–21, Aug. 1981.
89. Scholle, R. H. Poor timing. Edit. Am. Dent. A. J., 98:1062, June 1979.
90. Schulz, Donna. Out-on-a-limb and lovin' it. RDH, n.v.:14–6, May–June 1981.
91. Selden, W. K. Study of accreditation of selected health educational programs: Part one: working papers. Washington, National Commission on Accrediting, c1971. Various pagings.
92. Six dental schools reject capitation. Bul. Dent. Educ., 11:1–2, Oct. 1978.
93. Soricelli, D. A. Implementation of the delivery of dental services by auxiliaries: the Philadelphia experience. Am. J. Pub. Health, 62:1077–87, Aug. 1972.
94. State population changes during the 1970s. Statistical Bul. Metropolitan Life Insurance Co., 62:14–5, Jan.–Mar. 1981.
95. Stevens, Rosemary. Trends in medical specialization in the United States. Inquiry, 8:9–19, Mar. 1971.
96. Study shows decline in dental applicants. ADA Leadership Bul., 8:n.p., Mar. 27, 1978.
97. Tillman, Randi Sue. Women in dentistry—a review of the literature. Am. Dent. A. J., 91:1214–20, Dec. 1975.
98. United Nations, Department of Economic and Social Affairs. Demographic yearbook, 1972. 24th ed. New York, U.N. Publishing Service, 1973. viii + 664 p.
99. U.S. Congress. National Health Planning and Resources Development Act of 1974. PL 93–641, 93rd Congress, 2nd sess., 1974. S.2994. Washington, D.C., Government Printing Office, 1975. 52 p.
100. U.S. Department of Commerce, Bureau of the Census. Population of the United States: trends and prospects, 1950–1990. Current Pop. Rep. Spec. Studies Ser. P-23 No. 49. Washington, D.C., Government Printing Office, 1974. iv + 221 p.
101. ______. Current population reports: estimates of the population of states by age; July 1, 1971 to 1979. Series P-25, No. 875. Washington, D.C., Government Printing Office, Jan. 1980. 14 p.
102. U.S. Department of Health, Education, and Welfare. Health; United States 1978. DHEW Publ. No. (PHS) 78–1232. Washington, D.C., Government Printing Office, 1978. xviii + 488 p.
103. U.S. Department of Health, Education, and Welfare, Public Health Service. Health manpower shortage areas: criteria for designation (Part II). Fed. Register, 43:1586–96, Jan. 10, 1978.
104. ______. National Health Service Corps. Fed. Register, 43:33265–8, July 31, 1978.
105. U.S. Department of Health and Human Services, Public Health Service. Health manpower shortage areas: criteria for designation. Appendix B. Criteria for designation of areas having shortages of dental manpower. Fed. Register, 45:76003–5, Nov. 17, 1980.
106. U.S. Public Health Service, Division of Dental Health, Manpower Studies Branch. Manpower supply and educational statistics for dentists and dental auxiliaries. Bethesda, Division of Dental Health, 1972. v + 51 p.

107. U.S. Public Health Service, Division of Health Professions Analysis. Unpublished data on dental personnel. June 1979–Feb. 1981.
108. U.S. Public Health Service, Health Resources Administration. Health Service Areas designated under the National Health Planning and Resources Development Act of 1974. DHEW Publ. No. (HRA) 78–14014. Washington, D.C., Government Printing Office, n.d. 49 p.
109. U.S. Public Health Service, National Center for Health Statistics. Decennial census data for selected health occupations: United States, 1970, by Handler, Aaron. DHEW Publ. No. (HRA) 76–1231. Rockville, Maryland, Government Printing Office, 1975. vi + 93 p.
110. U.S. Public Health Service, Division of Dentistry. Unpublished data.
111. ———. Projections of national requirements for dentists 1980, 1985, and 1990. DHEW Publ. No. (HRA) 77–48. Washington, D.C., Government Printing Office, 1977. v + 87 p.
112. U.S. Public Health Service. A report to the President and Congress on the status of health professions personnel in the United States. DHEW Publ. No. (HRA) 78–93. Washington, D.C., Government Printing Office, 1978. xxi + 315 p.
113. U.S. Public Health Service, Bureau of Health Manpower. Foreign dental graduates in the United States. DHEW Publ. No. (HRA) 79–24. Washington, D.C., Government Printing Office, 1978. 16 p.
114. U.S. Public Health Service, National Center for Health Statistics. Current estimates from the Health Interview Survey, United States, 1979, by Jack, S. R., and Ries, P. W. DHHS Publ. No. (PHS) 81–1564, Ser. 10, No. 136. Washington, D.C., Government Printing Office, 1981. iv + 121 p.
115. U.S. Public Health Service, Bureau of Health Manpower. Dental manpower fact book, by Ake, J. N., and Johnson, D. W. DHEW Publ. No. (HRA) 79–14. Washington, D.C., Government Printing Office, 1979. iii + 106 p.
116. Whiteside, D. F. Training the nation's health manpower—the next four years. Pub. Health Rep., 92:99–107, Mar.–Apr. 1977.
117. Woodall, Irene R., and Bentley, Marvin. Independent contracting as an alternative financial arrangement. RDH, n.v.:46–50, May–June 1981.
118. World Health Organization. Report of an expert committee on auxiliary dental personnel. Geneva, World Health Organization Tech. Rep. Series No. 163, 1959. 32 p.
119. ———. Inter-regional seminar on the training and utilization of dental personnel in developing countries. New Delhi, Dec. 5–11, 1967. Geneva, World Health Organization Document DH/68.2, 1968. 43 p. duplicated.
120. Young, W. O. Dental health. p. 5–94. (In Hollinshead, B. S., dir. The survey of dentistry: the final report. Washington, D.C., American Council Education, c1961. xxxiv + 603 p.)

VI EDUCATION FOR ORAL HEALTH

CHAPTER 15

Education for Oral Health

To the Reader: *Several comments about terms used in the following chapter are appropriate. First, "dental health professional" refers to the person conducting the educational efforts, inasmuch as the process and principles that apply are the same whether that person is a dentist, dental hygienist, dental assistant, dental laboratory technician, or spouse of a dental professional. Second, the terms "client" and "patient" are used as synonyms. Many health educators prefer the former word, because they think it connotes a more nearly equal partner, free to accept or reject the health professional's recommendations. The client may, of course, be one individual, a key person within the community, a group, or the entire community. For most dental health professionals, the majority of educational efforts will occur within the office or clinic—therefore, many examples in this chapter stem from that clinical orientation rather than an exclusive focus on community health education. Finally, the title of the chapter has been changed from "Dental Health Education," its designation in this book's first and second editions. Although the change may appear to be merely a rearrangement of words, its intent was to focus attention on the outcome of educational efforts, which is—or should be—improvement or maintenance of the health of the entire oral cavity.*

CHAPTER 15

EDUCATION FOR ORAL HEALTH

Dolores M. Malvitz

INTRODUCTION

Americans seem to have great expectations of education. When one reads of problems facing the country or a segment of its population, one also usually reads that at least a part of the solution is to "educate" people about the problem and about ways in which their actions can contribute to solving it. For example, hopes of preventing teenage pregnancies rely heavily on dispelling myths about sexuality and on "educating" teens regarding effective contraceptive methods.

Reliance on education and faith in its outcome have often been translated into teaching people how they must behave if they are to prevent illness or its untoward consequences. The elimination of most infectious diseases as serious public health problems has strengthened this educational emphasis in the United States. Current attention is directed mostly to chronic diseases, the prevention of which requires substantially greater and more long-term alterations in behavior than does prevention of infectious diseases, which may require only infrequent or one-time immunizations. Furthermore, employers and third-parties (e.g., insurance companies) are well aware that, if they are to reduce the soaring costs of health services, long-term changes in behavior are essential. Recent changes in lifestyles in the United States reflect, perhaps, both past educational efforts and the current emphasis on chronic health problems. At least a segment of the population is willing to alter current behavior, with the expectation of reward at some point in the future, for example, longer life or improved resistance to cardiovascular disease.

For years, dental health professionals have been aware of the chronic nature of most oral diseases. Dental health professionals have noted how education in regard to oral health is special because oral diseases are cumulative, do not heal themselves, and are perceived as inevitable. In addition, oral diseases usually require years of neglect before they become symptomatic.

They often result in expensive, extensive treatment, and they might be prevented entirely if an individual received optimum amounts of fluoride and elected to follow practices recommended by dental professionals. Increasingly, diseases treated by physicians can be described using many of these same phrases. More and more conditions affecting the general health of the public can be prevented entirely, or their severity reduced, by alterations in behavior, e.g., exercise and reduced smoking or alcohol consumption. In a frequently quoted California study,[3, 9, 10] behaviors within the control of the individual were found to be most highly correlated with both mortality and morbidity.

Two national agencies—one public, the other private—have been established in recent years to concentrate on health education as a mechanism for reducing disease and improving health. The Center for Health Promotion and Education, of the Department of Health and Human Services, is housed within the Centers for Disease Control in Atlanta and publishes a newsletter called *Focal Points*. The National Center for Health Education, the private-sector agency, is headquartered in San Francisco. In spite of the recent emphasis on health education, a relatively small portion of the health care dollar has gone for nontherapeutic services. The President's Committee on Health Education[56] estimated that preventive measures have consumed approximately 2 percent of total expenditures for health, while only one half of 1 percent of such funds have been spent for health education.

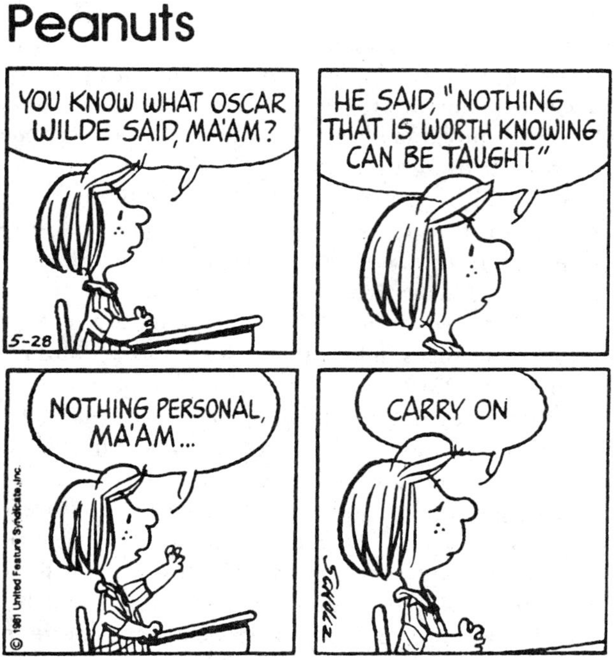
Peanuts
YOU KNOW WHAT OSCAR WILDE SAID, MA'AM?
5-28
HE SAID, "NOTHING THAT IS WORTH KNOWING CAN BE TAUGHT"
NOTHING PERSONAL, MA'AM...
© 1981 United Feature Syndicate, Inc.
CARRY ON
SCHULZ

Figure 15–1. The teacher does not really "teach" unless the learner wishes to learn. (Copyright 1981 United Features Syndicate, Inc.)

Health Education Defined

If there is agreement that the need for "health education" is likely to increase, there is substantially less agreement about what "health education" *is*. The term connotes different things to different people and becomes more complex the more carefully it is examined. Certainly from the point of view of intended learners, Peppermint Patty (see Fig. 15–1) is correct—one cannot successfully "teach" that which learners do not view as worth knowing.

Since dental health education is but one example of health education in general, it is useful to define the latter term. Health education was defined in a past edition of this textbook ". . . simply as the provision of health information to people in such a way that they apply it in everyday living."[92] Recent attention directed to health education has resulted in several attempts to agree on a definitive meaning for the term, so that all groups will understand and use it in a similar way. The goal is to include in the definition all activities that conceivably can be considered as health education. In this broadened view of health education, the provision of information—the traditional definition—may or may not be part of the strategy. Indeed, the health professional may simply listen, establish a climate of trust, then ask a few strategic questions in order to help clients identify their own health priorities. Such a health education activity supplies no new information at all.

One effort to establish comprehensive definitions for terms included representatives of seven health organizations* and resulted in the following definition of health education as:

> A process with intellectual, psychological and social dimensions relating to activities which increase the abilities of people to make informed decisions affecting their personal, family and community well-being. This process, based on scientific principles, facilitates learning and behavioral change in both health personnel and consumers, including children and youth.[56]

While this definition is obviously longer and more comprehensive than Young and Striffler's, significant differences in the committee's view of health education are apparent, including (1) greater, more specific attention to the psychosocial and cultural aspects of health behaviors; (2) emphasis on the contributions of the social and behavioral sciences to the underlying scientific foundation for understanding and influencing health actions; (3) acknowledgement that decisions relating to health are made by individuals, by health professionals, or by governmental officials; and (4) emphasis on the process of education, perhaps at the expense of attention to its outcome. The committee's definition is focused less on the individual and can accommodate the education of a community's leaders as well as their subsequent decisions to enhance the health of the people to whom they are responsible. For example, a city

---

*American Academy of Pediatrics; American Association of Health, Physical Education, and Recreation; American College Health Association; American School Health Association; Public Health Education and School Health Sections, American Public Health Association; and Society for Public Health Education.

council's decision to fluoridate the water supply might be the result of the "health education" of a few strategic persons.

One definition of health education has gained prominence in the literature of the discipline in recent years. Green and his co-workers define health education as ". . . any combination of learning experiences designed to facilitate voluntary adaptations of behavior conducive to health."[34, 35] Green's definition includes several elements common to the committee's more detailed one: (1) a focus on the individual's or group's own decision-making as the key to health, (2) an emphasis on changes in the behavior of the learner, and (3) the implication that learning experiences have been planned specifically to alter or enhance behaviors related to health. Incidental learnings that do not improve health knowledge or behavior would seem to be excluded from both definitions. Individuals may, indeed, conclude from watching television commercials that they should use "sex-appeal" toothpaste or that candy provides needed food energy (Fig. 15–2). Those incidental learnings, however, would not be considered health education because they neither "increase the abilities of people to make informed decisions affecting their personal . . . well-being"[56] nor "facilitate voluntary adaptations of behavior conducive to health."[35]

Distinctions should be made among terms related to health education. Health promotion refers to advocacy efforts that attempt to enhance the probability that personal, private, and public support of positive health practices will become a social norm. Disease prevention efforts are aimed at the prevention of a specific disease or its untoward consequences (see the description of levels of prevention, Chapter 8, p. 203) and are therefore usually narrower in focus than health promotion. Either effort may—and

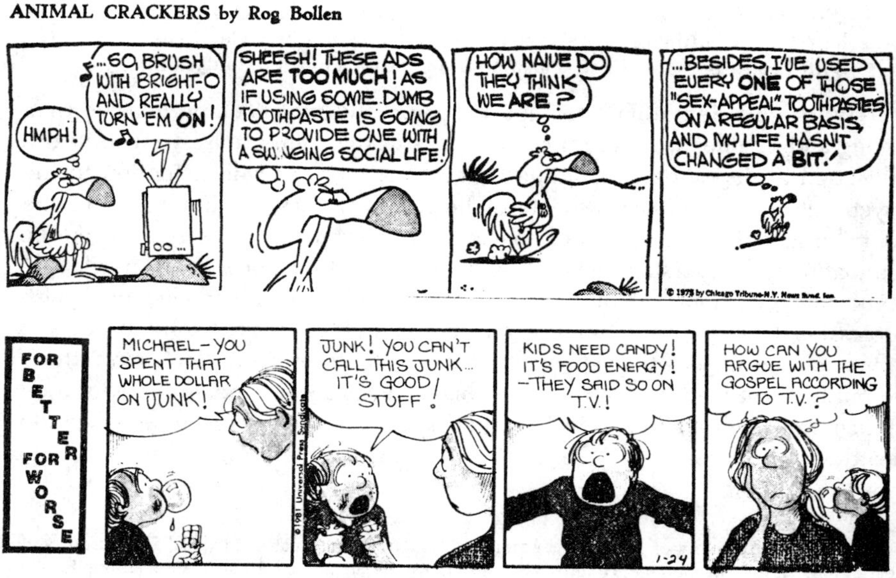
ANIMAL CRACKERS by Rog Bollen
...SO, BRUSH WITH BRIGHT-O AND REALLY TURN 'EM ON!
HMPH!
SHEESH! THESE ADS ARE TOO MUCH! AS IF USING SOME DUMB TOOTHPASTE IS GOING TO PROVIDE ONE WITH A SWINGING SOCIAL LIFE!
HOW NAIVE DO THEY THINK WE ARE?
...BESIDES, I'VE USED EVERY ONE OF THOSE "SEX-APPEAL" TOOTHPASTES ON A REGULAR BASIS, AND MY LIFE HASN'T CHANGED A BIT!
FOR BETTER FOR WORSE
MICHAEL-YOU SPENT THAT WHOLE DOLLAR ON JUNK!
JUNK! YOU CAN'T CALL THIS JUNK... IT'S GOOD STUFF!
KIDS NEED CANDY! IT'S FOOD ENERGY! -THEY SAID SO ON T.V.!
HOW CAN YOU ARGUE WITH THE GOSPEL ACCORDING TO T.V.?
1-24

Figure 15–2. Television advertising affects behavior, but it is not "health education." (Top, reprinted by permission of Tribune Company Syndicate, Inc.; bottom, reprinted by permission of Universal Press Syndicate, copyright 1981. All rights reserved.)

probably should—include health education as defined by Green. Efforts to exclude highly sugared snacks from school vending machines, for example, fit more into the realm of health promotion. Such products are associated with many health problems in addition to dental caries, and their removal from school vending machines is an attempt to promote positive health practices among students. A self-applied fluoride mouthrinse program conducted in a school aims specifically at preventing or reducing dental caries. Both programs should include efforts to inform key persons, as well as the general community, regarding probable benefits to schoolchildren from the recommended activities. Seldom, however, would a dental program consist only of education.

THE THEORETICAL BASIS FOR HEALTH EDUCATION

Because the theoretical basis for health education lies in the social and behavioral sciences, the dental health professional who wishes to encourage patients to adapt their behavior would be well advised to learn as much as possible about those concepts and principles. One observer has noted how often they have been disregarded:

> . . . past history has been replete with simplistic approaches to very complex educational problems. Millions of dollars have been spent on program efforts and activities which have been labeled health education when they have embodied no behavioral science concepts nor health education principles in their planning, implementation, or assessment of results.[83]

This blithe disregard of theoretical foundations was exemplified recently in dentistry by plaque-control programs in which patients were asked to adapt to the existing teaching program rather than the program's being adapted to their particular needs, values, and priorities. Often an evaluation of results—especially an assessment of disease levels—does not occur. Seldom, if ever, do learners help plan what they wish to learn or help decide what they will be willing to do at home. In the words of Peppermint Patty (or rather, of Oscar Wilde), they may not perceive what is being taught as "worth knowing." Dental health professionals responsible for the teaching may have neither diagnosed the educational problem carefully nor helped the learner perceive what was worth knowing before the "dental health education" occurred.

A number of recent publications[21, 31, 50, 71, 73, 89] by dental professionals with advanced education in the social and behavioral sciences or by social scientists working in the area of oral health emphasize these underlying principles as well as their application in dentistry. Although this chapter cannot include exhaustive treatment of all pertinent subjects, a brief review of important behavioral science concepts and educational principles seems warranted. This review is exceptionally superficial, treating complex theories as though they were simple; the dental health professional can benefit greatly from more thorough study of these concepts as well as of other theories not described here.

Communication

Before one can facilitate adaptations in oral health behaviors, one must be able to communicate successfully with clients—either one-to-one or with groups of varying sizes. Figure 15–3 illustrates the process of communication between two individuals. Given the number of steps in the process and the number of factors influencing communication, it should be clear that messages are seldom decoded exactly as senders intend. Figure 15–4 exemplifies communication problems that might have been avoided had the communicators checked to be sure their messages had been received accurately. Because words have different meanings to different persons and in different contexts, communicators (including dental professionals) must assume responsibility for verifying that their messages have been decoded accurately.

The one-to-one communication of the usual dental office setting can be an ideal situation, because the dental professional is able to monitor the patient's verbal and nonverbal responses while the message is being sent and check specifically to see that the information is understood. Words appropriate to the patient's level of understanding can be chosen, while dental jargon should almost always be avoided. Using a greatly simplified description of plaque with a microbiologist and a complex, highly technical one with a nonscientist would both be inappropriate. If a patient appears confused, the dental professional can choose other words or explain a second time, using a new example or simile. Nonverbal communication, including the patient's posture, facial expressions, and movements, can provide valuable clues to

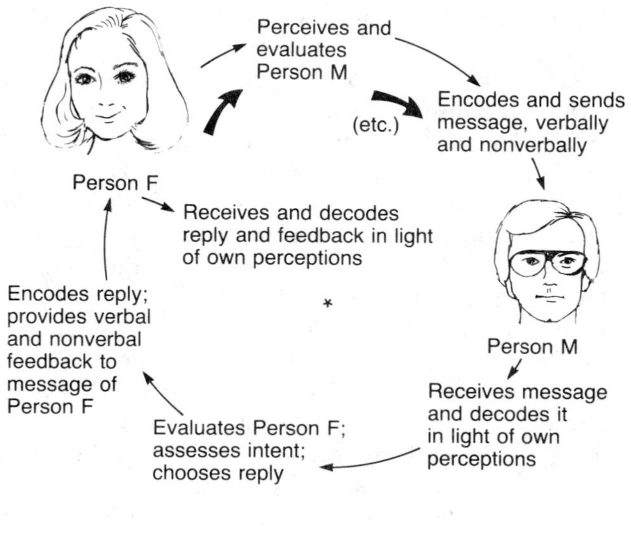

*At any point in the process, "noise" (e.g., frame of reference, attitudes, beliefs, or faulty perceptions) may intrude and distort the message.

Figure 15–3. The process of communication between two persons is a complex one.

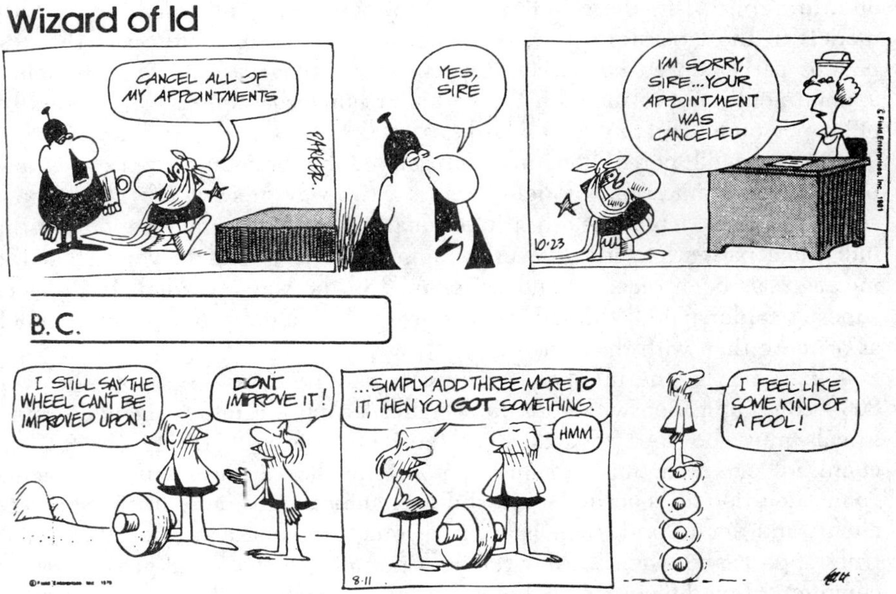
Wizard of Id
CANCEL ALL OF MY APPOINTMENTS
YES, SIRE
I'M SORRY, SIRE...YOUR APPOINTMENT WAS CANCELED
B.C.
I STILL SAY THE WHEEL CAN'T BE IMPROVED UPON!
DON'T IMPROVE IT!
...SIMPLY ADD THREE MORE TO IT, THEN YOU GOT SOMETHING.
HMM
I FEEL LIKE SOME KIND OF A FOOL!

Figure 15–4. Feedback must occur in order to make certain that the message was received accurately. (Reprinted by permission of Johnny Hart and Field Enterprises, Inc.)

underlying feelings. Of course, the dental professional's own nonverbal messages also may be affecting the process of communication either positively or negatively. Some have said that 93 percent of communication is nonverbal, while only 7 percent occurs through spoken messages.

Often verbal and nonverbal messages may conflict, as when patients assure the dental professional that they're "not nervous," while their hands clutch the arms of the dental chair and their knuckles turn white. Awareness of such subtleties, of course, requires that the dental health professional observe carefully. Time must be allowed for questions and for patients to fit new information into existing knowledge and attitudes. The patients' perceptions and biases must be identified if they are to be accommodated. For this level of understanding to occur, the dental professional must read previous entries in charts, provide opportunities for and listen to the patients' statements, and withhold value judgements relating to the patients' beliefs. In addition, it is helpful simply to ask patients to provide feedback, by explaining the concept just described in their own words or by using new information in the next level of comprehension (e.g., "Avoiding decay-producing foods means that you'll need to identify some new between-meal snacks. What are some you like that would be good?").

"Noise" may intrude on interchanges between patients and dental professionals; "noise" is any extraneous information that interferes with the accurate communication of a message. Examples abound, e.g., the array of strange-looking equipment in the operatory seen by a child (or adult for that matter) on a first-time visit, the grinding sounds produced by the trimming of study models in the laboratory next to the consultation room, or the fact that the patient parked in a "no parking" space because he was late for this dental appointment—not to mention the verbal or nonverbal messages provided by office personnel reacting to the tardiness.

Because all perceptions are determined by previous experiences and because communication, by definition, is a two-way process, it is the responsibility of the dental health professional to tailor communication to the individual patient, to identify and eliminate "noise," and to verify that the message has been received and understood in the way intended. If a patient "doesn't understand," the failure rests with the dental professional as much as or more than with the patient.

Inasmuch as the number of receivers may be 8, or 18, or 80—or even 800—communication with a group becomes far more complex. Dental professionals must be alert to signs that their messages are falling on deaf (or confused) ears and must assume responsibility for ensuring that successful communication does occur. Successful communication is more likely when the clients and dental professionals are free from interruptions, when they enjoy true rapport, and when the environment permits psychological privacy. Many communication difficulties can be prevented by careful preliminary assessment and planning, which will be discussed later in this chapter.

Motivation

Perhaps the most misused term among dental professionals is "motivation." It is much easier to explain failures to alter clients' behaviors by "they were not motivated" than to assume one's own share of the responsibility. Yet with such frequent and vague use of the term, much of its meaning has been lost. Dental professionals may find themselves in the same position as those sportscasters who overwork the term (Fig. 15–5) yet have no understanding of its precise meaning. "Motivation" is used to refer to the reasons or forces

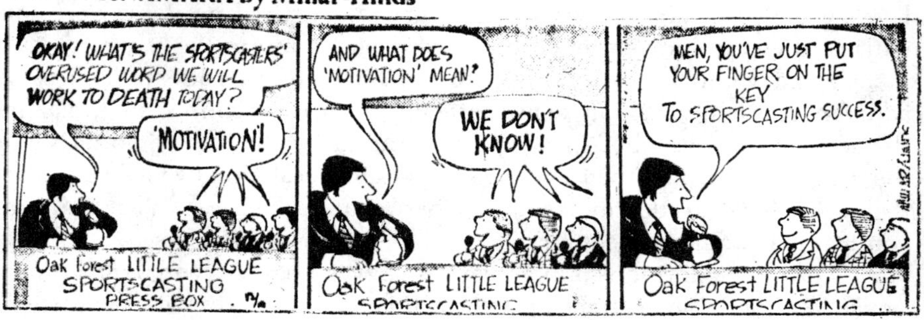
TANK McNAMARA by Millar-Hinds
OKAY! WHAT'S THE SPORTSCASTERS' OVERUSED WORD WE WILL WORK TO DEATH TODAY?
'MOTIVATION'!
Oak Forest LITTLE LEAGUE SPORTSCASTING PRESS BOX
AND WHAT DOES 'MOTIVATION' MEAN?
WE DON'T KNOW!
Oak Forest LITTLE LEAGUE
MEN, YOU'VE JUST PUT YOUR FINGER ON THE KEY TO SPORTSCASTING SUCCESS.
Oak Forest LITTLE LEAGUE

Figure 15–5. "Motivation" may be as overworked in educational efforts as it is in sportscasting. (Reprinted by permission of Universal Press Syndicate, copyright 1975. All rights reserved.)

that produce a given behavior. Many psychologists caution, however, that motives may not be inferred from observed behavior. Two individuals may share the underlying goal of saving money in regard to oral health care. One may seek regular, routine care, believing that those services ultimately will prevent additional, more extensive services and thus reduce costs. Another person, sharing a similar goal of reducing costs, may simply not seek dental care at all, thereby reducing current expenditures for dental care. The behaviors exhibited are quite different, but the underlying "motive" is the same. Of course, not seeking care may be associated with other factors having nothing to do with money. The point is that observing behavior does not necessarily provide accurate answers to *why* the individual engages in that particular behavior; furthermore, assumptions made by observers from their own individual frames of reference can be very wrong.

Different psychological theories explain the concept of motivation in different ways, though the term "motive" may not actually be used. Freud assumed that much behavior could be traced to underlying sexual motives and described the stages of development through which all individuals progress within that framework. Because the oral cavity assumes prominence in Freudian theory, the dental professional might derive great benefit from examining Freud's theories in greater detail.[40]

Another theory, relying on the internal status and perceptions of the individual, is Atkinson's definition of intrinsic motives.[6, 67, 86] Whether individuals receive their internal rewards from achievement or from affiliation will produce significant differences in their responses to the same opportunities to act. Using this theory, an appeal to the need to be loved and accepted when urging teenagers to care for their teeth would likely be unsuccessful if those particular teens possess low affiliation motives.

Lewin, although viewing behavior as an internally directed process, postulated that behavior resulted from an interaction of forces. His force-field theory suggests that some forces drive the individual toward, for example, voting for water fluoridation and some forces restrain such behavior. It is the individuals' perceptions of the balance of those forces that determine their behavior.[19] In the example, the individuals in whom positive forces outweigh negative forces will vote for water fluoridation; those for whom the weight falls on the negative side will oppose fluoridation.

Maslow postulated a hierarchy of individual needs, with more basic physiological and safety needs at lower or more basic levels and social, esteem, and self-actualizing needs at progressively higher levels. He theorized that higher levels of need do not emerge until lower levels are satisfied and that a need that has been met no longer "motivates" an individual. Thus, an appeal to the social benefits of oral health to a person with neither a steady job nor adequate housing would probably fail because lower needs are unmet and, therefore, needs higher in the hierarchy receive no attention from that person. Similarly, an appeal based on the dentition's role in social approval to one who has achieved status and recognition by peers would be equally likely to fall short of the desired outcome because the need for social approval has already been met and therefore will not "motivate" that person.[73]

Behavioral psychologists trace behaviors to external reinforcement of the same or similar behaviors. According to this theory, people brush their teeth because they receive some reward for doing so. As long as they continue to receive periodic reinforcement for that behavior, for example, praise for brushing or a fresh feeling in the mouth afterward, they will engage in the behavior. When, however, behavior results in punishment—or worse, no reinforcement—individuals will cease engaging in it. Much learning theory is an elaboration and extension of Skinner's work. To behavioralists, the concept of internalized attitudes and values is of limited utility. Because all is learned, one need only reinforce desired behaviors appropriately to turn them into habits.[5]

All of the theories cited are attempts to explain why given behaviors occur. Obviously, multiple motives may be operating simultaneously, and no single approach explains behavior entirely. One theory, specific to preventive health actions, is of special value in considering most oral health behaviors—those that require consistent, sustained, daily practice to be effective. One of the more generally accepted health belief models, which has been tested by considerable retrospective research (including attention to oral health practices),[39] was developed by Hochbaum, Rosenstock, and their colleagues.[2] The model postulates that in order for individuals to engage in preventive health behaviors (e.g., monthly breast self-examination, daily flossing of teeth, limitation of saturated fats in the diet) several beliefs must prevail. First, individuals must believe that they are susceptible to the particular disease or condition that the behavior is to prevent. In addition, they must believe that, should that disease or condition occur, the consequences would be serious. Finally, individuals must believe that there are actions that will prevent or lessen the severity of the condition; these measures must be perceived as no worse than the disease to be prevented.

In applying this model to dental health behaviors, several problem areas become apparent. While most individuals may believe they are susceptible to dental caries, few perceive the consequences of the disease as serious. Even loss of all one's teeth may not be viewed as an undesirable outcome. Furthermore, few individuals are aware of the role that optimum levels of fluoride and the application of occlusal sealants (for example) can play in preventing dental caries almost entirely or in lessening its severity. In examining beliefs about other oral conditions, even the first tenet of the model may not be met. Persons may not believe (or even know) that they are susceptible to periodontal diseases or oral cancer, much less be aware of or engage in the behaviors that can prevent those conditions.

Learning

Learning theory is, or should be, the basis for health education practice, including that education designed to improve oral health. Although educational philosophers have created descriptions of what they perceive learning to be and how it might best be enhanced, the term is difficult to define. Several principles or conditions can be drawn from these theories, however. In addition, students can illustrate the principles with their own learning experiences, both planned (learning experiences in professional school are but the most recent example) and incidental. The latter type of learning occurs as a result of an experience planned primarily for another purpose; for example, advertising designed to sell fluoride toothpaste also depicts oral health, defined as few cavities, as desirable. A useful summary of these widely accepted learning principles, adapted by Mico and Ross,[69] is abstracted here.

1. Learning is an experience that occurs inside the learner and is activated by the learner. No one directly teaches anyone anything of significance. People forget most of the content taught to them and retain only the content that is relevant to them personally. (Figures 15–1 and 15–2 are representations of this principle.)
2. Learning is the discovery of the personal meaning and relevance of ideas. People more readily adopt concepts and ideas that are relevant to their needs and problems.
3. Learning (behavioral change) is a consequence of experience.
4. Learning is a cooperative and collaborative process.
5. Learning is an evaluating process.
6. Learning is sometimes a painful process (giving up old comfortable ways of believing, thinking, and valuing).
7. One of the richest resources for learning is the learner.
8. Learning is an emotional as well as an intellectual process. It is affected by the total state of the individual. (Maximum learning occurs when thoughts and feelings are in harmony.)
9. The process of problem solving and learning is highly unique and individual.

These principles place the focus on the learner rather than the content or the teacher. Although the simplest definition of learning is a change in behavior, several levels of altered behavior can be identified. At the lowest level, *compliance*, individuals who are forced to engage in a given behavior will comply with that external demand. For example, children will brush their teeth at school during a formal program in which their brushing behavior is monitored. Once the program and the external demands for brushing end, brushing behavior will probably end as well. When people engage in behaviors because of the examples of others who are significant to them, *identification* is occurring. While identification is one step higher than compliance, individuals still are not responding for internal reasons. The highest level of behavior is *internalization*, when individuals have incorporated the new information and have made it consistent with their own values. Obviously, such accommodations make the behavioral change much more lasting and the internalized behaviors much more difficult to alter at a later time. While changes in behavior can be elicited using the process of compliance or identification, internalization will probably occur more often when learning opportunities are established consistent with the principles just enumerated.

These principles suggest conditions under which individual learning can be enhanced. It should be apparent (and one's own experiences probably support the fact) that a "canned" lecture on a subject selected by the lecturer, during which no opportunity for interaction between teacher and student exists, has little hope of producing lasting behavior change, or internalization. Yet that format is what often passes for education in regard to health. The patient or the community group is told what, where, when, why, and how either by a filmstrip or by a rushed professional who has rattled through the speech many times. Professionals may be impatient with what they perceive as the patients' lack of cooperation; they may have identified the problem themselves, consistent with their own values, rather than those of the patients; they may leave no time for questions—or may ask "Do you have questions?" in a condescending, hurried tone of voice that effectively precludes questions. (Just think of a recent medical visit or an experience when you had to deal with a professional in an area about which you knew little, e.g., the TV repairman, the insurance salesman, the sports physiologist.)

Mico and Ross[69] use the principles listed previously to clarify conditions that are likely to enhance individual or group learning. They suggest that internalization, learning that results in a sustained behavior change, is facilitated by conditions that

1. Encourage people to be active.
2. Help and promote the individual's discovery of personal meaning of ideas.
3. Emphasize the uniquely personal and subjective nature of learning.
4. Consistently recognize people's right to make mistakes.
5. Tolerate ambiguity.
6. Encourage openness of self rather than concealment of self.
7. Permit confrontation.

and in an atmosphere in which

8. Difference is good and desirable.
9. Evaluation is a cooperative process that emphasizes self-evaluation.
10. People are encouraged to trust themselves as well as external sources.
11. People feel they are respected.
12. People feel they are accepted.

Using these suggestions, the following behaviors of dental professionals would be preferred: (1) accepting patients' remarks that they have not been removing plaque as instructed without scolding and without negative feedback; (2) teaching interested patients to assess the health of their gingiva themselves rather than relying only on the dental professional's word; (3) teaching patients who want to learn to floss to do so in their own mouths rather than on models; and (4) accepting that there are a number of ways, other than the ideal choices outlined by the dental professional, to reach oral health goals.

THE APPLICATION OF THEORY

Although education for oral health may—and should—occur in many settings, certain activities should occur whatever the locale. Whether the client is a three-year-old accompanied by her father at a first dental appointment in a pedodontic practice, an entire troop of girl scouts, nursing home employees at an inservice session, or a group of Kiwanians attending their regular meeting, the educational process should follow the same format.

Identifying Needs

First, the needs of the learners must be identified and the problem must be diagnosed. Green and his co-workers have described a comprehensive framework for this diagnosis (see Fig. 15–6). This step includes not only that which the dental health professional identifies as needed, given the oral health status of the individual or group, but also that which patients themselves define as their oral health problems. (Green's framework acknowledges that some health problems can be traced to nonbehavioral causes and are, therefore, not amenable to solution by educational interventions.) It is a joint process, during which professionals may need to compromise on their ideal answers. In order to identify needs, something must be learned of the patients' current beliefs, values, attitudes, and practices related to health, specifically oral health. One is reminded of the old public health maxim, "Start where the people are." Often medical histories and information sheets completed for patient records, as well as progress notes and plaque scores recorded at prior visits, can provide valuable clues for the educator in a clinical setting. Group members simply may be asked to define oral health problems as they view them. The educator must be willing to listen to and accommodate the perceived needs of learners, for only then is the cooperative, collaborative, and personal nature of learning fully realized. Perhaps consumerism in health matters ultimately may result in program planning efforts that automatically take into account the perceived needs of the people.

The frame of reference from which issues are evaluated often determines how the "facts" are interpreted (see Fig. 15–7). An example is the group of nursing home aides who viewed the most pressing dental problem as the need to mark patients' dentures so those appliances would no longer be mixed up or distributed incorrectly. The dental hygienist, who initially had assessed the problem as the need to provide the aides information on how daily care of appliances and natural teeth should be accomplished, soon modified priorities to place marking dentures first. If one expects others to carry out actions, these individuals must be part of the planning process. Only after the same aides identified daily attention to patients' oral health as a problem could the hygienist expect to alter the aides' behavior in any significant way. Linking the professional's ideal desired behaviors to a problem identified or owned by the patient is a way to achieve long-term success, or internalization of the behavior.

Establishing Objectives

Once the needs have been identified and the problem defined, objectives for learning can be established. Patients should again participate in determin-

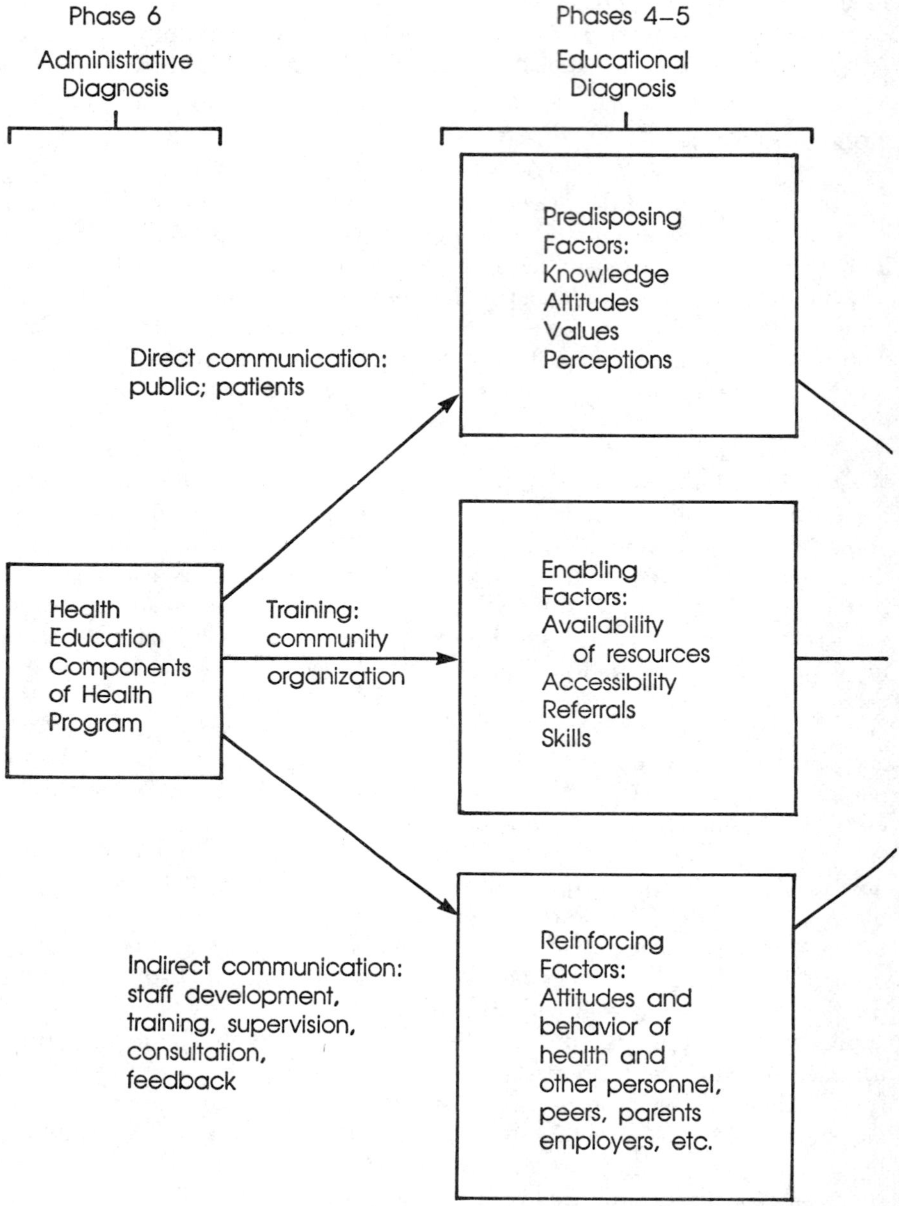

Figure 15–6. Framework recommended by Green and his co-workers for a complete diagnosis of a health problem, including those aspects that might be related to education. (From Green, L. W., et al. Health education planning; a diagnostic approach. Palo Alto, Mayfield, c1980. xvi + 306 p.)

Illustration continued on opposite page

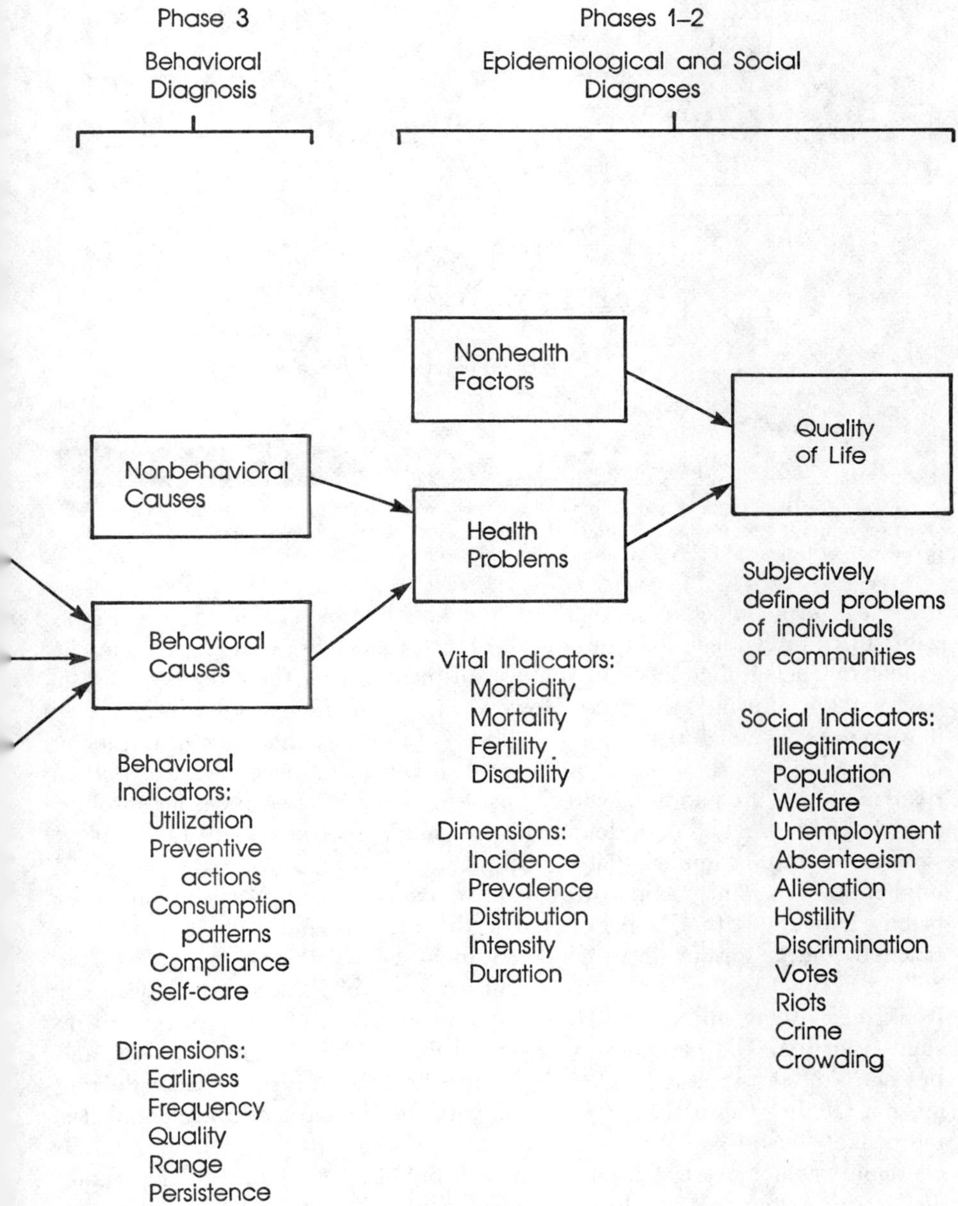

***Figure 15–6** Continued*

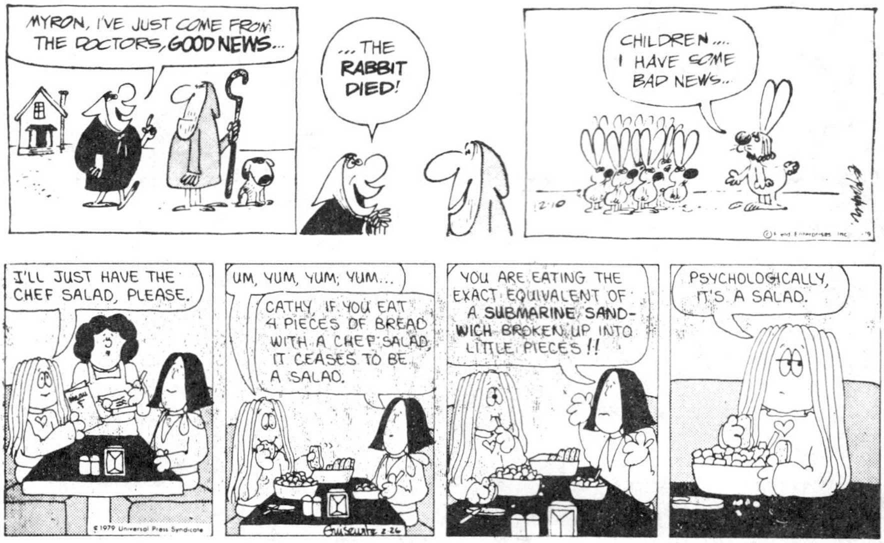
MYRON, I'VE JUST COME FROM THE DOCTORS, GOOD NEWS...
...THE RABBIT DIED!
CHILDREN.... I HAVE SOME BAD NEWS..
I'LL JUST HAVE THE CHEF SALAD, PLEASE.
UM, YUM, YUM, YUM...
CATHY, IF YOU EAT 4 PIECES OF BREAD WITH A CHEF SALAD, IT CEASES TO BE A SALAD.
YOU ARE EATING THE EXACT EQUIVALENT OF A SUBMARINE SANDWICH BROKEN UP INTO LITTLE PIECES!!
PSYCHOLOGICALLY, IT'S A SALAD.

Figure 15–7. The participant's frame of reference will determine how an event is perceived. (*Top*, reprinted by permission of Johnny Hart and Field Enterprises, Inc.; bottom, reprinted by permission of Universal Press Syndicate, copyright 1979. All rights reserved.)

ing short-term objectives and the dental health professional again must be willing to modify ideal, long-term goals of instruction. For example, one might expect that all individuals will remove all plaque from their teeth once per day, without injuring soft tissue. However, if a patient currently brushes once per week, does not use floss, and expresses the belief that such a frequency is quite adequate, the dental professional should not expect miracles. Rather than admonish the patient severely, insisting that once per day is an absolute minimum to prevent periodontal disease and then proceeding to teach all skills needed to accomplish that level of plaque removal, the dental professional might establish jointly as partners with the patient a compromise plan. After briefly explaining to the patient what the ideal is and why it should be reached, the dental health professional might ask what the patient would be willing to do. Eventually the two might agree on an objective that twice per week the patient will stain with a disclosing preparation and brush until no stain is visible. The patient is not berated for doing less than the ideal, and but one skill at a time is taught. Technics for sulcular brushing or for flossing are not taught. The oral contract made with the dental health professional is more likely to be kept because it seems reasonable to the patient, because coercion was not exercised, and because a public commitment to that action was made. At the next recall, new objectives may be established jointly *if* the patient has perceived the need for additional attention to oral hygiene practices.

Of course, those persons who do not have access to or who do not seek regular dental care have special needs. The dental professional working with a group of such individuals may find it difficult, if not impossible, to guide the attention of the group to primary preventive methods, especially if needs for treatment are widespread and of severe magnitude in the group. A compromise might include attention both to immediate treatment needs and to cost-beneficial methods of preventing future disease.

In this regard, it is worth noting that the goal of most educational efforts to improve oral health should focus on the ultimate improvement of oral health status. Children should experience smaller increments of new carious lesions, or diagnosis of oral malignancies in persons at high risk should occur earlier in the course of the disease, so the probability of successful treatment is increased. Seldom, if ever, will a public health program consist of educational components alone. Likewise, it will almost always be necessary to measure oral health status to determine the success of the program. It is not enough that plaque scores are lower at the end of a program—there should also be evidence that periodontal health has improved since the program's initiation. The educational diagnosis, short-term objectives, and a *tentative* long-term plan should be recorded in patient progress notes or in a program plan—just as a treatment plan for care needed or a program budget is recorded. The long-term plan should remain flexible and open to alteration as needs of the learners change. When identifying needs and establishing objectives, one must take care to avoid stereotyping patients, e.g., a teenager is concerned about appearance, a business executive about money, a disadvantaged person has a "low dental IQ." The individual or group must be treated individually, without condescension and with regard for unique characteristics. Such a statement appears to be a truism, yet a difference exists between genuine regard and poorly disguised efforts to manipulate the patient to do what the dental professional has already identified as necessary—and patients can tell the difference in an instant.

Objectives for instruction should be written in such a way that both clients and dental health professionals can determine when they have been achieved. Mager has provided a simple, entertaining description of the entire process,[63] and other volumes,[8, 37, 41, 60] are useful in learning to write clear, precise objectives. At this stage, mechanisms for evaluation of these objectives, and hence of instruction, should be identified. At least one researcher[46] has insisted that the impact of instruction cannot be assessed unless the criteria for reduced incidence of disease or improved or maintained health are measured. Certainly, such long-term measurement should be part of many more plans for instruction but should not be so far removed from instruction that confounding variables affect findings. Both short- and long-term assessments need to be built into evaluations.

There is one additional suggestion that all dental health professionals might heed: Many needs for learning about oral health exist, other than how and why to brush and floss the teeth and other than with only those patients who come to the dental office. For example, a second-grade teacher, after reading information about the replantation of an avulsed permanent incisor, remarked, "Why hasn't anyone told me this before?" Elementary school teachers should know specifics about such procedures, since they come into frequent contact with children and are apt to be present when accidents occur.

Sometimes, simply asking whether the client knows a given bit of information is enough to establish the need to know.

Dental professionals are reminded that learning may be within the cognitive, affective, or psychomotor domain[8, 41, 60] and that an ethical obligation exists to teach only information that is scientifically accurate. Many dental health professionals, in their zeal to convince the client about "the right way," stretch the truth. In the early years of plaque-control programs, many clients were promised that if they followed instructions and carefully maintained their mouths in a plaque-free state, they would never again experience dental caries. While research evidence supported the belief that periodontal disease could largely be prevented in that way and while logic underlaid the statement about dental caries, at that time no clinical research evidence existed that would have warranted making such promises. It is the responsibility of dental health professionals to make certain their knowledge is up-to-date and consistent with the findings of current, careful research. Professionals must read and evaluate information themselves without simply taking the word of the latest "expert" on the continuing education circuit. Principles of critical evaluation of the literature based on statistics, research design, and epidemiology can serve the dental professional well in making decisions about the scientific accuracy of information. Earlier sections of this book (see Chapters 5 and 10, especially) will be helpful in developing such evaluative skills, which are crucial to the selection of objectives and content that are scientifically accurate.

Designing Learning Experiences

After both client and professional are satisfied that the learning objectives established contribute to solving the problem or problems identified in the needs-assessment phase, resources can be identified, and then learning experiences can be designed and conducted for the particular client and objectives. Temptation may be great to use packages (e.g., *Learning About Your Oral Health*, published by the American Dental Association; *Toothtown, USA*, by the National Dairy Council; or commercial filmstrip/tape series) because they contain large amounts of information and seem appealing. The educator must exercise care that such materials are selected only when appropriate to accomplish the specific learning objectives that have been established for that particular learning experience. Similarly, the temptation to hand the client a pamphlet or to show a film must be resisted unless these activities seem clearly the best among possible ways of reaching the outcome desired or unless they support attainment of the unique objectives established. As one group of observers stated:

> All media used should have a clear purpose related to attaining a specific objective; media should not be used solely for diversional purposes or as the only means of education.[18]

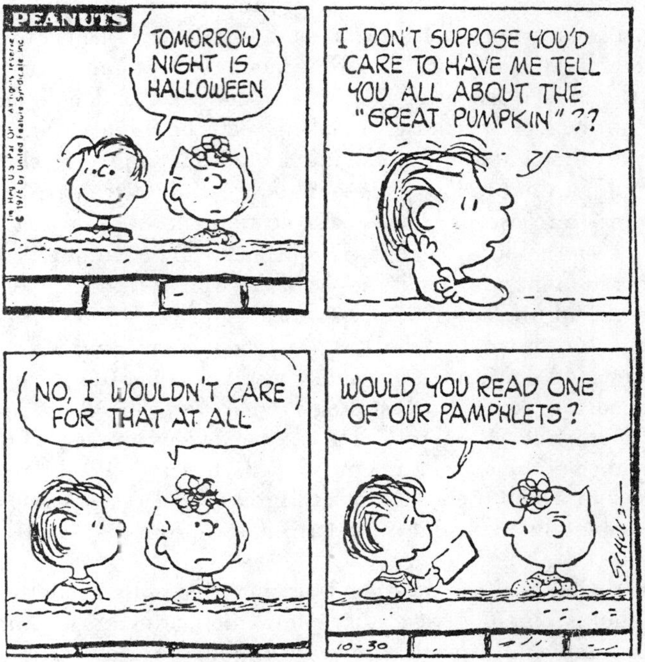
PEANUTS
TOMORROW NIGHT IS HALLOWEEN
I DON'T SUPPOSE YOU'D CARE TO HAVE ME TELL YOU ALL ABOUT THE "GREAT PUMPKIN"??
NO, I WOULDN'T CARE FOR THAT AT ALL
WOULD YOU READ ONE OF OUR PAMPHLETS?
10-30

Figure 15–8. Too often, dental health pamphlets are used in this way. (Copyright 1976 United Feature Syndicate, Inc.)

Previewing materials is the only way to develop familiarity with their content and approach so the dental professional can decide whether materials are appropriate for particular objectives. Materials should never be used without previewing or without such familiarity. Because materials should address particular objectives, simply placing a rack of pamphlets or a slide/tape "canned" message in the reception room is of questionable educational validity, and little should be expected from such arrangements. (Too often the use of dental health materials bears much resemblance to that shown in Fig. 15–8.)

Often the best learning aid can be the patient's own mouth and a hand mirror or existing knowledge, attitudes, and values. In addition, group processes operating in intact groups (e.g., neighborhood associations, service clubs, and 4–H groups) have not been explored to the extent they might as methods to alter behaviors related to oral health. The current gimmick may do nothing more than create a temporary distraction, or it may go so far as to alienate the patient—such as the businessman who expressed relief that the hygienist did not plan to have him watch "those ridiculous filmstrips." He clearly resented that he had been forced to spend valuable time during previous office visits listening to such messages.

Because underlying values so greatly affect behaviors related to health—

in fact, decisions may have been made without consideration of the health consequences—one approach used recently is that of "values clarification."[74] Clients are helped to identify what they value, to examine alternative choices as well as the consequences of each choice, and then to decide on a course of action themselves. Care must be taken that the professional's own value judgments are not imposed upon the client. For example, a statement such as "You wouldn't want to lose your teeth now, would you, Mrs. Jones?" would be inappropriate to use in a values clarification approach, because it imposes a "correct" belief upon the client. The primary objective of this technic is to assist clients in identifying what they value as well as the behaviors that might be consistent with their own value systems.

The greater the dental health professional's awareness of the client's existing knowledge, attitudes or values, and behavior, the greater the likelihood of choosing educational strategies that will contribute to producing change in one or all of the three.[35] Such enhanced awareness, when combined with acceptance of the learner as a person with inherent worth,[78] can minimize the instances in which the dental health professional's message is distorted or rejected completely because it is too far removed from the clients' perceptions and priorities.

Often, dental health professionals assume that appropriate behaviors will follow the clients' receipt of necessary information; attempts to alter knowledge dominate among educational efforts. It should be clear that provision of knowledge, while it may or may not be necessary, seldom is sufficient to produce behavioral changes. Clients' perceptions, attitudes, and values also must be examined; skill development and maintenance must receive attention. Mager[64, 66] has much to offer in understanding the limitations of educational efforts confined to providing information. His comment, especially in the context of this chapter and the process it describes, is a helpful reminder of the complex nature of education: "If telling were the same as teaching, we'd all be so smart we could hardly stand it."[64] Indeed, one writer[13] has suggested that relatively few dental behaviors are readily susceptible to alteration.

Information from unplanned sources may be a factor in existing knowledge, attitudes, and behavior, and the educator must be aware that these messages often are inaccurate or misleading. Frazier and her co-workers[27] examined content related to oral health, including advertisements of products in magazines and newspapers as well as on television. By their criteria, they found that 76 percent of broadcast advertising was fallacious or misleading. Magazines contained the highest proportion of accurate information (27 percent), yet 53 percent of the messages in magazines still were inaccurate. The frequency with which individuals are exposed to such messages, in comparison to the frequency of planned educational interventions, should make the scope of the problem clear. It should also emphasize the importance of learning (in a diplomatic way, of course) what the patient already believes, knows, and does *before* programs are planned.

Name ______________
Special Characteristics
Affecting Instruction:

( ) Brush
( ) Floss
( ) Yarn
( ) Gauze

( ) Perio Aid
( ) Floss Aid
( ) Mirror
( ) Disc Sln

( ) Proxabrush
( ) Bridge Loop
( ) __________
( ) __________

DATE	OBJECTIVES PLANNED	COMMITMENT BY PATIENT	STATUS OF SKILL	EVALUATION

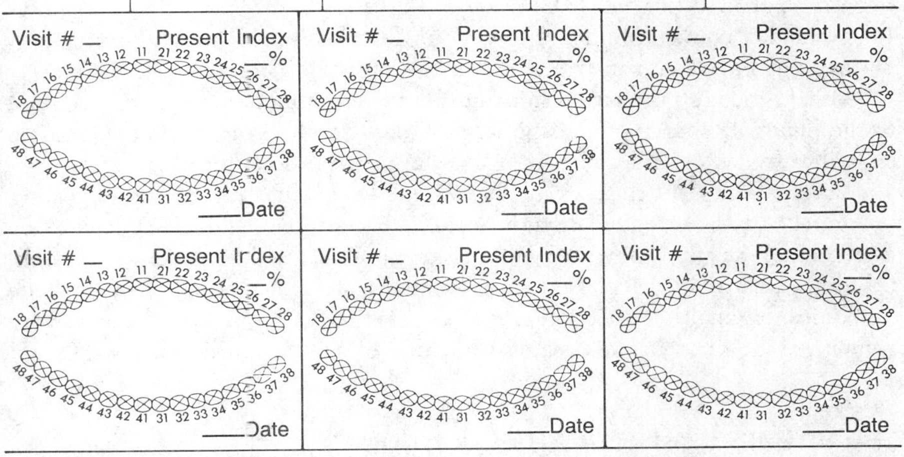

Plaque-containing surfaces / Available surfaces = % Index   Total number of available surfaces ________

Figure 15–9. A separate sheet, on which information related to education is recorded, can be a useful addition to the patient's chart.

Evaluation

Once the educational experience has been conducted and adequate time has elapsed, appropriate evaluation of the learning objectives must occur. In practice, this process is almost continuous with that of identifying needs. It is important that all steps in the process—needs, objectives, learning experiences, results of evaluation—be recorded in the chart or in a program plan, so others know what has been accomplished. A sheet such as that illustrated in Figure 15–9 may be useful in a clinical practice to condense and facilitate the recording of essential educational information.

The importance—and difficulty—of evaluation cannot be overstated.[33] Because so many variables contribute to whether clients actually choose to act on the basis of what they have been taught, one can almost never state with certainty that education alone was responsible for changes observed. Yet, seldom is the level of disease—or improved or maintained health status—part of the evaluation. Because reduction of oral disease and maintenance of oral health are the ultimate goals, such measures should be included in the evaluation when there is evidence that the measure does, in fact, reduce disease. Furthermore, dental health professionals often seem satisfied when a group of schoolchildren, for example, has a mean plaque score that is lower than it was before the program began. Although such a measure *may* reflect improvement, much detail (e.g., the number of individuals who improved, worsened, or stayed the same) is masked by the average.

Another error often made during before-and-after evaluations is the assumption that because a change occurred during the program, the program caused the change. Other factors not associated with the program may have been responsible for the alteration observed. A program undertaken to influence city council members to vote for fluoridation of the city's water may or may not have been instrumental in the outcome. Perhaps the availability of federal funds to purchase water fluoridation equipment was more important to the final vote than the educational program. Careful examination of possible contributory factors is a must in evaluation of educational programs.

Evaluation, as well as carefully designed research, must assume greater prominence in health education; in spite of the inherent difficulty in achieving documented results, they are essential for progress. Although some researchers, e.g., Warner,[88] have used sophisticated statistical methods to assess the outcomes of health education, findings have been equivocal. Much work remains to be done in the area of evaluation of health education.

THE SITE OF ORAL HEALTH EDUCATION

In the Office or Clinic

Although the process of education for oral health just described applies in the one-to-one setting with a patient, there are special aspects of that interchange that should be noted. First, of course, is the advantage in working with one person at a time. Second, the dental professional often sees these same persons periodically over longer periods of time, perhaps for many years, permitting the development of high levels of trust and allowing reinforcement and gradual refinement of desirable skills, knowledge, and attitudes. It is not necessary to teach everything at once, and a reasonable long-range educational plan can be developed and implemented for each patient.

It is important that all personnel in the office or clinic agree on the priority that education will assume for that setting and on its specific content. Otherwise, patients are likely to receive conflicting messages from different personnel, and disagreements may develop over time spent helping patients learn. While some insist that separate consultation or "plaque-control" rooms are required for proper education, others note that learning can occur in any setting, as long as the patient perceives a need and the professional demonstrates a genuine regard for the patient's dignity and psychological privacy and a true acceptance of the patient's key role in decisions relating to health.

In the School

The school would appear to provide numerous advantages for the dental health professional desiring to influence individuals' behavior related to oral health.[38, 51] An atmosphere in which the pursuit of knowledge prevails would seem the ideal location to bring about extensive changes in oral health behaviors, attitudes, and knowledge. While such efforts in prior years emphasized the functions and anatomy of teeth, including the universally hated "drawing a picture of a tooth," recent teaching has focused on developing the knowledge and skills needed to brush and floss the teeth. Attention also has been directed to establishing desired habits by including supervised plaque removal in the classroom. Although changes in knowledge and skill levels may have occurred in these programs, the new behaviors may not have been internalized. The frequent finding[32, 45] that gains in oral hygiene status achieved during a school-based plaque-control program are lost shortly after the program ends can be explained by the distinction among levels of behavior noted earlier in this chapter. Unless behaviors are internalized into the clients' value patterns, they most likely will not continue—which is why care must be taken in the needs-identification and objective-setting phases to elicit clients' actual values, beliefs, and practices in regard to oral health, rather than the ones they think the professional wants to hear. This distinction also emphasizes why primary preventive measures that work are preferred over scientifically questionable ones.[44]

Although the potential for education in the school is great, the dental health professional is cautioned that such bright promise may not be realized. A variety of reasons may contribute, such as (1) competing demands for school time by many special interest groups; (2) pressures to emphasize the basics rather than to implement programs that address areas perceived as "frills" during school time (Iverson[51] notes that programs addressing quiet problems, such as oral diseases, are especially likely to elicit that label); (3) resentment among school personnel of the trend to use the school as a social laboratory; (4) lack of reinforcement of oral health behaviors by parents and peers; and (5) conflicting messages in other aspects of school life. For example, one wonders how a child can reconcile the message, "Don't eat sweets between meals," with the band's vigorous campaign to sell candy bars in order to purchase new uniforms.

Dental health professionals, when asked to come into the classroom to "give a talk about teeth," may be tempted to comply by giving a lecture focused on that which they think important, by conducting a "brush-in," or by showing a clever movie. However, one could respond in several more appropriate ways by following the process delineated earlier. During the problem-identification phase, it may be discovered that the real problem is the level of dental health knowledge of the teacher. Or it may be a lack of priority given to oral health by parents or a lack of availability of oral health care services in the community. If any of these is the primary problem to be solved, such a visit to the classroom is not likely to be an effective educational intervention. More appropriate choices might include consulting or inservice sessions with teachers, a values-clarification exercise at a PTA meeting, or the mobilization of community resources to obtain needed care.

Should a classroom session be planned, several factors must be remembered. First, the visit should be cleared with all persons who have responsibility for monitoring instruction by nonschool personnel. They may include, for example, the curriculum coordinator, school nurse, classroom teacher, principal, or health specialist within the school or system. The initial contact with school personnel should provide the dental professional with specifics regarding the protocol for notifying appropriate personnel within that particular school system about the proposed program. Prior to the visit, the process of planning, including a careful identification of needs for instruction, should be conducted and appropriate objectives established—preferably jointly with the teacher and with students. Rather than trying to accommodate the group to existing materials, resources must be chosen with objectives in mind. (Obviously, more than one visit to the school may be required to accomplish these tasks.) Finally, after instruction has been conducted, it should be evaluated against the objectives, not just on the basis of whether the teacher was pleased or the students "seemed interested."

In many states or school districts, curricular guidelines exist to delineate content of health instruction at each grade level. In addition, dental health guidelines or guides to resources have been developed by health departments, by dental societies, or by interdisciplinary committees of health professionals. While these guidelines may be helpful in planning instruction, it is important to recognize that they are but one resource. Further, caution must be exercised in reminding oneself that what is *taught* may not necessarily be *learned.* While standardized objectives can provide a reasonable framework for planning, the unique needs of the group must assume priority and specific objectives, learning strategies, and evaluation mechanisms must be developed for and with that particular group. Assistance may be available from dental health consultants employed by school districts, by health departments, or by dental organizations.

In the Community

Education for oral health in the community often seems limited to activities such as puppet shows in shopping malls or smile contests during National Children's Dental Health Month, public service announcements on TV or radio, or newspaper question-and-answer columns related to oral health. While these activities may on occasion be appropriate components of community education for oral health, the dental health professional should pursue the planning process prior to deciding on specific activities or resources—or, indeed, on whether educational activities will solve the problem. It may well be that other solutions are better choices for achieving the group's needs, particularly when the objective is improved oral health status. In addition, it is difficult to evaluate the effectiveness of some community-based activities because clear objectives were not established prior to the decision to implement a particular activity. For example, what are the objectives of a smile or poster contest? How might these objectives be evaluated?

Expectations of what might be accomplished by mass media education for oral health are based on dental health professionals' experience as observers of commercial advertising. Because the comparison is not a valid one, expectations are often unrealistic. There are several major differences between the two. Commercial advertising may be considered successful if an increase of 1 or 2 percent in purchasers of the product can be achieved. Furthermore, it may be unnecessary for those consumers to continue purchasing the product if additional one-time buyers can be enticed by future advertising. However, oral diseases cannot be prevented by engaging in recommended behaviors just once. Sustained behavior at a high level of discipline and skill is required—once is not enough to attain success. In addition, few health professionals would be satisfied with a 1 or 2 percent increase in those complying with recommendations. The ideal in health matters, of course, would be 100 percent compliance (or better yet, 100 percent internalization).

Another detriment to achieving results with mass media comparable to results achieved by commercial advertising is often overlooked. While those selling products usually are able to appeal to values already held by potential consumers, those recommending health practices may have to compensate for attitudes or practices that are contrary to the desired behavior. It is difficult to convince children that they should eat noncariogenic snacks between meals when they have become accustomed to consuming high-sugar foods and beverages at snack times or to receiving high-sugar items as rewards from parents, teachers, physicians, or merchants. The extent of the challenges, of course, should not prevent exploring mass media as a way of attracting attention to an issue, of providing cues for desired actions, or of supplementing other instruction related to health promotion or disease prevention.

Effecting health education in the community is complicated by the often extreme diversity of the group. Some have suggested that efforts in community health education should be broadened from the focus of most individual instruction and that the content of education in the community should not be limited to personal behaviors such as oral hygiene practices or diet instruction. Griffiths states the case succinctly:

> In attempting to close [the gap between what is known about optimum health practice and that which is actually practiced], health education is concerned not only with individuals and their families, but also with the institutions and social conditions that impede or facilitate individuals toward achieving optimum health.[36]

Efforts in the community to accomplish fluoridation of the public water supply, which produces the greatest improvement in oral health status for the greatest number (see Chapter 7), would be consistent with this view of health education.

Frazier[25, 26] has argued convincingly that educational problems and target populations in education for oral health must be redefined to focus on adult decision-makers and opinion leaders in the community and that objectives of dental health professionals should not pay exclusive attention to individual motivation. She maintains that the latter is a more expensive, less productive way of solving problems than altering the environment in which those individuals' decisions are made. In addition, she suggests that content should emphasize known effective preventive measures, e.g., fluorides and sealants, and that educational methods should be redefined to encompass such activities as community organization and community development. In her comprehensive review of dental health educational programs (including those that are school based), she has broadened—or narrowed—the definition of health education in dental public health programs to the following:

> A process of organizing and involving groups of decision-makers and opinion leaders in active decision-making with regard to the selection and implementation of organized community dental programs which: (a) are designed to prevent or control oral diseases; (b) have been shown to be effective and practical at the community level; and (c) operate independently of individual performance or habit.[25]

By Frazier's definition and standards, it would be more desirable to use funds donated by the Rotary Club to finance a supervised fluoride mouthrinse program among all second-graders than to distribute toothbrushes to those same children. Obviously, if both can be accomplished, no dilemma exists. However, if funds are available for only one activity, it is the dental health professional's responsibility to provide the information and guidance necessary to help key persons make choices that will prevent the most oral disease in the target group. Obviously, the fluoride mouthrinse program would best accomplish this goal, while simultaneously minimizing the need for individual alteration of habits. Clear responsibilities exist in educating communities to the benefits of water fluoridation, and challenges in this area will multiply as environmental and antigovernmental groups increase the public's reservations about water fluoridation.

SUMMARY

It should be clear from this chapter's focus that education for oral health ought to be an integral part of preventive efforts at all levels—primary, secondary, and tertiary. Furthermore, while educational efforts are often necessary, seldom are they sufficient to accomplish improvement in health promotion or disease prevention efforts of individuals or groups. Rather than posing a simple solution to health—especially oral health—problems, educational efforts often become complex solutions, requiring specialized knowledge of the behavioral and social sciences, just as clinical diagnosis and treatment decisions require a solid foundation in the basic biological sciences.

In all educational efforts with individuals and groups, dental professionals should (1) assess needs *with* clients carefully *before* acting, (2) plan objectives and carry out educational activities consistent with the needs identified, (3) evaluate what has been accomplished in terms of improved oral health, if possible, and (4) maintain their enthusiasm, imagination, realism, and patience. Those latter qualities, combined with the process outlined in this chapter, should serve the professional well in implementing educational efforts that have the best potential for preventing oral disease and promoting oral health. Improving oral health status to the optimum possible for individuals and groups is the responsibility of all dental health professionals. In light of the almost universal prevalence of oral diseases, efforts to educate patients so that oral disease prevention and oral health promotion are enhanced will remain a challenge to dental health professionals far into the future. No matter what the level, *someone* will be making decisions that will affect oral health. Dental health professionals bear the responsibility for using their special knowledge in order to influence those decisions positively. Their goal should be optimum oral health for the largest number possible. In attempting to reach that goal, dental health professionals would do well to recall the lessons of this chapter and the warning by Carlyon:

> . . . it would appear that progress in dental health education will more likely come from careful planning to achieve realistic goals, than from frantic, futile searching for fashionable, simplistic answers.[12]

References

1. Ayer, W. A. Motivating people to oral health. Dent. Hyg., 53:221–4, May 1979.
*2. Becker, M. H., ed. The health belief model and personal health behavior. Health Educ. Monogr., 2:326–473, Winter 1974.

*Recommended for further reading.

3. Belloc, Nedra B., and Breslow, Lester. Relationship of physical health status and health practices. Preven. Med., 1:409–21, Aug. 1972.
*4. Bennis, W. G., et al. The planning of change. 3rd ed. New York, Holt, c1976. ix + 517 p.
5. Berger, S. M., and Lambert, W. W. Stimulus-response theory in contemporary social psychology. p. 81–178. (In Lindzey, Gardner, and Aronson, Elliot, eds. The handbook of social psychology. 2nd ed. Vol. 1. Historical introduction; systematic positions. Reading, Mass., Addison-Wesley, c1968. xv + 653 p.)
6. Berkowitz, Leonard. Social motivation. p. 50–135. (In Lindzey, Gardner, and Aronson, Elliot, eds. The handbook of social psychology. 2nd ed. Vol 3. The individual in a social context. Reading, Mass., Addison-Wesley, c1968. xiii + 978 p.)
*7. Bernstein, Lewis, Bernstein, Rosalyn S., and Dana, R. G. Interviewing; a guide for health professionals. 2nd ed. New York, Appleton-Century-Crofts, c1974. xix + 197 p.
8. Bloom, B. S., ed. Taxonomy of educational objectives; the classification of educational goals. Handbook I; cognitive domain. New York, McKay, c1956. 207 p.
9. Breslow, Lester. Policy assessment of preventive health practice. Preven. Med., 6:242–51, June 1977.
10. ———. Risk factor intervention for health maintenance. Science, 200:908–12, May 26, 1978.
11. Brill, Naomi I. Working with people; the helping process. Philadelphia, Lippincott, c1973. x + 202 p.
*12. Carlyon, W. H. Creative, innovative, vital, and dynamic health education programs that fail. Mich. Dent. A.J., 57:92–7, Feb. 1975.
*13. Chambers, D. W. Susceptibility to preventive dental treatment. J. Pub. Health Dent., 33:82–90, Spring 1973.
14. Cohen, A. R. Attitude change and social influence. New York, Basic Books, c1964. xv + 156 p.
15. Cohen, Lois K., and Lucye, Helen. A position on school dental health education. J. School Health, 40:361–5, Sept. 1970.
*16. Corah, N. L., ed. Behavioral science symposium; preventive dental behavior. Health Educ. Monogr., 2:197–245, Fall 1974.
17. Cormier, Patricia P., and Levy, Joyce I. Community oral health; a systems approach for the dental health profession. New York, Appleton-Century-Crofts, c1981. xiii + 237 p.
18. Deeds, Sigrid G., Hebert, Barbara J., and Walle, Joan M. A model for patient education programming; report of the APHA Public Health Education Section. Washington, D.C., American Public Health Association, Feb. 1979. iv + 29 p.
19. Deutsch, Morton. Field theory in social psychology. p. 412–87. (In Lindzey, Gardner, and Aronson, Elliot, eds. The handbook of social psychology. 2nd ed. Vol. 1. Historical introduction; systematic positions. Reading, Mass., Addison-Wesley, c1968. xv + 653 p.)
20. Dunning, J. M. Principles of dental public health. 3rd ed. Cambridge, Harvard University Press, c1979. xiv + 598 p. (p. 338–66)
21. Dworkin, S. F., Ferrence, T. P., and Giddon, D. B. Behavioral science and dental practice. St. Louis, Mosby, 1978. xii + 291 p.
*22. Fabun, Don, ed. Communications; the transfer of meaning. Beverly Hills, Calif., Glencoe Press, c1968. 39 p.
23. Fodor, J. T., and Dalis, G. T. Health instruction; theory and application. 3rd ed. Philadelphia, Lea & Febiger, 1981. xiii + 150 p.
24. John E. Fogarty International Center for Advanced Study in the Health Sciences and the American College of Preventive Medicine. Preventive medicine USA; health promotion and consumer health education. New York, Prodist, 1976. viii + 255 p.
25. Frazier, P. Jean. The effectiveness and practicality of current dental health education programs from a public health perspective; a conceptual appraisal. Presented as part of symposium, Methods for the Prevention of Dental Disease: Effectiveness and Practicality, at annual meeting of the Dental Health Section, American Public Health Association, Miami Beach, Florida, Oct. 20, 1976. 28 p. duplicated.
*26. ———. A new look at dental health education in community programs. Dent. Hyg., 52:176–86, Apr. 1978.
27. Frazier, P. Jean, et al. Quality of information in mass media; a barrier to the dental health education of the public. J. Pub. Health Dent., 34:244–57, Fall 1974.
*28. Frazier, P. Jean, and Horowitz, Alice M. Priorities in planning and evaluating community oral health programs. Fam. & Comm. Health, 3:103–13, Nov. 1980.

*Recommended for further reading.

*29. Freed, J. R., and Matthias, Ruth E. Evaluation of dental health education programs. J. Pub. Health Dent., 40:39–46, Winter 1980.

*30. Freudenberg, Nicholas. Shaping the future of health education; from behavior change to social change. Health Educ. Monogr., 6:372–7, Winter 1978.

31. Froelich, R. F., Bishop, F. M., and Dworkin, S. F. Communication in the dental office; a programmed manual for the dental professional. St. Louis, Mosby, 1976. viii + 151 p.

32. Graves, R. C., et al. A comparison of the effectiveness of the "toothkeeper" and a traditional dental health education program. J. Pub. Health Dent., 35:85–90, Spring 1975.

*33. Green, L. W. Evaluation and measurement; some dilemmas for health education. Am. J. Pub. Health, 67:155–61, Feb. 1977.

34. ———. First health education distinguished lecture. Presented at the Program in Health Education, School of Public Health, Columbia University, May 3, 1978. New York City, The University, 20 p. printed.

*35. Green, L. W., et al. Health education planning; a diagnostic approach. Palo Alto, Mayfield, c1980. xvi + 306 p.

36. Griffiths, William. Health education definitions, problems and philosophies. Health Educ. Monogr., 31:7–12, 1972.

37. Gronlund, N. E. Stating behavioral objectives for classroom instruction. New York, Macmillan, c1970 vi + 58 p.

*38. Haefner, D. P. School dental health programs. Health Educ. Monogr., 2:212–9, Fall 1974.

*39. ———. The health belief model and preventive dental behavior. Health Educ. Monogr., 2:420–32, Winter. 1974.

40. Hall, C. S., and Lindzey, Gardner. The relevance of Freudian psychology for the social sciences. p. 245–319. (In Lindzey, Gardner, and Aronson, Elliot, eds. The handbook of social psychology, 2nd ed. Vol. 1. Historical introduction; systematic positions. Reading Mass., Addison-Wesley, c1968. xv + 653 p.)

41. Harrow, Anita J. A taxonomy of the psychomotor domain; a guide for developing behavioral objectives. New York, McKay, c1972. x + 190 p.

*42. Havelock, R. G., et al. Planning for innovation through dissemination and utilization of knowledge. Ann Arbor, Center Utilization Scientific Knowledge, Institute Social Research, University Michigan, c1975. n.p.

*43. Hellman, Sandra. The dentist and preventive health information. Health Educ. Monogr., 4:132–76, Summer 1976.

*44. Horowitz, Alice M., and Frazier, P. Jean. Effective public education in achieving oral health. Fam. & Comm. Health, 3:91–101, Nov. 1980.

*45. Horowitz, Alice M., et al. Effect of supervised dental plaque removal by children after 3 years. Community Dent. Oral Epidemiol., 8:171–6, Aug. 1980.

46. Horowitz, H. S. Can we measure impact of communication information in terms of reduced incidence of dental disease? Edit. J. Pub. Health Dent., 38:131–5, Spring 1978.

47. ———. Promotion of oral health and prevention of dental caries. J. Pub. Health Dent., 41:92–5, Spring 1981.

48. ———. Pit and fissure sealants in private practice and public health programmes; analysis of cost-effectiveness. Internat. Dent. J., 30:117–26, June 1980.

49. Hunt, Sonja M. The teaching and practice of social psychology in health education. Presented at the symposium on the preparation of health personnel in health education, Cologne, Germany, November 1974. Regional Office for Europe, World Health Organization, 9 p. duplicated.

50. Ingersoll, Barbara D. Behavioral aspects in dentistry. New York, Appleton-Century-Crofts, c1982. xiii + 223 p.

*51. Iverson, D. C., ed. Promoting health through the schools; a challenge for the eighties. Health Educ. Quar., 8:5–117, Spring 1981.

52. Jaccard, James. A theoretical analysis of selected factors important to health education strategies. Health Educ. Monogr., 3:152–67, Summer 1975.

53. Jackson, Eric. Effective persuasion in dental practice. Am. Soc. Prev. Dent. J., 5:15–8, May-June 1975.

54. Jenkins, C. D. An approach to diagnosis and treatment of problems of health-related behaviour. Internat. J. Health Educ., 22:1–24 (supplement). Apr.-June 1979.

*55. Jenny, Joanna. Preventing dental disease in children; an ecological approach. Am. J. Pub. Health, 64:1147–55, Dec. 1974.

56. Joint Committee on Health Education Terminology. Report. Health Educ. Monogr., 33:63–70, 1973.

*Recommended for further reading.

*57. Kegeles, S. S. Adequate oral health; blocks and means by which they may be overcome. p. 73–128. (In Brown, W. E., ed. Oral health, dentistry, and the American public; the need for an improved oral care delivery system. Norman, Okla., University Oklahoma Press, c1974. vii + 372 p.)
*58. Keisler, C. A., Collins, B. F., and Miller, Norman. Attitude change; a critical analysis of theoretical approaches. New York, Wiley, c1969. xii + 386 p.
*59. Knutson, A. L. The individual, society, and health behavior. New York, Russell Sage Foundation, 1965. 533 p.
60. Krathwohl, D. R., Bloom, B. S., and Masia, B. B. Taxonomy of educational objectives; the classification of educational goals. Handbook II; affective domain. New York, McKay, c1964. xiv + 196 p.
61. Larry, R. H., chairman. The report of the President's Committee on Health Education. New York, The Committee, 1973. 71 p.
*62. Lau, Richard, et al. Channeling health; a review of the evaluations of televised health campaigns. Health Educ. Quar., 7:56–89, Spring 1980.
*63. Mager, R. F. Preparing instructional objectives. 2nd ed. Palo Alto, Fearon, c1975. 136 p.
*64. ______. Developing attitude toward learning. Belmont, Calif., Fearon, c1968. vii + 104 p.
65. ______. Goal analysis. Belmont, Calif., Fearon, c1972. vi + 136 p.
*66. Mager, R. F., and Pipe, Peter. Analyzing performance problems, or "you really oughta wanna." Belmont, Calif., Fearon, c1970. v + 111 p.
67. Marlowe, David, and Gergen, K. J. Personality and social interaction. p. 590–665. (In Lindzey, Gardner, and Aronson, Elliot, eds. The handbook of social psychology. 2nd ed. Vol. 3. The individual in a social context. Reading, Mass., Addison-Wesley, c1968. xiii + 978 p.)
68. McGuire, W. J. The nature of attitudes and attitude change. p. 136–314. (In Lindzey, Gardner, and Aronson, Elliot, eds. The handbook of social psychology. 2nd ed. Vol. 3. The individual in a social context. Reading, Mass., Addison-Wesley, c1968. xiii + 978 p.)
*69. Mico, P. R., and Ross, Helen S. Health education and behavioral science. Oakland, Calif., Third Party Associates, c1975. xxiii + 207 p.
70. Milio, Nancy. A framework for prevention; changing health-damaging to health-generating life patterns. Am. J. Pub. Health, 66:435–40, May 1976.
71. Morton, Judy C., et al. Dental teamwork strategies; interpersonal and organizational approaches. St. Louis, Mosby, 1980. xiii + 181 p.
72. Nyswander, Dorothy B. Education for health—some principles and their application. Calif. Health, 14:65–70, Nov. 1, 1956.
*73. Pipe, Peter, et al. Developing a plaque control program; a motivational approach to involving patients in dental care. Berkeley, Praxis, c1972. 80 p.
*74. Raths, L. E., Harmin, Merrill, and Simon, S. B. Values and teaching; working with values in the classroom. Columbus, Ohio, Merrill, c1966. ix + 275 p.
75. Rayner, Jeannette F. Communication between the public and the dental profession. Am. J. Pub. Health, 63:21–32, Jan. 1973.
76. Rayner, Jeannette F., and Cohen, Lois K. School dental health education. p. 275–307. (In Richards, N. D., and Cohen, Lois K., eds. Social sciences and dentistry; a critical bibliography. The Hague, Fédération Dentaire Internationale, c1971. 381 p.)
77. Richards, Ruth F., and Kalmer, Howard, eds. Patient education. Health Educ. Monogr., 2:1–92, Spring 1974.
*78. Rogers, C. A. Freedom to learn. Columbus, Ohio, Merrill, c1969. x + 358 p.
79. Rogers, K. D. Making school health education effective. Edit. Am. J. Pub. Health, 71:5–6, Jan. 1981.
*80. Ross, Helen S., and Mico, P. R. Theory and practice in health education. Palo Alto, Mayfield, c1980. xii + 338 p.
81. Simonds, S. K. Emerging challenges in health education. Internat. J. Health Educ., 19(Suppl.):2–19, Oct.–Dec. 1976.
*82. Simmons, Jeannette, ed. Making health education work. Am. J. Pub. Health, 65(Suppl.):1–49, Oct. 1975.
*83. Simmons, Jeannette. Complex issues facing health education. Edit. Am. J. Pub. Health, 66:429–30, May 1976.

*Recommended for further reading.

*84. Smith, L. W., et al. Teachers as models for programs for school dental health; an evaluation of "the toothkeeper." J. Pub. Health Dent., 35:75–80, Spring 1975.
*85. Stamm, J. W., Kuo, H. C., and Neil, D. R. An evaluation of the "toothkeeper" program in Vermont. J. Pub. Health Dent., 35:81–4, Spring 1975.
86. Tagiuri, Renato. Person perception. p. 395–449. (In Lindzey, Gardner, and Aronson, Elliot, eds. The handbook of social psychology. 2nd ed. Vol. 3. The individual in a social context. Reading, Mass., Addison-Wesley, c1968. xiii + 978 p.)
87. Tajfel, Henri. Social and cultural factors in perception. p. 315–94. (In Lindzey, Gardner, and Aronson, Elliot, eds. The handbook of social psychology. 2nd ed. Vol. 3. The individual in a social context. Reading, Mass., Addison-Wesley, c1968. xiii + 978 p.)
*88. Warner, K. F. Cigarette smoking in the 70's; the impact of the anti-smoking campaign on consumption. Science, 211:729–31, Feb. 13, 1981.
*89. Weinstein, Philip, and Getz, Tracy. Changing human behavior; strategies for preventive dentistry. Chicago, Science Research Associates, c1978. xviii + 134 p.
90. World Health Organization, Expert Committee on Dental Health Education. A report on dental health education; report of a WHO expert committee. WHO Techn. Rep. Ser. No. 449. Geneva, The Organization, 1970. 28 p.
91. Young, Marjorie A.C. Dental health education of adults. p. 241–74. (In Richards, N. D., and Cohen, Lois K., eds. Social sciences and dentistry; a critical bibliography. The Hague, Fédération Dentaire Internationale, c1971. 381 p.)
92. Young, W. O., and Striffler, D. F. The dentist, his practice, and his community. 2nd ed. Philadelphia, Saunders, 1969. xvi + 346 p. (p. 293–321).
93. Zander, Alvin. Influencing people in the face-to-face setting; research findings and their application. Health Educ. Monogr., 13:3–17, 1962.

INDEX

Page numbers in *italics* refer to illustrations; page numbers followed by "t" refer to tables.